# SELECTED TOPICS IN DNA REPAIR

Edited by **Clark C. Chen**

**Selected Topics in DNA Repair**
Edited by Clark C. Chen

**Published by InTech**
Janeza Trdine 9, 51000 Rijeka, Croatia



**Publishing Process Manager** Alenka Urbancic

**Technical Editor** Teodora Smiljanic

**Cover Designer** InTech Design Team

Additional hard copies can be obtained from orders@intechopen.com

Selected Topics in DNA Repair, Edited by Clark C. Chen
p. cm.
ISBN 978-953-307-606-5

For EU product safety concerns:
IN TECH d.o.o., Prolaz Marije Krucifikse Kozulić 3, 51000 Rijeka, Croatia,
info@intechopen.com or visit our website at intechopen.com.

# Meet the editor

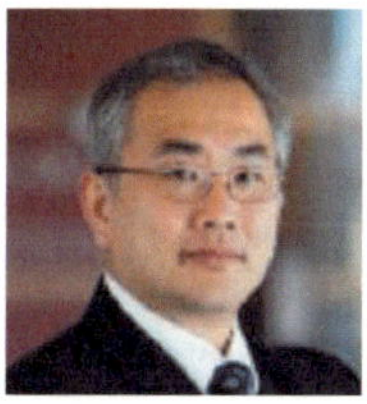

Dr. Clark C. Chen received his B.S. from Stanford University in 1992, M.S. from Columbia University in 1993, and his M.D.-Ph.D. from Harvard Medical School in 2001. He completed his neurosurgery training at the Massachusetts General Hospital and subsequently completed independent fellowships in stereotactic neurosurgery and radiosurgery. Dr. Chen previously served as the director of Clinical Neuro-Oncology at the Beth Israel Deaconess Medical Center before his current role as the Director of Stereotactic and Radiosurgery and Co-Director of Surgical Neuro-Oncology at the University of California, San Diego. Dr. Chen's research is directed at identifying alterations in DNA repair pathways as they relate to brain cancer therapy. Dr. Chen is the recipient of the Damon Runyon Fellowship Award, the James Kerr Award, American Brain Tumor Association Investigator Award, Paul Calabresi Scholar Award, Burroughs Wellcome Career Award, William Guy Forbeck Scholar Award, the Doris Duke Clinical Scientist Award, and the Kimmel Scholar Award.

# Contents

# Preface

In previous decades, we have seen a rapid advancement in our fundamental understanding of DNA repair, as well as translational application to medicine in general. In this context, a comprehensive review of key concepts in DNA repair is well beyond the scope of the presented text. Instead, select topics pertinent to the field are selected for presentation, with the goal of highlighting paradigmatic advances.

This book is divided into 26 chapters, and compartmentalized into four parts: DNA Damaging Agents, Mechanistic Insights, Methods in DNA Repair, and Insights into Therapeutic Strategies. Each component discusses key concepts in DNA repair. Selected articles are further meant to demonstrate how scientific ideas are developed, tested, dialogued and matured. It is my sincere hope that the articles presented will stimulate and inspire thoughts that, in turn, contribute to this critically important field.

**Clark C. Chen, M.D., Ph.D.**
University of California, San Diego
USA

# Part 1

## DNA Damaging Agents

# 1

# The DNA-Damage Response to Ionizing Radiation in Human Lymphocytes

Maddalena Mognato, Mauro Grifalconi, Sabrina Canova,
Cristina Girardi and Lucia Celotti
*University of Padova, Department of Biology,
Italy*

## 1. Introduction

The human genome is constantly subjected to DNA damage derived from endogenous and exogenous sources. Normal cellular metabolism can give raise to DNA damage through free radicals production and replication errors, whereas environmental agents, such as ultraviolet (UV) and ionizing radiation (IR), induce specific types of lesions. DNA damage can ultimately lead to genomic instability and carcinogenesis if not properly addressed, thus an elaborate network of proteins has evolved in cells to maintain genome integrity through a pathway termed the DNA-damage response (DDR). DDR allows DNA damage detection, signal propagation and transduction to a multitude of effector proteins, which promote cell survival and activate cell cycle arrest to allow DNA repair. When cells are unable to properly repair DNA, apoptosis or senescence pathways may be triggered, thus eliminating the possibility of passing on damaged or unrepaired genetic material to its progeny. The ultimate goal of DDR is to protect the integrity of genetic information and its faithful transmission, either to DNA by replication or to mRNA by transcription. Therefore, dysregulation of DDR pathway can contribute to carcinogenesis and developmental defects. Ionizing radiation represents a mutagen agent to which human population is exposed due to environmental, professional or accidental reasons. The biological effects of IR depend on the quality and the dose of radiation and on the cell type. Linear energy transfer (LET) represents the energy lost per unit distance as an ionizing particle travels through a material, and it is used to quantify the effects of IR on biological specimens. High-LET radiation (i.e. alpha-particles, neutrons, protons) are densely IR since they lose the energy throughout a small distance, causing dense ionization along their track with high localized multiple DNA damage. Low-LET radiation, such as X and $\gamma$-rays, are sparsely IR since they produce ionizations sparsely along their track and, hence, almost homogeneously within a cell. The biological effect of high-LET radiations are in general much higher than those of low-LET radiations with the same energy. This is because high-LET radiation deposits most of its energy within the volume of one cell and the damage to DNA is therefore larger (Anderson et al., 2002; Brenner & Ward, 1992; Prise et al., 2001). Radiation is potentially harmful to humans, because the ionization it produces can significantly alter the structure of molecules within a living cell.The exposure to ionizing radiation elicits a complex cell response to overcome the dangerous effects of DNA-radiation interaction, such as reactive oxygen species (ROS) production, base oxidation and DNA breaks formation (i.e. single-strand breaks, SSBs and double-strand breaks, DSBs ). In particular, DSBs represent the most severe form of damage, since an inefficient or inaccurate repair may lead to cell death or genomic instability (Wyman & Kanaar, 2006). The presence of DSBs leads to a cascade of post-translational modifications of a wide variety of proteins, including phosphorylation, ubiquitinylation, sumoylation, poly(ADP-ribosylation), acetylation and methylation (Huen & Chen, 2010). The early DSB response utilizes phosphorylation-dependent protein–protein interactions to coordinate DNA damage recognition and signal amplification. Following DSB formation the histone H2AX, a histone H2A variant that comprises 10-15% of total cellular H2A in higher eukaryotes, is rapidly phosphorylated on its serine residues 139 (γ–H2AX) (Rogakou et al., 1998) by members of the phosphatidylinositol-3-OH kinase (PI(3)K)-like family, such as ataxia telangiectasia mutated (ATM), DNA-PK and ataxia telangiectasia and Rad3 related (ATR) (Kinner et al., 2008). γ-H2AX formation occurs within minutes after damage, and extends for up to 1-2 megabases from the site of the break in mammalian cells, providing a platform for subsequent DNA repair protein recruitment and amplification at DSBs (Harper & Elledge, 2007). The phosphorylation of H2AX creates a signal recognized by many proteins of the DNA damage response, which are recruited to the sites of DSBs, forming the ionizing radiation-induced foci (IRIF, Lukas et al., 2004). The biological function of IRIF is thought to shelter the broken DNA ends from decay and prevent illegitimate repair processes, to amplify the DNA damage signal and to provide a local concentration of DDR factors relevant for DNA repair and metabolism. Stabilization of DDR factor recruitment to γ-H2AX nucleosomes is achieved through the recruitment of a wide variety of proteins regulating ubiquitylation, sumoylation, acetylation, methylation. The mediator of DNA damage checkpoint 1 (MDC1) is the major protein to localize to the sites of DNA breaks in a γ-H2AX-dependent pathway (Riches et al., 2008; Stucki, 2009) MDC1 has a role in controlling the assembly of multiple repair factors at DNA breaks and in amplifying the DNA damage signal. MDC1 orchestrates the recruitment of IRIF-associated proteins, specifically the MRN complex (MRE11, RAD51, NBS1) and many DNA damage repair proteins, including p53-binding protein 1 (53BP1) and BRCA1 (breast cancer 1). DDR is characterized by the synthesis of ubiquitin conjugates at the sites of damage-induced repair foci (Tanq & Greenberg, 2010). Recently, there has been intense interest regarding the role of ubiquitin and ubiquitin-like molecules in DNA damage repair and signalling, along with its interplay with phosphorylation (Al-Hakim et al., 2010). Protein ubiquitylation has emerged as an important regulatory mechanism that impacts almost every aspect of the DNA damage response, in particular in concentrating DNA repair proteins at the sites of DNA damage. The ubiquitylation cascade involves the activities of at least three enzymes: (i) the ubiquitin-activating enzyme (E1); (ii) the ubiquitin-conjugating enzyme (E2); and (iii) the ubiquitin ligase (E3) (Ciechanover et al.,1982; Hershko et al., 1983). E1 employs ATP to adenylate ubiquitin at its C-terminus, which then forms a thioester bond with the E1 active-site cysteine. The modified ubiquitin is then passed on to the E2 enzyme to form another thioester intermediate (the E2~Ub). Finally, ubiquitin is conjugated to its substrate with the aid of an E3 ubiquitin ligase (Al Hakim et al., 2010). The first E3 ubiquitin ligase that acts in this cascade is RING finger protein 8 (RNF8), which accumulates at DSBs via phospho-dependent interactions between its N-terminal fork head associated (FHA) domain and ATM-phosphorylated TQXF motifs on MDC1 (Huen et al., 2007; Kolas et al., 2007; Mailand et al., 2007). At damaged chromatin, RNF8 cooperates with the E2 conjugating enzyme UBC13 to ubiquitylate histones that likely include H2A and H2AX (Huen, et al., 2007; Mailand et al., 2007, Wu et al., 2008). The ubiquitin ligase RNF8 plays an instrumental role in promoting the maturation of DSB-associated chromatin (Huen et al., 2007; Mailand et al., 2007; Kolas et al., 2007; Wang et al., 2007). Through its direct interaction with MDC1, RNF8 is recruited to DSB sites along with the other factors in the initial wave of protein accumulation at IRIF (Mailand et al., 2007). Here, RNF8 initiates a complex and tightly regulated ubiquitylation cascade of histones H2A and H2AX at the DSB-flanking chromatin, which causes chromatin restructuring (through incompletely understood mechanisms) associated with the generation of binding sites for protein complexes that accumulate downstream of these early factors (Huen et al., 2007; Mailand et al., 2007).The covalent attachment of small ubiquitin-like modifier (SUMO) proteins to specific lysine residues of target proteins, a process termed sumoylation, is a recently discovered protein modification that plays an important role in regulating many diverse cellular processes. Sumoylation is a signalling mechanism which, analogous to and in parallel with ubiquitination, plays an important role in chromatin remodelling at DSB sites. Sumoylation is catalyzed by SUMO-specific E1, E2, E3s and is reversed by a family of Sentrin/SUMO-specific proteases, SENPs. The SUMO E3 ligases PIAS1 and PIAS4 are required for recruitment of proteins BRCA1 and 53BP1 to IRIF, respectively, and both SUMO1 and SUMO2/3 accumulate at IRIF (Galanty et al., 2009; Morris et al., 2009). Moreover, replicating protein A (RPA70) sumoylation facilitates recruitment of RAD51 to the DNA damage foci to initiate DNA repair through homologous recombination (Dou et al., 2010).

## 2. Cellular effects of ionizing radiation in human lymphocytes

### 2.1 Surviving fraction, *HPRT* mutant frequency and molecular characterization of mutations in irradiated human lymphocytes

To contribute to the understanding of the DDR pathway following radiation-induced damage, we studied the effects of IR on human peripheral blood lymphocytes (PBL) irradiated *in vitro* with different doses of γ-rays and low-energy protons (0.88 MeV; LET: 28keV/μm). Irradiated PBL were assayed for cell viability, for mutant frequency at the hypoxanthine-guanine phosphoribosyl transferase (*HPRT*) gene, and for molecular characterization of mutations. The *HPRT* gene, which in humans covers 44 kb and encodes a non-essential protein, allows a wide variety of mutations, from point mutation to total gene deletion, to be detected by using the *HPRT* mutation assay. Deletion of DNA segments is the predominant form of radiation damage in cells that survive irradiation and the mechanisms for producing deletion mutations appear to be very complex and dependent on target cell, gene studied, dose, dose-rate and radiation quality (Schwartz et al., 2000). Large deletions are thought to derive from two DNA double strand breaks close enough to interact each other. Thus, deletion frequency should be dependent on radiation dose and dose-rate. All PBL samples, irradiated either with γ-rays or protons, showed a dose-dependent cell survival decrease and a *HPRT* mutant frequency increase. In Table 1 we report the data of survival and *HPRT* mutant frequency in human PBL irradiated with different doses of γ-rays and low-energy protons.

Molecular analyses of *HPRT* mutants were carried out in clones derived from PBL exposed to γ-rays (1-4 Gy) and to low-energy protons (0.5-2Gy), and in non-irradiated clones of the same donors. Among the mutant clones obtained from γ-irradiated PBL, point mutations were the only kind of mutation in 1Gy irradiated clones, whereas deletions were the prevalent mutations among clones irradiated at 4Gy. In contrast, no partial or total deletions of the *HPRT* gene were detected in mutant clones isolated after proton irradiation. Figure 1 shows the percentages of mutation types calculated over the total number of mutations derived from human PBL irradiated with both radiation qualities. The difference of the mutational spectrum between γ-rays and protons probably depends on the nature of IR. Complex gene rearrangements and deletions are assumed to be a specific signature of exposure to high-LET radiation in mammalian cells. Nevertheless, the absence of these kind of mutations in PBL irradiated with protons could be due to their lower survival in comparison with γ-irradiated PBL, as a consequence of the more cytotoxic than mutagenic lesions induced.

| | SF (%) ± S.E. | HPRT MF ($x10^{-6}$) ± S.E. |
|---|---|---|
| γ-rays | | |
| 0.5 Gy | 99.5 ± 0 | 2.8 ± 0 |
| 1.0 Gy | 83.85 ± 11.36 | 10.5 ± 3.8 |
| 2.0 Gy | 44.7 ± 7.36 | 29.2 ± 3.7 |
| 3.0 Gy | 13.7 ± 4.56 | 50.6 ± 17.9 |
| 4.0 Gy | 6.2 ± 2.4 | 24.7 ± 11.1 |
| Protons | | |
| 0.5 Gy | 60.84 ± 7.82 | 5.33 ± 2.18 |
| 1.0 Gy | 39.87 ± 6.28 | 9.25 ± 2.8 |
| 1.5 Gy | 38.42 ± 11.35 | 16.72 ± 4.86 |
| 2.0 Gy | 35.5 ± 0 | 11.7 ± 1 |
| 2.5 Gy | 29.9 ± 11.35 | 5.06 ± 0 |

Table 1. Surviving fraction (SF) and *HPRT* mutant frequency (± standard error, S.E.) in human PBL irradiated with γ-rays and low-energy protons.

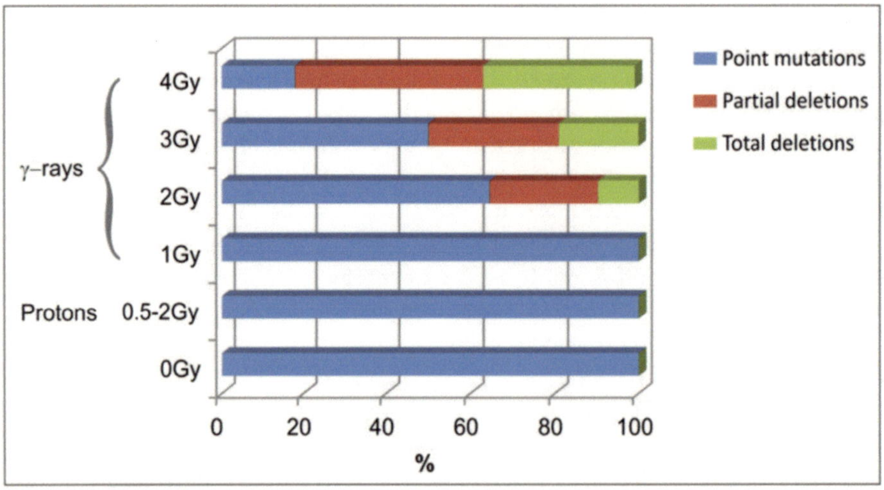


Fig. 1. Characterization of *HPRT* mutant clones derived from PBL irradiated with γ-rays and protons or non-irradiated (0Gy).

**2.2 Double strand break repair in irradiated human lymphocytes**

To evaluate the repair of DSBs in PBL irradiated with γ-rays or low-energy protons, we analyzed γ-H2AX kinetics through foci formation and disappearance. The presence of nuclear foci was monitored by *in situ* immunofluorescence at different time points after IR. Figure 2 shows the different γ-H2AX foci pattern at 2h after IR with high- and low-LET radiation, reflecting the sparsely and densely nature of IR.

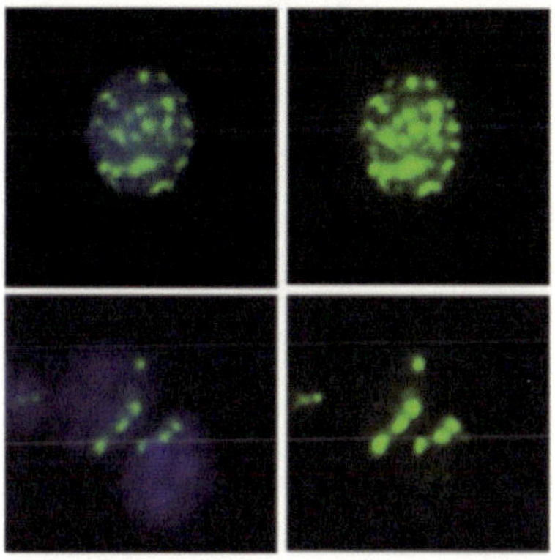


Fig. 2. Visualization by *in situ* immunofluorescence of γ-H2AX foci in human PBL irradiated with γ-rays or low-energy protons. The pattern of γ-H2AX localization within the nucleus is strictly dependent on the quality of radiation. Low-LET radiation, such as γ-rays, hit the cells throughout all directions, and DSBs are sparsely distributed; on the contrary, high-LET radiation such as protons, give raise to clustered DNA damage along tracks.

In irradiated PBL the kinetics of DSB repair was different according to the quality of radiation. In particular, the fraction of foci-positive cells was higher in γ-irradiated than in proton-irradiated lymphocytes at all times, except at 24h after IR. Early after irradiation (30 min and 2h) γ-H2AX foci were present in 80% and 43% of PBL, irradiated respectively with γ-rays and protons (Fig. 3A). This difference is mainly due to the quality of radiation: while sparsely IR as γ-rays lose their energy throughout all directions thus hitting all nuclei, densely IR as protons, hits the fraction of cells along their track. The preferential production of complex aberrations is related to the unique energy deposition patterns produced by densely ionizing radiation, causing highly localized multiple DNA damage. At 6h after IR the percentage of foci-positive cells decreased, revealing the repair capacity of DSBs in both kind of irradiated lymphocytes, although the repair kinetics was faster in γ-irradiated PBL. At 24h after IR the percentage of γ-H2AX foci positive cells tended to reach the value of non-irradiated PBL, either in γ- and in proton-irradiated PBL.

The mean number of γ-H2AX foci per nucleus was higher in PBL irradiated with γ-rays than with protons, at all times after IR (Fig. 3B). In our experiments, most of PBL displayed 10-20 or more γ-H2AX foci/nucleus 30 min after irradiation, giving a maximum yield of 4 foci/Gy, a number similar to that reported for human PBL irradiated with X-rays (about 10 foci/Gy) (Sak et al., 2007; Schertan et al., 2008), but much lower than that determined in human fibroblasts (32.2 foci/Gy) (Hamada et al., 2006). It has been reported that the number of γ-H2AX foci is well consistent with the number of theoretically calculated DSB/Gy of sparsely ionizing radiation (i.e. about 40) (Ward, 1991), if one DSB is contained per focus.

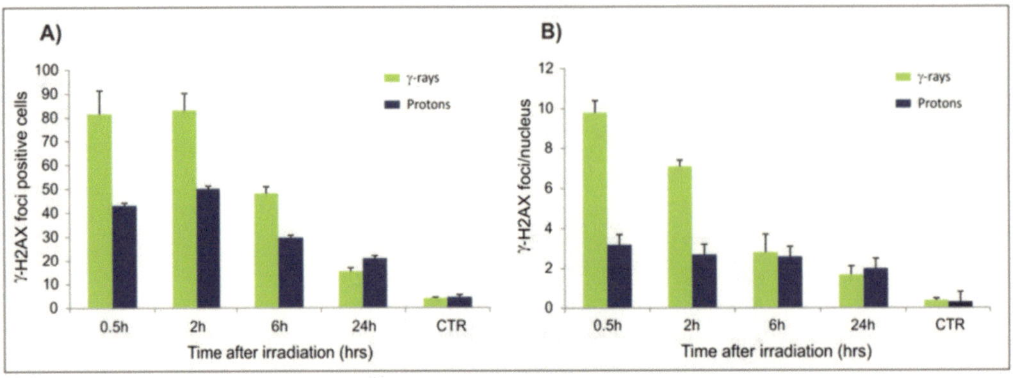


Fig. 3. Kinetics of γ-H2AX foci in PBL irradiated with γ-rays and low energy protons during the time after irradiation. A) Fraction of cells positive for γ-H2AX foci and B) mean number of γ-H2AX foci per nucleus.

The lower number of foci detected in peripheral lymphocytes could depend on the large amount of heterochromatin of resting cells, from which γ-H2AX foci are mostly excluded (Cowell et al., 2007) as well as on the small nuclear volume, where overlapping foci are difficult to detect separately. Thus, in accordance with the observations of Scherthan et al., (2008) we hypothesize that γ-H2AX foci detected very early after irradiation contained more than one DSB; later on, the number of foci decreased and probably each foci contained only one DSB. Furthermore , we found a size increase of γ-H2AX foci in cells irradiated with protons, as compared with gamma irradiations, probably as a consequence of DSBs clusters induced by high-LET radiation. Our results are in accordance with those in melanoma cells exposed to low- and high-LET radiation (Ibañez et al., 2009).

## 3. Cellular effects of ionizing radiation in human lymphocytes cultured in microgravity condition

The cellular response to ionizing radiation besides on genetic and physiological features of the biological systems, depends also on environmental conditions occurring during DNA repair. Space missions expose humans to an exogenous environment not encountered within our biosphere, in particular the contemporary presence of radiation and a condition of weightlessness called microgravity ($10^{-4}$–$10^{-6}$g). One of the important aspects of risk estimation during space flights, is whether the effects of radiation on astronauts are influenced by microgravity. The combination of microgravity and ionizing radiation has been demonstrated to have a synergistic action on human cells, both *in vivo* and *in vitro*. The effects of space environment experienced by astronauts include loss of calcium and minerals from bone, decreased skeletal muscle mass and depressed immune function (Longnecker et al., 2004). *Ex vivo* astronaut studies, in-flight cell cultures, and ground models of microgravity studies, have consistently demonstrated inhibition of lymphocyte proliferation and suppressed or altered cytokine secretion (Lewis et al., 1998; Grimm et al., 2002). Among the biological effects of the reduced gravity in human cell cultures, were described apoptosis induction, cytoskeletal alteration, cell growth inhibition and increased frequency of chromosome aberrations (Lewis et al., 1998; Grimm et al., 2002; Cubano et al., 2000; Sytkowski et al., 2001; Mosesso et al., 2001; Durante et al., 2003). Gene expression analyses on human cells grown in microgravity during space flights or in modeled microgravity (MMG) on Earth, report changes among genes involved in apoptosis induction, cell adhesion, cytoskeletal features and cell differentiation, even if large differences in culture conditions, cell types and methods to simulate microgravity were adopted in those experiments (Hammond et al., 2000; Lewis et al., 2001, Torigoe et al., 2001, Infanger et al., 2007). While the genotoxic effects of ionizing radiation have been intensely studied, the consequence of the reduced gravity together with radiation is still unclear. Therefore, it is of special importance to verify whether DDR is affected by the combined effects of IR and microgravity, in view of the prolonged permanence of man in future space missions. To analyze the possibility that a reduced gravitational force impairs the DDR pathway, increasing the risk of the exposure to conditions occurring during spaceflight, we studied the DDR to ionizing radiation in human PBL incubated in MMG and in parallel static conditions. Microgravity was simulated by culturing PBL in the Rotating Wall Vessel bioreactor (Synthecon, Cellon, Fig. 4) placed inside a humidified incubator, vertically rotating at 23 rpm.

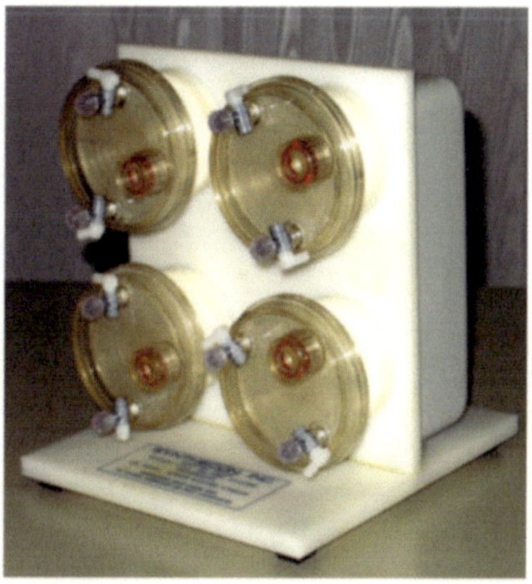

Fig. 4. Rotating Wall Vessel Bioreactor (Synthecon).

The Rotating Wall Vessel was developed at the NASA Johnson Space Center (Houston, TX) to simulate, as accurately as possible, culture conditions predicted to occur during experiments in space. In the rotating system, the gravity is balanced by equal and opposite mechanical forces (centrifugal, Coriolis and shear components), and the gravitational vector is reduced to about $10^{-2}$ g. In these conditions, single cells are nearly always in suspension, rotating quasi-stationary with the fluid, in a low-shear culture environment (Unsworth 1998, Maccarone et al., 2003). Ground based (1 g) PBL cultures, both irradiated and non-irradiated, were kept at the same cell density in flasks inside a humidified incubator for 24 h.

### 3.1 The DNA-damage response of human peripheral lymphocytes cultured in microgravity after γ-irradiation

The DNA-damage response was investigated in human PBL irradiated *in vitro* with different doses of gamma rays and incubated for 24 h in 1 g or in modeled microgravity (MMG). While cell survival was only slight affected by MMG, the *HPRT* mutant frequency significantly increased in PBL incubated in MMG after irradiation compared with those maintained in 1 g. Given the increase of *HPRT* mutants in MMG, we investigated whether the reduced gravity affected the progression of the rejoining of double strand breaks (DSBs) in human PBL irradiated with γ-rays and incubated in MMG or in 1g. The kinetics of γ-H2AX foci was monitored during the repair incubation, showing that DSBs rejoining was slower in MMG than in 1g at 6 and 24 h after irradiation. In addition, the mean number of γ-H2AX foci per nucleus was significantly higher in MMG than in 1g at the same time-points (Fig. 5).

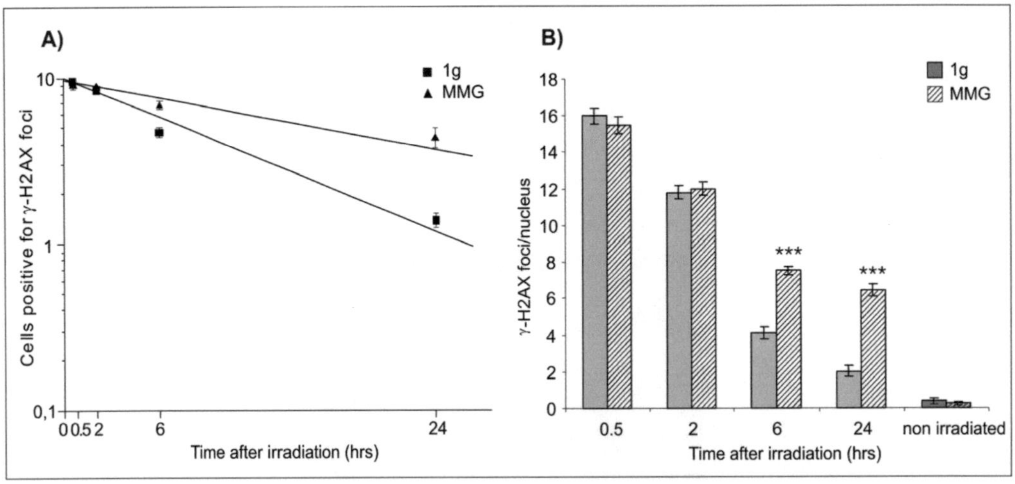


Fig. 5. Kinetics of γ-H2AX foci in PBL irradiated with 5Gy of γ-rays and incubated in 1g or MMG during the repair time. A) Fraction of PBL positive for γ-H2AX foci. B) Mean number of γ-H2AX foci/nucleus (****P*<0.001, *t*-test).

To verify whether the disappearance of γ-H2AX foci correlated with the rejoining of double strand breaks, we subjected irradiated lymphocytes to a non-radioactive PFGE assay (Gradzka et al., 2005). The fraction of DNA released (FR) from the plug after PFGE was considered a measure of DSB level. The kinetics of DSB removal in lymphocytes irradiated and incubated in 1g exhibits a typical fast initial component and a decreasing rate at longer repair intervals, in accordance with data from other authors (Stenerlow et al., 2000; Gradzka et al., 2005). Both the methods we used to quantify DNA fragmentation, reported a lower rate of DSB rejoining in lymphocytes incubated in MMG compared to those in 1g, in agreement with the kinetics of γ-H2AX foci. Our results provide evidences that MMG incubation during DNA repair delayed the rate of radiation-induced DSB rejoining, and increased, as a consequence, the genotoxic effects of ionizing radiation.

We then assessed whether MMG incubation affected IR-induced apoptosis. Human lymphocytes, irradiated and non-irradiated, were scored for the presence of fragmented nuclei and apoptotic bodies. Apoptotic index (A.I.) increased with time after irradiation and at 24 h it was significantly higher in PBL incubated in MMG compared to those in 1g (19.3% vs. 13.7% respectively, $P < 0.001$). Since DSBs can be induced, besides radiation, also by DNA fragmentation during early apoptosis, we measured caspase-3 activation at the same time-points by the cleavage of the peptide substrate DEVD-AFC. Caspase-3 activation was only slightly higher in PBL maintained in MMG than in 1g, in contrast to the high persistence of foci-positive cells ($P < 0.01$), and foci number/nucleus ($P < 0.001$), suggesting that the level of H2AX phosphorylation was principally correlated to a delayed DSB resolution rather than apoptosis induction.

We then tested for the possibility that MMG incubation affects DNA damage response by altering the recruitment of the signaling proteins, 53BP1, NBS1-p343 and ATM-p1981, which co-localize with γ-H2AX foci to DSB sites (Fig. 6A). After irradiation ~90% of cells became foci-positive for the three proteins in both gravity conditions (not shown). In contrast to γ-H2AX, the fraction of foci-positive cells persisted high up to 24 h after irradiation in 1g and no differences between the two culture conditions were detected. The number of foci/nucleus significantly decreased during post-irradiation incubation from 14–16 foci/nucleus at 30 min to 4–5 foci/nucleus at 24 h (Fig. 6B), without differences between samples in 1g and MMG. The discrepancies with the kinetics of γ-H2AX foci suggest that these proteins could represent the remaining scaffold structure used for DSB repair that persisted after the repair has been completed (Markova et al., 2007, van Veelen et al., 2005).

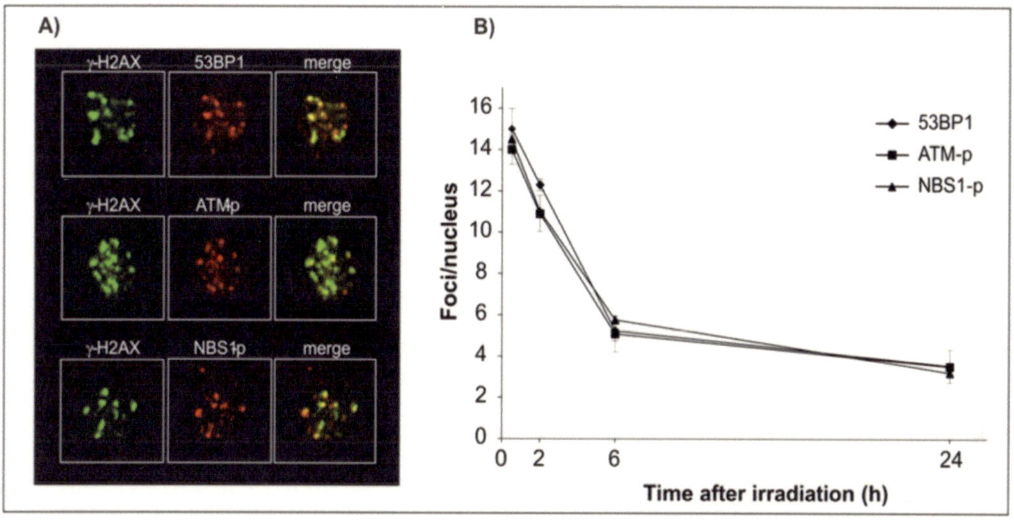


Fig. 6. Kinetics of 53BP1, ATM-p1981, NBS1-p343 foci in PBL irradiated with γ-rays and incubated in 1g. A) Co-localization with γ-H2AX foci to form the ionizing radiation-induced foci (IRIF). B) Mean number of foci per nucleus.

### 3.2 The DNA-damage response of human tumoral lymphocytes cultured in microgravity after γ-irradiation

We analyzed the DNA damage response to radiation also in human tumoral lymphocytes (TK6 cells, lymphoblastoid B cells) irradiated with γ–rays (1, 2, 4 Gy) and incubated in 1g or in MMG during the repair time. In irradiated TK6 cells, we observed a higher survival in MMG than in 1g, and the difference was significant at 4Gy. In addition, in cells maintained in MMG rather than in 1g after γ-irradiation, higher frequency of HPRT mutants was observed at all irradiation doses, particularly at 4Gy (Figure 7A). Remarkably, at this dose, mutant frequency may often be underestimated, since cells with many and severe mutations are unable to repair DNA damage and die. Instead, in TK6 cells cultured in MMG after irradiation, mutant frequency increased with doses up to 4Gy (Figure 7A). The frequency of micronucleated cells was measured in both gravity conditions after irradiation. At the end of post-irradiation incubation (24 h time-point), the percentage of micronuclei (MN) was significantly higher in both non-irradiated and in irradiated cells incubated in MMG compared with 1g (Fig.7B). Eighteen hours later (42 h from irradiation), the percentage of MN in cultures incubated in MMG was higher than in 1g only at 2Gy γ-ray dose. At 48 h time-point, MN frequencies observed in 1g or MMG were comparable. As expected, MN significantly increased after irradiation in both gravity conditions with respect to non-irradiated cells; a significant difference was still observed at 48 h after irradiation at both 1 and 2Gy. The significant increase of micronucleated cells in MMG suggested that MMG itself was able to induce chromosome damage.

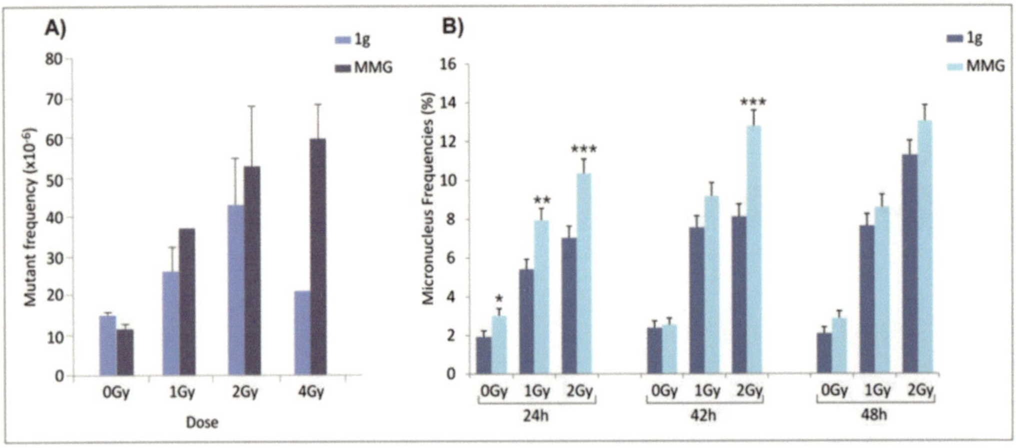


Fig. 7. A) Mutant frequency at the HPRT locus of irradiated and non-irradiated TK6 cells incubated for 24h in 1g or in modeled microgravity. B) Micronucleus frequencies (%) in irradiated and non-irradiated TK6 cells incubated in 1g of MMG for the first 24h after irradiation and then cultured in 1g up to 48 h. *$P$<0.05; **$P$<0.01; ***$P$<0.001 (*G* test).

The effect of MMG incubation on cell cycle alteration induced by γ−ray exposure was assessed by flow cytometry analysis. Figure 8 shows the cell cycle distribution of TK6 cells at various time-points from irradiation and incubation in MMG or 1g by representative DNA histograms. γ-ray irradiation induced an increase in G2/M-phase cells and a reduction in S-phase cells, both in TK6 maintained in 1g and MMG after irradiation. At the end of MMG or 1g incubation (24 h time-point), the percentages of cells in G1-phase were higher in cultures irradiated with 2-4 Gy and incubated in MMG compared with cells maintained in 1g. Moreover, the G2/M block after irradiation was less evident in MMG than in 1g condition. Also radiation-induced apoptosis was affected in TK6 cells by MMG incubation. Induction of apoptosis was significantly lower in irradiated TK6 cells incubated in MMG compared with cells irradiated with the same dose and incubated in 1g. The differences were more pronounced in cells analyzed at long post-incubation times (72 h time-point).
The observed decrease of apoptotic response in MMG incubated cultures could allow severely damaged cells, which in 1g condition should be eliminated by selection, to survive, with negative consequences on genomic integrity. Alterations in cell response to ionizing radiation due to MMG incubation during the DNA repair period may be caused by the reduced activity of some proteins, which play a crucial role in damage signaling. Previous data have shown that absence or reduction of gravity can alter gene expression (Walther et

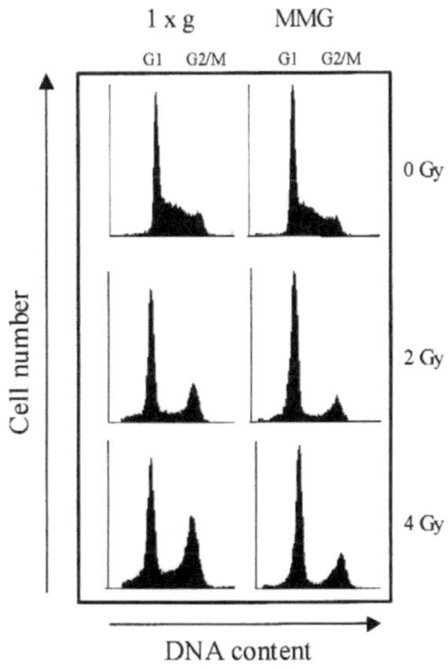


Fig. 8. Cell cycle distribution of irradiated and non-irradiated TK6 cells at the end of 24h incubation in 1g or in MMG.

al., 1998; Hughes-Fulford 2001; Kita et al., 2000), which in turn may explain the results reported here. It remains to be determined if one upstream or several downstream genes belonging to the pathway of the radiation response are involved in the effects induced by MMG incubation.

### 3.3 Gene expression changes in human lymphocytes cultured in microgravity during the DNA-damage response to radiation

Gene expression changes represent an early bio-indicator of radiation exposure. Given the increase of *HPRT* mutants observed in human lymphocytes incubated in modeled microgravity, we investigated whether this gravity condition can alter the transcription of 14 genes representative of the main DNA repair pathways. The genes analyzed are representative of the major DNA repair pathways: four genes (*Ku70, Ku80, DNA-ligase IV, XRCC4*) are involved in non-homologous end joining processes (NHEJ), three genes (*BRCA1, BRCA2, RAD51*) in homologous recombination (HR), four genes (*XRCC1, PCNA,GADD45A, p21Cip1/Waf1*) in base excision repair (BER) and two genes (*DDB2, XPC*) in nucleotide excision repair (NER). *DNA-ligase I*, involved in both BER and NER repair pathways, was analyzed too. Analyses were carried out in three pools of three donor, each by quantitative real time PCR. Results show that almost all BER and NER genes were up-regulated in irradiated PBL, whereas the expression of HR and NHEJ genes was only slightly or not affected by radiation (Fig.9). Incubation in modeled microgravity after irradiation did not significantly change the expression of genes involved in DNA repair, suggesting that transcriptional impairment was not responsible for the increase of mutant frequency observed in irradiated cells incubated in microgravity in comparison to the static 1 g condition. These findings in agreement with previous studies on gene expression of non-irradiated space flown and RWV cultured cells, showing that DNA repair genes were unaffected by low-gravity whereas intracellular signaling, growth regulatory, cytoskeletal and tumor suppressor genes were altered (Lewis et al., 2001; Hammond et al., 2000; Pardo et al., 2005).

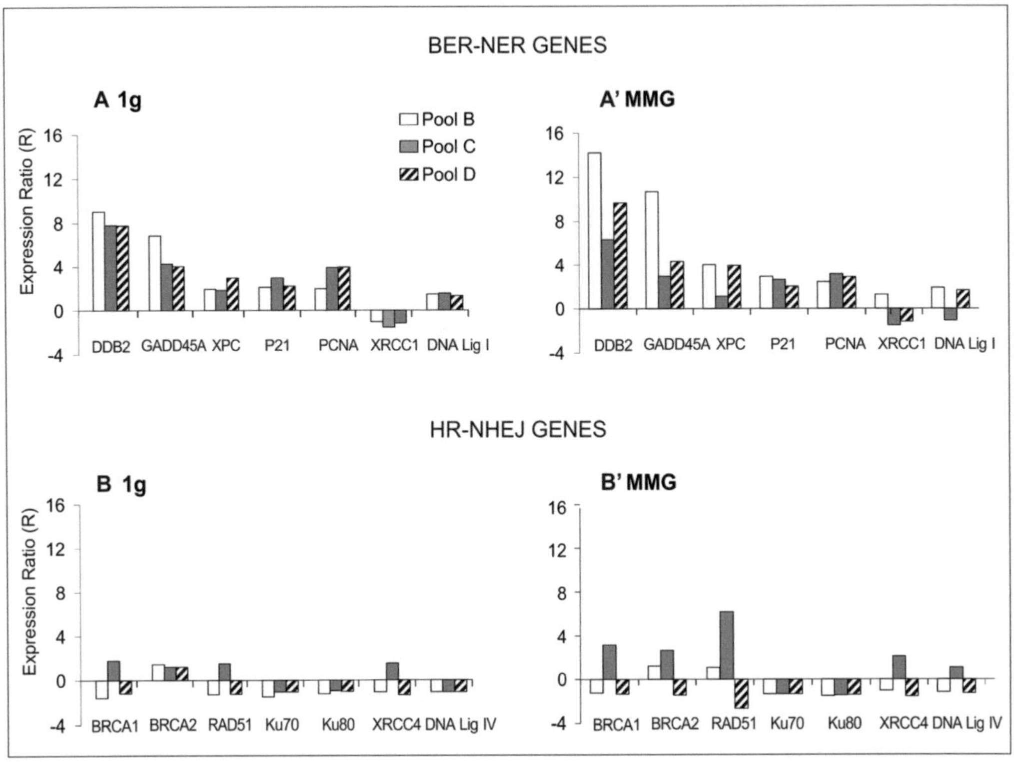


Fig. 9. Expression ratios in PBL of pools B–D incubated in 1 g and modeled microgravity after X-irradiation. (A) *R* values of BER and NER genes in 1g; (A) *R* values of BER and NER in MMG; (B) *R* values of HR and NHEJ genes in 1g; (B) *R* values of HR and NHEJ genes in MMG.

Recently, a new class of important gene modulators has been discovered: microRNAs. They are a large family of small non-coding RNAs of 18-24 nucleotides that negatively regulate gene expression levels by binding to microRNA-binding elements in the 3′ untranslated-region (3′UTR) of target mRNAs thereby triggering decreased protein translation mainly through mRNA degradation (Guo et al., 2010). A single miRNA may have broad effects on gene expression networks, such as regulating cell lineage specificity, cellular functions or stress response. By considering the complexity of the DNA-damage response (DDR), addressed to maintain genome integrity through cell cycle arrest, DNA repair and/or apoptosis, it is expected that miRNAs have an important role in this cellular process. Whilst miRNA-mediated DDR has been studied after UV radiation and hypoxic stress (Pothof et al., 2009; Crosby et al., 2009) that of radiation combined with microgravity has not been studied yet and should give important information about risk assessment in space environment. MicroRNAs profiling were carried out by using the platform "Human miRNA Microarray kit (V2)" (Agilent), according to the Agilent miRNA protocol. For mRNA expression profile we used the "Whole Human Genome Oligo Microarray" (Agilent), consisting of ~41.000 (60-mer) oligonucleotide probes, which span conserved exons across the transcripts of the targeted full-length genes. Identification of differentially expressed genes and miRNAs was performed with one and two class Significance Analysis of Microarray (SAM) program (Tusher et al., 2001) with default settings. Figure 10A shows a dendrogram relative to some miRNAs differentially expressed following ionizing radiation in human PBL.

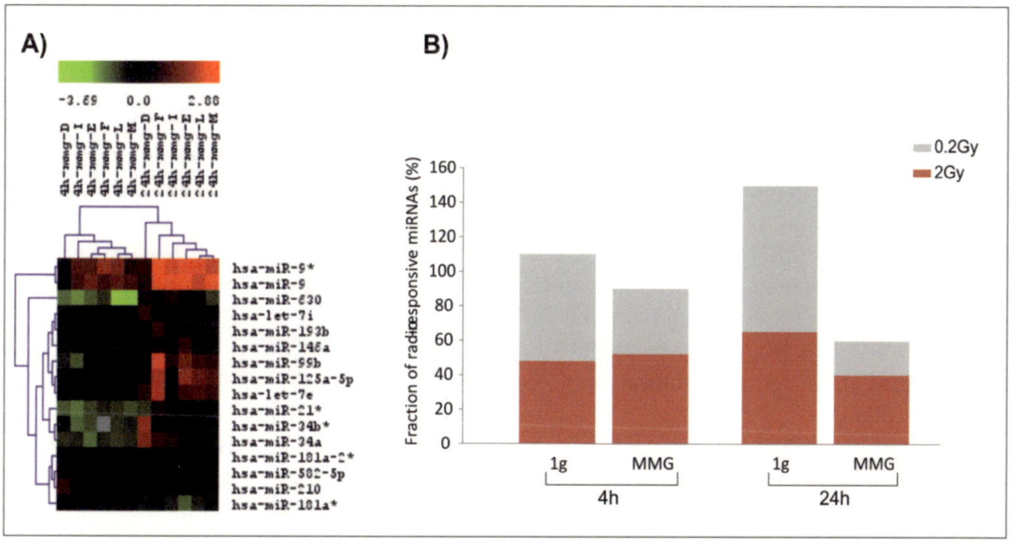


Fig. 10. A) Dendrogram showing several miRNAs differentially expressed in human PBL at 4 and 24h after irradiation with 0.2Gy. Range of expression value is determined as the log2 ratio of irradiated/non-irradiated sample. Down-regulated and up-regulated miRNAs correspond to green and red boxes, respectively. B) Fraction of radio-responsive miRNAs (%) in human PBL irradiated with 0.2 and 2Gy and incubated for 4 and 24h- in 1g or in modeled microgravity (MMG).

MiRNA expression profile was carried out at 4h and 24h after irradiation with 0.2Gy and 2Gy and incubation in 1g and MMG and compared to that of non-irradiated PBL maintained in parallel conditions. Results showed that in both gravity conditions the miRNA expression profile was dose-specific, as indicated by the low percentage of common miRNA responsive to both doses; moreover, the effects of the higher dose predominated at the late time point. Interestingly, MMG tended to decrease the number of radio-responsive miRNAs respect to 1g condition, in particular at 24h after irradiation (Figure 10B).

To predict the target genes of differentially expressed miRNAs we first performed a computational analyses using PITA algorithm available on line (Kertesz et al., 2007). However, all available software for target prediction are characterized by a large fraction of false positives, thus to identify the most likely targets, we have integrated mRNA and miRNA expression data, obtained on the same lymphocyte samples, using MAGIA (MiRNA And Genes Integrated Analysis) web tool (Sales et al., 2010). We used a non-parametric index (Spearman correlation coefficient), the most indicated statistical coefficient for a small number of measures, to estimate the degree of anti-correlation (e.g. up-regulated miRNA and corresponding down-regulated mRNA target) between any putative pairs of miRNA and mRNA (Xin et al., 2009; Wang and Li 2009). The anti-correlated transcripts were then classified according to DAVID (Database for Annotation, Visualization and Integrated Discovery) web tool (Huang et al. 2009), to determine which Gene Ontology (GO) terms were significantly enriched in our set of genes. Results of G0 analysis of anti-correlated genes showed that in MMG-incubated PBL were not enriched the categories of response to stress, to DNA damage and to apoptosis. miRNA-mRNA anti-correlations of DDR pathway were visualized by using Cytoscape software package (Shannon et al., 2003; Cline et al., 2007) (Figure 11). The results showed that, in most cases, the same mRNA was targeted by different miRNA species according to the different condition of gravity.

Future research is addressed to validate several of the anti-correlations highlighted with our analyses as important in DDR pathway. In particular, we will perform a functional assay to demonstrate the regulatory effect of a particular miRNA on its putative target mRNA. The luciferase assay represents the most efficient approach to evaluate the activity of a miRNA on its anti-correlated mRNA. This assay allows to demonstrate the activity of a miRNA on its anti-correlated mRNA by the quantification of the luminescent signal derived from the luciferase reporter enzyme. Cells are co-transfected with a reporter vector containing the firefly luciferase gene together with the 3'UTR target sequence predicted for that miRNA and the miRNA precursor (pre-miRNA) or inhibitor (anti-miRNA), which respectively mimics and inhibits the endogenous miRNA. The binding of pre-miRNA to the complementary target sequence will cause the repression of luciferase gene expression, whereas the binding of anti-miRNA to the endogenous miRNA will induce the expression of luciferase gene. The quantification of the luminescent signal derived from the luciferase reporter enzyme thus allows to demonstrate the activity of a miRNA on its putative target mRNA. In addition to the luciferase assay, it would be interesting to study the role of selected miRNAs in DDR pathway by a biological approach. Usually, several end points such as cell survival, DNA repair, cell cycle progression and apoptosis induction are analyzed in cells over-or under-expressing the miRNA of interest.

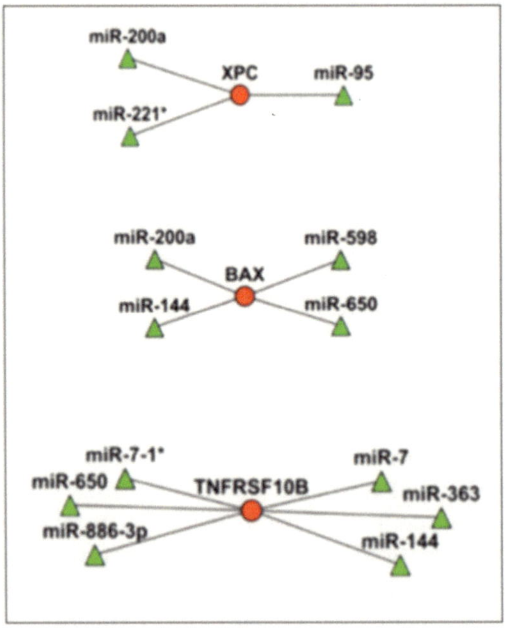


Fig. 11. Example of visualization of inversely correlated miRNA-mRNA relationships in irradiated human PBL. Circles represent transcripts and triangles miRNAs, shown with the color corresponding to the expression value.

## 4. The DNA-damage response of human lymphocytes to indirect effect of ionizing radiation

In addition the cellular effects arising as a direct response to ionizing radiation, in the last decade it has been suggested that extranuclear or extracellular targets can contribute to the genetic damage in non-irradiated (bystander) cells. The bystander effect (BE) is the biological response of non-irradiated cells induced by contact with irradiated cells. The contact with bystander factors may occur by direct cell–cell interaction or be mediated by the fluid surrounding the cells. It has been reported that the BE causes cell death, cell cycle arrest, apoptosis, changes in gene expression, and increases micronucleus induction, chromosomal aberrations, mutation frequency, and DNA damage in cells neighboring hit cells. In contrast to DNA damage induced by direct irradiation, bystander cell DNA damage is still poorly understood. Many data showed that early events of the radiation induced bystander effect are rapid calcium fluxes and generation of reactive oxygen species in bystander cells. Mitochondria seem to play a central role in bystander signaling: irradiated cell conditioned media can cause changes of mitochondrial distribution, loss of mitochondrial membrane potential, increases in ROS, and increase in apoptosis among the medium receptor cells, which can be blocked by treatments with antioxidants (Chen et al., 2008). Experiments carried out in hepatoma cell lines provide evidence that the BE can be modulated by the p53 status of irradiated cells and that a p53-dependent release of cytochrome-c from mitochondria may be involved in producing BE (He et al., 2011).

We investigated on the mechanisms of the medium-mediated bystander response induced by low doses of $\gamma$-rays in human tumoural lymphocytes (TK6 cells), a cell line growing in suspension, in which gap-junction communications are not involved in transferring bystander signals and only medium-mediated molecules may be responsible for BE induction. Cell cultures were irradiated and the culture medium discarded immediately after irradiation and replaced with a fresh one to eliminate ROS originating during irradiation. Irradiated cells were incubated for 6h in fresh medium, which, at the end of incubation time, is referred as conditioned medium (CM) and used to incubate non-irradiated TK6 cells for different times (2-48 h). In bystander cultures, cell mortality at the fixed incubation times ranged between 24 and 19%, very similar values to that of directly irradiated cells (28 and 20%). The mortality percentages for all incubation times were significantly higher with respect to that of the controls (0Gy and 0Gy CM). The survival fraction of directly 1Gy irradiated or CM incubated cells was determined by the clonogenic assay. The data show that both irradiated and bystander TK6 cells had a lower cloning efficiency than their respective controls. Figure 12 reports the results about cell mortality and survival (given as the ratio of the cloning efficiency of treated vs. untreated control cells) in TK6 cells exposed directly to IR or to CM. Apoptosis induction was tested by the presence of fragmented nuclei and apoptotic bodies at 2, 24 and 48h after 1Gy irradiation or CM incubation. The apoptotic index (A.I.) ranged between 7 and 9 % in irradiated cells and between 6 and 7.5 % in bystander cells, and was significantly higher than the relative controls at all times (Figure 13). The induction of apoptosis was also analyzed by the activation of caspase-3, the principal effector caspase, assayed by the cleavage of the peptide substrate DEVD-AFC, at 1, 2, 24 and 48h after irradiation or CM incubation. In bystander cells caspase-3 activation increased from 1.4- to 2.7-fold during the 48h of CM incubation, suggesting that bystander apoptosis increases after 48h. Bystander apoptosis in TK6 cells was sensitive to the inhibitor of caspase-8, the Z-IETD-fmk, added during CM treatment or

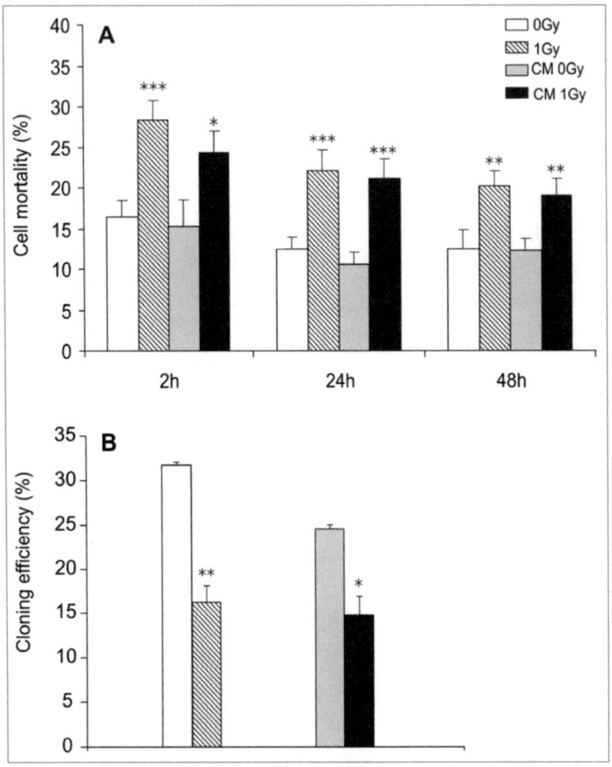


Fig. 12. Cell mortality determined by Trypan blue staining (A) and cloning efficiency (B) in non-irradiated control cells (0Gy), in irradiated cells (1Gy), in cells incubated with conditioned medium from non-irradiated cells (CM 0Gy) and in cells incubated with conditioned medium from irradiated cells (CM 1Gy). Results are the means of 3-5 independent experiments ± S.E. (*$P$< 0.05, **$P$<0.01, ***$P$<0.001, *t* test).

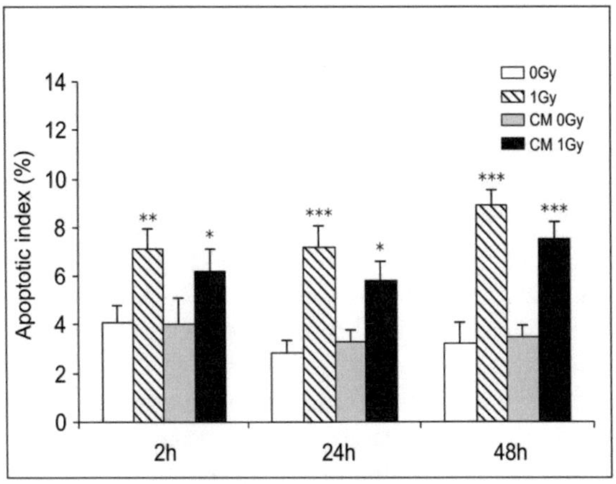


Fig. 13. Apoptotic index (A) in irradiated and bystander cells. Results are the means ± S.E. of 5-8 independent experiments. Significant differences were observed in 1Gy and CM 1Gy vs 0Gy and CM 0Gy, respectively (*$P$<0.05, **$P$<0.01, ***$P$<0.001, *t* test).

post-irradiation incubation. The presence of the inhibitor significantly decreased the induction of apoptosis to the control level, but it did not significantly decrease the level of apoptosis in either irradiated or non-irradiated controls (Figure 14). These results suggest that caspase-8 activation is triggered by signaling molecules present in the conditioned medium. The addition of the ROS scavenger Cu-Zn superoxide dismutase and N-acetylcysteine to the conditioned medium allowed to investigate the involvement of oxidative stress in inducing bystander apoptosis. ROS scavengers did not significantly decrease the apoptotic index in CM cultures; by treating non-irradiated TK6 cells with medium irradiated without cells (IM), we evaluated the contribute of ROS produced by irradiation in inducing bystander apoptosis.

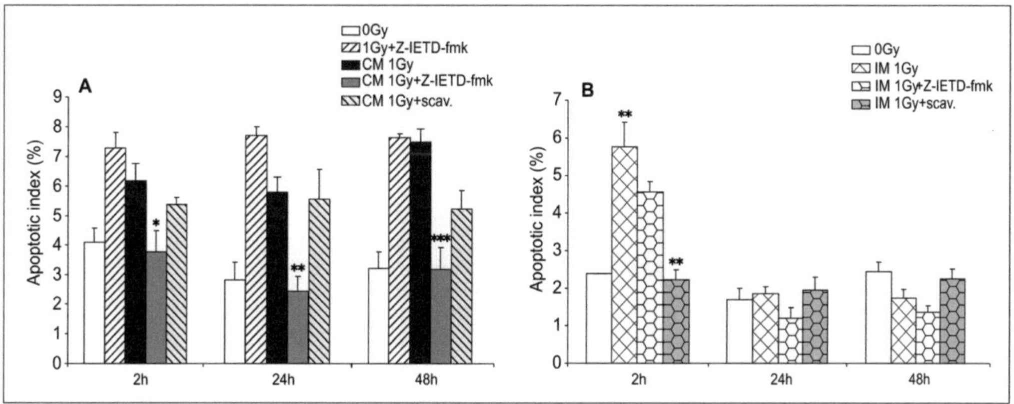


Fig. 14. Apoptotic index in irradiated cells (1Gy), in irradiated cells incubated with caspase-8 inhibitor (1Gy + Z-IETD-fmk), in bystander cells incubated with caspase-8 inhibitor (CM 1Gy + Z-IETD-fmk), and with ROS scavengers SOD and NAC (CM 1Gy + scav.). Results are the means of 3-5 independent experiments ± S.E. Significant differences were observed in CM 1Gy vs CM 1Gy + Z-IETD-fmk at all times. **B**. Apoptotic index in cells incubated with irradiated medium (IM 1Gy), with irradiated medium in the presence of caspase-8 inhibitor (IM 1Gy + Z-IETD-fmk), and ROS scavengers (IM 1Gy + scav.). The values are the means of 3 independent experiments ± S.E. Significant differences were observed at 2 h of incubation with IM 1 Gy vs IM 1Gy + Z-IETD-fmk (*$P<0.05$, **$P<0.01$, ***$P<0.001$, *t*-test).

IM incubation for 2h increased the apoptotic index which was totally inhibited by ROS scavengers and little affected by incubation with the caspase-8 inhibitor, whereas at 24 and 48h no significant differences among samples incubated with IM were observed. DSBs induced by ionizing radiation can easily be detected by the extensive H2AX phosphorylation occurring near DNA lesions, forming foci that co-localize with several repair proteins (Fernandez-Capetillo et al., 2003). 85% of TK6 were γ-H2AX foci positive at 2h after irradiation with 1Gy, then this percentage decreased to the level of non-irradiated cells 24h later, fitting DNA repair kinetics. The incubation of cells with CM for 2h significantly increased the percentage of γ-H2AX foci positive cells (9-11%) but, when the CM was kept in contact with bystander cells for 24h the number of positive cells decreased to control levels, suggesting that DNA lesions induced at the beginning of CM incubation are repaired and no new damage accumulates later. Data from other human cells show that γ-H2AX foci induction in bystander cells persists in time, probably as a consequence of the formation of bystander factors that themselves generate ROS, leading to a self-sustaining system responsible for long-lasting effects (Yang 2005, Sokolov 2005, Kashino 2004, Lyng 2006). In irradiated TK6 cells both 53BP1 and NBS1p343 proteins co-localized with γ-H2AX foci, whereas in bystander cells co-localization was partial or absent (Figure 15).

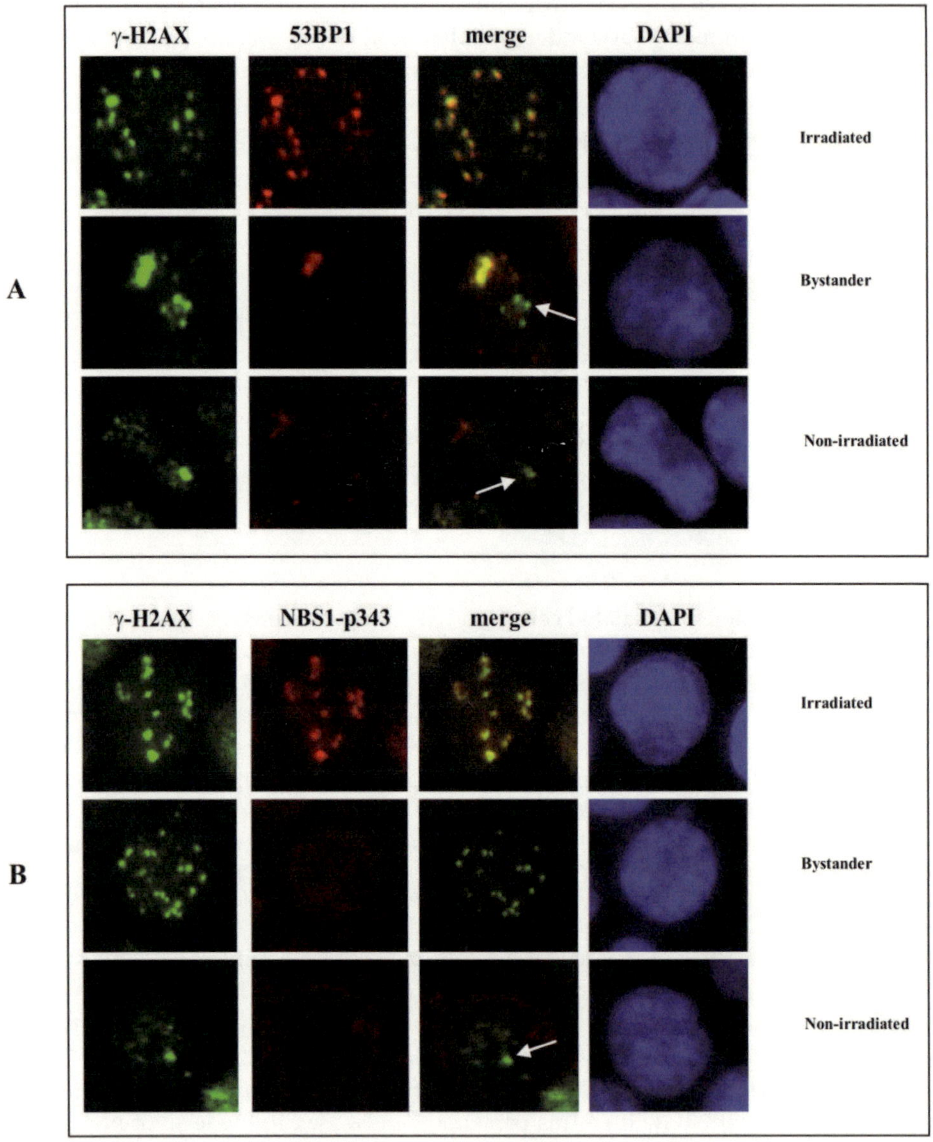


Fig. 15. Non-irradiated, irradiated and bystander TK6 cells were fixed and co-stained with anti- γH2AX (green), anti-53BP1 and anti-NBS1-p343 (red), at 2 h from irradiation or CM incubation. The red and green images were merged and subjected to co-localization analysis. Arrows indicate γH2AX foci without co-localization of 53BP1and NBS1-proteins. Nuclei were counterstained with DAPI.

We suggest that the short-lived ROS released in the medium by irradiated cells are responsible for DNA lesions, unlike double strand breaks, which activate H2AX phosphorylation but do not require the 53BP1 and NBS1p343 proteins to be repaired. It is possible that in our experiments DNA damage induced by CM treatment consisted of a few DSBs, the repair of which requires the recruitment of 53BP1 and NBS1p343 proteins and mainly in other types of DNA lesions, in which repair occurs without these proteins. Recent studies suggest that there are important differences between the DNA damage response in directly irradiated cells and non-targeted cells via bystander signals. The DNA damage in bystander cells seems to persist for a prolonged time (Burdak-Rothkamm et al., 2007), differently from DNA damage induced directly by irradiation which is repaired completely within few hours depending on radiation dose. Studies carried out in p53 wild-type (TK6), p53 null (NH32),and p53 mutant (WTK1) lymphoblastoid cells using siRNA to knockdown DNA PKcs demonstrated the central role of non-homologous end-joining in processing bystander damage, in contrast to the role of homologous recombination which seems to be essential only in inducing sister chromatid exchanges in bystander cells (Zhang et al., 2008). ATM- and Rad3-related (ATR) protein kinases have a central role into DNA damage signaling in bystander cells, with ATM activation occurring downstream of ATR. DNA-PK is not essential in mortality inducing in bystander cells neither for bystander γH2AX foci induction (Burdak-Rothkamm et al., 2007). These differences between bystander and direct DNA damage response offer new potential targets for repair inhibitors, with the aim to protect bystander normal tissues during cancer radiotherapy.

## 5. Conclusions

The DNA-damage response pathway relies on the recruitment and modification of many different proteins that sense and signal the damage, activate transducer and effector proteins involved in cell cycle arrest, DNA repair and apoptosis. A correct DDR safeguards cells, whereas perturbations/defects in this pathway might contribute to the occurrence or to the acceleration of carcinogenesis. Our results have contributed to highlight cell response of human lymphocytes to DNA damage induced directly or indirectly by ionizing radiation. In particular, novel aspects of low- and high-LET radiation effects on human lymphocytes have been described, such as double strand break repair kinetics, mutational effects, micronuclei induction, apoptosis induction, cell cycle alterations, gene and microRNA expression changes. In addition, we have reported new findings about the cell response of human lymphocytes when ionizing radiation exposure occurred in microgravity, condition which has been experimentally simulated by the Rotating Wall Vessel. The results clearly indicate that modeled microgravity affects the cell response to radiation, thus contributing to increase the risk of radiation exposure during space missions. By considering that the levels of DNA repair genes were not significantly changed in MMG condition, we suppose that perturbations in the cell response to ionizing radiation are due to the altered activity of proteins playing an important role in DDR pathway. Evidences are accumulating on the strict dependence between efficiency in DNA repair and chromatin structural organization (Gontijo et al., 2003, Rübe et al., 2011). The elaborate higher-order organization of chromatin appears to be important in assembling the repair machinery, improving the accessibility of DNA lesions to repair complexes. Modifications of cell structure and perturbations of nuclear architecture induced by microgravity may affect the accessibility in chromatin to DNA repair machinery. The preliminary results obtained from miRNA-mRNA profiling

represent new insights about the radio-responsiveness in MMG. They seem promising to clarify the role of miRNAs in DNA-damage response to radiation in microgravity, thus improving the scientific approach towards environmental exposure risk.
The studies on molecular mechanisms of bystander effect could have great implications in evaluating radiation risk of IR exposures, and also have the potential to reassess radiation damage models currently used in radiotherapy. The radiation-induced bystander effect was shown to occur in a number of experimental systems both *in vitro* and *in vivo* and it is supposed to be realized through several pathways of transmission of the stress signal: a direct cellular contact, interaction through gap-junctions and through the culture medium of the irradiated cells. In our experimental system the conditioned medium was the main way by which the irradiated cells communicate their stressed condition to the non-irradiated cells. ROS released by irradiated TK6 cells into the culture medium were short-lived and probably other soluble molecules are necessary to maintain high the level of cell mortality in bystander cells. Recent studies, investigating on the nature of such molecules, suggest that fragments of extracellular genomic DNA, probably released from the apoptotic irradiated cells in the culture medium, are able to induce the bystander effects (Ermakov et al., 2011). Such DNA fragments bind to the Toll-like receptors family, leading to a signaling mechanism whose outcome is the dynamic transformation of the cytoskeleton and alteration in the spatial localization of chromatin portions in the nucleus. Thus, in bystander cells, as for microgravity-incubated lymphocytes, modifications in the nuclear structural organization may affect the assembly of the DNA repair machinery.

## 6. Acknowledgment

We gratefully acknowledge Dr. Cristiano De Pittà and Dr. Chiara Romualdi of the Department of Biology, University of Padova, for miRNA and mRNA expression profiling and statistical assistance. We acknowledge Dr. Vito Barbieri of the Department of Oncological and Surgical Sciences of Padova's University for cell irradiation with γ-rays and Roberto Cherubini of the INFN, Laboratori Nazionali di Legnaro, Padova, for cell irradiation with low-energy protons.

## 7. References

Al-Hakim, A.; Escribano-Diaz, C.; Landry, MC.; O'Donnell, L.; Panier, S.; Szilard, RK.; Durocher, D. (2010). The ubiquitous role of ubiquitin in the DNA damage response. *DNA Repair,* Vol. 9, No. 12, pp.1229-40, ISSN 1568-7864.

Anderson, RM.; Marsden, SJ.; Wright, EG.; Kadhim, MA.; Goodhead, DT.; Griffin, CS. (2000). Complex chromosome aberrations in peripheral blood lymphocytes as a potential biomarker of exposure to high-LET alpha-particles. *Int J Radiat Biol,* Vol. 76, pp. 31–42, ISSN 1362-3095.

Anderson, RM.; Stevens, DL.; Goodhead, DT. (2002). M-FISH analysis shows that complex chromosome aberrations induced by alpha -particle tracks are cumulative products of localized rearrangements. *Proc Natl Acad Sci USA.,* Vol. 99, No.19, pp. 12167-72, ISSN 1091-6490.

Brenner, DJ. & Ward, JF. (1992). Constraints on energy deposition and target size of multiply damaged sites associated with DNA double-strand breaks. *Int J Radiat Biol.,* Vol. 61, No. 6, pp. 737-48, ISSN 1362-3095.

Burdak-Rothkamm, S.; Short, S.C.; Folkard, M.; Rothkamm, K.; Prise, K.M. (2007) ATR-dependent radiation-induced gamma H2AX foci in bystander primary human astrocytes and glioma cells. *Oncogene,* Vol. 26, No. 7 (Feb 2007) pp. 993-1002, ISSN 0950-9232.

Chen, S.; Zhao, Y., Han, W.; Zhao, G.; Zhu, L.; Wang, J.; Bao, L.; Jiang, E.; Xu, A.; Hei, TK.; Yu, Z.; Wu, L. (2008) Mitochondria-dependent signalling pathway are involved in the early process of radiation-induced bystander effects. *Br J Cancer,* Vol. 98, No. 11 (Jun 2008) pp. 1839-44, ISSN 0007-0920.

Ciechanover, A.; Elias, S.; Heller, H.; Hershko, A. (1982). "Covalent affinity" purification of ubiquitin-activating enzyme. *J. Biol. Chem.,* 257 (5) 2537–2542. ISSN 0021-9258.

Cline, MS.; Smoot, M.; Cerami, E.; Kuchinsky, A.; Landys, N.; Workman, C.; Christmas, R.; Avila-Campilo, I.; Creech, M.; Gross, B.; Hanspers, K.; Isserlin, R.; Kelley, R.; Killcoyne, S.; Lotia, S.; Maere, S.; Morris, J.; Ono, K.; Pavlovic, V.; Pico, AR.; Vailaya, A.; Wang, PL.; Adler, A.; Conklin, BR.; Hood, L.; Kuiper, M.; Sander, C.; Schmulevich, I.; Schwikowski, B.; Warner, GJ.; Ideker, T.; Bader, GD. (2007). Integration of biological networks and gene expression data using Cytoscape. *Nature Protocols,* Vol. 2, pp. 2366-82, ISSN 1754-2189.

Cowell, I.G.; Sunter, N.J.; Singh, P.B.; Austin, C.A.; Durkacz, B.W.; Tilby, M.J. (2007). gammaH2AX foci form preferentially in euchromatin after ionising-radiation. *PLoS ONE,* Vol. 2, No. 10, ISSN 1932-6203.

Crosby, ME.; Kulshreshtha, R.; Ivan, M.; Glazer, PM. (2009). MicroRNA regulation of DNA repair gene expression in hypoxic stress. *Cancer Research,* Vol. 69, pp. 1221-1229, ISSN 0008-5472.

Cubano, L.A. & Lewis M.L. (2000). Fas/APO-1 protein is increased in spaceflown lymphocytes (Jurkat). *Exp. Gerontol.,* Vol. 35, No. 3, pp. 389–400, ISSN 0531-5565.

Dou, H.; Huang, C.; Singh, M.; Carpenter, PB.; Yeh, ET. (2010). Regulation of DNA repair through deSUMOylation and SUMOylation of replication protein A complex. *Mol Cell.,* Vol. 39, No. 3, pp. 333-45, ISSN 1097-2765.

Durante, M.; Snigiryova, G.; Akaeva E., Bogomazova A., Druzhinin S., Fedorenko B., Greco O., Novitskaya N., Rubanovich A., Shevchenko V., Von Recklinghausen U., Obe G. (2003). Chromosome aberration dosimetry in cosmonauts after single or multiple space flights. *Cytogenet. Genome Res.,* Vol. 103, pp. 40–46, ISSN 1424-8581.

Ermakov A.V., Konkova M.S., Kostyuk S.V., Smirnova T.D., Malinovskaya E.M., Efremova L.V., Veiko N.N.(2011). An extracellular DNA mediated bystander effect produced from low dose irradiated endothelial cells. *Mutat Res.,* (Mar 2011). ISSN 0027-5107.

Galanty, Y.; Belotserkovskaya, R.; Coates, J.; Polo, S.; Miller, KM.; Jackson, SP. (2009). Mammalian SUMO E3-ligases PIAS1 and PIAS4 promote responses to DNA double-strand breaks. *Nature,* Vol. 462, No. 7275, pp. 935-9, ISSN 0028-0836.

Gontijo AM, Green CM, Almouzni G. (2003). Repairing DNA damage in chromatin. *Biochimie.*, Vol. 85, No. 11, pp. 1133-47, ISNN 0300-9084.

Gradzka, I.; Iwanenko, T. (2005). A non-radioactive, PFGE-based assay for low levels of DNA double-strand breaks in mammalian cells. *DNA Repair*, Vol. 4, pp. 1129–1139, ISSN 1568-7864.

Grimm, D., Bauer, J.; Kossmehl, P.; Shakibaei, M.; Schonberger, J.; Pickenhahn, H.; Schulze-Tanzil, G.; Vetter, R.; Eilles, C.; Paul, M.; Cogoli, A. (2002). Simulated microgravity alters differentiation and increases apoptosis in human follicular thyroid carcinoma cells. *FASEB J.*, Vol. 16, pp. 604–606, ISSN 0892-6338.

Guo, H.; Ingolia, NT; Weissman, JS.; Bartel, DP. (2010). Mammalian microRNAs predominantly act to decrease target mRNA levels. *Nature*, Vol. 466, No. 7308, pp. 835–840, ISSN 0028-0836.

Hamada, N.; Schettino, G.; Kashino, G.; Vaid, M.; Suzuki, K.; Kodama, S.; Vojnovic, B.; Folkard, M.; Watanabe, M.; Michael, B.D.; Prise, K.M. (2006). Histone H2AX phosphorylation in normal human cells irradiated with focused ultrasoft X rays: evidence for chromatin movement during repair. *Radiat. Res.*, Vol. 166, pp. 31–38, ISSN 0033-7587.

Hammond, T.G.; Benes, E.; O'Reilly, K.C.; Wolf, D.A.; Linnehan, R.M.; Taher, A.; Kaysen, J.H.; Allen, P.L.; Goodwin, T.J. (2000). Mechanical culture conditions effect gene expression: gravity induced changes on the space shuttle, *Physiol. Genom.*, Vol. 3 No. 3, pp. 163–173, ISSN 1094-8341.

Harper, JW. & Elledge SJ. (2007). The DNA damage response: ten years after. *Mol Cell.*, Vol. 28, No. 5, pp.739-45, ISSN 1097-2765.

He, M.; Zhao, M.; Shen, B.; Prise, KM.; Shao, C. (2011). Radiation-induced intercellular signaling mediated by cytochrome-c via a p53-dependent pathway in hepatoma cells. *Oncogene*, Vol. 30, No.16, pp. 1947-55, ISSN 0950-9232.

Hershko, A.; Heller, H.; Elias, S.; Ciechanover, A. (1983). Components of ubiquitin–protein ligase system, Resolution, affinity purification, and role in protein breakdown, *J. Biol. Chem.*, Vol. 258, No. 13, pp. 8206–8214, ISSN 0021-9258.

Huang, DW.; Sherman, BT.; Lempicki, R. (2009). Systematic and integrative analysis of large gene lists using DAVID bioinformatics resources. *Nature Protocols*, Vol. 4, pp. 44-57, ISSN 1754-2189.

Huen, M.S.; Grant, R.; Manke, I.; Minn, K.; Yu, X.; Yaffe, M.B.; Chen, J. (2007). RNF8 transduces the DNA-damage signal via histone ubiquitylation and checkpoint protein assembly, *Cell*, Vol. 131, pp. 901–914, ISSN 0092-8674.

Huen, M.S.Y. & Chen, J. (2010). Assembly of checkpoint and repair machineries at DNA damage sites. *Trends Biochem. Sci.*, Vol. 35, pp. 101-108, ISSN 0968-0004.

Hughes-Fulford, M., (2001). Changes in gene expression and signal transduction in microgravity. *Journal of Gravitational Physiology*, Vol. 8, pp. 1-4.

Ibañez, I.L.; Bracalente, C.; Molinari, B.L.; Palmieri, M.A.; Policastro, L.; Kreiner, A.J.; Burlón, A.A.; Valda, A.; Navalesi, D.; Davidson, J.; Davidson, M.; Vázquez, M.; Ozafrán, M.; Durán, H. (2009). Induction and rejoining of DNA double strand breaks assessed by H2AX phosphorylation in melanoma cells irradiated with proton and lithium beams. *Int J Radiat Oncol Biol Phys.,* Vol. 74, pp. 1226-35, ISSN 0360-3016.

Infanger, M.; Ulbrich, C.; Baatout, S.; Wehland, M.; Kreutz, R.; Bauer, J.; Grosse, J.; Vadrucci, S.; Cogoli, A.; Derradji, H.; Neefs, M.; Küsters, S.; Spain, M.; Paul, M.; Grimm, D. (2007). Modeled gravitational unloading induced downregulation of endothelin-1 in human endothelial cells. *J. Cell. Biochem.,* Vol. 101 pp. 1439–1455, ISSN 0730-2312.

Kashino, G.; Prise, K.M.; Schettino, G.; Folkard, M.; Vojnovic, B.; Michael, B.D.; Suzuki, K.; Kodama, S.; Watanabe, M. (2004). Evidence for induction of DNA double strand breaks in the bystander response to targeted soft X-rays in CHO cells. *Mutat. Res.,* Vol. 556, pp. 209–215, ISSN 0027-5107.

Kertesz, M.; Iovino, N.; Unnerstall, U.; Gaul, U.; Segal, E. (2007). The role of site accessibility in microRNA target recognition. *Nat Genet,* Vol. 39, pp. 1278-84, ISSN 1061-4036.

Kinner, A.; Wu, W.; Staudt, C.; Iliakis, G. (2008). Gamma-H2AX in recognition and signaling of DNA double-strand breaks in the context of chromatin. *Nucleic Acids Res.,* Vol. 36, No.17, pp. 5678-5694, ISSN 0305-1048.

Kita, K.; Moriya, T.; Wu, Y.P.; Sugaya, S.; Takahashi, S.; Nomura, J.; Suzuki, N. (2000). Search for gravity-responsive genes by PCR-based mRNA differential display in human cells. *Journal of gravitational physiology,* Vol. 7, pp. 75-76.

Kolas, N.K.; Chapman, J.R.; Nakada, S.; Ylanko, J.; Chahwan, R.; Sweeney, F.D.; Panier, S.; Mendez, M.; Wildenhain, J.; Thomson, T.M.; Pelletier, L.; Jackson, S.P.; Durocher, D. (2007). Orchestration of the DNA-damage response by the RNF8 ubiquitin ligase. *Science,* Vol. 318, pp. 1637–1640, ISSN 0036-8075.

Lewis, M.L.; Reynolds, J.L.; Cubano, L.A.; Hatton, J.P.; Lawless, B.D.; Piepmeier, E.H. (1998). Spaceflight alters microtubules and increases apoptosis in human lymphocytes (Jurkat). *FASEB J.,* Vol. 12, pp.1007–1018, ISSN 0892-6338.

Lewis, M.L.; Reynolds, J.L.; Cubano, L.A.; Hatton, J.P.; Lawless, B.D.; Piepmeier, E.H. (2001). cDNA microarray reveals altered cytoskeletal gene expression in space-flown leukemic T lymphocytes (Jurkat). *FASEB J.,* Vol. 18, pp. 1783–1785, ISSN 0892-6338.

Longnecker, D.E.; Manning, F.J.; Worth Jr. M.H. (Eds.) (2004). Review of Nasa's Longitudinal Study of Astronaut Health, *National Academies Press,* Washington, DC.

Lukas, J.; Lukas, C.; Bartek, J. (2004). Mammalian cell cycle checkpoints: signalling pathways and their organization in space and time. *DNA Repair,*Vol. 3, No. 8-9, pp. 997–1007, ISSN 1568-7864.

Maccarone, M.; Battista, N.; Meloni, M.; Bari, M.; Galleri, G.; Pippia, P.; Cogoli, A.; Finazzi-Agr`o, A. (2003). Creating conditions similar to those that occur during exposure of cells to microgravity induces apoptosis in human lymphocytes by 5-lipoxygenase mediated mitochondrial uncoupling and cytochrome *c* release. *J. Leukocyte Biol.,* Vol. 73, pp. 472–481, ISSN 0741-5400.

Mailand, N.; Bekker-Jensen, S.; Faustrup, H.; Melander, F.; Bartek, J.; Lukas, C.; Lukas, J. (2007). RNF8 ubiquitylates histones at DNA double-strand breaks and promotes assembly of repair proteins. *Cell,*Vol. 131, pp. 887–900, ISSN 0092-8674.

Markova, E.; Schultz, N.; Belyaev, I.Y. (2007). Kinetics and dose-response of residual 53BP1/γ-H2AX foci: co-localization, relationship with DSB repair and clonogenic survival. *Int. J. Radiat. Biol.*, Vol. 83, pp. 319–329, ISSN 0955-3002.

Morris, J.R. (2010). SUMO in the mammalian response to DNA damage. *Biochem. Soc Trans*, Vol. 38, pp. 92-97, ISSN 0300-5127.

Mosesso, P.; Schuber, M.; Seibt, D.; Schmitz, C.; Fiore, M.; Schinoppi, A.; Penna, S.; Palitti, F. (2001). X-ray-induced aberrations in human lymphocytes in vitro are potentiated under simulated microgravity conditions (Clinostat), *Phys. Med.* XVII (Supplement 1).

Pardo, S.J.; Patel, M.J.; Sykes, M.C.; Platt, M.O.; Boyd, N.L.; Sorescu, G.P.; Xu, M.; van Loon, J.J.; Wang, M.D.; Jo, H. (2005). Simulated microgravity using the random positioning machine inhibits differentiation and alters gene expression profiles of 2T3 rre-osteoblasts. *Am. J. Physiol. Cell Physiol.*, Vol. 288, No.6, pp. 1211–1221, ISSN 0363-6143.

Pothof, J.; Verkaik, N.S.; van IJcken, W.; Wiemer, E.A.; Ta, V.T.; van der Horst, G.T.; Jaspers, N.G.; van Gent, D.C.; Hoeijmakers, J.H.; Persengiev, S.P. (2009). MicroRNA-mediated gene silencing modulates the UV-induced DNA-damage response. *EMBO J*, Vol. 28, pp. 2090-9, ISSN 0261-4189.

Prise, K.M.; Pinto, M.; Newman, H.C.; Michael, B.D. (2001). A review of studies of ionizing radiation-induced double-strand break clustering. *Radiat Res*, Vol. 156, pp. 572–576, ISSN 0033-7587.

Riches, L.C.; Lynch, A.M.; Gooderham, N.J. (2008). Early events in the mammalian response to DNA double-strand breaks. *Mutagenesis*, Vol. 23, No. 5, pp. 331–339, ISSN 0267-8357.

Rogakou, E.P.; Pilch, D.R.; Orr, A.H.; Ivanova, V.S.; Bonner, W.M. (1998). DNA double stranded breaks induce histone H2AX phosphorylation on serine 139, *J. Biol. Chem.*, Vol. 273, pp. 5858–5868, ISSN 0021-9258.

Rübe, C.E.; Lorat, Y.; Shuler, N.; Schanz, S.; Wennemuth, G.; Rübe, C. (2011). DNA repair in the context of chromatin: new molecular insights by the nanoscale detection of DNA repair complexes using transmission electron microscopy. *DNA Repair*, Vol. 10, pp. 427-437, ISSN 1568-7864.

Sales, G.; Coppe, A.; Bisognin, A.; Biasiolo, M.; Bortoluzzi, S.; Romualdi, C. (2010). MAGIA, a web-based tool for MiRNA and Genes Integrated Analysis. *Nucleic Acid Research*, Vol. 38 Suppl: W352-9, ISSN 0305-1048.

Sak, A.; Grehl, S.; Erichsen, P.; Engelhard, M.; Grannaß, A.; Levegrün, S.; Pöttgen, C.; Groneberg, M.; Stuschke, M. (2007). gamma-H2AX foci formation in peripheral blood lymphocytes of tumor patients after local radiotherapy to different sites of the body: dependence on the dose-distribution, irradiated site and time from start of treatment, *Int. J. Radiat. Biol.*, Vol. 83, pp. 639–652, ISSN 0955-3002.

Schwartz, J.L.; Jordan, R.; Sun, J.; Ma, H.; Hsie, A.W. (2000). Dose-dependent changes in the spectrum of mutations induced by ionizing radiations, *Radiat. Res.*, Vol. 153, pp. 312–317, ISSN 0033-7587.

Scherthan, H.; Hieber, L.; Braselmann, H.; Meineke, V.; Zitzelsberger H. (2008). Accumulation of DSBs in gamma-H2AXdomains fuel chromosomal aberrations. *Biochem. Biophys. Res. Commun.*, Vol. 371, pp. 694–697, ISSN 0006-291X.

Shannon, P.; Markiel, A.; Ozier, O.; Baliga, N.S.; Wang, J.T.; Ramage, D.; Amin, N.; Schwikowski, B.; Ideker, T. (2003). Cytoscape: a software environment for integrated models of biomolecular interaction networks. *Genome Research,* Vol. 13, pp. 2498-504, ISSN 1088-9051.

Sokolov, M.V.; Smilenov, L.B.; Hall, E.J.; Panyutin, I.G.; Bonner, W.M.; Sedelnikova, O.A. (2005). Ionizing radiation induces DNA double-strand breaks in bystander primary human fibroblasts. *Oncogene* Vol. 24, pp. 7257–7265, ISSN 0950-9232.

Stucki, M. (2009 ). Histone H2A.X Tyr142 phosphorylation: a novel sWItCH for apoptosis? *DNA Repair,* Vol. 8, No. 7, pp. 873-6, ISSN 1568-7864.

Sytkowski, A.J. & Davis, K.L. (2001). Erythroid cell growth and differentiation in vitro in the simulated microgravity environment of the Nasa Rotating Wall Vessel Bioreactor. *In Vitro Cell Dev. Biol. Anim.*, Vol. 37, pp. 79–83.

Tanq, J.B. & Greenberg (2010). Connecting the Dots: Interplay Between Ubiquitylation and SUMOylation at DNA Double Strand Breaks. *Genes Cancer,* Vol. 1, No. 7, pp. 787-796.

Torigoe, T.; Ichinohe, T.; Sato, N.; Yano, S. (2001). Analysis of gene expression of lymphocytes in microgravity. *Biol. Sci. Space*, Vol. 15, pp. 306–307.

Tusher, V.G.; Tibshirani, R.; Chu, G. (2001). Diagnosis of multiple cancer types by shrunken centroids of gene expression. *Proc Natl Acad Sci U S A,* Vol. 98, pp. 5116-121, ISSN 1091-6490.

Unsworth, B.R. & Lelkes, P.I. (1998). Growing tissues in microgravity, *Nat. Med.* Vol. 4, pp. 901–907, ISSN 1078-8956.

van Veelen, L.R.; Cervelli, T.; van de Rakt, M.W.M.M.; Theil, A.F.; Essers, J.; Kanaar, R. (2005). Analysis of ionizing radiation-induced foci of DNA damage repair proteins. *Mutat. Res.*, Vol. 574, pp. 22–33, ISSN 0027-5107.

Walther, I.; Pippia, P.; Meloni, M.A.; Turrini, F.; Mannu, F.; Cogoli, A. (1998). Simulated microgravity inhibits the genetic expression of interleukin-2 and its receptor in mitogen-activated T lymphocytes. *FEBS lett., Vol.* 436, pp. 115-118, ISSN 0014-5793.

Ward, J.F. (1991). DNA damage and repair. *Basic Life Sci.*, Vol. 58, pp. 403–415.

Wu, J.; Huen, M.S.; Lu, L.Y.; Ye, L.; Dou, Y.; Ljungman, M.; Chen, J.; Yu, X. (2008). Histone ubiquitination associates with BRCA1-dependent DNA damage response. *Mol. Cell Biol.*, Vol. 29, No. 3, pp. 849–860, ISSN 0270-7306.

Wyman C., & Kanaar, R. (2006). DNA double strand break repair: all's well that ends well. *Annu. Rev. Genet.*, Vol. 40, pp. 363-383, ISSN 0066-4197.

Xin, F.; Li, M.; Balch, C.; Thomson, M.; Fan, M.; Liu, Y.; Hammond, S.M.; Kim, S.; Nephew, K.P. (2009). Computational analysis of microRNA profiles and their target genes suggests significant involvement in breast cancer antiestrogen resistance. *Bioinformatics,* Vol. 25, pp. 430-434, ISSN 1367-4803.

Yang, H.; Asaad, N.; Held, K.D. (2005). Medium-mediated intercellular communication is involved in bystander responses of X-ray-irradiated normal human fibroblasts, *Oncogene* Vol. 24, pp. 2096–2103, ISSN 0950-9232.

Zhang, Y.; Zhou, J.; Held, K.D.; Redmond, R.W.; Prise, K.M.; Liber, H.L. (2008). Deficiencies of double-strand break repair factors and effects on mutagenesis in directly gamma-irradiated and medium-mediated bystander human lymphoblastoid cells. *Radiat. Res.*, Vol. 169, No. 2, pp. 197–206, ISSN 0033-7587.

# 2

# Interactions by Carcinogenic Metal Compounds with DNA Repair Processes

Simona Catalani and Pietro Apostoli
*Department of Experimental and Applied Medicine,*
*Section of Occupational Health and Industrial Hygiene,*
*University of Brescia,*
*Italy*

## 1. Introduction

Some metal compounds, including arsenic, beryllium, cadmium, chromium and nickel have long been recognized as human and animal carcinogens, while for other as antimony, cobalt, lead and vanadium their carcinogenic action are probable or possible. Except chromium (VI), carcinogenic metals are only weak mutagens in mammalian cells and often inactive in bacterial assays. Since the mutagenicity in bacterial assays indicates reactivity with DNA, metals are thought to exert genotoxicity mainly by indirect mechanisms. The four main, partly overlapping, DNA repair pathways operating in mammalian cells are base excision, mismatch, nucleotide excision and recombinational repair; each of repair pathways is involved in the removal of the specific DNA lesions. In addition, many carcinogenic metal compounds at low concentrations have been identified as inhibitors of the repair of DNA damage caused by other xenobiotics or endogenous factor. Furthermore, DNA is not only damaged by environmental mutagens including UV-light and polycyclic aromatic hydrocarbons, but also by reactive oxygen species generated from the same metallic elements. Failure to repair DNA damage can result in the accumulation of damaged DNA, mutation and carcinogenesis.

## 2. Mechanism of action

The potential target of metallic elements on DNA repair proteins are the zinc finger structures in their DNA binding motifs. Within these structures, zinc is complexed to four cysteines and/or histidines, folding different structural domains mediating DNA-protein as well as protein-protein interactions. It is estimated that about 1% of all mammalian genes encode zinc finger proteins, which are involved in many processes maintaining genomic integrity (Mackay & Crossley, 1998). The zinc ions do not participate in interactions conveyed by zinc finger domains, but are necessary for their function since they maintain their three-dimensional structures. In the case of transcription factors and DNA repair proteins, the absence of metal ions lead to loss in DNA-binding capacity. The functions of individual zinc finger include recognition of structures and sequences of nucleic acids and proteins. The majority of identified zinc finger may be classified as transcription factors. Another well known function of various zinc finger motifs, is the assembly of multiprotein complexes having structural or enzymatic functions. The main zinc finger proteins involved are the bacterial formamidopyrimidine-DNA glicosylase (fpg), the xeroderma pigmentosum A (XPA) protein, the poly(ADP-ribose) polymerase (PARP) and tumor suppression protein p53. The studies about of metal ions interaction indicated that apparently similar zinc finger domains may have different reactivity and suggested to draw a sort of list of possible mechanisms of zinc finger damage (Hartwig, 2001). Among these mechanisms, the most important are isostructural substitution, substitution with altered geometry, mixed complex formation, and catalysis of thiol oxidation. Many studies showed that different concentrations are needed to observe an inhibition and wide differences were observed for example when comparing the results obtained with Fpg and XPA (Witkiewicz-Kucharczyk & Bal., 2006). Regarding XPA, arsenic and lead did not decrease its binding to a UV-irradiated oligoucleotide, whereas cadmium, cobalt and nickel interfere with its DNA binding ability. A simultaneous treatment with zinc largely prevented this inhibition (Asmuß et al., 2000). Structural investigations by different spectroscopic methods revealed a tetrahedrally co-ordination of all three metal ions with no major distortion of XPA while for cadmium an increased Cd-S bond length was observed. Poly(ADP-ribosyl)ation of various proteins is one of the earliest nuclear events following DNA strand break induction. Yager & Wiencke (1997) and Hartwig et al., (2002) demonstrated an inhibition of $H_2O_2$-induced PARP activity in intact cells by nickel, cobalt, cadmium and very low concentration of arsenic in HeLa cells, while no effect was observed with lead. One other zinc-dependent protein with great impact on the processing of DNA damage and genomic stability is the p53 suppressor protein. Zinc has been shown to be required for proper folding in wild type conformation, and exposure to either isolate p53 protein or human breast cancer cells to cadmium resulted in disruption of native p53 conformation and inhibition of DNA binding (Meplan et al., 1999). Witkiewicz-Kucharczyk & Bal (2006) assessed the different metal binding properties of zinc finger and reported that cobalt is practically isostructural with zinc in zinc finger peptides and proteins, regardless of the number of cysteine residues involved. However, there is a strong, although quantitative variable thermodynamic preference for zinc over cobalt in tetrahedral environments provided by zinc finger. This effect is due to the ligand field stabilization effect, modulated by entropic contributions (Lachenmann et al., 2004). The substitution of nickel into zinc finger can also be achieved, but it results in distortions of the binding geometry and alterations of the peptide fold. A distorted tetrahedral coordination was found for cysteine$_2$-Histidine$_2$ zinc fingers (Posewitz & Wilcox, 1995), while a nearly square planar arrangement of donors was demonstrated in a cysteine$_4$ environment (Bal et al., 2003). Also the efficacy of cadmium binding is related to the number of coordinated thiolates (Krizek et al., 1993). Zinc seems to be preferred in the cysteine$_2$-histidine$_2$ environment, the affinities of zinc and cadmium may be comparable for cysteine$_3$-histidine, and cadmium is strongly preferred in cysteine$_4$ zinc finger peptides (Kopera et al., 2004). This preference is due to the high enthalpy of the cadmium-S bond. The cadmium ion fits into tetrahedral environments with little strain, however, it is significantly larger than zinc and cobalt ions, which results in local distortions of zinc finger geometries (Buchko et al., 2000). Finally lead, element with high affinities to thiolates, can replace zinc in zinc finger domains and disrupt their fold. Arsenic too is known to have a high affinity to -SH groups and it is demonstrated by arsenic-mediated repair inhibition not related with a direct mechanism of one or more specific repair proteins, but rather with changes in gene expression and/or signal transduction (Asmuß et al., 2000). Finally redox regulation has been *in vitro* and *in vivo* demonstrated in several DNA-binding zinc finger proteins. The metal ions can oxidize the essential cysteines and/or other residues in zinc finger structures interfering in metal binding domain. Taken together, the above mentioned mechanisms indicate that DNA repair, zinc homeostasis, oxidative assault and the redox status of the cell are all interconnected (Fig 1). The toxic/carcinogenic metals with sufficiently high affinities to thiols may interfere at all stages of zinc homeostasis and signaling, but specific ways of their actions can only be understood in appropriately complicated experimental designs. Yet each zinc finger protein exerts its own structural function toward metallic compounds but no general prediction about this phenomenon appear to be possible.

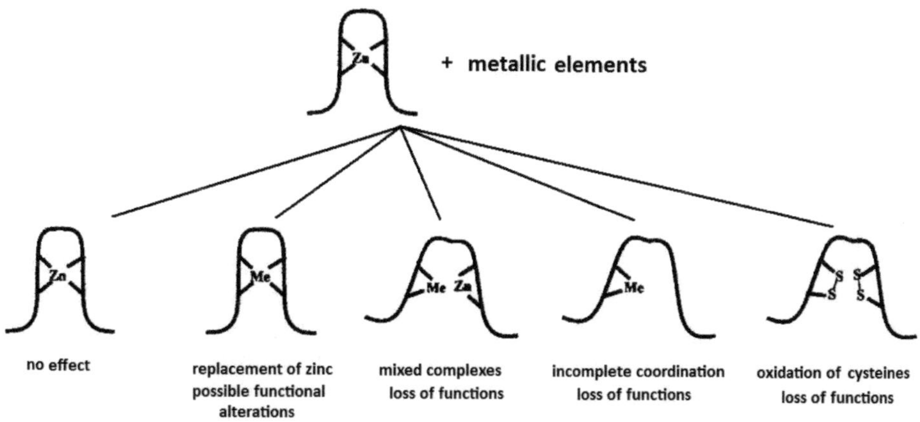


Fig. 1. Schematic representation of potential interactions of metallic elements with zinc-binding structures in transcription factors and DNA repair protein (modified from Hartwig et al.,2001).

## 3. Arsenic

Different mechanism of action have been suggested for arsenic carcinogenicity including the induction of oxidative stress, induction of genetic damage, altered DNA methylation patterns, enhanced cell proliferation, inhibition of the tumor suppressor protein p53, DNA repair alteration and recently biomethylation (Aposhian & Aposhian 2006). A possible molecular mechanism for arsenic toxicity may lie in its ability to react with thiols, for example, in zinc binding structures of transcription factors, cell cycle control and DNA repair proteins (Kitchin & Wallace, 2008). Nucleotide excision repair (NER) in particular is strongly inhibited by arsenic. NER is capable of removing a wide variety of bulky, DNA helix distorting lesions, caused, e.g., by UV-irradiation or environmental mutagens. Arsenic is known to enhance the persistence of bulky DNA lesions and consequently the mutagenicity induced by UV and benzo[a]pyrene (Hartmann & Speit 1996; Gebel, 2001). Since bulky lesion formation is the possible responsible for their carcinogenicity, genetic integrity depends largely on NER efficiency. Many studies have shown that inorganic arsenic inhibits repair of bulky DNA adducts induced by UV-irradiation (Hartwig et al., 1997; Danaee et al., 2004) or benzo[a]pyrene in cultured cells and laboratory animals (Schwerdtle et al., 2003; Shen et al., 2008); additionally arsenite has been shown to down-regulate expression of some NER genes in cultured human cells (Hamadeh et al., 2005). In humans, arsenic exposure via drinking water was correlated with a dose relationship dependent to decreased expression of some NER genes and reduced repair of lesions in lymphocytes (Andrew et al., 2006). Human lymphoblastoid cells were pre-exposed to arsenite (As(III)) alone and in combination with UV, the pre-treatment with As(III) specifically inhibited the repair of UV-induced pyrimidine dimer-related DNA damage and leads to enhanced UV mutagenesis. Hartwig et al (1997) investigated the effects of arsenite in removal of benzo[a]pyrene-induced DNA damage. When damaged DNA is replicated prior to repair, these adducts can lead to mutations and cancer. This study was carried out in A549 human lung cancer cells; in absence of arsenite, about 45% of benzo[a]pyrene diolepoxide–DNA adducts were repaired within 6–8 h, in presence of arsenite, there was a significant increase of adduct formation. Additionally, the repair capacity towards the stable lesions was decreased in a concentration-dependent shape reaching about 25% of the control at 75 μM, a still slightly cytotoxic effect for this cell line (Schwerdtle et al., 2003b). Similar results have been obtained *in vivo*. Thus, in rats the frequency of benzo[a]pyrene-induced DNA adducts quantified by $^{32}P$ post-labeling was drastically reduced in the presence of arsenite (Tran et al., 2002). Interesting was the evidence in the human study, arsenic exposure was associated with decreased expression of excision repair cross-complement 1 (ERCC1) in isolated human lymphocytes at the mRNA and protein levels. The mRNA levels of ERCC1 expression were positively associated with water arsenic concentration and nail arsenic concentration and significantly correlated with the amount of OGG1, a base pair excision repair gene (Mo et al., 2009). More detailed studies have been undertaken to assess the potential effects of the trivalent and pentavalent methylated metabolites on DNA repair processes. In humans and many other mammals, inorganic arsenic is converted into trivalent and pentavalent methylated metabolites, monomethylarsonous (MMA(III)) and dimethylarsinous (DMA(III)) acid, monomethylarsonic (MMA(V)) and dimethylarsinic (DMA(V)) acid. Biomethylation has long been thought to be a sort of detoxification process, yet nowadays it is reasonable to conclude that some adverse health effects seen in humans chronically exposed to inorganic arsenic are in fact caused by these metabolites. When considering MMA(III) and DMA(III) been demonstrated in some investigations as toxic, or even more toxic, compared to inorganic arsenic with an increase in benzo[a]pyrene diolepoxide–DNA adducts formation and repair inhibition for MMA(III), at much lower concentrations than arsenite (Schwerdtle et al., 2003). Repair inhibition was also observed at 5 μM DMA(III), but no effect on adduct generation was evident. Nevertheless, the cytotoxicity of the trivalent metabolites was also higher as compared to arsenite (Hartwig et al., 2003). Moreover, significant but less repair inhibition was mediated by 250 and 500μM of DMA(V) or MMA(V). Altogether, the results demonstrate that arsenite as well as the methylated metabolites interfere with cellular repair systems; the strongest effects with respect to inhibitory concentration were found for the trivalent metabolites (Schwerdtle et al., 2003b). Shen et al. (2009) investigated the difference manifested by DMA(III) compared to other trivalent arsenic species on the formation of benzo[a]pyrene diolepoxide–DNA adducts. At concentrations comparable to those used in the study by Schwerdtle et al. (2003) they found that each of the three trivalent arsenic species were able to enhance the formation of benzo[a]pyrene diolepoxide–DNA adducts with the potency in a decreasing order of MMA(III) > DMA(III) > As(III), well related with their cytotoxicity. Similar to As(III), DMA(III) the modulation of reduced glutathione (GSH) or total glutathione S-transferase (GST) activity could not account for its enhanced effect on DNA adduct formation. Additionally, similar effects elicited by the trivalent arsenic species were demonstrated to be highly time-dependent. Nollen et al. (2009) investigated the gene expression, total protein level and localization of proteins during NER and comparing inorganic arsenite and MMA(III). Arsenite and MMA(III) strongly decreased expression and protein level of the main initiator of global genome NER, i.e. Xeroderma pigmentosum complementation group C (XPC). This led to diminished association of XPC to sites of local UVC damage, resulting in decreased recruitment of further NER proteins. These data demonstrate that in human skin fibroblasts arsenite and MMA(III) more interacts with XPC expression, resulting in decreased XPC protein level and diminished assembly of the NER. The observed stronger impact on XPC by MMA(III) may explain the more potent NER inhibition by MMA(III) as compared to arsenite (Schwerdtle et al., 2003; Shen et al., 2008). Finally, these data provide further evidence that in the case of DNA repair inhibition the biomethylation of arsenic increases inorganic arsenic induced genotoxicity and probably contributes to its carcinogenicity. With respect to DNA repair inhibition, several studies point to an interaction of arsenic with various DNA repair pathways, which may in turn decrease genomic integrity. The effect of arsenic on the extent of poly(ADP-ribosyl)ation has been investigated previously in two studies with controversial conclusion. Yager & Wiencke (1997) observed a decreased amount of poly(ADP-ribose) in human T-cell lymphoma-derived at arsenite concentrations above 5 μM. In contrast, an increase of poly(ADP-ribosyl)ation reaction was reported at higher concentrations in CHO-K1 cells (Lynn et al., 1998). Hartwig et al., 2003b investigated the effects of arsenite on poly(ADP-ribosyl)ation stimulated by $H_2O_2$ in intact cells by applying an anti-poly(ADP-ribose) monoclonal antibody. The experiments demonstrated a clear reduction of poly(ADP-ribosyl)ation level just evident at the extremely low and non-cytotoxic concentration of 10nM arsenite and reaching about 40% of residual activity at 0.5 μM arsenite. There was an increase in induced DNA single strand break formation by arsenite in agreement with the assumed role of poly(ADP-ribosyl)ation in DNA strand break repair (Hartwig et al., 2003b). Also the effect of the arsenicals on the activity of the isolated formamidopyrimidine glycosylase (Fpg) was examined. Fpg is a glycosylase initiating base excision repair in Escherichia coli: it recognizes and removes a lot of DNA base modification including 7,8-dihydro-8-oxoguanine (8-oxoguanine). Even though Fpg is a bacterial repair protein, the recent discovery of human homologues suggests its relevance for mammalian cells too (Hazra et al., 2003). After 30 min preincubation MMA(III) and DMA(III) inhibited Fpg activity in dose-dependent shape, yielding 48 and 15% of the Fpg activity at 1 mM, respectively. In contrast, arsenite and the pentavalent metabolites did not show any effects on Fpg activity up to 10mM (Schwerdtle et al., 2003b). Finally, we describe the effects of arsenic compounds on the zinc finger structure of XPA. Different arsenicals promote the release of zinc from a peptide consisting of 37 amino acids representing the zinc finger domain of the human XPA protein (XPAzf). All trivalent arsenic compounds induced zinc release from XPAzf, starting at low micromolar concentrations, with MMA(III) and DMA(III) more active than arsenite. In contrast, MMA(V) and DMA(V) showed no or only slight effects up to 10mM (Schwerdtle et al., 2003b). Moreover there are some evidence about the influence of arsenic on BER, the predominant repair pathway for DNA lesions caused by reactive oxygen species (ROS) (Liu et al., 2001). Some studies have shown that low doses of arsenic can also cause an hormetic response in DNA polymerase β (Pol β), as well as telomerase activity (Zhang et al., 2003; Snow et al. 2005). DNA polymerase β is not only responsible for the incorporation of nucleotides in BER, but also excises the 5'-deoxyribose-5-phosphate (dRP) moiety prior to completion of repair (Wilson, 1998). Sykora et al. (2008) investigated the regulation of DNA polymerase β (Pol β) and AP endonuclease (APE1), in response to low but physiologically relevant doses of arsenic. Lung fibroblasts and keratinocytes were exposed to As(III), and mRNA, protein levels and BER activity were assessed. Both Pol β and APE1 mRNA exhibited significant dose-dependent down regulation at doses of As(III) above 1 μM. However, at lower doses Pol β mRNA and protein levels, and consequently, BER activity were significantly increased. In contrast, APE1 protein levels were only marginally increased by low doses of As(III) and there was no correlation between APE1 and overall BER activity. Enzyme supplementation of nuclear extracts confirmed that Pol β was rate limiting. These changes in BER are related to the overall protective against sunlight UV-induced toxicity at low doses of As(III) while at high doses there is a synergistic toxicity action. The results provide evidence that changes in BER due to low doses of arsenic could contribute to a non-linear, threshold dose response for arsenic carcinogenesis. The primary function of APE1 in BER is to act as an endonuclease responsible for the excision of apurinic/apyrimidinic (AP) sites. However, APE1 is also a redox factor responsible for signal transduction in response to oxidative stress (Hsieh et al., 2001). Arsenic has the potential to affect both the endonuclease and the functions of APE1, through its increase in ROS levels and inhibition of DNA repair (Hamadeh et al., 2002).

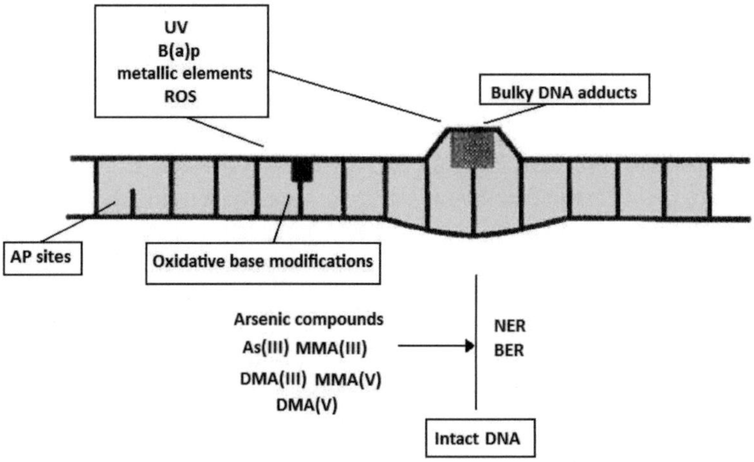


Fig. 2. Schematic outline of DNA repair inhibition by arsenite and its methylated metabolites(modified from Hartwig et al., 2003).

## 4. Beryllium

Beryllium does not directly damage the DNA but it can lead to morphological cell transformation and inhibition of DNA repair synthesis. However, the effects observed on DNA repair are not specific for beryllium since similar findings are reported for other metallic compounds. A possible hypothesis is that the mechanism of genotoxicity is unlikely to be a non-threshold mechanism. A practical threshold can be postulated for beryllium since both direct DNA repair enzyme inhibition or DNA/protein expression-mediated effects do definitely require more than one ion to inhibit all DNA repair enzyme molecules (Strupp, 2011a). Dylevoĭ (1990), using four strains of E. coli with different DNA repairing capacities, established that beryllium efficacy in the DNA repair test depended on pH of medium and ions concentration. The DNA of rat primary hepatocytes was treated by incubation with 2-acetylaminofluorene, a known DNA damaging agent, and co-incubated with beryllium metal extracts (Strupp, 2011b). They observed that, the DNA repair synthesis were reduced by co-incubation with beryllium metal extract. However, it should be noted that this effect was observed only when the concurrent DNA damage was massive (>80% cells in repair), while no effects were observed in cells with lower DNA damage. These findings deserve however further investigations about their relevance in vivo.

## 5. Cadmium

Several reports suggested that cadmium genotoxicity is not direct but rather mediated by reactive oxygen free radicals and resulting oxidative stress. In spite of being a weak genotoxic chemical, cadmium exhibits remarkable potential to inhibit DNA damage repair, and this has been identified as a major mechanism for its carcinogenicity (Giaginis et al., 2006). Cadmium is comutagenic and increases the mutagenicity of UV radiaton, alkylation and oxidation in mammalian cells. These effects may be explained by cadmium inhibition on several types of DNA repair: base excision repair, nucleotide excision repair, mismatch repair and the elimination of the premutagenic DNA precursor 8-oxodGTP. Regarding base excision repair, low concentrations of cadmium which did not generate oxidative damage as such, inhibited the repair of oxidative DNA damage in mammalian cells (Dally & Hartwig 1997; Fatur et al. 2003). Exposure of human cells to sub-lethal concentrations of cadmium leads to a time and concentration dependent decrease in hOGG1 activity, i.e. of the main DNA glycosylase activity responsible for the initiation of the base excision repair of 8-oxoguanine, an abundant and mutagenic form of oxidized guanine. The study of Bravard et al. (2010) confirms that part of the inhibitory effect of low dose cadmium on the cellular 8-oxoguanine DNA glycosylase activity can be attributed to an already described reduced hOGG1 transcription (Youn et al., 2005). This moderate inhibitory effect of cadmium on hOGG1 mRNA levels cannot explain the dramatic decrease observed in the levels and activity of hOGG1 protein. Indeed, inhibition of the ectopically expressed hOGG1-GFP in cells exposed to the metal confirmed the post-transcriptional effect of cadmium on hOGG1 protein and activity levels. A different response of the second enzyme in the cellular BER pathway has been described. Bravard et al (2010) found that in vivo treatment of human cells with cadmium has no effect on the APE1 activity, suggesting that in their experimental conditions most cadmium is complexed within the cells and therefore the intracellular concentrations of free cadmium do not reach the levels required for the inhibition of APE1. These results, taken together with the indirect inhibition of hOGG1 by oxidation, support the hypothesis that the effects on the BER pathway are in the consequence of the cellular redox imbalance rather than the direct interaction with proteins. Candelas et al. (2010) showed that cadmium inhibits the repair of uracile (U) in DNA, resulting both from mis-incorporation and cytosine (C) deamination. These lesions, as those on AP sites, are common in any cell, and must constantly be repaired to avoid mutagenic events. The necessity to continuously repair these lesions is underscored by the high levels of expression of UNG2 and APE1 (Cappelli et al., 2001). This genotoxic consequence of cadmium exposure might participate in the deregulation of physiological cellular processes by altering the pattern of gene expression on the one hand (U), and increasing the mutation rate on the other hand (on

AP site), thereby interfering with the normal control of cell growth and division. Moreover cadmium exposure inhibits and modifies some proteins of BER such as formamidopyrimidine glycosylase (Fpg): the substitution of a cysteine in the zinc finger localized in the C terminal of Fpg protein may inhibit the binding of the protein to DNA (O' Connor et al., 1993). With respect to nucleotide excision repair, cadmium interferes with the removal of thymine dimers after UV irradiation by inhibiting the first step of this repair pathway (Hartwig & Schwerdtle 2002; Fatur et al. 2003). Also both association and dissociation of essential NER proteins are disturbed in presence of cadmium. Because of decreased of XPC nuclear protein levels, a reduced XPC localization to UVC-induced DNA damage in cells was observed after incubation with a non cytotoxic concentration of $CdCl_2$. Interestingly, the tumor suppressor protein p53 also contain a zinc binding domain, which is essential for DNA binding and p53 function in transcription mechanism. In this context, Meplan et al. (1999) demonstrated that cadmium chloride alters p53 conformation in MCF7 cells, inhibits its DNA binding and down regulates transcriptional activation of a reporter gene. As p53 has been shown to act as a transcription factor for two important NER genes XPC and P48 and cadmium induced p53 conformational change may also result in altered p53 NER downstream effects (Adimoolam & Ford 2002). Cadmium exposure inhibits the xeroderma pigmentosum A (XPA) protein. XPA contains a typical four-cysteine zinc finger, which is not directly involved in DNA binding of the protein. The DNA binding capacity of XPA is strongly reduced after intoxication with cadmium (Hartmann et al., 1998; Hartwig et al., 2002). Another aspect is that cadmium found in liver and kidney cortex is bound to metallothioneins (MT), small, cystein-rich metal-binding proteins which are considered to be protective from cadmium toxicity (Klaassen et al., 1999; Nordberg 2009; Chang et al., 2009). Nevertheless, Hartwig et al 2002 demonstrated that the inhibitory cadmium effect for fpg proteins were comparable independent of whether CdCl2 or MT-bound Cd(II) was applied. Thus, metal ions complexed to MT may still be available for toxic reactions. In a recent study Schwerdtle et al., (2010) compared genotoxic effects of particulate CdO and soluble $CdCl_2$ in cultured human cells and reported that both cadmium compounds inhibited the nucleotide excision repair of benzo[a]pyrene diol epoxide-induced bulky DNA adducts and UVC-induced photolesions in a dose-dependent shape at non-cytotoxic concentrations. This agreement with the similar carcinogenic effects of both water-soluble and water insoluble cadmium compound indicates that $Cd^{2+}$ is the most common species responsible for indirect genotoxicity of the element (Oldiges et al., 1989).

## 6. Chromium

Among the carcinogenic metal compounds, only chromium (VI) has been clearly defined mutagenic in bacterial and mammalian test systems and its carcinogenic activity is thought to be due to the induction of DNA damage generated by reactive intermediates arising in its intracellular reduction to chromium (III) (Klein, 1996). Cr(VI)-carcinogenesis may be initiated or promoted through several mechanistic processes including, the intracellular metabolic reduction of Cr(VI) producing chromium species capable of interacting with DNA to yield genotoxic and mutagenic effects, Cr(VI)-induced inflammatory/immunological responses, and alteration of survival signaling pathways. The intracellular reduction of Cr(VI) produces a broad spectrum of DNA lesions including binary DNA adducts, DNA interstrand crosslinks (ICLs), DNA-protein adducts, DNA double-strand breaks and oxidized bases (Nickens et al., 2010). On the contrary the knowledge about the role of DNA repair system in this process is lacking. Several lesions generated by Cr(VI) reduction (i.e. oxidized bases) are substrates for base excision repair (BER). In BER, damaged (alkylated or oxidized) bases are recognized by specific DNA glycosylases and are excised, resulting in the formation of apurinic/ apyrimidinic (AP) sites. Interesting to note that chromium(VI) can be reduced in body fluids, which results in its detoxification, due to the poor ability of chromium(III) to cross cell membranes. Infact chromium(VI), when introduced by the oral route, is efficiently detoxified up reduction by saliva and gastric juice and sequestration by intestinal bacteria (De Flora, 2000). Administration of up to 20 mg chromium (VI), either in drinking water or by gavage, failed to produce any effect in the mouse bone marrow micronucleus assay or in the rat hepatocyte DNA rapair assay (Mirsalis et al., 1996).The results of studies carried out by O'Brien et al (2002; 2005) suggested that NER functions is essential in the protection of cells from Cr(VI) lethality and for the removal of Cr(III)-DNA adducts. Brooks et al., (2008) suggest that NER and BER are required for Cr(VI) genomic instability and postulate that, in the absence of excision repair, DNA damage is directed an error-free system of DNA repair or damage tolerance.

## 7. Nickel

Epidemiological studies in exposed workers identified some species of nickel as carcinogenic for upper respiratory tract and lung (Polednak 1981; Roberts et al. 1984; Roberts et al. 1989). The carcinogenic potency depends largely on properties such as solubility and kind of salts, which influence its bioavailability. Water soluble nickel salts are taken up only slowly by cells, while particulate of nickel compounds are phagocytosed and, due to the low pH, gradually dissolved in lysosomes, yielding high concentrations of nickel ions in the nucleus (Costa et al., 2005). Using in vitro cells and animal models, nickel compounds have been found to generate various types of adverse effects, including chromosomal aberrations, DNA strand breaks, high reactive oxygen species production, impaired DNA repair, hypoxia-mimic stress, aberrant epigenetic changes, and signaling cascade activation (Lu et al., 2005). Nickel has been shown to interfere with the repair mechanisms involved in removing UV-, platinum-, mitomycin C, g-radiation- and benzo[a]pyrene-induced DNA damage (Dally et al., 1997; Hartmann et al., 1998; Schwerdtle et al., 2002). These comutagenic effects are explained by the inhibition of all major types of DNA repair processes. Potentially sensitive targets for the toxic action of nickel(II) are zinc finger structures present in several DNA repair enzymes, including the bacterial Fpg protein and the mammalian XPA protein, DNA ligase III and poly(ADP-ribose) polymerase (PARP). Some studies investigated the effects of nickel compounds on the repair of DNA and showed that both soluble and particulate nickel can inhibit repair of benzo[a]pyrene DNA adducts in human lung cells (Schwerdtle et al., 2002). Low doses of nickel chloride (1 µmol/L) inhibited repair of UV or N-Methyl-N-nitro-N'-nitrosoguanidine -induced DNA damage as indicated by accumulating strand breaks, and 1–5 µm nickel chloride inhibited the formamidopyrimidine-DNA glycosylase (Fpg), 3-methyladenine-DNA glycosylase II (Alk A) and endonuclease III (Endo III) enzymes involved in DNA excision repair (Wozniak and Blaziak, 2004). The mechanisms of this action may include interactions with a specific structure containing zinc or the –SH groups of repair proteins. Because nickel compounds, such as NiS, $Ni_3S_2$, NiO (black and green), and soluble $NiCl_2$, have been shown to be active inducers of reactive oxygen species (ROS) in Chinese hamster ovary cells, the involvement of reactive oxygen species has been implicated in the inhibition of DNA repair (Lynn, 1997). Inhibition of glutathione synthesis or catalase activity increased the enhancing effect of nickel on the cytotoxicity of ultraviolet light. Inhibition of catalase and glutathione peroxidase activities also enhanced the retardation effect of nickel on the rejoining of DNA strand breaks accumulated by hydroxyurea plus cytosine-beta-D-arabinofuranoside in UV-irradiated cells. Lynn et al., (1997) showed that nickel, in the presence of $H_2O_2$, exhibited a synergistic inhibition on both DNA polymerization and ligation and caused protein fragmentation. In addition, glutathione could completely repair the inhibition by nickel or $H_2O_2$ alone but only partially the inhibition by nickel when associated with $H_2O_2$. Therefore, nickel may bind to DNA-repair enzymes and generate oxygen-free radicals to cause protein degradation in situ. Schwerdtle et al., (2002) studied the effect of soluble and particulated nickel compounds on the formation and repair of stable benzo(a)pyrene DNA adducts in human lung cells. With respect to adduct formation, NiO, but not $NiCl_2$, reduced the generation of DNA lesions by ~30%. Regarding their repair in the absence of nickel compounds most lesions were removed within 24h; nevertheless, between 20 and 35% of induced adducts remained longer than 48h after treatment; $NiCl_2$ (100μM) led to ~80% residual repair capacity; after 500μM the repair was reduced to ~36%. Also, even at the completely non-cytotoxic concentration of 0.5 μg/cm² NiO, lesion removal was reduced to ~35% of control and to 15% at 2.0 μg/cm². Nevertheless, under the same experimental conditions, the extent of DNA strand breaks and oxidative DNA base modifications were increased only at highly cytotoxic concentrations of both compounds (Hartwig et al., 2002). Repair inhibition by nickel appears therefore to be independent from metal compounds, and the results do not provide an explanation for the marked differences in carcinogenic potencies between soluble and particulated nickel species. However when considering the carcinogenicity in human or in experimental animals the retentions times in the body have to be taken into account. Thus, analysis of nickel contents in rat lungs after inhalation of different nickel species, especially for NiO, an impaired clearance and up to 1000-fold higher and persistent nickel lung burdens have been shown when compared to water-soluble nickel sulphate (Dunnick et al., 1995). Therefore, exposure to particulate nickel compounds may give rise to continuous DNA repair impairment and thus the biological consequences may be far more severe. The overall data add further evidences that the inhibition of DNA repair processes is an important mechanism in nickel genotoxicity, especially, because these effects are observed at low, non-cytotoxic concentrations. Since oxidative DNA damage is continuously induced during aerobic metabolism, an impaired repair of these lesions might explain the carcinogenic action of nickel(II).

## 8. Interaction on DNA repair processes of metallic elements classified as a possible or probable human carcinogen

### 8.1 Antimony

Trivalent antimony is a known genotoxic agent and it is classified as a possible human carcinogen by the International Agency for Research on Cancer (1989) and as an animal carcinogen by the Deutsche Research Foundation (DFG 2008). The chemico-toxicological characteristics of antimony are similar to those of arsenic: their trivalent species are responsible for toxicological properties, and they have carcinogenic potential. In contrast to arsenic, however, informations about the toxicity of antimony and its possible mechanisms are limited. Tkahashi et al., (2002) investigated the effects of antimony trichloride ($SbCl_3$) and antimony potassium tartrate ($C_4H_4KO_7Sb$) on the repair of DNA double strand breaks induced by γ-radiation. Antimony compounds inhibited repair of DNA double strand breaks in a dose dependent manner. Both in trichloride, 0.2 mM antimony significantly inhibited the rejoining of double strand breaks, while 0.4 mM was necessary in potassium antimony tartrate. The mean lethal doses ($D_0$) for the treatment with antimony trichloride and antimony potassium tartrate, were approximately 0.21 and 0.12 mM, respectively. This indicates that the repair inhibition by antimony trichloride occurred in the dose range near $D_0$, but the antimony potassium tartrate inhibited the repair mechanism at doses where most cells lost their proliferating ability. This relationship is consistent with the general tendency of their respective toxicity: trivalent antimony compounds are less toxic than trivalent arsenic compounds, but more toxic than bismuth compounds (Leonard & Gerber, 1996; Huang et al., 1998). Grosskopf et al., (2010) show that trivalent antimony interferes with proteins involved in nucleotide excision repair and partly impairs this pathway, pointing to an indirect mechanism in the genotoxicity of trivalent antimony. After irradiation of human lung carcinoma cells with UVC, a higher number of cyclobutane pyrimidine dimers (CPD) remained in the presence of $SbCl_3$, whereas processing of the 6–4 photoproducts and benzo[a]pyrene diol epoxide (BPDE)-induced DNA adducts were not impaired. Nevertheless, cell viability was reduced more than in additive mode after combined treatment of $SbCl_3$ with UVC as well as with BPDE. A decrease in gene expression and protein level of XPE was found and moreover, trivalent antimony was shown to interact with the zinc finger domain of XPA with concentration dependent release of zinc from peptide of this domain. Compared to the data on arsenite, antimony is more effective in zinc releasing from XPA, yielding 50% zinc release at 10 times lower concentration (Schwerdtle et al., 2003). Antimony might be able to interact with proteins involved in DNA repair, via their cysteine or histidine side chains. Complexes between antimony(III) and glutathione via sulphur binding site of the tripeptide have already been confirmed (Burford et al., 2005).

### 8.2 Cobalt

The carcinogenic potential of cobalt and its compounds was evaluated in 1991 by the International Agency for Research on Cancer (1991, 2006), the Commision concluded that cobalt and its compounds are possibly carcinogenic to humans (group 2B). Also the Deutsche Research Foundation (DFG 2008) has classified cobalt among the carcinogens of Category 2. Production of active oxygen species and inhibition of DNA repair appear to be the predominant mechanism of action in cobalt genotoxicity (Lison et al., 2001). Specifically by nucleotide excise repair pathway, in fact cobalt inhibits the removal of UV-induced cyclobutane pyrimidine dimers in mammalian cells but did not inhibit DNA strand rejoining after X-irradiation (Hartwig et al., 1991). Furthermore, by applying the nucleoid sedimentation assay in HeLa cells, Snyder et al (1989) demonstrated that cobalt causes an accumulation of DNA strand breaks after UV irradiation, indicating an impairment of the polymerization and/or the ligation step of nucleotide excision repair. Kasten et al. (1992) provided further evidence that cobalt at low non-cytotoxic concentration, inhibits both the incision and polymerization step of nucleotide excision repair in human fibroblasts. De Boeck et al., (1998) assessed the interference of cobalt compounds with the repair of primarily-induced DNA damage and showed that cobalt was able to cause persistence of methylmethanesulphonate-induced DNA lesions by interference its repair. In particular, cobalt inhibited the Xeroderma pigmentosum group A (XPA) protein, a zinc finger protein involved in nucleotide excision repair (Asmuß et al. 2000) where it substituted for the zinc ion (Kopera et al. 2004). Cobalt at low, non-cytotoxic concentrations interferes with the incision step of UV-induced DNA repair, but the removal of lesions may not be uniformly affected (Kasten et al., 1997). This effect may be related to differences in processing these lesions. Regarding the effect of cobalt on the incision frequency, a potentially preferential inhibition of incisions at 6-4-photoproducts could be due to either the disruption of the highly effective damage recognition at the site of this lesion or to a enhanced inhibition of the global genome repair system, while the transcription-coupled repair is unaffected at low doses. In addition to the incision step, the polymerization is inhibited by cobalt as well, while the ligation of repair patches is not affected by this element. A possible mechanism of the interference of cobalt with DNA polymerases could be the competition with magnesium; in fact the inhibition of the polymerization step was completely reversed in the presence of magnesium ions (Kasten et al. 1992, 1997). Sirover and Loeb (1976) demonstrated a dose-dependent reduction of the catalytic activity as well as the fidelity of isolated DNA polymerases from different organisms after substitution of magnesium ions by cobalt. Taken together, the data indicate that cobalt belongs to a group of metal compounds which enhance the genotoxicity of direct mutagens.

### 8.3 Lead

The toxicity of lead and its compounds is well known for many centuries for anaemia, effects on nervous system and developmental disorders above all. Nevertheless, during the last years potential carcinogenic effects have been focused, leading to the classification of inorganic lead compounds as "Probably carcinogenic to humans" (Group 2A) by IARC (1987; 2006) and in the Group 2 by the Deutsche Research Foundation (DFG 2008). Although inorganic lead compounds exhibit only a weak mutagenic potential, they show more pronounced co-mutagenic activities in combination with DNA alkylating and oxidizing agents (Roy & Rossman, 1992; Hartwig et al., 1994). These effects were due to an interference with DNA repair processes, following an accumulation of DNA strand breaks, as shown in human HeLa cells after UV irradiation. Lead enhanced the frequencies of UV-induced mutations and sister chromatid exchanges at very low, nontoxic concentrations. Mutations as well as DNA strand breaks occurred only after long-term treatment at doses much higher than cytotoxic ones (Roy & Rossman, 1992). Considering the base excision repair, lead has been shown to inhibit the apurinic/apyrimidinic endonuclease (APE1) in micromolar concentration range both in an isolated enzymic test and in cells leading to an accumulation of apurinic sites in DNA and to an increase in methyl methansulfonate-induced mutagenicity (McNeill et al. 2007). Current evidences suggest that inactivation of APE1 is mediated by an unique and specific interaction of metal with active site residues then disrupting the in magnesium-dependent catalytic reaction. Furthermore, lead interferes with the repair of DNA double strand breaks via interaction with the stress response pathway induced by a phosphoinositol-3-kinase (PIKK) related kinase (Gastaldo et al. 2007). Due to its high affinity for sulfhydryl groups, a mechanism for lead interaction with proteins could be the displacement of zinc from zinc binding structures. In support of this assumption, in cell-free systems lead has been shown to reduce DNA binding of transcription factors (TFIIIA) and Sp1 (Huang et al. 2004). No impact was however described on the zinc-containing DNA repair proteins Fpg or XPA (Asmuß et al. 2000).

### 8.4 Vanadium

The International Agency for Research on Cancer has classified vanadium pentoxide ($V_2O_5$) as a possible carcinogen (Group 2B) (2006) while the Deutsche Research Foundation included vanadium among the carcinogens of Category 2 (DFG, 2008). The genotoxicity of vanadium compounds is explained by mechanisms of induction of oxidative stress, inhibition of DNA repair and interference with the activity of protein phosphatases and kinases. Only few studies have been carried out about the genotoxic action of vanadium compounds; Ivancsits et al. (2002) tested the impact of vanadate(V) on DNA repair kinetics of UV and bleomycin treated human fibroblasts. They observed a significant increase of DNA migration in the alkaline comet assay accompanied by persistent double-stranded breaks after exposure to vanadate in combination with UV-light or bleomycin, as compared to vanadate treatment alone. This indicates that vanadate may act as an indirect genotoxic agent by converting repairable single-stranded breaks into non-repairable double-stranded breaks. This effect was confirmed by the strong differences between lymphocytes of workers exposed to vanadium pentoxide after bleomycin treatment and controls. Bleomycin-induced DNA migration was higher in the exposed group (25%), whereas the repair of bleomycin-induced lesions was reduced (Erlich et al., 2008).

## 9. Conclusion

The carcinogenic action of some metallic elements includes different mechanism such as induction of oxidative stress, inhibition of DNA repair, activation of mitogenic signalling, and epigenetic modification of gene expression. Nevertheless, each metallic elements and also each metal species exert characteristic interactions, and even though similar cellular pathways are affected, the underlying mechanisms are quite different. A relevant factor in metal carcinogenesis is the bioavailability of different metal species and the capacity to penetrate the cell barrier. The DNA does not appear to be the primary binding site for carcinogenic metal ions. This suggests that an inhibition of DNA repair processes may be a predominant mechanism in metal-induced genotoxicity. In addition, most carcinogenic metal compounds have been shown to increase the cytotoxicity, mutagenicity, and clastogenicity in mammalian cells when combined with different types of DNA-damaging agents (UV-light and/or alkylating agents). For most metal compounds, interactions with proteins appear to be more relevant for carcinogenicity as compared to direct DNA damage, and several targets have been identified, such as DNA repair, tumor suppressor and signal transduction proteins. Since metal ions can bind in principle to many electron rich centers in proteins the existence of particularly metal-sensitive protein structures may be suggested. The zinc finger proteins have been identified as potential molecular targets for toxic metal compounds and are involved not only in DNA binding but also in protein-protein interactions. Thus, there is an increasing evidence for zinc binding as structures very sensitive for toxic metal compounds. Significant factors appear to be not only the physicochemical properties but also accessibility and the protein microenvironment. The efficient repair of DNA lesions induced by endogenous processes and by environmental factors are an important prerequisite to maintain DNA integrity; if repair is not efficient, cells may accumulate DNA damage, leading to increased probabilities of genes instability and alteration in cellular cycle control and thus to tumor formation. The study and elaboration of metallic elements carcinogenicity should be conducted in parallel with dose-response studies in order to have a real idea of exposures especially when considering the possibility of co-exposures to other carcinogenic organic.

## 10. Abbreviations

APE1: Apurinic/apyrimidinic endonuclease
As(III): Arsenite
BER: Base excision rapair
BPDE: Benzo[a]pyrene diol epoxide
CPD: Cyclobutane pyrimidine dimers
DFG: Deutsche Forschungsgemeinschaft, German Research Foundation
DMA(III): Dimethylarsinous acid
DMA(V): Dimethylarsinic acid
dRP: 5'-deoxyribose-5-phosphate
ERCC1: Excision repair cross-complement 1
Fpg: Formamidopyrimidine-DNA glicosylase
GSH: Reduced glutathione
GST: Total glutathione S-transferase
IARC: International Agency for Research on Cancer
MMA(III): Monomethylarsonous acid
MMA(V): Monomethylarsonic acid
MMR: Mismatch repair
MT: Metallothioneins
NER: Nucleotide excision repair
PARP: Poly(ADP-ribose) polymerase
Pol β: Polymerase β
ROS: Reactive oxygen species
XPA: Xeroderma pigmentosum A
XPAzf: Zinc finger domain of the human XPA protein
XPC: Xeroderma pigmentosum complementation group C

## 11. References

Adimoolam, S. & Ford, J.M. (2002). p53 and DNA damage-inducible expression of the xeroderma pigmentosum group C gene. *Proceedings of the National Academy of Sciences of the U.S.A.* Vol. 99, pp. 12985-12990

Andrew, A. S., Burgess, J. L., Meza, M. M., Demidenko, E., Waugh, M.G., Hamilton, J.W. & Karagas, MR. (2006). Arsenic exposure is associated with decreased DNA repair in vitro and in individuals exposed to drinking water arsenic. Environ Health Perspectives.Vol.114, pp.1193-1198

Aposhian, H. V. & Aposhian, M. M. (2006). Arsenic toxicology: Five questions. *Chemical Research in Toxicology*. Vol. 19, pp. 1–15

Asmuß, M., Mullenders, L.H. & Hartwig, A. (2000). Interference by toxic metal compounds with isolated zinc finger DNA repair proteins. *Toxicology Letters*. Vol. 112-113, pp. 227-231

Bravard, A., Campalans, A., Vacher, M., Gouget, B., Levalois, C., Chevillard, S. & Radicella JP. (2009). Inactivation by oxidation and recruitment into stress granules of hOGG1 but not APE1 in human cells exposed to sub-lethal concentrations of cadmium. *Mutation Research*. Vol. 685, pp. 61–69

Brooks, B., O'Brien, T.J., Ceryak, S., Wise, J.P. Sr, Wise, S.S., Wise, J.P. Jr, Defabo, E. & Patierno SR. (2008). Excision repair is required for genotoxin-induced mutagenesis in mammalian cells. *Carcinogenesis*. Vol.29, pp. 1064-1069

Buchko, G.W., Hess, N.J. & Kennedy, M.A. ( 2000). Cadmium mutagenicity and human nucleotide excision repair proteinXPA: CD,EXAFS and (1)H/(15)N-NMR spectroscopic studies on the zinc(II)- and cadmium(II)-associated minimal DNA-binding domain (M98- F219). *Carcinogenesis*. Vol. 21, pp. 1051–1057

Burford, N., Eelman, M.D. & Groom, K. (2005). Identification of complexes containing glutathione with As(III), Sb(III), Cd(II), Hg(II), Tl(I), Pb(II) or Bi(III) by electrospray ionization mass spectrometry. Journal of Inorganic Biochemistry. Vol. 99, pp. 1992-1997

Candéias, S., Pons, B., Viau, M., Caillat, S. & Sauvaigo, S. (2010). Direct inhibition of excision/synthesis DNA repair activities by cadmium: analysis on dedicated biochips. *Mutation Research*. Vol.694, pp. 53-59

Cappelli, E., Hazra, T., Hill, J.W., Slupphaug, G., Bogliolo, M. & Frosina G. (2001). Rates of base excision repair are not solely dependent on levels of initiating enzymes. *Carcinogenesis*. Vol. 22, pp. 387–393

Chang, X., Jin, T., Chen, L., Nordberg, M. & Lei, L. (2009). Metallothionein I isoform mRNA expression in peripheral lymphocytes as a biomarker for occupational cadmium exposure. *Experimental and Biological Medicine (Maywood)*. Vol. 234:666-672

Commission for the Investigation of Health hazards of Chemical Compounds in the Work Area, DFG (2008) *List of MAK and BAT values 2008, report no. 44*. Wiley. VCH, Weinheim

Costa, M., Davidson, T.L., Chen, H., Ke, Q., Zhang, P., Yan, Y., Huang, C. & Kluz, T. (2005). Nickel carcinogenesis: epigenetics and hypoxia signaling. *Mutation Research*. Vol.592, No.1-2, pp.79-88

Dally, H. & Hartwig, A. (1997). Induction and repair inhibition of oxidative DNA damage by nickel(II) and cadmium(II) in mammalian cells. *Carcinogenesis*. Vol. 18, pp. 1021-1026

Danaee, H., Nelson, H.H., Liber, H., Little, J.B. & Kelsey, K.T. (2004). Low dose exposure to sodium arsenite synergistically interacts with UV radiation to induce mutations and alter DNA repair in human cells. *Mutagenesis*. Vol. 19, pp. 143–148

De Boeck, M., Lison, D. & Kirsch-Volders, M. (1998). Evaluation of the in vitro direct and indirect genotoxic effects of cobalt compounds using the alkaline comet assay. Influence of interdonor and interexperimental variability. *Carcinogenesis*. Vol.19, pp. 2021-2029

De Flora, S. (2000). Threshold mechanisms and site specificity in chromium(VI) carcinogenesis. *Carcinogenesis*. Vol.21: 533-541

Dunnick, J.K., Elwell, M.R., Radovsky, A.E., Benson, J.M., Hahn, F.F., Nikula, K.J., Barr, E.B. & Hobbs, C.H. (1995). Comparative carcinogenic effects of nickel subsulfide, nickel oxide, or nickel sulfate hexahydrate chronic exposures in the lung. *Cancer Research*. Vol. 55, No. 22, pp. 5251-5256

Dylevoĭ, MV. (1990). An evaluation of the DNA-damaging action of the metal carcinogen beryllium using a bacterial repair test. *Mikrobiologicheskiĭ zhurnal*.Vol.52, pp. 34-38

Ehrlich, V.A., Nersesyan, A.K., Atefie, K., Hoelzl, C., Ferk, F., Bichler, J., Valic, E., Schaffer, A., Schulte-Hermann, R., Fenech, M., Wagner, K.H. & Knasmüller, S. (2008).

Inhalative exposure to vanadium pentoxide causes DNA damage in workers: results of a multiple end point study. *Environmental Health Perspective*. Vol.116, pp. 1689-1693

Fatur, T., Tusek, M., Falnoga, I., Scancar, J., Lah, T.T. & Filipic, M. (2003). Cadmium inhibits repair of UV-, methyl methanesulfonate- and Nmethyl- N-nitrosourea-induced DNA damage in Chinese hamster ovary cells. *Mutation Research*. Vol. 529, pp. 109-116

Gastaldo, J., Viau, M., Bencokova, Z., Joubert, A., Charvet, A.M., Balosso, J. & Foray, N. (2007). Lead contamination results in late and slowly repairable DNA double-strand breaks and impacts upon the ATM-dependent signaling pathways. *Toxicology Letters*. Vol. 173, pp. 201-214

Gebel, T. W. (2001). Genotoxicity of arsenical compounds. International Journal of Hygiene and Environmental Health. Vol. 203, pp. 249–262

Giaginis, C., Gatzidou, E. & Theocharis, S. (2006). DNA repair systems as targets of cadmium toxicity. *Toxicology and Applied Pharmacology*. Vol. 213, pp. 282–290

Grosskopf, C., Schwerdtle, T., Mullenders, L.H. & Hartwig, A. (2010). Antimony impairs nucleotide excision repair: XPA and XPE as potential molecular targets. *Chemical Research in Toxicology*. Vol.23, pp. 1175-1183

Hamadeh, H. K., Trouba, K. J., Amin, R. P., Afshari, C. A. & Germolec, D. (2002). Coordination of altered DNA repair and damage pathways in arsenite-exposed keratinocytes. *Toxicology Science*. Vol. 69, pp. 306–316

Hartmann, M. & Hartwig, A. (1998). Disturbance of DNA damage recognition after UV-irradiation by nickel(II) and cadmium(II) in mammalian cells. *Carcinogenesis*. Vol. 19, pp. 617-621

Hartwig, A., Groblinghoff, U.D., Beyersmann, D., Natarajan, A. T., Filon, R. & Mullenders, L.H.(1997). Interaction of arsenic(III) with nucleotide excision repair in UV-irradiated human fibroblasts, *Carcinogenesis*. Vol. 18, pp. 399–405

Hartwig, A., Snyder, R.D., Schlepegrell, R. & Beyersmann, D. (1991). Modulation by Co(II) of UV-induced DNA repair, mutagenesis and sister-chromatid exchanges in mammalian cells. *Mutation Research*. Vol. 248, pp. 177-185

Hartwig, A., Mullenders, L.H., Schlepegrell, R., Kasten, U. & Beyersmann, D. (1994). Nickel(II) interferes with the incision step in nucleotide excision repair in mammalian cells. *Cancer Research*. Vol. 54, pp.4045-4051

Hartwig, A. (2001). Zinc finger proteins as potential targets for toxic metal ions: differential effects on structure and function. *Antioxidant & Redox Signaling*. Vol. 3, pp. 625-634

Hartwig, A. & Schwerdtle, T. (2002). Interactions by carcinogenic metal compounds with DNA repair processes: toxicological implications. *Toxicology Letters*. Vol. 127, pp. 47-54

Hartwig, A., Asmuß, M., Blessing, H., Hoffmann, S. , Jahnkem, G., Khandelwal, S., Pelzer, A. & Bürkle, A. (2002). Interference by toxic metal ions with zinc-dependent proteins involved in maintaining genomic stability. *Food and Chemical Toxicology*. Vol.40, pp. 1179-1184

Hartwig, A., Blessing, H., Schwerdtle, T. & Walter, I. (2003). Modulation of DNA repair processes by arsenic and selenium compounds. Toxicology. Vol. 193, pp. 161–169

Hartwig, A., Pelzer, A., Asmuß, M. & Bürkle, A. (2003b). Very low concentrations of arsenite suppress poly(ADP-ribosyl)ation in mammalian cells. *International Journal of Cancer*. Vol. 104, pp. 1-6

Hazra, T.K., Izumi, T., Kow, Y.W. & Mitra, S. (2003). The discovery of a new family of mammalian enzymes for repair of oxidatively damaged DNA, and its physiological implications. *Carcinogenesis*. Vol. 24, pp. 155–157

Hsieh, M., Hegde, V., Kelley, M. & Deutsch, W. (2001). Activation of APE/Ref-1 redox activity is mediated by reactive oxygen species and PKC phosphorylation. *Nucleic Acids Research*. Vol. 29, pp. 3116–3122

Huang, H., Shu, S.C., Shih, J.H., Kuo, C.J. & Chiu, I.D. (1998). Antimony trichloride induces DNA damage and apoptosis in mammalian cells. *Toxicology*. Vol. 129, pp. 113-123

IARC (1989). Some Organic Solvents, Resin Monomers and Related Compounds, Pigments and Occupational Exposures in Paint Manufacture and Painting. *Monographs on the Evaluation of Carcinogenic Risks to Humans*. Vol. 47

IARC (1991). Chlorinated Drinking-water; Chlorination By-products; Some Other Halogenated Compounds; Cobalt and Cobalt Compounds. *Monographs on the Evaluation of Carcinogenic Risks to Humans*. Vol.52.

IARC (2006). Cobalt in Hard Metals and Cobalt Sulfate, Gallium Arsenide, Indium Phosphide and Vanadium Pentoxide. *Monographs on the Evaluation of Carcinogenic Risks to Humans*. Vol. 86

IARC (2006). Inorganic and Organic Lead Compounds. *Monographs on the Evaluation of Carcinogenic Risks to Humans*. Vol. 87

Ivancsits, S., Pilger, A., Diem, E., Schaffer, A. & Rüdiger, H.W. (2002). Vanadate induces DNA strand breaks in cultured human fibroblasts at doses relevant to occupational exposure. *Mutation Research*. Vol. 519, pp. 25-35

Kasten, U, Hartwig, A. & Beyermann, D. (1992). Mechanisms of cobalt(II) uptake into V79 Chinese hamster cells. *Archives of Toxicology*. Vol. 66, pp. 592–597

Kasten, U., Mullenders, L.H. & Hartwig, A. ( 1997). Cobalt(II) inhibits the incision and the polymerization step of nucleotide excision repair in human fibroblasts. *Mutation Research*. Vol. 383, pp. 81-89

Kitchin, K. T. & Wallace, K. (2008). The role of protein binding of trivalent arsenicals in arsenic carcinogenesis and toxicity, *Journal of inorganic biochemistry*. Vol. 102, pp. 532–539

Klaassen, C.D., Liu, J. & Choudhuri, S. (1999). Metallothionein: an intracellular protein to protect against cadmium toxicity. *The Annual Review of Pharmacology and Toxicology*. Vol. 39, pp. 267-294

Klein, C.B. (1996). Carcinogenicity and genotoxicity of chromium. In *Toxicology of Metals,* Chang, L.W. pp. 205-219, Ed. Lewis, Boca Raton

Kopera, E., Schwerdtle, T., Hartwig, A. & Bal, W. (2004). Co(II) and Cd(II) substitute for Zn(II) in the zinc finger derived from the DNA repair protein XPA, demonstrating a variety of potential mechanisms of toxicity. *Chemical Research in Toxicology*. Vol.17, pp.1452-1458

Krizek, B.A., Merkle, D.L. & Berg, J.M. (1993). Ligand variation and metal ion binding specificity in zinc finger peptides. *Inorganic Chemistry*. Vol. 32, pp. 937–940

Lachenmann, M.J., Ladbury, J.E., Dong, J., Huang, K., Carey, P. & Weiss, M.A.( 2004). Why zinc fingers prefer zinc: ligand-field symmetry and the hidden thermodynamics of metal ion selectivity. *Biochemistry*. Vol. 43, pp. 13910–13925

Leonard, A. & Gerber, G.B. (1996). Mutagenicity, carcinogenicity and teratogenicity of antimony compounds. *Mutation Research*. Vol. 366, pp. 1-8

Lison, D., De Boeck, M., Verougstraete, V. & Kirsch-Volders M. (2001). Update on the genotoxicity and carcinogenicity of cobalt compounds. *Occupational Environmental Medicine*. Vol. 58, No. 10, pp. 619–625

Liu, S.X., Athar, M., Lippai, I., Waldren, C. & Hei, T.K. (2001). Induction of oxyradicals by arsenic: implication for mechanism of genotoxicity. *Proceedings of the National Academy of Sciences of the U.S.A*. Vol. 98, pp. 1643–1648

Lu, H., Shi, X., Costa, M. & Huang, C. (2005) Carcinogenic effect of nickel compounds. *Molecular Cellular Biochemistry*. Vol. 279, pp. 45–67

Lynn, S., Yew, F.H., Chen, K.S. & Jan, K.Y. (1997). Reactive oxygen species are involved in nickel inhibition of DNA repair. *Environmental and Molecular Mutagenesis*. Vol.29, pp. 208-216

Lynn, S., Shiung, J.N., Gurr, J.R. & Jan, K.Y. (1998). Arsenite stimulates poly(ADP-ribosylation) by generation of nitric oxide. *Free Radical Biology & Medicine*. Vol. 24, pp. 442–449

Mackay, J.P. & Crossley, M. (1998). Zinc fingers are sticking together. *Trends in Biochemical Science*. Vol. 23, pp. 1–4

McNeill, D.R., Wong, H.K., Narayana, A. & Wilson, D.M. 3rd. (2007). Lead promotes a basic site accumulation and co-mutagenesis in mammalian cells by inhibiting the major abasic endonuclease Ape1. *Molecular Carcinogenesis*. Vol. 46, pp. 91 - 99

Meplan, C., Richard, M.J. & Hainaut P. (1999). Redox signalling and transition metals in the control of the p53 pathway. *Biochemical Pharmacology*. Vol.59, pp. 25-33

Mirsalis, J.C., Hamilton, C.M., O'Loughlin, K.G., Paustenbach, D.J., Kerger, B.D. & Patierno, S. (1996). Chromium (VI) at plausible drinking water concentrations is not genotoxic in the in vivo bone marrow micronucleus or liver unscheduled DNA synthesis assays. *Environmental and Molecular Mutagenesis*. Vol. 28: 60-63

Mo, J., Xia, Y., Ning, Z., Wade, T.J. & Mumford, J.L. (2009). Elevated ERCC1 gene expression in blood cells associated with exposure to arsenic from drinking water in Inner Mongolia. *Anticancer Research*. Vol. 29, pp. 3253-3259

Nickens, K.P., Patierno, S.R. & Ceryak, S. (2010). Chromium genotoxicity: A double-edged sword. *Chemico Biological Interactions*. Vol.188, pp.276-288

Nordberg, G.F. (2009). Historical perspectives on cadmium toxicology. *Toxicology and Applied Pharmacology*. Vol. 238:192-200.

O'Brien, T.J., Fornsaglio, J.L., Ceryak, S. & Patierno, S.R. (2002). Effects of hexavalent chromium on the survival and cell cycle distribution of DNA repair-deficient S. cerevisiae. *DNA Repair (Amst)*. Vol.1, pp.617-627

O'Brien, T.J., Brooks, B.R. & Patierno, S.R. (2005). Nucleotide excision repair functions in the removal of chromium-induced DNA damage in mammalian cells. *Molecular and Cellular Biochemistry*. Vol.279, pp. 85-95

Oldiges, H., Hochrainera, D. & Glasera, U. (1989). Long-term inhalation study with Wistar rats and four cadmium compounds. *Toxicological & Environmental Chemistry*. Vol. 19, pp. 217-222

Polednak, A.P. (1981). Mortality among welders, including a group exposed to nickel oxides. Archive of Environmental Health. Vol. 36, pp. 235–242

Posewitz, M.C. & Wilcox, D.E. (1995). Properties of the Sp1 zinc finger 3 peptide: coordination chemistry, redox reactions, and metal binding competition with metallothionein. *Chemical Research in Toxicology*. Vol. 8, pp. 1020–1028

Roberts, R.S., Julian, J.A., Muir, D.C. & Shannon, H.S. (1984) Cancer mortality associated with the high-temperature oxidation of nickel subsulfide. *IARC Scientific Publications*. Vol. 53, pp. 23–35

Roberts, R.S., Julian, J.A., Muir, D.C. & Shannon, H.S. (1989) A study of mortality in workers engaged in the mining, smelting, and refining of nickel. II: mortality from cancer of the respiratory tract and kidney. *Toxicology Industrial Health*. Vol. 5, pp. 975–993.

Roy, N.K. & Rossman, T.G. (1992). Mutagenesis and comutagenesis by lead compounds. *Mutation Research*. Vol. 298, pp.97-103

Schwerdtle, T., Ebert, F., Thuy, C., Richter, C., Mullenders, L.H. & Hartwig, A. (2010). Genotoxicity of soluble and particulate cadmium compounds: impact on oxidative DNA damage and nucleotide excision repair. *Chemical Research in Toxicology*. Vol.23, pp. 432-442

Schwerdtle, T., Walter, I. & Hartwig, A. (2003). Arsenite and its biomethylated metabolites interfere with the formation and repair of stable BPDE-induced DNA adducts in human cells and impair XPAzf and Fpg. *DNA Repair (Amst)*. Vol. 2, pp. 1449-1463

Schwerdtle, T., Walter, I., Mackiw, I. & Hartwig, A. (2003b). Induction of oxidative DNA damage by arsenite and its trivalent and pentavalent methylated metabolites in cultured human cells and isolated DNA. *Carcinogenesis*. Vol. 24, pp. 967–974

Shen, S., Lee, J., Weinfeld, M. & Le, X. C. (2008). Attenuation of DNA damage-induced p53 expression by arsenic: A possible mechanism for arsenic co-carcinogenesis. *Molecular Carcinogenesis*. Vol. 47, pp.508–518

Shen, S., Lee, J., Cullen, W.R., Le, X.C. & Weinfeld, M. (2009). Arsenite and its mono- and dimethylated trivalent metabolites enhance the formation of benzo[a]pyrene diol epoxide-DNA adducts in Xeroderma pigmentosum complementation group A cells. *Chemical Research in Toxicology*. Vol. 22, pp.382-390

Sirover A. & Loeb, L.A. (1976). Infidelity of DNA synthesis in vitro: screening for potential metal mutagens or carcinogens. *Science*. Vol. 194, pp. 1434–1436

Snow, E.T., Sykora, P., Durham, T.R. & Klein, C.B. (2005). Arsenic, mode of action at biologically plausible low doses: what are the implications for low dose cancer risk? *Toxicology and Applied Pharmacology*. Vol. 207, pp. S557–S564

Snyder, R.D., G.F. Davis & P.J. Lachmann. (1989) .Inhibition by metals of X-ray and ultraviolet-induced DNA repair in human cells. *Biological Trace Element Research*. Vol. 21, pp. 389–398

Strupp, C. (2011a). Beryllium metal II. a review of the available toxicity data. *The Annals of Occupational Hygiene*. Vol.55, No.1, pp. 43-56

Strupp, C. (2011b). Beryllium metal I. experimental results on acute oral toxicity, local skin and eye effects, and genotoxicity. *The Annals of Occupational Hygiene*. Vol.55, pp.30-42

Sykora, P. & Snow, E.T. (2008). Modulation of DNA polymerase beta-dependent base excision repair in cultured human cells after low dose exposure to arsenite. *Toxicology and Applied Pharmacology*. Vol. 228, pp. 385-394

Takahashi, S., Takeda, E., Kubota, Y. & Okayasu, R. (2000). Inhibition of repair of radiation-induced DNA double-strand breaks by nickel and arsenite. *Radiation Research.*Vol.154, pp. 686-691.

Tran, H.P., Prakash, A.S., Barnard, R., Chiswell, B. & Ng, J.C. (2002). Arsenic inhibits the repair of DNA damage induced by benzo(a)pyrene, *Toxicology Letters.* Vol.133, pp. 59–67

Wilson, S. (1998). Mammalian base excision repair and DNA polymerase beta. *Mutation Research.* Vol. 407, pp. 203–215

Witkiewicz-Kucharczyk, A & Bal, W. (2006). Damage of zinc fingers in DNA repair proteins, a novel molecular mechanism in carcinogenesis. *Toxicology Letters.* Vol.162, pp. 29-42

Yager, J.W. & Wiencke, J.K. (1997). Inhibition of poly(ADP-ribose) polymerase by arsenite. *Mutation Research.* Vol. 386, pp. 345–351

Youn, C.K., Kim, S.H., Lee do, Y., Song, S.H., Chang, I.Y., Hyun, J.W,. Chung, M.H & You H.J. (2005). Cadmium down-regulates human OGG1 through suppression of Sp1 activity. *Journal of Biological Chemistry.* Vol. 280, pp. 25185–25195.

Zhang, T., Schmitt, M. & Mumford, J. (2003). Effects of arsenic on telomerase and telomeres in relation to cell proliferation and apoptosis in human keratinocytes and leukemia cell in vivo. *Carcinogenesis.* Vol. 24, pp. 1811–1817

# 3

# Effect of Oxidative Stress on DNA Repairing Genes

Bedia Cakmakoglu, Zeynep Birsu Cincin and Makbule Aydin
*Istanbul University, Institute for Experimental Medicine Research, Turkey*

## 1. Introduction

Oxidative DNA damage has been thought to contribute to the general decline in cellular functions that are associated with a variety of diseases including Alzheimer disease, amyotrophic lateral sclerosis (ALS), Parkinson's disease, atherosclerosis, ischemia/reperfusion neuronal injuries, degenerative disease of the human temporomandibular-joint, cataract formation, macular degeneration, degenerative retinal damage, rheumatoid arthritis , multiple sclerosis , muscular dystrophy, diabetes mellitus, human cancers as well as the aging process itself. Oxidative stress occurs when the production of the reactive oxygen species (ROS) exceeds natural antioxidant defence mechanisms. There are several sources that form the ROS. Most of ROS come from the endogenous sources as by-products of normal and essential metabolic reactions, such as energy generation from mitochondria or the detoxification reactions involving the liver cytochrome *P-450* enzyme system. There are also exogenous ROS sources including exposure to cigarette smoke, environmental pollutants such as emission from automobiles and industries, consumption of alcohol in excess, asbestos, exposure to ionizing radiation, and bacterial, fungal or viral infections. ROS cause damage to biomolecules such as lipid, proteins and DNA by attaching. ROS may directly attack DNA, either the sugar, phosphate or purine and pyrimidine bases. On the other hand, oxidative damage may be indirect by rising of intracellular $Ca^{+2}$ ions. Free radical-mediated reactions can cause structural alterations in DNA (e.g., nicking, base-pair mutations, rearrangement, deletions insertions and sequence amplification). Degradation of the bases will produce numerous products, including 8-OH-Gua, hydroxymethylurea, urea, thymine glycol; thymine and adenine ring opened and saturated products. Most oxidized bases in DNA are repaired by base excision repair (BER). BER consists of four main steps. The first step involves the removal of the oxidised base by a specific DNA glycosylase, yielding an apurinic/apyrimidinic (AP) site. In the second step, an AP endonuclease removes the deoxyribose phosphate group from the AP site generating a single nucleotide gap. A DNA polymerase, thought to be predominantly DNA polymerase b, fills this gap. Finally, a DNA ligase, probably DNA ligase III, seals the stand break and completes the repair process.

This chapter mainly deals with: (i) formation of ROS in physiological and pathological conditions, (ii ) ROS-mediated DNA damage, leading to cellular pathology and ultimately to cell death (iii) Oxidative DNA damage repair systems, (iv) The molecular mechanism of ROS-mediated diseases such as cancer, cardiovascular disease, neurodegenerative diseases, inflammatory disease, ischemia-reperfusion injury and aging.

If the mechanisms of oxidative DNA damage and DNA repairing system are well understood, the diseases resulting from oxidative DNA damage or inefficient DNA repairing could be treated in future and a better understanding of these mechanisms would also allow biomarkers of DNA damage to become potentially useful clinical tools.

## 2. Formation of reactive oxygen species

**Oxygen** ($O_2$) is an element obligatory for life and living systems have evolved to survive in the presence of molecular $O_2$. Oxidative properties of $O_2$ play a vital role in diverse biological phenomena. $O_2$ has double-edged properties, being essential for life; it can also aggravate the damage within the cell by oxidative events. This situation is referred to as the "Oxygen Paradox" [Sen et al., 2010; Khanna & Shiloh, 2009].

Aerobic organisms are constantly subjected to a variety of reactive entities derived from molecular $O_2$, often collectively referred to as reactive oxygen species (ROS). Some ROS contain unpaired electrons and are therefore referred to as free radicals. A radical is an atom or group of atoms that have one or more unpaired electrons. Radicals can have positive, negative or neutral charge. A prominent feature of radicals is that they have extremely high chemical reactivity, which explains not only their normal biological activities, but also how they inflict damage on cells. There are many types of radicals, but in biological systems most significant are those derived from $O_2$ [Khanna & Shiloh, 2009, Colton & Gilbert, 1999]. The radicals derived from the reduction of molecular oxygen: superoxide/hydroperoxyl radicals hydrogen peroxide and the hydroxyl radical ($^{\bullet}OH$) the species derived from the reaction of carbon-centered radicals with molecular oxygen: peroxyl radicals alkoxyl radicals and organic hydroperoxides (ROOH); and other oxidants resulting in free radical formation such as hypochlorous acid (HOC1), peroxynitrite and singlet $O_2$ [Khanna & Shiloh, 2009, Colton & Gilbert, 1999].

The **diatomic oxygen** molecule qualifies as a radical, because it possesses two unpaired electrons, each located at a different orbital. Since both electrons have the same quantum spin number, $O_2$ itself has relatively low reactivity. Another radical derived from $O_2$ is singlet oxygen, $^1O_2$. This is an excited form of $O_2$ in which one of the electrons jumps to a superior orbital following absorption of energy. For $O_2$ to oxidize a molecule directly, it would have to accept a pair of electrons with a spin opposite to that of the $O_2$. In biological systems, $O_2$ can accept an electron and form one of the following species: superoxide anion ($^{\bullet}O_2^-$), $^{\bullet}OH$, or hydrogen peroxide ($H_2O_2$). These molecules possess various degrees of reactivity with nonradical compounds [Colton & Gilbert, 1999, Kohen & Nyska, 2002].

The mitochondrial respiratory chain is the major source of $^{\bullet}O_2-$, [Colton & Gilbert, 1999, Kohen & Nyska, 2002, Bielski & Cabelli, 1995, Halliwell & Gutteridge, 1999, Schafer & Buettner, 2001, Forman & Boveris, 1982]. $^{\bullet}O_2-$ is abundant and can reach an intracellular concentration of about $10^{-11}$ M [Halliwell & Gutteridge, 1999, Schafer & Buettner, 2001, Forman & Boveris, 1982, Babior, 2000, Nohl & Hegner, 1978]. $^{\bullet}O_2-$ is not highly reactive for biological molecules however once formed it quickly undergoes dismutation to generate hydrogen peroxide, which is highly reactive. This reaction is markedly accelerated by a family of enzymes, the superoxide dismutases (SODs). $^{\bullet}O_2^-$ can react with H+ to form $HO_2^{\bullet}$ (hydroperoxy radical) which is much more reactive than $^{\bullet}O_2^-$. NADPH oxidase, primarily located in phagocytes, neutrophils and monocytes, can generate $^{\bullet}O_2^-$ and other reactive oxidants that are used for fighting invading microorganisms [Sohal, 1997].

The •**OH** is an extremely reactive oxidant [Halliwell & Gutteridge, 1999, Khanna & Shiloh, 2009]. It is also a short-lived molecule with an estimated half-life of nanoseconds at 37°C, traveling only a few Ångstroms. Despite its short life span, •OH is capable of inducing considerable damage to nuclear and mitochondrial DNA. This radical alone can cause over 100 types DNA modifications [Khanna & Shiloh, 2009, Michalik et al., 1995]. In addition, •OH can lead to lipid peroxidation and oxidation of amino acids, sugars, and metals. The •OH is a major product of irradiation due to radiation-induced dissociation of water molecules.

Although $\mathbf{H_2O_2}$ itself is not a radical, it is included in ROS due to producing highly reactive free radical, •OH. $H_2O_2$ is one of the most stable ROS and acts as a messenger in cellular signaling pathways [Khanna & Shiloh, 2009, Kamata & Hirata, 1999]. There are some enzymes that can produce $H_2O_2$ directly or indirectly, including SOD, monoamine oxidase (MAO), diamine and polyamine oxidase, and glycolate oxidase. Under normal conditions, $H_2O_2$ is not toxic up to a cellular concentration of about $10^{-8}$ M [Imlay et al., 1988] $H_2O_2$ molecules are freely dissolved in aqueous solution and can easily penetrate biological membranes. Their deleterious chemical effects can be divided into the categories of direct activity, originating from their oxidizing properties, and indirect activity in which they serve as a source for more deleterious species, such as OH· or HClO. In the presence of transition metals such as $Fe^{2+}$ or $Cu^{+}$, $H_2O_2$ it can be converted to highly reactive •OH, either by Fenton or Harber- Weiss reactions [Yamasaki & Piette, 1991, Halliwell & Gutteridge, 1999, Khanna & Shiloh, 2009]. $H_2O_2$ is detoxified by a set of enzymes that includes the selenium-dependent glutathione peroxidase (GPx) and catalase.

**The nitric oxide (NO), or nitrogen monoxide**, which is a radical (NO• ), is produced by the oxidation of one of the terminal guanido nitrogen atoms of L-arginine. In this reaction, L-arginine is converted to NO and L-citrulline by nitric oxide synthase (NOS) which has three isoforms: neuronal NOS, endothelial NOS (eNOS), and inducible NOS (iNOS). NO is quite stable and benign for a free radical, with a lifetime of several seconds. Under normal conditions, NO has many physiological functions such as a neuronal messenger and modulator of smooth muscle contraction. NO can interact with $^{\bullet}O_2^{-}$ to form the peroxynitrite anion (ONOO−) that induces a cascade of events that can eventually lead to cell death [Radi et al., 1991a]. This molecule accounts for much of the NO toxicity. The reactivity of ONOO− is roughly the same as that of •OH and $N\ O_2^{\bullet}$. Its toxicity is derived from its ability to directly nitrate and hydroxylate the aromatic rings of amino acid residues [Schafer & Buettner, 2001] and to react with sulfahydryls [Beckman et al., 1992], lipids [Radi, 1991b], proteins [Moreno & Pryor, 1992] and DNA [King et al., 1992]. Under physiological conditions, ONOOH can react with other components present in high concentrations, such as $H_2O_2$ or $CO_2$, to form an adduct that might be responsible for many of the deleterious effects seen in biological sites. Peroxynitrite anion can also affect cellular energy status by inactivating key mitochondrial enzymes [Radi et. Al, 1994], and it may trigger calcium release from the mitochondria [Packer & Murphy, 1994].

## 3. Classification of reactive oxygen species

ROS generated in response to both endogenous and exogenous stimuli can be divided into Endogenous ROS and exogenous ROS. (Figure 1) [Ziech et al., 2010, Fukai & Nakamura, 2008, Klaunig & Kamendulis, 2004, Galaris et al., 2008].

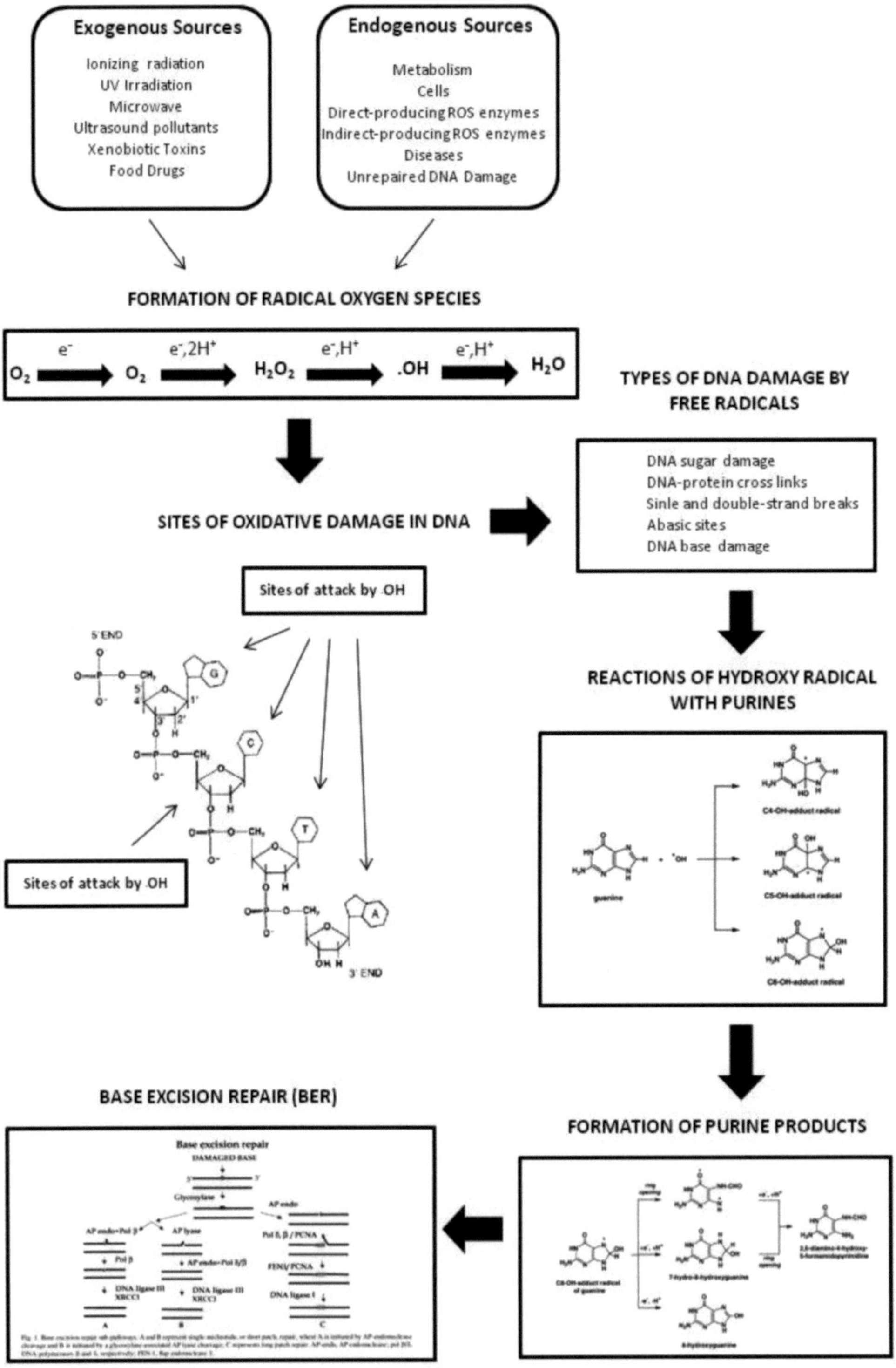


Fig. 1. Oxidative damage and repair of DNA.

### Endogenous ROS

In eukaryotic cells, aerobic respiration in the mitochondria is the main source for the generation of ROS. ROS are also produced by peroxisomal oxidation of fatty acids, microsomal cytochrome P450 metabolism of xenobiotic compounds, stimulation of phagocytosis by pathogens or lipopolysaccharides, arginine metabolism and tissue specific enzymes [Adly, 2010]. Enzymes in the cytosol, such as oxygenases, peroxidases and oxidases, generate small amounts of ROS. It is estimated that more than 95% of $^{\bullet}O_2^-$ produced during normal metabolism are generated as a by-product from the electron transfer reactions at the inner mitochondrial membrane. Approximately 1-2% of the $O_2$ consumed by mitochondria is converted into $^{\bullet}O_2^-$ [Cadenas & Davies, 2000, Hashiguchi et al., 2004].Because of such a highly oxidative environment, mitochondria are also one of the main cellular targets of ROS induced damage, and in fact relatively high levels of oxidized proteins, lipids and nucleic acids are detected in mammalian mitochondria under normal metabolic conditions [Hashiguchi et al., 2004, Raha & Robinson, 2000].

Another significant endogenous source of ROS production is via the reduction of molecular $O_2$ by inflammatory cells [Klaunig & Kamendulis, 2004, Ziech et al., 2010, Fukai & Nakamura, 2008]. In this reaction, phagocytes produce $^{\bullet}O_2^-$ via oxygen's monovalent reduction. In order to counterbalance ROS-mediated injury, endogenous antioxidant defense systems exist and function by quenching and clearing intracellular ROS activity and accumulation and maintaining redox equilibrium [Ziech et al., 2010, Dizdaroğlu et al., 1993]. Generated chronic oxidative stress damage to cellular macromolecules like DNA, lipids and proteins [Klaunig & Kamendulis, 2004, Ziech et al., 2010]. The endogenous enzymatic antioxidant defenses (SOD, GPx and catalase) can counterbalance oxidative microenvironments by chelating superoxide and various other peroxides. Also, the non-enzymatic endogenous antioxidants (Vitamins E and C, coenzyme Q, B-carotene and glutathione) have the ability to eliminate ROS activity. Thus, ROS can be considered as critical determinants of intracellular redox states and thus serve as important cellular regulatory mechanism(s) in both health and disease [Klaunig & Kamendulis, 2004, Ziech et al., 2010].

### Exogenous ROS

Environmental agents like radiation, xenobiotics and chlorinated compounds are significant inducers of cellular damage via ROS mediated toxicity [Galaris et al., 2008]. In addition, anticancer drugs, anesthetics, analgesics, trauma; radiation; electromagnetic fields; alcohol; cigarette smoke; medications; stress; allergens; cold, excessive exercise; dietary factors such as excess sugar, saturated fat and fried oils; malnutrition and various disease states have been considered as most established environmental sources of ROS [Cadenas & Davies, 2000]. Furthermore, exposure to ionizing and ultraviolet radiations also induces ROS-mediated alterations in major pathways associated with the control of cellular growth and survival. For instance, ultraviolet B rays can damage DNA directly and also increase ROS concentrations in epidermal cells [Mena et al., 2009]. In addition, urban air contains a mixture of oxidizing gases and particulates arising from a variety of sources, such as power plants, motor vehicles, wildfires and waste incinerators. Chronic exposure to polluted air induces irreversible damage to cellular macromolecules (DNA, proteins, lipids etc.) via ROS production and their accumulation in cells and tissues [Moller et al., 2008]. Metabolism of exogenous sources of ethanol and phenobarbital contributes to ROS generation through changes in the cytochrome P450 pathway [Wu & Cederbaum, 2003].

## 4. ROS-mediated DNA damage

Although DNA is a stable and well-protected molecule, ROS can interact with it and cause several types of damage: modification of DNA bases, single- and double-DNA breaks, loss of purines (apurinic sites), damage to the deoxyribose sugar, DNA-protein cross-linkage, and damage to the DNA repair system (Figure 1) [Kohen & Nyska, 2002].

Of the ROS, the highly reactive •OH reacts with DNA by addition to double bonds of DNA bases and by abstraction of an H atom from the methyl group of thymine and each of the C-H bonds of 2′-deoxyribose. Addition of •OH to the C5-C6 double bond of pyrimidines leads to C5-OH and C6-OH adduct radicals of cytosine and thymine and H atom abstraction from thymine results in the allyl radical. Adduct radicals differ in terms of their redox properties, C5-OH- and C6-OH-adduct radicals of pyrimidines possess reducing and oxidising properties, respectively [Sonntag, 1987, Steenken, 1987, Teoule, 1987, Cooke et al., 2003].

Pyrimidine OH-adduct radicals and the allyl radical are oxidised or reduced depending on their redox environment, redox properties and reaction partners, yielding a variety of products [Dizdaroglu, 1992, Evans et al., 2004]. Product types and yields depend on absence and presence of $O_2$ and on other conditions [Cooke et al., 2003, Breen & Murphy, 1995]. In the absence of $O_2$, the oxidation of C5-OH adduct radicals, followed by addition of OH_ (or addition of water followed by deprotonation), leads to cytosine glycol and thymine glycol. The oxidation of the allyl radical of thymine yields 5-hydroxymethyluracil (5-OHMeUra) when molecular $O_2$ adds to C5-OH-adduct radicals at diffusion-controlled rates generating C5-OH-6-peroxyl radicals, which subsequently eliminate $O_2$•− followed by reaction with water (addition of $OH^-$) to yield thymine and cytosine glycols [Evans et al., 2004, Sonntag, 1987, Teoule, 1987].

Addition of $O_2$ to the allyl radical leads to 5-OHMeUra and 5-formyluracil (5-FoUra). Pyrimidine peroxyl radicals are also reduced and then protonated to give hydroxyhydroperoxides [Teoule, 1987], which decompose and yield thymine glycol, 5-OHMeUra, 5-FoUra, and 5-hydroxy-5-methylhydantoin [Wagner et al., 1994, Dizdaroglu et al., 1993a].

Cytosine products may deaminate and dehydrate. Cytosine glycol deaminates to give uracil glycol, 5-hydroxycytosine (5-OH-Cyt), and 5-hydroxyuracil (5-OH-Ura) that are unique in that they can deaminate and dehydrate. However, there is evidence that these four compounds (cytosine glycol, uracil glycol, 5-OH-Cyt, and 5-OH-Ura) may simultaneously be existed damaged DNA [Wagner et al., 1994, Dizdaroglu et al., 1993a]. In the absence of $O_2$, C5-OH adduct radicals may be reduced, followed by protonation to give rise to 5-hydroxy-6-hydropyrimidines. 5-Hydroxy-6-hydrocytosine (5-OH-6-HCyt) readily deaminates into 5-hydroxy-6-hydrouracil (5-OH-6-HUra). Similarly, C6-OH adduct radicals of pyrimidines are reduced yielding 6-hydroxy-5-hydropyrimidines. Formation of these products are inhibited in the presence of $O_2$, because $O_2$ reacts with their precursors C5-OH- and C6-OH-adduct radicals at diffusion-controlled rates to yield peroxyl radicals and then other products.

Further reactions of C5-OH-6-peroxyl and C6-OH-5-peroxyl radicals of cytosine result in formation of 4-amino-5-hydroxy-2, 6(1H, 5H)-pyrimidinedione and 4-amino-6-hydroxy-2, 5(1H, 6H)-pyrimidinedione, respectively. The former deaminates to give dialuric acid, which is readily oxidised to yield alloxan [Dizdaroglu et al., 1993a, Behrend et al., 1989, Dizdaroglu 1993b]. The presence of alloxan in damaged DNA has been shown by its release from DNA by *E. coli* Nth [Dizdaroglu et al., 1993a].

Decarboxylation of alloxan yields 5-hydroxyhydantoin (5-OH-Hyd) upon acidic treatment. Isodialuric acid is formed by deamination of 4-amino-6-hydroxy-2, 5(1H, 6H)-pyrimidinedione. However, these two compounds may simultaneously exist in DNA as evidenced from the detection of their enol forms (5, 6-dihydroxycytosine (5, 6-diOH-Cyt) and 5, 6-dihydroxyuracil (5, 6-diOH-Ura), respectively) [11, 13]. 5-OH-6-hydroperoxide of cytosine undergoes intramolecular cyclisation to yield *trans*-1-carbamoyl-2-oxo-4, 5-dihydroxyimidazolidine as a major product in cytosine [Kohen & Nyska, 2002] However, this compound is formed as a minor product in DNA [Dizdaroglu et al., 1993a, Behrend et al., 1989, Dizdaroglu 1993b].

Hydroxyl adduct radicals of guanine are formed by addition of •OH to the C4-, C5- and C8-positions of guanine, generating C4-OH-, C5-OH- and C8-OH-adduct radicals [O'Neill, 1983, Steenken, 1989, Candeisas & Steenken, 2000]. The 6-substituted purines such as adenine undergo analogous reactions, yielding at least two OH adducts, are formed: C4-OH and C8-OH adduct radicals [Steenken, 1989, Candeisas & Steenken, 2000]. C4-OH and C5-OH adduct radicals of purines differ in their redox properties, with C4-OH-adduct radicals being oxidising, and C5-OH- and C8-OH-adduct radicals being primarily reducing.

On the other hand, different mesomeric structures of these radicals may be oxidizing or reducing, a phenomenon called "redox ambivalence" [Vieira & Steenken, 1990]. Dehydration of C4-OH- and C5-OH-adduct radicals of purines reconstitutes the purine by first yielding a purine (–H)• radical, followed by reduction and protonation [Melvin et al., 1996]. The C4-OH-adduct radical of guanine also eliminates OH− to give rise to the guanine radical cation (guanine•+), which may deprotonate depending on pH to give guanine(-H)• [Moreno & Pryor, 1992]. Furthermore, on the basis of product analysis, the radical cation does not hydrate to lead to the C8-OH adduct radical and then to 8-hydroxyguanine by oxidation. However, it may react with 2′-deoxyribose in DNA by H abstraction, leading to DNA strand breaks [O'Neill & Chapman, 1985].

This diversity has been explained by the notion that the hydration of guanine•+ in ds-DNA may be much faster than that of monomeric guanine•+ [Candeias & Steenken, 2000]. $O_2$ readily reacts with guanine(-H)•; however, its reaction with the C4-OH-adduct radical of guanine is rather slow [Candeias & Steenken, 2000]. The reaction of guanine(-H)• with $O_2$ leads to imidazolone and oxazolone derivatives [Cadet et al., 1991]. However, this suggestion has not been confirmed by pulse radiolysis data and an alternative mechanism has been proposed [Melvin et al., 1996]. The C4-OH-adduct radical of adenine readily reacts with $O_2$, however, final products of this reaction are not known [O'Neill & Chapman, 1985]. C8-OH adduct radicals of purines may be oxidized by oxidants including $O_2$. In contrast to C4-OH adduct radicals, their reaction with $O_2$ is diffusion controlled [Vieira & Steenken, 1990].

8-Hydroxypurines are formed in DNA by the one-electron oxidation of C8-OH-adduct radicals [Bielski & Cabelli, 1995, Halliwell & Gutteridge, 1999] This reaction competes with the unimolecular opening of the imidazole ring by scission of the C8–N9 bond [Steenken, 1989, Candeias & Steenken, 2000]. The one-electron reduction of the ring-opened radical leads to 2, 6-diamino-4-hydroxy-5-formamidopyrimidine (FapyGua) from guanine and 4, 6-diamino-5-formamidopyrimidine (Fapy- Ade) from adenine [O'Neill, 1983, Breen & Murphy, 1995]. The C8-OH adduct radicals may also be reduced without ring opening to give rise to 7-hydro-8-hydroxypurines, which, as hemiorthoamides, are converted into formamidopyrimidines. However, 8-Hydroxypurines and formamidopyrimidines are unique in that they are formed in DNA both in the absence and presence of $O_2$, although $O_2$ increases the yields of 8-hydroxypurines. Moreover, other experimental conditions highly affect the yields of these compounds, such as the presence of reducing or oxidizing agents [Dizdaroglu, 1992, Breen & Murphy, 1995]. In the case of adenine, the •OH attack at the C2-position has also been proposed to take place and yield 2-hydroxyadenine (2-OH-Ade) when oxidation of the thus-formed C2-OH-adduct radical [Nackerdien et al., 1991]. Reactions of pyrimidines and purines result in multiple products in DNA. Most of these modified bases were identified in DNA in vitro and in vivo upon exposure to free radical generating systems [Dizdaroglu, 1998].

Reactions of •OH with the sugar moiety of DNA by H abstraction give rise to sugar modifications. Some sugar products are released from DNA as free modified sugars, whereas others remain within DNA or constitute end groups of broken DNA strands. A unique reaction of the C5′-centered sugar radical is the addition to the C8- position of the purine ring of the same nucleoside. This intramolecular cyclisation followed by oxidation yields 8, 5′-cyclopurine-2′-deoxynucleosides [Dizdaroglu, 1986, Dirksen et al., 1988]. Both 5′R- and 5′S-diastereomers of 8, 5′-cyclo-2′-deoxyguanosine (cyclo-dG) and 8, 5′-cyclo-2′-deoxyadenosine (cyclo-dA) are generated in DNA[Dizdaroglu, 1986, Dirksen et al., 1988]. (5′R)-and (5′S)- cyclo-dGs were also identified in human cells exposed to ionizing radiation [Dizdaroglu, 1987]. These tandem lesions represent a concomitant damage to both the base and sugar moieties of DNA. $O_2$ inhibits their formation by reacting with the C5′ centered sugar radical before cyclization.

Another reaction of base radicals is the addition to an aromatic amino acid of proteins or combination with an amino acid radical, leading to DNA–protein cross-linking [Dizdaroglu, 1988]. Covalent DNA–protein cross-links are formed in cells in vivo or in chromatin in vitro by exposure to free radical-generating systems, e.g., ionising radiation. The formation of a thymine–tyrosine cross-link has been observed in mammalian chromatin in vitro and in living cells upon exposure to ionising radiation, $H_2O_2$, metal ions and carcinogenic compounds [Dizdaroglu et al. 1989, Nackerdien et al., 1991, Olinski et al., 1992, Altman et al., 1995]. The formation mechanism of DNA–protein cross-link has been proposed to involve the addition of the allyl radical of thymine in DNA to tyrosine in a protein, followed by oxidation. Chemical structures of other DNA base-amino acid cross-links have been identified in mammalian chromatin in vitro, but not in vivo [Dizdaroglu, 1998]

## 5. Mechanism of oxidative DNA base damage: The BER pathway

As mentioned above, excess ROS may induce oxidative DNA damage, DNA strand breaks, base modifications and chromosomal aberrations [Marnett, 2000]. For repair of the DNA damage, human cells have five DNA repair systems: Direct reversal, mismatch repair, double-strand break repair, base excision repair (BER) and nucleotide excision repair (NER) [Wood et al., 2001]. DNA lesions resulting from oxidative stress, as well as single strand breaks, are repaired via the BER pathway in organisms ranging from E. coli to mammals (Figure 1) [Hazra et al., 2007, Krokan et al., 2003].

It is believed that DNA-BER is the major pathway for repairing deaminated bases and bases with oxidative damage generated by ROS and can be used to repair alkylated bases [Hazra et al., 2007, Hedge et al., 2008]. BER has 4 main steps (i.e. base removal, AP site incision, synthesis, and ligation) and involves 4 major classes of DNA repair enzymes: DNA glycosylases, APE, DNA polymerases, and DNA ligases.

The proteins involved in this reaction function in concert to remove a damaged DNA base and replace it with the correct base. A currently accepted model for the BER pathway reveals five distinct enzymatic steps for the repair of damaged bases.

Glycosylases at the initial step of BER. DNA glycosylases make BER possible - glycosylases recognize specific damaged bases and excise them from the genome, effectively initiating both longpatch and short-patch BER. To date, 11 different mammalian glycosylases have been characterized. The primary function of most DNA glycosylases is to recognize their substrate (the damaged base) and catalyze the cleavage of an N-glycosidic bond, releasing a free base and creating an abasic site [Lindahl, 1974]. In addition to catalyzing the cleavage of N-glycosydic bonds, some glycosylases are bifunctional having an additional AP lyase activity [O'Connor & Laval, 1989]. The uracil-DNA glycosylase (UNG) was the first DNA glycosylase identified and cloned [Lindahl, 1974]. MPG, N-methylpurine-DNAglycosylase, and 8-oxoguanine-DNA glycosylase (OGG1)represent some extensively studied DNA glycosylases [Sedgwick et al., 2007, Kavli et al., 2007, Klungland & Bjelland, 2007, Robertson et al., 2009]. After recognition of the damaged base by the appropriate DNA glycosylase, this glycosylase catalyzes the cleavage of an N-glycosidic bond, effectively removing the damaged base and creating an apurinic or apyrimidinic site (AP site). The DNA backbone is cleaved by either a DNA AP endonuclease or a DNA AP lyase - an activity present in some glycosylases. AP endonuclease activity creates a single-stranded DNA nick 5′ to the AP site, contrasting with the nick being created 3′ to the AP site as a result of activity (β-elimination or β, δ-elimination).

Repair can then proceed through one of two subpathways: short or long-patch BER. The short-patch BER involves the incorporation of a single nucleotide into the gap by DNA polymerase followed by strand ligation by DNA ligase. The long-patch BER involves incorporation of several nucleotides, typically two to seven, followed by cleavage of the resulting 5′ flap and ligation. Mitochondria possess independent BER machinery, the components of which are coded by nuclear genes.

Most DNA glycosylases have broad substrate specificities but can have preferences for either purines or pyrimidines. The major bifunctional glycosylase for purines is 8-oxoguanine DNA glycosylase 1, which removes OHdG and 8-oxoG. Most oxidized pyrimidines are removed by endonuclease III-like protein, uracil DNA glycosylase (UNG), and Nei-like DNA glycosylase (NEIL-1 and NEIL-2). In human cells, there are at least 2 isoforms of OGG1 (α and β) that arise from alternative splicing of products of the OGG1 gene [Boeiteux & Radicella, 2000]. α-OGG1 is a 345-amino acid (~39 kd) protein that localizes to the nucleus and mitochondria, whereas β-OGG1 is a 424-amino acid protein (47 kd) that seems to localize exclusively to mitochondria [Boeiteux & Radicella, 2000]. Because of the absence of an αO helix domain, β-OGG1 seems to lack glycosylase activity [Hashiguchi et al., 2004]. Endonuclease III-like protein 1 is a 312-amino acid (~34 kd) protein that localizes to the nucleus. OGG1 and endonuclease III-like protein require duplex DNA for efficient repair. After the glycosylase reaction, the newly created nick is processed by the Apurinic/apyrimidinic endonuclease (APE), creating a single-nucleotide gap in the DNA. Importantly, the gap created contains a 3′- hydroxyl and a 5′-phosphate, substrates compatible with the downstream enzymatic reactions in BER.

APE cleaves intact AP sites by making a single nick 5′ to the AP site to create 3′-OH and 5′-deoxyribose phosphate termini that are removed by the activity of 3′-OH and 5′-deoxyribose phosphatase proteins such as DNA Polβ. The 3-phosphate removal activity of APE is, however, approximately 70-fold lower than the AP endonuclease activity of APE [Winters et al., 1994], suggesting that other enzymes are important for the processing of damaged 3′ ends [Takahashi et al., 2007] APE is a 317-amino acid (~37 kd) multifunctional protein localized to the nucleus [Demple et al., 1991]. In addition to its role in BER, APE is required for the redox activation of transcription factors (e.g. p53) spontaneously oxidized at cysteine residues in DNA binding domains to establish DNA binding activity [Jayaraman et al., 1997]. Deletion of APE in mice causes embryonic lethality [Jayaraman et al., 1997]. Cells from mice with APE haploinsufficiency respond poorly to oxidative stress [Meira et al., 2001].

The nick generated by the cleavage of the abasic site is filled in by either Pol β or Pol δ/ε in the nucleus, and Pol γ in the mitochondria. Pol γ is the only DNA polymerase identified so far in vertebrate mitochondria and functions both as the replicative and the repair polymerase [Weissman et al., 2007, Kaguni, 2004]. Relevant to its role in BER, Pol γ has a dRP-lyase activity and can catalyze the 3′-end-processing necessary for short-patch BER [Longley et al., 1998].

The final step in the BER pathway is ligation of the nick with the correct nucleotide by DNA polymerases. An adenosine triphosphate-dependent DNA ligase (Ligase [Lig]I or III) completes the repair process and restores the integrity of the helix by sealing the nick. In the nucleus, two distinct DNA ligases participate in BER, ligase I, which has been implicated in long-patch BER, and ligase III, implicated in short-patch. The human ligase III gene (*LIG3*) also encodes for a mitochondrial variant, with a putative MTS generated by an alternative downstream translation initiation site [Lakshmipathy & Campbell, 1999, Lakshmipathy & Campbell, 2001]. The localization of ligase III protein to mitochondria suggests, then, that this enzyme may perform the ligation step in mtBER. Accordingly, reduction of ligase III expression using an antisense strategy resulted in an increase in breaks in mtDNA [Lakshmipathy & Campbell, 2001].

## 6. Diseases associated with defects of oxidative DNA damage repair systems

It is quite new and non conclusive that oxidative DNA damage might result in diseases. Increasing numbers of oxidatively modified DNA lesions are proposed to be appropriate, intermediate biomarkers of a disease endpoint. For this reason alone, the association between oxidative DNA damage and disease should be determined. As seen above , it is clear that oxidative DNA damage has effects upon cells other than mutation. Nevertheless, DNA mutation is perhaps one of the most important consequences of lesion persistence, evidenced by the presence of multiple systems to prevent lesion formation and, should damage occur, ensure rapid lesion removal; with the DNA repair systems responsible for the latter having much overlap of substrates, as discussed previously [Evans et al., 2004].

Cumulative oxidative DNA damage have a significant effect of the impairment on normal cellular repair mechanisms. In fact, one of the main etiological hypotheses linking genomic instability, mutagenesis and tumorigenesis is that of deficient cellular repair mechanisms due to extensive oxidative DNA damage and cellular injury [Ziech, 2011]. Clearly, reduced repair will result in elevated lesions and an increased risk of disease [Cooke et al., 2003]. ROS-mediated DNA damage in addition to ineffective DNA repair mechanisms are well established lesions common to many life threatening human diseases, including neurodegenerative diseases, atherosclerosis, cancer, and aging has invoked free radical reactions as an underlying mechanism of injury [Ziech, 2011]. Given the importance of mutation in carcinogenesis, cancer will be the first disease in which a role for oxidative DNA damage in its aetiology is considered [Evans et al., 2004].

**Cancer**

The carcinogenicity of oxidative stress is primarily attributed to the genotoxicity of ROS in diverse cellular processes [ Ziech, 2011]. Oxidative mechanisms have been demonstrated to possess a potential role in the initiation, promotion, and malignant conversion (progression) stages of carcinogenesis [Cooke et al., 2003] . It has been suggested that some signaling system induces ROS that exhibit dual roles, cancer promoting and cancer suppresing, in tumorogenesis. ROS participate simultaneously in two signaling pathways that have inverse functions in tumorigenesis, Ras-Raf-MEK1/2-ERK1/2 signaling and the p38 mitogen-activated protein kinases (MAPK) pathway. Ras-Raf-MEK1/2-ERK1/2 signaling plays a role in oncogenesis, while the p38 MAPK pathway contributes to cancer suppression. The accumulation of intracellular ROS induced by oncogenic Ras is ERK-dependent during the activation of p38a [Pan et al., 2009)

Increased intracellular levels of ROS, induced by the Ras-Raf-MEK-ERK signaling cascade, may mediate the activation of the p38 pathway and act as an intermediate signal between the MEK-ERK and MKK3/6-p38 pathways. On the one hand, the activation of p38 mitogen-activated protein kinase (MAPK) is a prerequisite for ROS-mediated functions such as apoptotic cell death in cancer cells. On the other hand, inhibiting or scavenging ROS may attenuate the activation of p38-dependent pathways. Human cancer cell lines with high ROS levels display enhanced tumorigenicity and impaired p38α activation by ROS [Pan et al., 2009].

The effect of ROS by Ras may occur at the transcription level. GATA-6 is a component of the specific protein-DNA complexes at the nicotinamide adenine dinucleotide phosphate oxidase (Nox) 1 promoter, and is able to trans-activate the Nox1 promoter. GATA-6 is phosphorylated at serine residues by MEK-activated extracellular signal regulated kinase (ERK), which enhances GATA-6 DNA binding. The activity of the ROS-generating enzyme Nox1 is required for vascular endothelial growth factor (VEGF), a potent stimulator of tumor angiogenesis. Ras signaling enhances the transcription of Nox1 [Adachi et al., 2008]. A regulatory subunit, Rac, of the NADPH oxidase complex also involves the regulation of ROS [Heyworth et al., 1993, Kadara et al., 2008]. However, if extracellular signal-regulated kinase (ERK)-dependent phosphorylation of the transcription factor Sp1 and Sp1 binding to a VEGF promoter is inhibited, this activity does not occur [Pan et al., 2009].

Although some studies suggested that increased intracellular ROS elevate the activation of p38, these results have not been confirmed yet by the other researchers. It seems that further studies are needed to understand the mechanism of ROS in cancer.

Since the main purpose of this chapter is not to deal with the effect of ROS in tumorogenesis, we will explain the effect of ROS on DNA and DNA repair enzymes. ROS can cause direct oxidative DNA damage by increasing a cell's mutation.

Major oxidative DNA damage products including those of 8-oxo-7, 8-dihydroadenine (8-oxoAde), 8-oxo-7, 8-dihydroguanine (8-oxoGua), 8-oxo-7, 8-dihydro-2'-deoxyguanosine (8-oxodG), and 5, 6-dihydroxy-5, 6-dihydrothymine as well as the ring-open lesions of 4, 6-diamino-5-formamido-pyrimidine and 2, 6-diamino-4-hydroxy-5-formamido-pyrimidine [Kohen & Nyska, 2002]. Of these oxidative products, 8-oxoGua is known to be a biomarker of oxidative stres and its mutagenicity in mammalian cells demonstrates an additional potential as an intermediate marker of a disease endpoint (e.g. cancer). Elevated levels of such DNA lesions have been noted in many tumor types and are strongly implicated in the etiology of cancer [Valko et al., 2006]. Approximately 50%

higher rates of 8-oxoGua levels have been observed in lung, breast or prostate cancer patients when compared to otherwise healthy individuals [Tudek et al., 2010]. In addition, recent investigations have showed higher endogenous levels of 8-oxoGua in tumor tissues when compared to controls, thus suggesting oxidative DNA damage as a contributing factor in cancer development [Trachootham et al., 2009]. In addition, high levels of 8-oxoGua and possibly other DNA lesions are suggested as reliable risk factors associated with the transformation of benign to malignant tumors [Chen et al., 2007]. Furthermore, 8-oxoGua lesions are known to induce aberrant modifications in adjacent DNA a hypothesized mechanism that significantly contributes to the genetic instability and metastatic potential of tumor cells [Valko et al., 2006]. For example, formation of 8-oxoGua lesions has been shown to induce a cascade of adjacent DNA base mutations, such as GC → TA transversions in the *ras* oncogene [Bos, 1988] and *p53* tumour suppressor gene in lung and liver cancer [Valko et al.2006, Mos, 1988, Takahashi et al., 1989]. Under normal conditions, DNA repair mechanisms include OGG1, nei-like glycosylase 1 (NEIL1), APE1, and MutY homologue (MUTYH) (Evans et al. 2004). In addition, nucleotide excision repair (NER) may also participate in the process of removing the 8-OHdG lesion [Klaunig, 2010]. Several genes involved in the processing of oxidative DNA damage have been analysed in relation to human cancer risk in molecular epidemiological studies . Among these genes, allele polymorphic variants have been found in OGG1, XRCC1, Pol b, APE1 and MUTYH, which are associated with a varying extent increased cancer risk [Canbay et al., 2010, Agachan et al., 2009, Narter et al., 2009, Attar et al., 2010]. Several SNPs within hOGG1 have been reported [Kohno et al., 1998]. As polymorphisms in this gene alter glycosylase function and an individual's ability to repair oxidatively damaged DNA, they may contribute to carcinogenesis [Boiteaux & Radicella, 2000, Ide & Kotera, 2004, Shao et al., 2006]. Epidemiologic studies investigating the association between the SNPs of OGG1 have led to conflicting results. The variant allele of this SNP was shown to be associated with significantly increased risk of a number of human cancers, including lung [Hung et al., 2005, Li & Kong, 2008], esophageal [Xing et al., 2001], prostate [Xu et al., 2002], and gastric [Farinati et al., 2008] cancer but not with squamous cell carcinoma of the head and neck (SCCHN) [Zhang et al., 2004] or pancreatic cancer [McWilliams et al., 2008]. A total of eighteen polymorphisms in APE1 have been reported, among which Gln51His and Asp148Glu are the two most common SNPs. Associations between polymorphisms in APE1 and increased risk of lung, colon, breast, SCCHN, prostate, and pancreatic cancer have been reported, but with mixed results [Hung et al., 2005, Zhang et al., 2004, Goode et al., 2002, Jiao et al., 2006].

Studies relating to lung cancer and smoking have supported a potential role for ROS in cancer. Cigarette smoking is strongly linked to the aetiology of lung cancer [Hoffman & Wynder, 1986], being shown to increase the generation of free radical species [Church & Pryor, 1985] and elevate levels of oxidative DNA damage in human lungs [Asami et al., 1997, Agachan et al., 2009, ] and white blood cells [Kiyosawa et al., 1990, Lodovici et al., 2000], as well as to increase the repair of 8-OH-Gua [Asami et al., 1996] and lead to an increased urinary excretion of 8-OH-dG and 5-OHMeUra in smokers compared to non-smokers [Loft et al., 1994, Pourcelot et al., 1999].

Recently ROS-mediated mutations in mitochondrial DNA (mtDNA) have emerged as an important contributor to human carcinogenesis [Freuhaug & Meyskens, 2007]. Mutations in mitochondrial genes encoding complexes I, III, IV and V, as well as within the hypervariable region of mtDNA, have been identified in various human cancers. In general, mtDNA is more susceptible to oxidative damage than nuclear DNA because (i) mitochondrial DNA is not protected by histones, (ii) mitochondrial DNA repair capacity is limited, and (iii) under physiological conditions, the mitochondria converts roughly 3-5% of $O_2$ consumed into $\bullet O_2-$ and subsequently $H_2O_2$. In addition, mtDNA is located in close proximity to the respiratory chain and thus is consequently readily exposed to ROS-induced oxidative damage. As a result, mtDNA has more than two orders of magnitude higher frequency of oxidative damage than that of nuclear DNA and significantly correlates with the development of cancer [Ralph et al., 2010].

**Cardiovascular disease**

It is known that DNA alterations exist in atherosclerotic tissues and may play a fundamental role in the pathogenesis of this disease [Olinski et al., 2002, De Flora et al., 1997, Lee et al., 2001]. Elevated level of 8-OH-Gua found in the lesion of the aorta wall in atherosclerotic patients may be one of the events directly involved in the development of the disease [De Flora et al., 1997]. Oxidized low-density lipoprotein (LDL) might play an important role in the development of atherosclerotic lesions [Ross, 1993]. Interestingly, it has been found that oxidized LDL downregulates enzymes that take part in the BER pathways [Chen et al., 2000]. This DNA repair mechanism is responsible for the removal of 8-OH-Gua from cellular DNA [Dianov et al., 1998]. Therefore, it is possible that oxidized LDL that contributes directly to the development of atherosclerosis, may also be responsible for the high level of 8-OH-Gua observed in blood lymphocytes [Chen et al., 2000].

**Neurodegenerative diseases**

Alzheimer's disease (AD), Huntington's disease and Parkinson's disease (PD) are neurodegenerative conditions, thought to be the result, in part, of chronic exposure to environmental neurotoxins, coupled with a genetic component. These diseases all have oxidative stress implicated in their pathogenesis [Lovell et al., 1999, Lezza et al., 1999, Alam et al., 1997, Zhang et al., 1999], and elevated levels of oxidative DNA damage have been measured in a broad range of neurological conditions [ Koppele et al., 1996, Alam et al., 2000]. Supportive of the studies showing elevated lesion levels are data derived from in vitro studies demonstrating that neurotransmitters such as dopamine and serotonin can generate DNA-damaging, free radical species [Spencer et. al., 1994, Wrona et al., 1998]. Overall, the role of oxidative stress in neurodegenerative disease appears undisputed. However, damage to lipid and protein, rather than DNA, appears to have been apportioned the greatest significance [Markesbery, 1999, Christen, 2000, Smith et al., 2000].

**Inflammatory disease**

The association between inflammation and oxidative stress is well documented [Wiseman et al., 1996, Khanna & Shiloh, 2009], with numerous studies of inflammatory conditions or infections reporting elevated levels of 8-OH-dG: hepatitis [Shimoda et al., 1994], hepatitis C infection [Farinati et al., 1999], and atopic dermatitis. An important source of the ROS are the bactericidal species ($O_2^{\bullet-}$ and $H_2O_2$), generated from the respiratory burst of invading neutrophils, macrophages, and eosinophils damaging surrounding tissue. Chronic inflammation, and the accompanying oxidative stress, has been closely linked to the pathogenesis of autoimmune diseases such as rheumatoid arthritis [Bashir et.al, 1993] and systemic lupus erythematosus [Lunec et.al., 1994], with free radical production resulting, not

only in connective tissue damage, but also modified biomolecules being exposed to the systemic circulation, postulated to be the antigen driving autoantibody production [Weitzman & Gordon, 1990].
Elevated DNA levels of 8-OH-dG have been reported in lymphocytes from patients with RA, SLE, vasculitis or Behcet's disease. These same lymphocytes, from RA and SLE patients, also display increased sensitivity to hydrogen peroxide-induced cytotoxicity [Bashir et al., 1993].

**Ischemia-reperfusion injury**

The literature provides a growing number of reports in which levels of oxidative DNA damage are elevated in post-ischaemia-reperfusion. Elevated levels of urinary 8-OH-dG or dTg were reported following liver transplantation, which proposed to be due to ischemia-reperfusion or reoxygenation injury [Thier et al., 1999, Loft et al., 1995]. Ischaemia-reperfusion injury is a significant factor affecting morbidity and mortality following bypass and transplantation surgery, haemorrhagic or septic shock, myocardial infarction and multiple organ failure. During the period of ischaemia, xanthine dehydrogenase is converted to xanthine oxidase. Upon reperfusion, there is a "burst" of xanthine oxidase activity which, rather than transferring electrons to NAD+, transfers them to $O_2$, generating superoxide, with the subsequent potential for generating other ROS and hence DNA damage. Endogenous levels of xanthine dehydrogenase vary from organ to organ and hence ischemia-reperfusion injury might be more relevant to some tissues than others. Human leukocytes appear to be sensitive to the genotoxic effects of ischemia-reperfusion (163) and therefore represent a potential surrogate tissue in which to study the effects of ischemia-reperfusion that have affected a less accessible tissue.

**Aging**

Major theories of aging are grouped under two categories: damage accumulation aging and developmentally programmed aging. However, a developing (emerging) hypothesis described as the free radical theory of aging appears to have adopted elements of the former theories. The basis of the Harman's theory [Harman, 1956] suggested that aging occurs through the gradual accumulation of free radical damage to biomolecules. With age, antioxidant defences fail to scavenge all potentially damaging radical species that result in the insidious accumulation of damage and gradual loss of function [Beckman et al., 1998]. One of the few focussing upon DNA damage, is a report of an age-related increase in serum 8-OH-dG in apparently disease-free individuals over an age range of 15–91 years [Rattan et al., 1995]. Although this same trend was not evident in the urinary 8-OH-dG output of infants, a gradual increase was noted over the first month postpartum, which mirrored the velocity growth curve [Drury et al., 1998].
The accumulation of lesions can, in part, be explained by the discovery that DNA repair capability correlates with species-specific life span [168]. Furthermore, repair activity appears to decline with age, resulting in the persistence of damage and a subsequent increase in replication errors [Hirano et al., 1995].

## 7. Conclusion

Although there is association between oxidative DNA damage and diseases, elucidation of the role of oxidative DNA damage requires much more work. It is well known that DNA repair enzymes are important for oxidative DNA damage. If individual spesific biomarkers related DNA repair enzyme are found, new treatmant strategies would be developed to cure disease related oxidative DNA damage.

## 8. References


Adachi Y, Shibai Y, Mitsushita J, Shang WH, Hirose K, Kamata T. 2008. Oncogenic Ras upregulates NADPH oxidase 1 gene expres s ion through MEK-ERK-dependent phosphorylation of GATA-6. *Oncogene* 27: 4921-4932

Adly, AAM. 2010. Oxidative stress and disease: An updated review. *Res. J. Immunol.*, 3: 129-145.

Agaçhan B, Küçükhüseyin O, Aksoy P, Turna A, Yaylim I, Görmüs U, Ergen A, Zeybek U, Dalan B, Isbir T. 2009. Apurinic/apyrimidinic endonuclease (APE1) gene polymorphisms and lung cancer risk in relation to tobacco smoking. *Anticancer Res.*, 29(6):2417-20.

Alam ZI, Jenner A, Daniel SE, Lees AJ, Cairns N, Marsden CD, Jenner P, Halliwell B. 1997. Oxidative DNA damage in the Parkinsonian brain: an apparent selective increase in 8-hydroxyguanine levels in substantia nigra, J. *Neurochem.* , 1196–1203.

Alam ZI, Halliwell B, Jenner P. 2000. No evidence for increased oxidative damage to lipids, proteins, or DNA in Huntington's disease. J. *Neurochem.*, 840–846

Altman SA, Zastawny TH, Randers-Eichhorn L, Cacciuttolo MA, Akman SA, Dizdaroglu M., Rao G. 1995. Formation of DNA-protein cross-links in cultured mammalian cells upon treatment with iron ions. *Free Radical Biol. Med.*, 897–902.

Asami S, Manabe H, Miyake J, Tsurudome Y, Hirano T, Yamaguchi R, Itoh H, Kasai H. 1997. Cigarette smoking induces an increase in oxidative DNA damage, 8-hydroxydeoxyguanosine, in a central site of the human lung. *Carcinogenesis,* 18;1763–1766.

Asami S, Hirano T, Yamaguchi R, Tomioka Y, Itoh H, Kasai H. 1996. Increase of a type of oxidative DNA damage, 8-hydroxyguanine, and its repair activity in human leukocytes by cigarette smoking. *Cancer Res.*, 56; 2546–2549.

Attar R, Cacina C, Sozen S, Attar E, Agachan B. 2010. DNA repair genes in endometriosis. *Genet Mol Res.*, 6;9(2):629-36.

Babior BM.2000. The NADPH oxidase of endothelial cells. *IUBMB Life,* 50;267–269.

Bashir S, Harris G, Denman MA, Blake DR, Winyard PG. 1993. Oxidative DNA damage and cellular sensitivity to oxidative stress in human autoimmune diseases. *Ann. Rheum. Dis.*, 52; 659–666.

Beckman JS, Ischiropoulos H, Zhu L, van der Woerd M, Smith C, Chen J, Harrison J, Martin JC, Tsai M.1992. Kinetics of superoxide dismutase- and iron-catalyzed nitration of phenolics by peroxynitrite. *Arch Biochem Biophys.*, 298:438–445.

Beckman KB and Ames BN. 1998. The free radical theory of aging matures. *Physiol. Rev.*, 78, 547–581.

Behrend, R. and Roosen, O. 1889. Synthese der Harnsa¨ure. *Liebigs Ann.Chem.*, 251, 235–256.

Bielski BHJ and Cabelli DE. 1995. Superoxide and hydroxyl radical chemistry in aqueous solution. In: *Active Oxygen in Chemistry*, Foote CS, Valentine JS, Greenberg A, Liebman JF (eds). Chapman and Hall, London, pp. 66–104.

Boiteux S and Radicella JP.2000. The human OGG1 gene: Structure, functions, and its implication in the process of carcinogenesis. *Arch Biochem Biophys.*, 377, 1–8.

Bos JL. 1988. The ras gene family and human carcinogenesis.*Mutat. Res.*, 195;255–271.

Breen AP and Murphy JA.1995. Reactions of hydroxyl radicals with DNA. *Free Radic. Biol. Med.*, 18, 1033–1077

Cadenas E and Davies KJ. 2000. Mitochondrial free radical generation, oxidative stress, and aging. *Free Radic Biol Med.*, 29(3-4):222-30.

Cadet J, Berger M, Decarroz C, Mouret JF, Vanlier JE, Wagner RJ. 1991.Photoinduced and radio-induced radical oxidation of the purine and pyrimidine bases of nucleic acids. *J. Chim. Phys. Phys.-Chim. Biol.* 88;1021–1042.

Cadet J, Berger M, Buchko GW, Joshi PC, Raoul S., Ravanat J-L. 1994.2, 2-Diamino-4-[3, 5-di-*O*-acetyl-2-deoxy-betad-erythrosepentofuranosyl) amino]-5-(2H)-oxazolone—a novel and predominant radical oxidation product of 3_, 5_-di-*O*-acetyl-2_-deoxyguanosine. *J. Am. Chem. Soc.* 116;7403–7404.

Canbay E, Agachan B, Gulluoglu M, Isbir T, Balik E, Yamaner S, Bulut T, Cacina C, Eraltan IY, Yilmaz A, Bugra D. 2010.Possible associations of APE1 polymorphism with susceptibility and HOGG1 polymorphism with prognosis in gastric cancer. *Anticancer Res.*, 30(4):1359-64.

Candeias LP, Steenken S. 2000. Reaction of HO. with Guanine Derivatives in Aqueous Solution: Formation of Two Different Redox-Active OH-Adduct Radicals and Their Unimolecular Transformation Reactions. Properties of G(-H).*Chemistry - A European Journal*, 6: 475–484

Chen HI, Liou SH, Ho SF, Wu KY, Sun CW, Chen MF, Cheng LC, Shih TS, Loh CH.2007. Oxidative DNA damage estimated by plasma 8-hydroxyxeoxyguanosine (8-OHdG): influence of 4, 4'-methylenebis (2-chloroaniline) exposure and smoking. *J. Occup. Health.* 49, pp. 389–398

Chen KH, Srivastava DK, Singhal RK, Jacob S, Ahmed AE, Wilson SH. 2000.Modulation of base excision repair by low density lipoprotein, oxidized low density lipoprotein and antioxidants in mouse monocytes. *Carcinogenesis*, 21:1017–1022.

Christen Y. 2000.Oxidative stress and Alzheimer disease. *Am. J. Clin. Nutr.* 71;621S–629S.

Church DF, Pryor WA. 1985. Free-radical chemistry of cigarette smoke and its toxicological implications. *Environ. Health Perspect.* 64;111–126.

Colton CA , Gilbert DL. 1999. Reactive Oxygen Species in Biological Systems: An Interdisciplinary Approach. *Springer US. 740. Hardcover*

Cooke MS, Evans MD, Dizdaroglu M, Lunec J. 2003.Oxidative DNA damage: mechanisms, mutation, and disease. *FASEB J.*, 17(10):1195-214.

De Flora S, Izzotti A, Walsh D, Degan P, Petrilli GL, Lewtas J. 1997.Molecular epidemiology of atherosclerosis. *FASEB J*, .11:1021–1031.

Demple B, Herman T, Chen DS. 1991.Cloning and expression of APE, the cDNA encoding the major human apurinic enodnuclease: Definition of a family of DNA repair enzymes. *Proc Natl Acad Sci U S A*, 88:11450–54.

Dianov G, Bischoff C, Piotrowski J, Bohr VA.1998. Repair pathways for processing of 8-oxoguanine in DNA by mammalian cell extracts. *J. Biol. Chem.*, 273:33811–33816.

Dirksen ML, Blakely WF, Holwitt E, Dizdaroglu, M.1988.Effect of DNA conformation on the hydroxyl radicalinduced formation of 8, 5_-cyclopurine 2_-deoxyribonucleoside residues in DNA. *Int. J. Radiat. Biol.*, 54, 195–204

Dizdaroglu M, Bauche C, Rodriguez H, Laval J. 2000.Novel substrates of *Escherichia coli* Nth protein and its kinetics for excision of modified bases from DNA damaged by free radicals. *Biochemistry*, 39;5586–5592.

Dizdaroglu M, Gajewski E, Reddy P, Margolis SA.1989. Structure of a hydroxyl radical induced DNA-protein cross-link involving thymine and tyrosine in nucleohistone.*Biochemistry*, 28; 3625–3628.

Dizdaroglu M.1998.Mechanisms of free radical damage to DNA, in: O.I. Aruoma (Ed.), DNA & Free Radicals: Techniques, Mechanisms & Applications, *OICA International, Saint Lucia*, pp. 3–26.

Dizdaroglu M.1993. Quantitative determination of oxidative base damage in DNA by stable isotope-dilution mass spectrometry, *FEBS Lett.*, 315;1–6.

Dizdaroglu M.1986.Free-radical-induced formation of an 8, 5_-cyclo-2_-deoxyguanosine moiety in deoxyribonucleic acid. *Biochem. J*, . 238, 247–254

Dizdaroglu M. 1992. Oxidative damage to DNA in mammalian chromatin. *Mutat. Res*, 275, 331–342.

Dizdaroglu M, Dirksen, ML, Jiang HX, Robbins JH. 1987. Ionizing-radiation-induced damage in the DNA of cultured human cells. Identification of 8, 5-cyclo-2-deoxyguanosine. *Biochem. J.*, 241, 929–932

Dizdaroglu M, Laval J, Boiteux S.1993.Substrate specificity of the *Escherichia coli* endonuclease III: excision of thymine- and cytosine-derived lesions in DNA produced by radiation-generated free radicals. *Biochemistry*, 32, 12105–12111.

Drury JA, Jeffers G, Cooke RW.1998.Urinary 8-hydroxydeoxyguanosine in infants and children. *Free Radic. Res.* 28, 423–428

Duarte V, Gasparutto D, Jaquinod M, Cadet J.2000. In vitro DNA synthesis opposite oxazolone and repair of this DNA damage using modified oligonucleotides. *Nucl. Acids Res.* 28;1555–1563.

Evans MD, Dizdaroglu M, Cooke MS. 2004.Oxidative DNA damage and disease: induction, repair and significance. *Mutat Res.* 567(1):1-61.

Farinati F, Cardin R, Bortolami M, Nitti D, Basso D., de Bernard M., Cassaro M., Sergio A, Rugge, M. 2008. Oxidative DNA damage in gastric cancer: CagA status and OGG1 gene polymorphism. *Int J Cancer.* , 123, 51–5.

Farinati, F., Cardin, R., Degan, P., De Maria, N., Floyd, R. A., Van Thiel, D. H., and Naccarato, R. (1999) Oxidative DNA damage in circulating leukocytes occurs as an early event in chronic HCV infection. *Free Radic. Biol., Med.* 27, 1284–1291

Forman HJ, Boveris A. 1982. Superoxide radical and hydrogen peroxide in mitochondria, in: WA Pryor (Ed.), *Free Radicals in Biology*, Vol. V, New York: Academic Press, pp. 65–90

Frenkel K. 1992. Carcinogen-mediated oxidant formation and oxidative DNA damage. *Pharmacol. Ther.* 53, 127–166

Fruehaug JP, Meyskens FL. 2007.Reactive oxygen species: a breath of life of death? *Clin. Cancer Res.* 13;789–794.

Galaris D, Skiada V, Barbouti A.2008. Redox signaling and cancer: the role of 'labile' iron, Cancer Lett. 266;21–29.

Goode EL, Ulrich CM, Potter JD.2002. Polymorphisms in DNA repair genes and associations with cancer risk. *Cancer Epidemiol Biomarkers Prev.*, 11, 1513–30.

Halliwell B, Gutteridge JM. 1999.Free Radicals in Biology and Medicine, third edition. *Oxford University Press,* Midsomer Norton, Avon, England.

Harman D.1956. Aging: a theory based on free radical and radiation chemistry. *J. Gerontol,* . 11, 298–300

Hart RW, Setlow RB.1974. Correlation between deoxyribonucleic acid excision-repair and life-span in a number of mammalian species. *Proc. Natl. Acad. Sci. USA,* 71;2169–2173.

Hashiguchi K, Bohr VA, de Souza-Pinto NC. 2004.Oxidative stress and mitochondrial DNA repair: implications for NRTIs induced DNA damage. *Mitochondrion.,* 4(2-3):215-22.

Hashiguchi K, Stuart JA, de Souza-Pinto NC, Bohr VA. 2004.The C-terminal αO helix of human Ogg1 is essential for 8-oxoguanine DNA glycosylase activity: The mitochondrial β-Ogg1 lacks this domain and does not have glycosylase activity. *Nucleic Acids Res.,* 32:5596–5608.

Hazra TK, Das A, Das S.2007.Oxidative DNA damage repair in mammalian cells: A new perspective. *DNA Repair,* 6: 470–480.

Hedge ML, Hazra TK, Mitra S. 2008.Early steps in the DNA base excision/single-strand interruption repair pathway in mammalian cells. *Cell Res.* 18:27–47.

Heyworth PG, Knaus UG, Settleman J, Curnutte JT, Bokoch GM. Regulation of NADPH oxidase activity by Rac GTPase activating protein(s). *Mol Biol Cell* 1993; 4: 1217-1223

Hirano T, Yamaguchi Y, Hirano H, Kasai H. 1995.Ageassociated change of 8-hydroxyguanine repair activity in cultured human fibroblasts.*Biochem. Biophys. Res.Commun.,* 214;1157–1162.

Hoffmann D, Wynder EL. 1986. Chemical constituents and bioactivity of tobacco smoke, *IARC Sci. Publ.,* 74; 145–165.

Hsu IC, Metcalf RA, Sun T, Welsh JA, Wang NJ, Harris CC.1991. Mutational hotspot in the p53 gene in human hepatocellular carcinomas.*Nature,* 350;427–428.

Hung RJ, Hall J, Brennan P, Boffetta P. 2005. Genetic polymorphisms in the base excision repair pathway and cancer risk: A HuGE review.*Am J Epidemiol,* 162, 925–42.

Ide H., Kotera M. 2004. Human DNA glycosylases involved in the repair of oxidatively damaged DNA. *Biol Pharm Bull,* 27, 480–5.

Imlay JA, Chin SM, Linn S. 1988. Toxic DNA damage by hydrogen peroxide through the Fenton reaction in vivo and in vitro. *Science,* 240; 640-642.

Jayaraman L, Murthy KGK, Zhu C.1997. Identification of redox/repair protein Ref-1 as a potent activator of p53. *Genes Dev.,* 11:558–70.

Jiao L., Bondy ML, Hassan MM, Wolff RA, Evans DB, Abbruzzese JL., Li D. 2006. Selected polymorphisms of DNA repair genes and risk of pancreatic cancer. *Cancer Detect Prev,* 30, 284–91

Kadara H, Tahara E, Kim HJ, Lotan D, Myers J, Lotan R. Involvement of Rac in fenretinide-induced apoptosis. *Cancer Res* 2008; 68: 4416-4423

Kaguni LS.2004. DNA polymerase gamma, the mitochondrial replicase.*Annu Rev Biochem,* 73:293–320.

Kamata H, Hirata H.1999.Redox regulation of cellular signalling. *Cell Signal,* 11:1–14.

Kavli B, Otterlei M, Slupphaug G, Krokan HE. 2007. Uracil in DNA – general mutagen, but normal intermediate in acquired immunity. *DNA Repair (Amst),* 6, 505–516.

Khanna KK, Shiloh Y.2009.The DNA Damage Response: Implications on Cancer Formation and Treatment. *Springer Publication.* XII, 449 p.

King PA, Anderson VE, Edwards JO, Gustafson G, Plumb RC, Sugas JW. 1992. A stable solid that generates hydroxyl radical upon dissolution in aqueous solution: reaction with proteins and nucleic acids. *J Am Chem Soc*, 114:5430 -5432.

Kiyosawa H, Suko M, Okudaira H, Murata K, Miyamoto T, Chung MH, Kasai H, Nishimura S.1990. Cigarette smoking induces formation of 8-hydroxydeoxyguanosine, one of the oxidative DNA damages in human peripheral leukocytes. *Free Radical Res. Commun.* 11;23–27.

Klaunig J, Kamendulis LM.2004. The role of oxidative stress in carcinogenesis.*Annu.Rev. Pharmacol. Toxicol.* 44; 239–267.

Klaunig JE, Kamendulis LM, Hocevar BA.2010. Oxidative stress and oxidative damage in carcinogenesis. *Toxicol Pathol.*, 38(1):96-109.

Klungland A, Bjelland S. 2007.Oxidative damage to purines in DNA: role of mammalian Ogg1. *DNA Repair (Amst),* 6, 481–488.

Kohen R, Nyska A. 2002. Oxidation of biological systems: oxidative stress phenomena, antioxidants, redox reactions, and methods for their quantification. *Toxicol Pathol.* , 30(6):620-50.

Kohno T, Shinmura K, Tosaka M, Tani M, Kim, SR, Sugimura H, Nohmi T, Kasai H, Yokota J. 1998. Genetic polymorphisms and alternative splicing of the hOGG1 gene, that is involved in the repair of 8-hydroxyguanine in damaged DNA. *Oncogene*, 16, 3219–25.

Koppele J, Lucassen PJ, Sakkee AN, van Asten JG, Ravid R, Swaab DF, van Bezooijen CFA.1996. 8-OHdG levels in brain do not indicate oxidative DNA damage in Alzheimer's disease. *Neurobiol. Aging,* 17, 819–826

Krokan HE, Nilsen H, Skorpen F, et al.2000 Base excision repair of DNA in mammalian cells. *FEBS Lett,* 476: 73–77.

Lakshmipathy U, Campbell C.1999.The human DNA ligase III gene encodes nuclear and mitochondrial proteins. *Mol Cell Biol*, 19: 3869–3876.

Lakshmipathy U, Campbell C.2001.Antisense-mediated decrease in DNA ligase III expression results in reduced mitochondrial DNA integrity. *Nucleic Acids Res.,* 29:668–676.

Lee KW, Lee HJ.2006. Biphasic effects of dietary antioxidants on oxidative stress- mediated carcinogenesis.*Mech. Ageing Dev.* 127; 424–431.

Lee SH, Blair IA.2001. Oxidative DNA damage and cardiovascular disease. *Trends Cardiovasc. Med.,* 11:148–155.

Lezza A, Mecocci P, Cormio A, Flint Beal M, Cherubini A, Cantatore P, Senin U, Gadaleta MN. 1999.Areaspecific differences in OH8dG and mtDNA4977 levels in Alzheimer disease patients and aged controls.J. Anti-aging Med. 2 ;209–215.

Li W, Kong AN. 2008. Molecular mechanisms of Nrf2-mediated antioxidant response. *Mol Carcinog*, 48, 91–104.

Lindahl T.1974. An N-glycosidase from Escherichia coli that releases free uracil from DNAcontaining deaminated cytosine residues. *Proc. Natl. Acad. Sci. USA*, 71, 3649–3653

Lodovici M, Casalini C, Cariaggi R, Michelucci L, Dolara P.2000.Levels of 8-hydroxydeoxyguanosine as a marker of DNA damage in human leukocytes.*Free Radical Biol. Med.,* 28;13–17.

Loft S, Astrup A, Buemann B, Poulsen HE.1994. Oxidative DNA damage correlates with oxygen consumption in humans, *Faseb J.* 8;534–537.

Loft S, Larsen PN, Rasmussen A, Fischer-Nielsen A, Bondesen S, Kirkegaard P, Rasmussen LS, Ejlersen E, Tornoe K, Bergholdt, R. 1995. Oxidative DNA damage after transplantation of the liver and small intestine in pigs. *Transplantation,* 59, 16–20

Longley MJ, Prasad R, Srivastava DK, Wilson SH, Copeland WC. 1998. Identification of 5=-deoxyribose phosphate lyase activity in human DNA polymerase gamma and its role in mitochondrial base excision repair in vitro. *Proc Natl Acad Sci U S A* , 95:12244-12248.

Lovell MA, Gabbita SP, . Markesbery WR.1999. Increased DNA oxidation and decreased levels of repair products in Alzheimer's disease ventricular CSF. *J. Neurochem.* 72; 771–776.

Lunec J, Herbert K, Blount S, Griffiths HR, Emery P.1994. 8-Hydroxydeoxyguanosine. A marker of oxidative DNA damage in systemic lupus erythematosus. *FEBS Lett.* 348 ; 131–138.

Markesbery WR. 1999.The role of oxidative stress in Alzheimer disease.*Arch. Neurol.* 56; 1449–1452.

Marnett LJ.2000. Oxyradicals and DNA damage. *Carcinogenesis,* 21:361–70.

McWilliams RR., Bamlet WR, Cunningham JM, Goode EL, de Andrade M, Boardman LA, Petersen, GM. 2008. Polymorphisms in DNA repair genes, smoking, and pancreatic adenocarcinoma risk. *Cancer Res.* 68, 4928–35.

Meira LB, Devaraj S, Kisby GE.2001.Heterozygosity for the mouse Apex gene result in phenotypes associated with oxidative stress. *Cancer Res,* 61:5552–57.

Mena S, Ortega A, Estrela J.2009. Oxidative stress in environmental-induced carcinogenesis. *Mutat. Res.* 674 ;36–44.

Michalik V, Spotheim Maurizot M, Charlier M.1995. Calculation of hydroxyl radical attack on different forms of DNA. *J Biomol Struct Dyn,* 13:565–575.

Moller P, Folkmann JK, Forchhammer L, Brauner EV, Danielsen P, Rison L, Loft S. 2008.Air pollution, oxidative damage to DNA, and carcinogenesis. *Cancer Lett.*;266;84–97.

Moreno JJ, Pryor WA (1992) Inactivation of alpha 1-proteinase inhibitor by peroxynitrite. Chem Res Toxicol 5:425–431.

Nackerdien Z, Rao G., Cacciuttolo MA, Gajewski E, Dizdaroglu M.1991. Chemical nature of DNA-protein cross-links produced in mammalian chromatin by hydrogen peroxide in the presence of iron or copper ions, *Biochemistry* 30; 4873–4879.

Nackerdien Z, Kasprzak KS, Rao G, Halliwell B, Dizdaroglu M.1991. Nickel(II)- and cobalt(II)-dependent damage by hydrogen peroxide to the DNA bases in isolated human chromatin. *Cancer Res.* 51, 5837–5842.

Narter KF, Ergen A, Agaçhan B, Görmüs U, Timirci O, Isbir T. 2009.Bladder cancer and polymorphisms of DNA repair genes (XRCC1, XRCC3, XPD, XPG, APE1, hOGG1). *Anticancer Res.,* 29(4):1389-93.

Nohl H, Hegner D.1978. Do mitochondria produce oxygen radicals in vivo? *Eur J Biochem,* 82:563-567.

O'Connor TR, Laval J. 1989. Physical association of the 2, 6-diamino-4-hydroxy-5N-formamidopyrimidine-DNA glycosylase of Escherichia coli and an activity nicking DNA at apurinic/apyrimidinic sites. *Proc. Natl. Acad. Sci. USA,* 86, 5222–5226.

O'Neill P.1983. Pulse radiolytic study of the interaction of thiols and ascorbate with OH adducts of dGMP and dG: implications for DNA repair processes. *Radiat. Res.*, 96 ; 198–210.

Olinski R, Gackowski D, Foksinski M, Rozalski R, Roszkowski K, Jaruga P.2002.Oxidative DNA damage: assessment of the role in carcinogenesis, atherosclerosis, and acquired immunodeficiency syndrome. *Free Radic Biol Med.* 33(2):192-200.

Olinski R, Nackerdien Z, Dizdaroglu M.1992. DNA-protein cross-linking between thymine and tyrosine in chromatin of gamma-irradiated or $H_2O_2$-treated cultured human cells.*Arch. Biochem. Biophys.* 297; 139–143.

O'Neill P, Chapman PW. 1985. Potential repair of free radical adducts of dGMP and dG by a series of reductants. A pulse radiolytic study. *Int. J. Radiat. Biol. Relat. Stud. Phys. Chem. Med.*, 47, 71–80

Packer MA, Murphy MP. 1994. Peroxynitrite causes calcium efflux from mitochondria which is prevented by Cyclosporin A. *FEBS Lett.*, 345:237–240.

Pan JS, Hong MZ, Ren JL. Reactive oxygen species: a double-edged sword in oncogenesis. World J Gastroenterol. 2009 Apr 14;15(14):1702-7.

Pourcelot S, Faure H, Firoozi F, Ducros V, Tripier M, Hee J, Cadet J, Favier A.1999. Urinary 8-oxo-7, 8-dihydro-2_-deoxyguanosine and 5-(hydroxymethyl) uracil in smokers. *Free Radical Res.*, 30; 173–180.

Radi R, Beckman JS, Bush KM, Freeman BA. 1991a. Peroxynitrite-induced membrane lipid peroxidation: the cytotoxic potential of superoxide and nitric oxide. *Arch Biochem Biophys.*, 288:481–487.

Radi R, Beckman JS, Bush KM, Freeman BA. 1991b. Peroxynitrite oxidation of sulfhydryls. The cytotoxic potential of superoxide and nitric oxide. *J Biol Chem.*, 266:4244–4250.

Radi R, RodriguezM, Castro L, Telleri R.1994. Inhibition of mitochondrial electron transport by peroxynitrite. *Arch Biochem Biophys.*, 308:89–95.

Raha S, Robinson BH. 2000. Mitochondria, oxygen free radicals, disease and ageing. *Trends Biochem. Sci.* 25, 502–508.

Ralph SJ, Enríquez SR, Neuzil J, Saavedra E, Sánchez RM. 2010. The causes of cancer revisited: "mitochondrial malignancy" and ROS-induced oncogenic transformation -Why mitochondria are targets for cancer therapy. *Mol. Aspects Med.* 31; 145–170.

Raoul S, Berger M, Buchko GW, Joshi PC, Morin B, Weinfeld M, Cadet J.1996. H-1, C-13 and N-15 nuclear magnetic resonance analysis and chemical features of the two main radical oxidation products of 2_-deoxyguanosine: oxazolone and imidazolone nucleosides. *J. Chem. Soc. Perkin Trans.*, 371–381.

Rattan S, Siboska GE, Wikmar FP, Clark BFC, Woolley P. 1995. Levels of oxidative DNA damage product 8-hydroxy-2_-deoxyguanosine in human serum increases with age. *Med. Sci. Res.* 23, 469–470

Robertson AB, Klungland A, Rognes T, Leiros I. 2009.DNA repair in mammalian cells: Base excision repair: the long and short of it. *Cell Mol Life Sci.*, 66(6):981-93.

Ross R. 1993. *Rous-Whipple Award Lecture.* Atherosclerosis: a defense mechanism gone awry. *Am J Pathol., 143: 987–1002*

Schafer FQ, Buettner GR. 2001. Redox environments of the cell as viewed through the redox state of the glutathione disulfide/glutathione couple. *Free Rad Biol Med.,* 30: 1191–1212.

Sedgwick B, Bates PA, Paik J, Jacobs SC, Lindahl T. 2007. Repair of alkylated DNA: recent advances. *DNA Repair* (Amst) 6, 429–442.

Sen S , Chakraborty R, Sridhar C, Reddy YSR, De B. 2010. Free Radicals, Antioxidants, Diseases and Phytomedicines: Current Status and Future Prospect. *International Journal of Pharmaceutical Sciences Review and Research,* Volume 3, Issue 1, p.91-100

Shao L, Hittelman WN, Lin J, Yang H, Ajani JA., Wu X. 2006.Deficiency of cell cycle checkpoints and DNA repair system predispose individuals to esophageal cancer. *Mutat Res.,* 602, 143–50.

Shimoda R, Nagashima M., Sakamoto M, Yamaguchi N, Hirohashi S, Yokota J, Kasai H. 1994. Increased formation of oxidative DNA damage, 8-hydroxydeoxyguanosine, in human livers with chronic hepatitis. *Cancer Res.,* 54, 3171–3172

Smith MA, Rottkamp CA, Nunomura A, Raina AK, Perry G.2000. Oxidative stress in Alzheimer's disease. *Biochim.Biophys. Acta,* 1502;139–144.

Sohal RS.1997. Mitochondria generate superoxide anion radicals and hydrogen peroxide. FASEB J 11:1269–1270.

von Sonntag C. 1987. The Chemical Basis of Radiation Biology. *Taylor* and *Francis,* London, *1987,* p. 57

Spencer JP, Jenner A, Aruoma OI, Evans P J, Kaur H., Dexter DT, Jenner P, Lees AJ, Marsden DC, Halliwell B. 1994.Intense oxidative DNA damage promoted by L-dopa and its metabolites. Implications for neurodegenerative disease. *FEBS Lett.,* 353, 246–250

Steenken S.1989. Purine bases, nucleosides, and nucleotides:aqueous solution redox Chemistry and transformation reactions of their radical cations and e− and OH adducts.*Chem. Rev.* 89;503–520.

Steenken S. 1987. Addition-elimination paths in electrontransfer reactions between radicals and molecules. *J. Chem. Soc. Faraday Trans. I,* 83, 113–124

Sultan SM, Ioannou Y, Isenberg DA. 2000. Is there an association of malignancy with systemic lupus erythematosus? An analysis of 276 patients under long-term review. *Rheumatology (Oxford),* 39, 1147–1152

Takahashi T, Tada M, Igarashi S, et al. Aprataxin, causative gene product for EAOH/AOA1, repairs DNA single-strand breaks with damaged 3'-phosphate and 3'-phosphoglycolate ends. Nucleic Acids Res 2007;35:3797–3809.

Takahashi T, Nau MM, Chiba I, Birrer MJ, Rosenberg RK, Vinocour M, Levitt M, Pass H, Gazdar AF, . Minna JD.1989. p53: a frequent target for genetic abnormalities in lung cancer.*Science,* 246 ;491–494.

Teoule R. 1987. Radiation-induced DNA damage and its repair. *Int. J. Radiat. Biol. Relat. Stud. Phys. Chem. Med.,* 51, 573–589

Thier R, Bruning T, Kocher K, Blaszkewicz M, Makropoulos V, Sundberg A, Bolt HM.1999. Determination of urinary thymidine glycol using affinity chromatography, HPLC and post-column reaction detection: a biomarker of oxidative DNA damage upon kidney transplantation. *Arch. Toxicol.,* 73, 479–484

Toyokuni S, Mori T, Hiai H, Dizdaroglu M.1995.Treatment of Wistar rats with a renal carcinogen, ferric nitrilotriacetate, causes DNA-protein cross-linking between thymine and tyrosine in their renal chromatin. *Int. J. Cancer,* 62;309–313.

Trachootham D, Alexander J, Huang P.2009. Targeting cancer cells by ROS-mediated mechanism: a radical therapeutic approach? *Nat. Rev.* 8;579–591.

Tudek B, Winczura A, Janik J, Siomek A, Foksinski M, Olinski R.2010. Involvement of oxidatively damaged DNA and repair in cancer development and aging. *Am. J. Transl. Res.*, 2; 254–284.

Ushio-Fukai M, Nakamura Y.2008. Reactive oxygen species and angiogenesis:NADPH oxidase as target for cancer therapy. *Cancer Lett.* 266; 37–52.

Valko M, Rhodes CJ, Moncol J, Izakovic M, Mazur M.2006. Free radicals, metals and antioxidants in oxidative stress-induced cancer, Chem. Biol. Interact. 160 ;1-40.

Vieira AJSC, Steenken S. 1990. Pattern of OH radical reaction with adenine and its nucleosides and nucleotides. Characterisation of two types of isomeric OH adduct and their unimolecular transformation reactions. *J. Am. Chem. Soc.*, 112, 6986–6994

Wagner JR, Van Lier JE, Berger M, Cadet, J. 1994. Thymidine hydroperoxides: structural assignments, conformational features and thermal decomposition in water. *J. Am. Chem. Soc*, . 116, 2235–2242

Weissman L, de Souza-Pinto NC, Stevnsner T, Bohr VA. 2007. DNA repair, mitochondria, and neurodegeneration. *Neuroscience*, 145(4):1318-29.

Weitzman SA, Gordon LI. 1990. Inflammation and cancer: role of phagocyte-generated oxidants in carcinogenesis. *Blood*, 76, 655–663

Willy C, Dahouk S, Starck C, Kaffenberger W, Gerngross H, Plappert UG. 2000. DNA damage in human leukocytes after ischemia/reperfusion injury. *Free Radic. Biol. Med*, . 28, 1–12

Winters TA, Henner WD, Russel PS, et al. 1994.Removal of 3'-phosphoglycolate from DNA strand-break damage in an oligonucleotide substrate by recombinant human apurinic/apyrimidinic endonuclease. *Nucleic Acids Res*, 22:18866–73.

Wiseman H, Halliwell B.1996. Damage to DNA by reactive oxygen and nitrogen species: role in inflammatory disease and progression to cancer. *Biochem. J.* , 313, 17–29

Wood RD, Mitchell M, Sgouros J, Lindahl T. 2001.Human DNA repair genes. *Science*, 291:1284–9.

Wrona MZ, Dryhurst G. 1998. Oxidation of serotonin by superoxide radical: implications to neurodegenerative brain disorders. *Chem. Res. Toxicol.*, 11, 639–650

Wu D, Cederbaum AI.2003.Alcohol, oxidative stress and free radical damage. *Alcohol Res. Health*, 27; 277–284.

Xing DY, Tan W, Song N, Lin DX. 2001. Ser326Cys polymorphism in hOGG1 gene and risk of esophageal cancer in a Chinese population.*Int J Cancer*, 95, 140–43.

Xu J, Zheng SL, Turner A, Isaacs SD, Wiley KE, Hawkins GA, Chang BL, Bleecker ER., Walsh PC, Meyers, DA, Isaacs WB.2002. Associations between hOGG1 sequence variants and prostate cancer susceptibility. *Cancer Res*, 62, 2253–57.

Yamasaki I, Piette LH.1991. EPR spin trapping study on the oxidizing species formed in the reaction of the ferrous ion with hydrogen peroxide. *J Am Chem Soc* , 113:7588–7593.

Zhang J, Perry G, Smith MA, Robertson D, Olson SJ, Graham DG, Montine TJ.1999. Parkinson's disease is associated with oxidative damage to cytoplasmic DNA and RNA in substantia nigra neurons. *Am. J. Pathol.* 154 ;1423- 1429.

Zhang Z, Shi Q, Sturgis EM, Spitz MR, Hong WK., Wei, Q.2004. Thymidylate synthase 5'- and 3'-untranslated region polymorphismsassociated with risk and progression of squamous cell carcinoma of the head and neck. *Clin Cancer Res*, 10, 7903–10.

Ziech D, Franco R, Georgakilas AG, Georgakila S, Malamou-Mitsi V, Schoneveld O, Pappa A, Panayiotidis MI. 2010.The role of reactive oxygen species and oxidative stress in environmental carcinogenesis and biomarker development. *Chem Biol Interact.* , 188(2):334-9.

Ziech D, Franco R, Pappa A, Panayiotidis MI.2011. Reactive Oxygen Species (ROS)--Induced genetic and epigenetic alterations in human carcinogenesis. *Mutat Res.*, Mar 16.

4

# UV Damaged DNA Repair & Tolerance in Plants

Ashwin L. Ganpudi and Dana F. Schroeder
*University of Manitoba,
Canada*

## 1. Introduction

In both natural and agricultural conditions, plants are frequently subjected to unfavourable environments, resulting in varying degrees of stress. UV irradiation, drought, heat shock, chilling/freezing, salinity and oxygen deficiency are a few of the major abiotic factors restricting plant growth and development. An important consequence of stratospheric ozone depletion is increased transmission of solar Ultra Violet (UV) radiation through the earth's atmosphere. This increased incidence of UV irradiation causes detrimental effects to all life forms on earth.

### 1.1 UV irradiation

The spectrum of solar electromagnetic radiation striking the earth's atmosphere ranges from 100 nm to 1 mm. This includes the UV spectrum (100-400 nm), visible spectrum (380-780 nm) and infrared spectrum (700 nm-1 mm). The UV spectrum is further subdivided into three catogories: UV-C (100-280 nm), UV-B (280-315 nm), and UV-A (315-400 nm) (Ballaré, 2003). The shortest of these wavelengths, UV-C, is blocked completely by the ozone layer and atmospheric oxygen. In contrast, UV-A is weakly absorbed and directly transmitted to the earth's surface. Wavelengths in the UV-B range are absorbed efficiently though not completely by ozone, as a very small percentage may pass through holes in the ozone. UV-C is extremely harmful, followed by UV-B, while UV-A has milder effects (Batschauer et al., 1999).

### 1.2 Plants and UV radiation

Plants, due to their non-motile nature, generally have a higher rate of UV tolerance than animals. Plant secondary metabolites aid in defence against both abiotic and biotic stress factors. Plants are capable of reflecting or absorbing harmful UV rays via thick layers of waxy cutin or submerin on the cell walls and intracellular accumulation of chemical substances such as flavanols or phenolics. The biological effects of UV radiation on plants include altered growth responses, reproductive deformities, epigenetic variations, plant susceptibly to biotic factors, premature senescence, damage to the photosynthetic apparatus, and altered conformation of membrane structures. A wide array of genes were found to be induced upon prolonged exposure to low doses of UV-B in the model plant *Arabidopsis thaliana* (Frohnmeyer & Staiger, 2003; Mackerness, 2000; Ries et al., 2000). Upregulated transcripts include: antioxidant/free radical scavenging enzymes, proteins involved in: DNA repair, translation, E3 ligase system, cell cycle, signal transduction, and secondary metabolites, as well as several other genes with unknown function (Brosché et al., 2002; Jansen et al., 2008). UV-B also results in numerous changes in plant morphology. This signalling cascade is well reviewed elsewhere (Jenkins, 2009). Here we focus on plant responses to UV-induced DNA damage.

### 1.3 UV induced DNA damage

UV-C/B radiation is directly absorbed by DNA, inducing lesions which inhibit vital cellular functions such as transcription and DNA replication. UV-A is comparatively less efficient in lesion induction but triggers the production of reactive oxygen species (ROS) (Kunz et al., 2006). The primary UV induced DNA lesions include cyclobutane pyrimidine dimers (adjacent pyrimidines covalently linked between C-5 and C-6 carbon atoms) and secondary lesions 6-4 pyrimidine-pyrimidone photoproducts (6-4 PP) (covalent linkage between the C-4 position of a pyrimidine to the C-6 position of an adjacent pyrimidine) (Fig. 1). In order to respond to this damage, plants employ specific mechanisms (Britt, 1999). In light conditions, photoreactivation catalyses dimer monomerizations while during dark conditions, Nucleotide Excision Repair (NER) excises these helix-distorting lesions. Finally, residual lesions are bypassed via translesion synthesis (TLS).

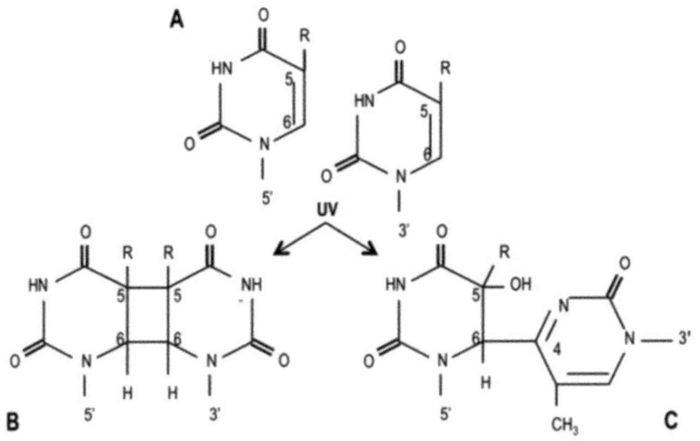


Fig. 1. A) Normal adjacent pyrimidine residues. B) UV-induced Cyclobutane Pyrimidine Dimer (CPD) and C) 6-4 Pyrimidine-Pyrimidone photoproduct (6-4 PP).

## 2. Photoreactivation

Photoreactivation is a blue light dependant DNA repair mechanism catalysed by the photolyase (E.C 4.1.99.3) class of enzymes. Pyrimidine dimers are split by the action of two photoactive damage specific DNA repair enzymes - CPD photolyase and 6-4 PP photolyase. Both classes of photolyase require two co-factors, one being the two electron reduced form of Flavin Adenine Dinucleotide (FAD) and the second chromophore, a blue light harvesting photoantenna, being either 5,10- methenyltretrahydrofolate (MTHF) or 8-hydroxy-7,8-didemethyl-5-deazariboflavin (8-HDF). FAD is an essential co-factor for regulating DNA binding and repair. In contrast, the second chromophore has a higher extinction co-efficient and an absorption maximum at longer wavelengths, hence regulates the rate of repair depending on the external light intensity. MTHF or 8-HDF absorbs the photoreactivating blue light photons and transfers this excitation energy to the reduced FAD. The FADH$^-$ in turn transfers electrons to the lesions, catalyzing the cleavage of the cyclobutane rings and dimer monomerization (Deisenhofer, 2000; Sancar, 2003, 2008). Multiple sequence alignment reveals that conserved homology between prokaryotic and eukaryotic CPD photolyases is limited to the C-terminal FAD binding site. It has been suggested that a common ancestor gave rise to both type I and type II photolyases but diverged at an early evolutionary stage (Yasui et al., 1994). CPD photolyases have been classified into Class I (microbial) and Class II (higher eukaryotes excluding placental mammals) groups, respectively. The 6–4 photolyases from *Drosophila* and *Arabidopsis* have strong sequence similarity to class I CPD photolyases (Nakajima et al., 1998; Todo et al., 1996). Similarly cryptochromes, the plant blue light photoreceptors, are 30% similar to the class I microbial photolyases, but demonstrate no photolyase activity (Ahmad & Cashmore, 1993). Thus, microbial Class I CPD photolyases, eukaryotic 6–4 photolyases, and blue light photoreceptors constitute the class I photolyase/photoreceptor family.

Genes encoding CPD photolyases and 6-4 PP photolyases have been identified and characterized in a range of prokaryotic and eukaryotic systems (Sancar, 2003). In plants genes encoding CPD photolyases have been identified in *Arabidopsis thaliana* (Ahmed et al., 1997), cucumber (Takahashi et al., 2002), rice (Hirouchi et al., 2003), spinach (Yoshihara et al., 2005), and soybean (Yamamoto et al., 2008). Genes encoding 6-4 PP photolyases have been identified in *Arabidopsis* and rice (Chen et al., 1994; Singh et al., 2010). In *Arabidopsis,* the highest levels of both photolyases are associated with floral tissues, which may presumably serve to minimize lesions in germline cells. While expression of the CPD photolyase is light/UV-B regulated, 6-4 PP photolyase is constitutively expressed (Takahashi et al., 2002; Waterworth et al., 2002). The *Arabidopsis* CPD photolyase gene (*AtPHR1*) encodes a class II CPD photolyase. An *Arabidopsis* mutant (*uvr2*) lacking this gene is hypersensitive to UV. AtPHR1 is efficient in CPD photoreactivation but deficient in 6-4 photoproduct repair (Ahmed et al., 1997; Landry et al., 1997). *AtPHR1* is upregulated several fold in a UV insensitive mutant of *Arabidopsis* (*uvi1*) irrespective of light conditions, conferring constitutive protection (Tanaka et al., 2002). Overexpression of CPD photolyase in *Arabidopsis* and rice resulted in enhanced CPD removal (Hidema et al., 2007; Kaiser et al., 2009; Ueda et al., 2005). Genetic complementation of photolyase deficient *E.coli* strains with soybean, rice, spinach and *Arabidopsis* CPD photolyase genes restored photoreactivation activity (Yamamoto et al., 2007, 2008; Yoshihara et al., 2005). CPD photolyase activity in *Arabidopsis* (Pang & Hays, 1991; Waterworth et al., 2002), soybean (Yamamoto et al., 2008) and rice (Hidema et al., 2000) has been reported to be temperature sensitive. Rice CPD photolyase, encoded by a single copy gene in the nuclear genome, translocates to chloroplasts, mitochondria and nuclei to repair UV-induced CPDs in all three genomes (Takahashi et al., 2011), a phenomenon not observed in spinach chloroplasts (Hada et al., 2000) or young *Arabidopsis* seedlings (Chen et al., 1996). However, upon exposure to photoreactivating blue light, *Arabidopsis* seedlings did exhibit efficient repair of CPDs in the extracellular organelles (Draper & Hays, 2000). The *Arabidopsis* 6-4 PP photolyase, encoded by the *UVR3* gene, encodes a 62 kDa protein with 45% identity to *Drosophila* 6-4 PP photolyase and 17% identity to the Class II CPD photolyases. AtUVR3 is proficient in 6-4 photoproduct removal but deficient in CPD repair. Both *uvr2* and *uvr3* are nonsense mutations, and the double mutants are extremely sensitive to UV relative to the single mutants (Nakajima et al., 1998). Photolyases appear to be the sole repair mechanism active in non-proliferating plant tissues (Kimura et al., 2004). Hence, photolyases play an important role in plant repair of UV damaged DNA.

## 3. Nucleotide excision repair

Nucleotide excision repair (NER) is a light independent repair process involving a series of reactions: initial damaged DNA recognition, DNA unwinding, dual incision bracketing the lesion, repair synthesis and final ligation to seal the repaired site. NER initiates with specific sub-pathways for transcriptionally active (Transcription Coupled Repair (TC-NER)) or silent (Global Genomic Repair (GG-NER)) DNA. TC-NER and GG-NER exhibit different damage recognition strategies followed by a common repair pathway (Gillet & Scharer, 2006) (Fig. 2). Defects in human NER genes result in the photosensitive syndromes Xeroderma pigmentosum (XP) or Cockayne syndrome (CS). Eight genetic complementation groups for XP have been identified (XPA-G, V) as well as two for CS (CSA and CSB). While XP-V mutation uniquely results in defects in translesion synthesis, XP -A, -B, -D, -F, and -G mutation results in both TC-NER and GG-NER defects, while XP –C and -E mutation results in GG-NER defects only. CSA and CSB mutation results exclusively in TC-NER defects (Hoeijmakers, 2001; Svejstrup, 2002). Bioinformatic analysis of the plant NER protein machinery suggests the molecular mechanisms are largely but not entirely conserved with that of the extensively studied yeast *S. cerevisiae* and mammalian cells (Kimura & Sakaguchi, 2006; Kunz et al., 2005, 2006). NER in plants has been studied primarily in rice and *Arabidopsis* (Singh et al., 2010). Many *Arabidopsis* NER related genes were initially isolated by analysis of UV hypersensitive (*uvh*) and UV repair defective (*uvr*) mutants which were subsequently mapped to homologues of the human XP genes (Table 1).

### 3.1 Global genomic repair
### 3.1.1 Damage recognition
#### 3.1.1.1 DDB1 & DDB2

In mammalian systems, damage detection in the GG-NER pathway involves UV-Damaged DNA Binding protein 1 and 2 (DDB1 and DDB2) followed by the XPC-HR23B-CEN2 complex. In humans DDB2 complements the *XPE* mutation and plays a role in recognition of the UV-induced lesion, while DDB1 is required for high affinity interaction of the DDB1-DDB2 complex (Groisman et al., 2003; Luijsterburg et al., 2007; Rapic-Otrin et al., 2002). *S. pombe* Ddb1 knockouts result in chromosomal segregation defects, UV sensitivity and slow S phase progression leading to defects in meiosis (Holmberg et al., 2005). DDB1 and DDB2 homologues have been identified in rice, where they are UV-induced in proliferating tissues (Ishibashi et al., 2003). *Arabidopsis thaliana* encodes two homologs of DDB1 - DDB1A and DDB1B. These proteins are 91% identical with redundant function. Although *ddb1b* null alleles appear lethal, a viable partial loss of function allele exhibits no developmental or UV sensitive phenotypes (Bernhardt et al., 2010; Schroeder et al., 2002). Overexpression of DDB1A in *Arabidopsis* confers enhanced UV resistance and *ddb1a* knockouts exhibit mild UV sensitivity (Al Khateeb & Schroeder, 2009; Molinier et al., 2008). *AtDDB2* encodes a 48 kDa nuclear localized protein with upregulated expression upon UV-induction. *AtDDB2* loss of function results in UV sensitivity while overexpression increases UV tolerance (Biedermann & Hellmann, 2010; Koga et al., 2006; Molinier et al., 2008).

#### 3.1.1.2 Cullin based E3 ligases

The 127 kDa DDB1 homologs function as substrate adaptors for CULLIN4 based E3 ubiquitin (Ub) ligases (Groisman et al., 2003). E3 Ub ligases are multimeric complexes that add ubiquitin moieties to target proteins and contain CULLIN proteins as scaffolding

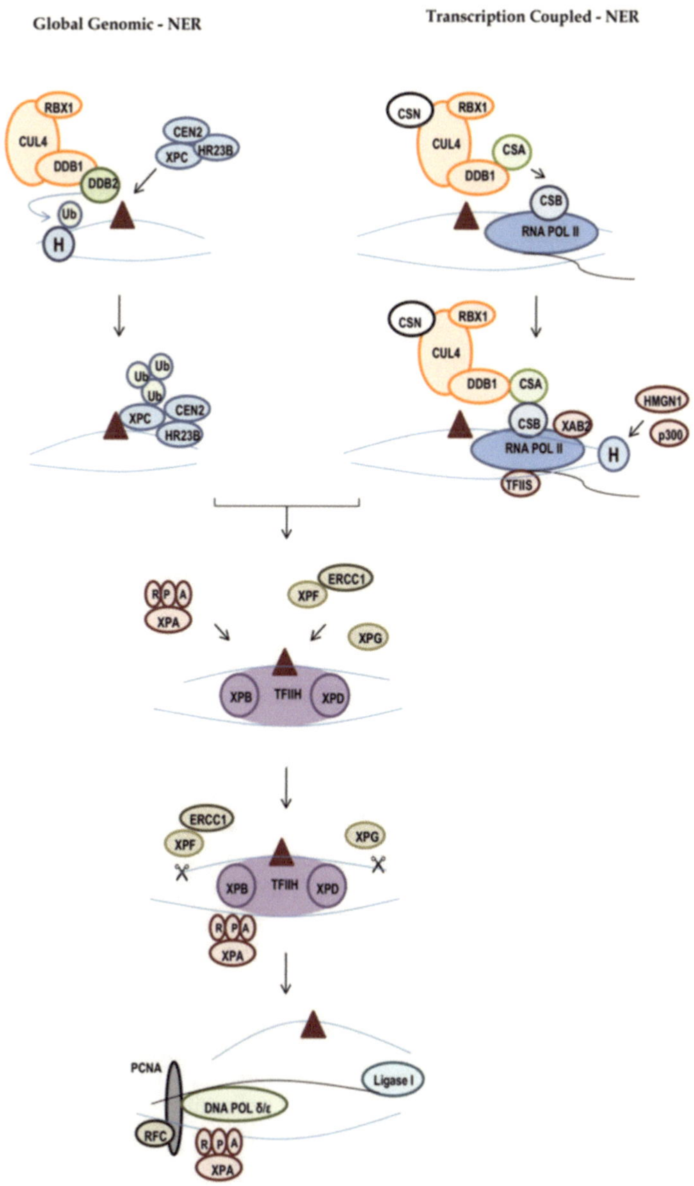


Fig. 2. Overview of mammalian nucleotide excision repair. In GG-NER, DDB2-CUL4 mediated histone (H) and XPC ubiquitination facilitates lesion binding. In TC-NER, stalled RNA POL II recruits CSB and the CSA-CUL4-CSN complex, followed by recruitment of other TC-NER specific factors. In both cases, NER core players follow suit: XPB and XPD helicases of the TFIIH complex, XPF-ERCC1 and XPG endonucleases, and the ssDNA binding XPA-RPA complex. The fragment encompassing the lesion is excised, followed by repair synthesis and ligation. Repair synthesis requires DNA POL δ/ε in concert with accessory proteins PCNA, RFC and RPA. See text for details.

subunits (Hua & Vierstra, 2011). CUL4 based E3 ubiquitin ligases consist of three core subunits: CULLIN4 (CUL4), RING finger protein REGULATOR OF CULLINS1 (ROC1)/RING-BOX1 (RBX1), and DDB1. The CUL4 - RBX1 - DDB1 complex interacts with a large number of proteins containing WD40 motifs referred to as DCAF proteins (DDB1-CUL4 Associated Factor) or DWD proteins (DDB1 binding WD40 proteins) (Lee & Zhou, 2007). DDB2 is an example of a WD40 domain containing DCAF protein. WD40 motifs are characterized by 40 amino acid repeats initiated by a glycine-histidine dipeptide and terminated by a tryptophan-aspartate (WD) dipeptide facilitating protein-protein interactions. DDB1 is composed of three β propeller domains (BPA, BPB and BPC) and DDB2, in addition to the WD40 domain, contains a helix loop helix (HLX) segment in the N terminal. While the clam shaped BPA-BPC of DDB1 mediates interaction with the HLX motif of DDB2 and other DCAF substrates, BPB exhibits exclusive interactions with CUL4 (Scrima et al., 2008).

AtCUL4 is a 91 kDa protein with a conserved CH motif and an extended N terminal region of 65 amino acids that shares close sequence similarity to its human/mouse orthologs. *AtCUL4* loss of function results in abnormal plant development (Bernhardt et al., 2006; Chen et al., 2006) and UV sensitivity (Molinier et al., 2008). Examples of DCAF proteins interacting with the *Arabidopsis* CUL4–DDB1A/B complex include AtDDB2 (Bernhardt et al., 2006), AtCSA-1&2 (Biedermann & Hellmann, 2010; Zhang et al., 2010), as well as the negative regulator of photomorphogenesis DET1 (De-etiolated1) (Schroeder et al., 2002), and many other DWD proteins (Lee et al., 2008). Recent results have shed light on the cross talk between photomorphogenesis regulation and repair of UV damaged DNA. HY5, a positive regulator of photomorphogenesis, has been shown to regulate gene sets connected to UV tolerance, such as the *UVR3* and *PHR1* photolyases, as well as secondary metabolite transcriptional regulators (Oravecz et al., 2006; Ulm et al., 2004). DET1, initially identified as a nuclear localized negative regulator of photomorphogenesis, exhibits a constitutively light grown phenotype in addition to increased levels of flavanoids (Pepper et al., 1994). Recent papers show that *det1* mutants exhibit enhanced UV tolerance through increased levels of secondary metabolites reflecting/absorbing UV irradiation as well as by upregulation of photolyase genes. Further it appears that DET1 protein dosage influences UV sensitivity of plants as DET1 overexpressing lines exhibit increased UV sensitivity (Castells et al., 2010, 2011).

#### 3.1.1.3 Histone ubiquitination facilitates NER machinery entry

In mammals, in the absence of UV irradiation, DDB2-DDB1-CUL4-RBX1 (DDB2 complex) was found to be associated with the COP9 Signalosome complex (CSN). CSN shares significant structural homology with the 19S lid of 26S proteosome. The CSN deconjugates neddylation (Nedd8) from CULLINs, thereby regulating the activation, stability or the disassembly of CULLIN based E3 ligase activity (Parry & Estelle, 2004; Schwechheimer & Deng, 2001). The DDB2 - CSN complex show no ubiquitin ligase activity, but upon UV irradiation, these complexes disassociate in parallel with increased neddylation and activation of CUL4 (Groisman et al., 2003). Core histone proteins have been identified as potential targets for DDB2-DDB1-CUL4-RBX1 mediated proteosomal degradation. Kapetanaki et al. (2006) and Wang et al. (2006) describe the ubiquitination of H2A, H3 and H4 histone proteins. Reduction of histone H3 and H4 ubiquitination by knockdown of *cul4* impairs recruitment of the repair protein XPC to the damaged foci and inhibits the repair process. Thus biochemical studies indicate that DDB-CUL4-RBX1-mediated histone

| Human | Yeast | Function | ATG no. | Arabidopsis |
|---|---|---|---|---|
| **Photoreactivation:** | | | | |
| *ND* | *ND* | 6-4 PP Photolyase | At3g15620 | *UVR3* |
| *ND* | *PHR1* | Class II CPD Photolyase | At1g12370 | *PHR1/UVR2* |
| **Nucleotide Excision Repair:** | | | | |
| *DDB1* | *ND* | Substrate adaptor for CUL4. Interacts with DCAF proteins | At4g05420<br>At4g21100 | *AtDDB1a*<br>*AtDDB1b* |
| *DDB2/XPE* | *ND* | Damaged DNA binding (DCAF) | At5g58760 | *AtDDB2* |
| *CUL4* | *CUL4* | Scaffolding subunit of E3 Ub ligase | At5g46210 | *AtCUL4* |
| *XPC* | *RAD4* | GG-NER damage recognition | At5g16630 | *AtXPC* |
| *HR23B* | *RAD23* | Binds to XPC | At1g79650<br>At1g16190<br>At3g02540<br>At5g38470 | *AtRAD23A*<br>*AtRAD23B*<br>*AtRAD23C*<br>*AtRAD23D* |
| *CEN2* | *CEN2* | Stabilizes XPC-HR23B complex | At3g50360 | *AtCEN2* |
| *XPB* | *RAD25* | Subunit of TFIIH. 3′->5′ helicase | At5g41370<br>At5g41360 | *AtXPB1*<br>*AtXPB2* |
| *XPD* | *RAD3* | Subunit of TFIIH. 5′->3′ helicase | At1g03190 | *AtXPD/UVH6* |
| *GTF2H1*<br><br>*GTF2H2*<br>*GTF2H3*<br>*GTF2H4*<br>*GTF2H5* | *TFB1*<br><br>*SSL1*<br>*TFB4*<br>*TFB2*<br>*TFB5* | Core TFIIH subunits | At1g55750<br>At3g61420<br>At1g05055<br>At1g18340<br>At4g17020<br>At1g12400<br>At1g62886 | *AtTFB1-1*<br>*AtTFB1-2*<br>*Atp44*<br>*AtTFB4*<br>*AtTFB2*<br>*AtTFB5-1*<br>*AtTFB5-2* |
| *XPA* | *RAD14* | ssDNA binding | ND | *ND* |
| *XPG* | *RAD2* | 3′ endonuclease | At3g28030 | *AtXPG/UVH3* |
| *ERCC1* | *RAD10* | 5′ endonuclease with XPF | At3g05210 | *AtERCC1/UVR7* |
| *XPF* | *RAD1* | 5′ endonuclease with ERCC1 | At5g41150 | *AtXPF/UVH1* |
| *PCNA* | *PCNA* | RFC dependant sliding clamp | At1g07370<br>At2g29570 | *AtPCNA1*<br>*AtPCNA2* |
| *RFC1*<br>*RFC2*<br>*RFC3*<br>*RFC4*<br>*RFC5* | *RFC1*<br>*RFC2*<br>*RFC3*<br>*RFC4*<br>*RFC5* | DNA-dependent ATPase required for DNA replication and repair | At5g22010<br>At1g21690<br>At1g77470<br>At1g63160<br>At5g27740 | *AtRFC1*<br>*AtRFC2*<br>*AtRFC3*<br>*AtRFC4*<br>*AtRFC5* |
| *RPA70*<br><br><br><br><br>*RPA32*<br><br>*RPA14* | *RFA1*<br><br><br><br><br>*RFA2*<br><br>*RFA3* | ssDNA binding protein required for architectural role in dual lesion incision and repair synthesis | At2g06510<br>At4g19130<br>At5g08020<br>At5g45400<br>At5g61000<br>At2g24490<br>At3g02920<br>At3g52630<br>At4g18590 | *AtRPA70A*<br>*AtRPA70B*<br>*AtRPA70C*<br>*AtRPA70D*<br>*AtRPA70E*<br>*AtRPA32A*<br>*AtRPA32B*<br>*AtRPA14A*<br>*AtRPA14B* |
| *CSA* | *RAD28* | TC-NER specific DCAF protein | At1g27840<br>At1g19750 | *AtCSA1A*<br>*AtCSA1B* |

| Human | Yeast | Function | ATG no. | Arabidopsis |
|---|---|---|---|---|
| *CSB* | *RAD26* | SWI/SNF2 like ATPase | At2g18760 | *AtCSB* |
| *XAB2* | *SYF1* | Complex stabilization | At5g28740 | *AtXAB2* |
| *TFIIS* | *TFIIS* | TC-NER elongation factor | At2g38560 | *AtTFIIS* |
| *HMGN1* | *ND* | Nucleosome binding | ND | *ND* |
| *EP300/CBP* | *ND* | Histone acetyl transferase | At1g79000<br>At1g67220<br>At1g55970<br>At3g12980<br>At1g16710 | *HAC1*<br>*HAC2*<br>*HAC4*<br>*HAC5*<br>*HAC12* |
| **Translesion Synthesis** | | | | |
| *POLH/XPV* | *RAD30* | Y-family DNA polymerase | At5g44740 | *AtPOLH* |
| *REV1* | *REV1* | Y-family DNA polymerase | At5g44750 | *AtREV1* |
| *POLZ* | *REV3* | B-family DNA polymerase | At1g67500 | *AtREV3* |
| *REV7* | *REV7* | REV3 accessory subunit | At1g16590 | *AtREV7* |
| *POLK* | *ND* | Y-family DNA polymerase | At1g49980 | *AtPOLK* |

Table 1. Genes involved in UV damaged DNA repair and tolerance. ND=not detected.

ubiquitination weakens the interaction between histones and DNA to further facilitate the recruitment of repair proteins to damaged DNA (Guerrero-Santoro et al., 2008; Higa et al., 2006). The activated DDB2 complex recruits XPC via protein-protein interactions, followed by ubiquitination of XPC and DDB2. Polyubiquitinated DDB2 exhibits reduced affinity for damaged DNA and is subsequently displaced from the damaged foci, whereas polyubiquitinated XPC enhances its binding to DNA (Sugasawa et al., 2005). In *Arabidopsis,* DDB2 turnover is abrogated in *cul4, ddb1a, atr* and *det1* mutants suggesting that ATR and DET1 may co-operate with the CUL4-DDB1 E3 ligase complex in regulating NER (Castells et al., 2011; Molinier et al., 2008).

#### 3.1.1.4 XPC-HR23B-CEN2

The next step in GG-NER involves the homologous heterodimers hXPC-hHR23B (in Humans) and RAD4-RAD23 (in yeast). In addition to hXPC-hHR23B, Araki et al. (2001) identified hCEN2, a $Ca^{2+}$ binding protein contributing to the stability of the hXPC-hHR23B complex. Hence in mammalian systems the identified protein recognition complex is hXPC-hHR23B-hCEN2, however neither hHR23B nor hCEN2 bind to damaged DNA but enhance both the affinity and specificity of hXPC binding to damaged DNA (Fitch et al., 2003; Nishi et al., 2005). AtCEN2 shares 49% identity with hCEN2, *Atcen2* mutants are UV sensitive, and AtCEN2 overexpression resulted in enhanced repair. Upon UV irradiation, AtCEN2 level increases and it rapidly translocates to the nucleus. AtCEN2-AtXPC interaction in *Arabidopsis thaliana* has also been demonstrated (Liang et al., 2006; Molinier et al., 2004). Potential homologs of HR23B/RAD23 have been identified in *Arabidopsis thaliana, Oryza sativa* and *Daucus carota* (Schultz & Quatrano, 1997; Sturm & Leinhard, 1998). The *Arabidopsis* genome has 4 loci encoding RAD23 homologs (RAD23a, RAD23b, RAD23c, RAD23d), and although mutants exhibit multiple pleotrophic developmental defects (Farmer et al., 2010), UV sensitivity or complex interactions with the *Arabidopsis* NER machinery have not yet been reported.

### 3.1.2 DNA unwinding complex assembly

Following recognition, the damaged region is unwound by the TFIIH transcription factor which joins the XPC-CEN2-HR23B complex. TFIIH is a complex of 10 proteins, seven of which are players in the NER pathway (helicases XPB and XPD, p62, p44, p34, p52, and p8). The last five proteins are encoded by GTF2H1, GTF2H2, GTF2H3, GTF2H4, GTF2H5 (Frit et al., 1999). TFIIH not only participates in NER of transcriptionally active and inactive DNA, but also in RNA POL II dependant transcription, cell cycle control and regulation of nuclear receptor activity (Chen & Suter, 2003). ATP dependant 5′->3′ and 3′->5′ helicase activities associated with XPD/RAD3 and XPB/RAD25 respectively unwind the DNA encompassing the lesion with the concomitant release of the recognition complex. Human XPB and the corresponding yeast RAD25 knockouts are lethal. *Arabidopsis thaliana,* unlike the sugarcane, rice or mammalian genomes, encodes two homologs of XPB - AtXPB1 and AtXPB2. These proteins are 95% identical with redundant functions and are expressed constitutively throughout plant development (Morgante et al., 2005; Ribeiro et al., 1998). Despite this redundancy, *xpb1* mutants exhibit delayed germination and flowering phenotypes but are not UV sensitive (Costa et al., 2001). Phenotypes of *Arabidopsis xpb2* or double mutants have not yet been reported. *Arabidopsis* XPD is 56% and 50% identical to human and yeast sequences. *Arabidopsis XPD/RAD3* null mutations are lethal, however viable point mutation alleles are UV sensitive and were identified as *uvh6* (*uv hypersensitive 6*) mutants. (Jenkins et al., 1997; Liu et al., 2003). Another component of the of TFIIH complex, p44, was identified in *Arabidopsis* as ATGTF2H2 and was found to interact in vivo with AtXPD (Vonarx et al., 2006).

### 3.1.3 Endonuclease recruitment following unwinding

TFIIH further recruits additional factors such as XPA and heterotrimeric Replication Protein A (RPA), composed of 70, 32 and 14 kDa subunits, to promote and stabilize the formation of an open intermediate essential for the dual incision by XPG and XPF-ERCC1 (Excision Repair Complementing defective repair in Chinese hamster 1) (RAD1/RAD10) endonucleases at the 3′ and 5′ sites respectively (Tapais et al., 2004). The RPA-XPA complex exhibits interactions with both endonucleases (He et al., 1995; Wold, 1997), however the specific function of XPA is still not evident. Initially it was thought to function as a lesion recognition complex in concert with XPC, but was later determined to be recruited after TFIIH entry and facilitate XPC complex departure (Hey et al., 2002; Volker et al., 2001). In addition, XPA homologues do not exist in plants (Kunz et al., 2005). The dual incisions catalyzed by the endonucleases excise oligonucleotides of about 20-30 bases containing the lesion (Reidl et al., 2003).

Potential homologs of ERCC1, XPF, XPG and RPA have been identified in plants. Although ERCC1 was first cloned from male germ line cells of *Lilium longiforum,* southern blots confirmed the presence of ERCC1 across diverse plant species such as *A. thaliana, B. napus, Z. mays, L. esculentum, N. tobacum,* and *O. sativa* (Xu et al., 1998). Hefner et al. (2003) mapped the *Arabidopsis uvr7* mutant to *AtERCC1. Atercc1* knockouts are phenotypically normal in contrast to the lethal mammalian counterparts (Weeda et al., 1997). *Atercc1* mutants are extremely sensitive to DNA damaging chemicals such as mitomycin and ionizing agents such as UV and $\gamma$ - radiation (Hefner et al., 2003). More recent studies in *Arabidopsis* indicate significant roles of *AtERCC1* in concert with *AtXPF* in homologous recombination and chromosomal stability (Dubest et al., 2002, 2004; Vannier et al., 2009). Gallego et al. (2000) and Liu et al. (2000) characterized the single copy AtXPF which is 37% and 29% identical to human XPF and *S. cerevisiae* RAD1 respectively. *AtXPF* is homogenously expressed, was mapped to the *uvh1* mutant in *Arabidopsis,* and partially complements the yeast *rad1* mutant (Gallego et al., 2000). *AtXPF* point mutations result in sensitivity to ionizing radiation and mitomycin C, and impaired removal of photoproducts (Fidanstef et al., 2000; Vonarx et al., 2002). *AtXPG* was mapped to the *UVH3* locus and knockouts result in UV sensitivity as well as premature senescence and reduced seed production (Liu et al., 2001). The *XPG* rice homolog, *OsSEND-1,* exhibits upregulated mRNA levels in response to UV and DNA damaging agents (Furukawa et al., 2003a).

ssDNA binding RPA proteins in plants were first identified in rice (Ishibashi et al., 2001). Unlike most eukaryotic organisms, *Arabidopsis* and rice possess multiple copies of the RPA homologs. In addition to participating in DNA repair, RPA proteins play a role in homologous recombination and DNA replication in humans and yeast (Sakaguchi et al., 2009). The rice genome encodes three OsRPA70 (OsRPA70A, OsRPA70B, OsRPA70C), three OsRPA32 (OsRPA32-1, OsRPA32-2, OsRPA32-3) and one OsRPA14. *In vivo* interactions in rice confirms three different complex formations: OsRPA70A-OsRPA32-2-OsRPA14 (Type1); OsRPA70B-OsRPA32-1-OsRPA14 (Type2); and OsRPA70C-OsRPa32-3-OsRPA14 (Type3). Subcellular localization of all three OsRPA32 was detected in both the nucleus and chloroplasts. OsRPA70A was only in the chloroplast whereas OsRPA70B and OsRPA70C were exclusively to the nucleus. This data suggest that while the Type1 complex may participate in chloroplast DNA repair, Type2 and Type3 complexes concentrate on nuclear DNA repair (Ishibashi et al., 2006). OsRPA70A and OsRPa70B share only 33% sequence homology and exhibit differences in expression pattern (Ishibashi et al., 2001). A T-DNA insertion in *OsRPA70A* resulted in partial male sterility, complete female sterility and hypersensitivity to DNA mutagens (Chang et al., 2009). OsRPA32 protein abundance is regulated by both UV irradiation and cell cycle phase (Marwedal et al., 2002). *Arabidopsis,* on the other hand, encodes five putative RPA70 genes and two copies each of RPA32 and RPA14 (Shultz et al., 2007). *Arabidopsis* RPA70A interacts preferentially with AtRPA32A rather than AtRPA32B. Knockouts of both AtRPA70A and AtRPA70B exhibited UV sensitivity when irradiated, but exhibited wildtype characteristics under normal conditions (Ishibashi et al., 2005; Takashi et al., 2009).

### 3.1.4 Repair synthesis and ligation

In mammals, the gap formed by the excision is filled via PCNA (Proliferating Cell Nuclear Antigen) and RFC dependant DNA synthesis by DNA POL δ/ε. These components are likely recruited by XPG and RPA as RFC exhibits interaction with RPA (Yuzhakov et al., 1999). RFC catalyzes the ATP dependant loading of PCNA to DNA at the 3′ OH. PCNA is a homotrimeric protein which forms a sliding clamp-like complex (Gulbis et al., 1996) and interacts with the DNA POL to ensure replication occurs processively (Mocquet et al., 2008). The final phase of NER is completed by phosphodiester backbone rejoining of the repaired DNA strand by DNA Ligase I.

Although PCNA and RFC homologues have been identified in plants, their specific role in nucleotide excision repair has not yet been elucidated (Furukawa et al., 2003b; Strzalka & Ziemienowicz, 2011). Recently, Roy et al. (2011) cloned and characterized a homolog of mammalian DNA POLλ in *Arabidopsis.* AtPOLλ was upregulated upon UV induction under dark conditions, and *Atpolλ* mutants exhibited UV sensitivity and decreased DNA repair. Thus, this report suggests a role for DNA POLλ in plant NER.

### 3.2 Transcription coupled repair

The emerging picture of mammalian TC-NER is of a complex mechanism requiring two essential assembly factors (CSA and CSB), certain TC-NER specific proteins (P300, HMGN1, XAB2 and TFIIS), as well as core NER proteins. UV induced DNA damage is initially recognised by RNA POL II, which stalls when it encounters helix-distorting lesions on the template strand during transcription. Stalled RNA POL II backtracks a few nucleotides and is recognised by the CSB protein which in turn co-ordinates the recruitment of the repair factors required to accomplish Transcription Coupled NER (Mellon, 2005).

Cloning and characterization of the mammalian CSB gene revealed a nuclear protein of 168 kDa with a region of homology to the SWI2/SNF2 family of helicases. CSB has been shown to interact with RNA POL II and this interaction is enhanced and prolonged by UV exposure (van den Boom et al., 2004). Studies propose that functional CSB in the absence of UV could also serve as a component of the transcriptional machinery promoting elongation (Fousteri & Mullenders, 2008; Hanawalt & Spivak, 2008). Further, CSB facilitates the entry of the core NER factors XPA, XPG and TFIIH through complex interactions (Laine & Egly, 2006; Saxowsky & Doetsch, 2006; Svejstrup, 2002). Mammalian CSA on the other hand is a 46 kDa DWD protein containing seven WD40 repeats that associates with DDB1-CUL4 type E3 ligases and is recruited to the damaged site after CSB. CSA physically interacts with the CSB-RNA POL II complex in a UV dependant manner (Groisman et al., 2003; Fousteri et al., 2006). Interestingly, unlike the DDB2 complex, the CSA-CUL4 Ub ligase complex is active under normal conditions but is rapidly inactivated upon UV irradiation by CSN. Hence CSN plays a differential and dynamic role in regulating both pathways of Nucleotide Excision Repair. The stable CSN-CSA-CSB complex is required for the recruitment of the other NER factors. Following repair, CSN dissociates, reactivating CSA Ub ligase activity and resulting in CSB degradation. Clearance of CSB is required for the reinitiation of transcription by RNA POL II (Groisman et al., 2003, 2006).

Several papers over the years propose the fate of RNA POL II during the coupling process: either ubiquitinated and degraded, translocated or bypassed from the lesion site, or simply stalled during the entire repair process, is still a matter of debate (Reviewed in Tornaletti, 2009). XAB2 (XPA binding protein 2) is a RNA-binding protein with 15 tetratricopeptide repeats. In addition to interacting with XPA, XAB2 is capable of interacting with CSA, CSB and RNA POL II (Nakatsu et al., 2000). XAB2 is thought to stabilize protein assemblies by functioning as a scaffolding subunit. XAB2 knockouts in mammalian cells exhibit hypersensitivity and decreased recovery of mRNA synthesis post UV irradiation (Kuraoka et al., 2008). Increased amounts of histone acetyl transferase p300 and High Mobility Group Nucleosome binding domain containing protein 1 (HMGN1) interact with RNA POL II in a CSB-dependant manner upon UV irradiation but exhibit weak interactions under normal conditions (Fousteri et al., 2006). Both HMGN1 and p300 are nucleosome interacting proteins which remodel the chromatin structure behind the arrested polymerase and facilitating the backward translocation of RNA POL II (Hanawalt & Spivak, 2008). TFIIS, functioning as a transcription elongation factor, stimulates the arrested RNA POL II to restart elongation. This TFIIS-RNA POL II interaction is significantly increased upon UV irradiation (Fousteri et al., 2006). Hence it is proposed that TFIIS facilitates resumption of transcription post DNA lesion removal in a CSA/B-dependent manner.

Elucidation of the TC-NER mechanism in plants is still at its infancy. While there is no plant homologue for HMGN1, the *Arabidopsis* genome encodes homologues of XAB2,

TFIIS, and five p300/CBP homologues, however the role of these genes in DNA repair has not been assessed (Grasser et al., 2009; Kunz et al., 2005; Pandey et al., 2002). Only recently was the homolog of human CSA cloned and characterized in *Arabidopsis*. In contrast to mammalian systems, the *Arabidopsis* genome encodes two homologs of CSA – AtCSA1A and AtCSA1B, 92% identical DWD proteins with overlapping subcellular localization and expression patterns. These proteins exist as heterotetramers in planta and are capable of interacting with the DDB1-CUL4 E3 complex. Knockouts of either gene result in UV sensitivity and decreased photoproduct removal (Zhang et al., 2010). Concurrently, another group overexpressed AtCSA1A, which surprisingly also resulted in increased UV sensitivity. This result is hypothesised to be due to competition between CSA and with other DWD proteins to interact with the DDB1-CUL4 complex. Interestingly AtCSA1A levels remained constant upon UV induction (Biedermann & Hellmann, 2010). RNAi of a putative *Arabidopsis* CSB homolog resulted in a UV sensitive phenotype (Shaked et al., 2006). Hence, taken as a whole, these results confirm the role of the CUL4-DDB1-CSA and CSB pathway in plants.

## 4. Translesion synthesis

Despite the available repair mechanisms, there are times when UV damage persists and DNA replication proceeds past UV lesions via translesion synthesis (TLS). This synthesis proceeds via one of several DNA polymerases: Polη, Rev1, Polζ, Polκ or Polι. Polη (eta) is encoded by the *POLH* locus in humans and is homologous to yeast RAD30. Polη performs error-free bypass of CPDs, and loss of function results in increased mutation and xeroderma pigmentosa (XP-V) in humans. REV1 exhibits dCMP transferase activity but is required for 6-4 PP bypass independent of this activity, suggesting its role may be in recruitment of other polymerases. Polζ is composed of REV3 and REV7 and exhibits error prone repair. REV3 is a B-family polymerase (unlike the other TLS polymerases which are all Y-family polymerases) and REV7 an accessory subunit that enhances REV3 activity (Waters et al., 2009). Polκ activity is specific to N2-dG lesions in both animals and plants, while plants do not have a Polι homologue (Garcia-Diaz & Bebenek, 2007; Garcia-Ortiz et al., 2007).

Homologues of REV1, REV3 and REV7 as well as Polη have been identified in *Arabidopsis* (Sakamoto et al., 2003; Santiago et al., 2006; Takahashi et al., 2005). Mutant alleles of *REV3*, *REV1* and *REV7* all result in UV sensitivity, although *rev1* only weakly and *rev7* only to long-term UV exposure (Sakamoto et al., 2003; Takahashi et al., 2005). Interestingly, AtREV1 cannot insert nucleotides across from UV-induced DNA lesions, suggesting that its role is primarily in the recruitment of other TLS polymerases (Takahashi et al., 2007). The UV sensitivity of the *rev1 rev3* double mutant is similar to that of *rev3*, additional evidence that the role of REV1 may be in REV3 recruitment (Takahashi et al., 2005). Analysis of mutation frequency in *rev1* and *rev3* mutants shows a reduction relative to wildtype rate, evidence that these genes contribute to error-prone repair (Nakagawa et al., 2011).

Polη is encoded by the *Arabidopsis POLH* gene. The *POLH* transcript is ubiquitously expressed and alternatively spliced, and AtPolη exhibits similar levels of activity *in vitro* as the human protein (Hoffman et al., 2008; Santiago et al., 2008a, 2009). *AtPOLH* overexpression results in increased UV tolerance, while *AtPOLH* loss of function results in weak UV sensitivity, but enhances the sensitivity of the *rev3* mutant, evidence that Polη is acting independently of Polζ (Curtis & Hays, 2007; Santiago et al., 2008b). *POLH* mutants exhibit an increased mutation frequency, indicating a role in error-free repair. Interestingly, this increased mutation rate is suppressed in the *rev3 polh* double mutant, indicating that REV3 is required for the increased mutations in *polh* (Nakagawa et al., 2011). AtPolη interacts with the *Arabidopsis* PCNA homologues PCNA1 and PCNA2. In yeast the interaction with PCNA2 was found to be functionally important and require the PCNA-interacting protein (PIP) box and Ubiquitin-binding motif (UBM) of AtPolη (Anderson et al., 2008).

In other systems, PCNA monoubiquitination by RAD6/RAD18 is implicated in polymerase switching during translesion synthesis (Waters et al., 2009). While the *Arabidopsis* genome contains *RAD6* homologues (*AtUBC1-3*), no obvious *RAD18* homologue exists (Kraft et al., 2005). Interestingly, in mammalian cells, the CUL4-DDB1-CDT2 E3 ubiquitin ligase was recently shown to also monoubiquitinate PCNA and promote translesion synthesis (Terai et al., 2010). The CUL4-DDB1-CDT2 complex also ubiquitinates Polη (Kim & Micheal, 2008; Soria & Gottifredi, 2010), suggesting that this complex may be a key regulator of translesion synthesis (Abbas & Dutta, 2011). All components of the CUL4-DDB1-CDT2 complex exist in plants (Lee et al., 2008), so it will be interesting to examine the role of this complex in translesion synthesis.

## 5. Other responses

In addition to DNA repair and TLS, UV-damaged DNA also triggers other cellular responses such as cell cycle arrest and cell death (Batista et al., 2009). In general, relatively little is known about the molecular basis of these responses in plants. As in mammalian systems, in plants the initial damage sensors include ATM (double strand breaks), ATR (ssDNA) and ATR-interacting protein ATRIP (Culligan et al., 2004; Furukawa et al., 2010; Sakamoto et al., 2009). Plants do not have a p53 homologue, in contrast damage signalling pathways converge on the SOG1 transcription factor, resulting in cell cycle arrest and cell death (Furukawa et al., 2010; Preuss & Britt, 2003; Yoshiyama et al., 2009). UV-induced cell death in plants also involves topoismerase I (Balestrazzi et al., 2010), metacaspase-8 and caspase-3-like activities (Danon et al., 2004; He et al., 2008; Zhang et al., 2009), as well as changes in reactive oxygen species and mitochrondria (Gao et al., 2008).

## 6. Conclusions

Thus, despite the barrage of damage resulting from solar UV exposure plants face every day, they have a variety of mechanisms which allow them to survive. UV induced DNA damage is repaired by direct photoreactivation via photolyases, or by dark repair (NER) in both transcribed (TC-NER) or non-transcribed regions (GG-NER). Finally, rather than repair UV damage, plants can tolerate its presence and proceed with DNA replication via translesion synthesis, although there can be mutagenic consequences of this activity. The continued study of these pathways and the interplay between them in plants is sure to bring additional insight.

## 7. Acknowledgements

Research in our laboratory is supported by a grant from the Natural Sciences & Engingeering Research Council of Canada (NSERC).

## 8. References

Abbas, T. & Dutta, A. (2011). CRL4Cdt2: master coordinator of cell cycle progression and genome stability. *Cell Cycle,* 10(2):241-9

Ahmad, M. & Cashmore, A.R. (1993). *HY4* gene of *A. thaliana* encodes a protein with characteristics of a blue-light photoreceptor. *Nature,* 366 (6451):162-6

Ahmad, M., Jarillo, J.A., Klimczak, L.J., Landry, L.G., Peng, T., Last, R.L. & Cashmore, A.R. (1997). An enzyme similar to animal type II photolyases mediates photoreactivation in *Arabidopsis*. *Plant Cell,* 9(2):199-207

Al Khateeb, W.M. & Schroeder, D.F. (2009). Overexpression of *Arabidopsis* damaged DNA binding protein 1A (DDB1A) enhances UV tolerance. *Plant Mol Biol.,* 70(4):371-83

Anderson, H.J., Vonarx, E.J., Pastushok, L., Nakagawa, M., Katafuchi, A., Gruz, P., Di Rubbo, A., Grice, D.M., Osmond, M.J., Sakamoto, A.N., Nohmi, T., Xiao, W. & Kunz, B.A. (2008). *Arabidopsis thaliana* Y-family DNA polymerase eta catalyses translesion synthesis and interacts functionally with PCNA2. *Plant J.,* 55(6):895-908

Araki, M., Masutani, C., Takemura, M., Uchida, A., Sugasawa, K., Kondoh, J., Ohkuma, Y. & Hanaoka, F. (2001). Centrosome protein centrin 2/caltractin 1 is part of the xeroderma pigmentosum group C complex that initiates global genome nucleotide excision repair. *J Biol Chem.,* 276(22):18665-72

Balestrazzi, A., Locato, V., Bottone, M.G., De Gara, L., Biggiogera, M., Pellicciari, C., Botti, S., Di Gesù, D., Donà, M. & Carbonera, D. (2010). Response to UV-C radiation in topo I-deficient carrot cells with low ascorbate levels. *J Exp Bot.,* 61(2):575-85

Ballaré, C.L. (2003). Stress under the sun: spotlight on ultraviolet-B responses. *Plant Physiol.,* 132:1725-1727

Batista, L.F., Kaina, B., Meneghini, R. & Menck, C.F. (2009). How DNA lesions are turned into powerful killing structures: insights from UV-induced apoptosis. *Mutat Res.,* 681(2-3):197-208

Batschauer, A. (1999). Light perception in higher plants. *Cell Mol Life Sci.,* 55:153-165

Bernhardt, A., Lechner, E., Hano, P., Schade, V., Dieterle, M., Anders, M., Dubin, M.J., Benvenuto, G., Bowler, C., Genschik, P. & Hellmann, H. (2006). CUL4 associates with DDB1 and DET1 and its downregulation affects diverse aspects of development in *Arabidopsis thaliana*. *Plant J.,* 47(4):591-603

Bernhardt, A., Mooney, S. & Hellmann, H. (2010). *Arabidopsis* DDB1a and DDB1b are critical for embryo development. *Planta,* 232(3):555-566

Biedermann, S. & Hellmann, H. (2010). The DDB1a interacting proteins ATCSA-1 and DDB2 are critical factors for UV-B tolerance and genomic integrity in *Arabidopsis thaliana*. *Plant J.,* 62(3):404-15

Biedermann, S. & Hellmann, H. (2011). WD40 and CUL4-based E3 ligases: lubricating all aspects of life. *Trends Plant Sci.,* 16(1):38-46

Britt, A.B. (1999). Molecular genetics of DNA repair in higher plants. *Trends Plant Sci.,* 4(1):20-25

Brosché, M., Schuler, M.A., Kalbina, I., Connor, L. & Strid, A. (2002). Gene regulation by low level UV-B radiation: identification by DNA array analysis. *Photochem Photobiol Sci.,* 1(9):656-64

Castells, E., Molinier, J., Drevensek, S., Genschik, P., Barneche, F. & Bowler, C. (2010). *det1-1*-induced UV-C hyposensitivity through *UVR3* and *PHR1* photolyase gene over-expression. *Plant J.,* 63:392–404

Castells, E., Molinier, J., Benvenuto, G., Bourbousse, C., Zabulon, G., Zalc, A., Cazzaniga, S., Genschik, P., Barneche, F. & Bowler, C. (2011). The conserved factor DE-ETIOLATED 1 cooperates with CUL4-DDB1(DDB2) to maintain genome integrity upon UV stress. *EMBO J.*, 30(6):1162-72

Chang, Y., Gong, L., Yuan, W., Li, X., Chen, G., Li, X., Zhang, Q. & Wu, C. (2009). Replication protein A (RPA1a) is required for meiotic and somatic DNA repair but is dispensable for DNA replication and homologous recombination in rice. *Plant Physiol.*, 151(4):2162-73

Chen, H., Shen, Y., Tang, X., Yu, L., Wang, J., Guo, L., Zhang, Y., Zhang, H., Feng, S., Strickland, E., Zheng, N. & Deng, X. W. (2006). *Arabidopsis* CULLIN4 Forms an E3 Ubiquitin Ligase with RBX1 and the CDD Complex in Mediating Light Control of Development. *Plant Cell*, 18(8):1991-2004

Chen, J.J., Mitchell, D.L. & Britt, A.B. (1994). A Light-Dependent Pathway for the Elimination of UV-Induced Pyrimidine (6-4) Pyrimidinone Photoproducts in *Arabidopsis*. *Plant Cell*, 6(9):1311-1317

Chen, J.J., Jiang, C.Z. & Britt, A.B. (1996). Little or no repair of cyclobutyl pyrimidine dimers is observed in the organellar genomes of the young *Arabidopsis* seedlings. *Plant Physiol.*, 111(1):19–25

Chen, J. & Suter, B. (2003). Xpd, a structural bridge and a functional link. *Cell Cycle*, 2(6):503-6

Costa, R.M., Morgante, P.G., Berra, C.M., Nakabashi, M., Bruneau, D., Bouchez, D., Sweder, K.S., Van Sluys, M.A. & Menck, C.F. (2001). The participation of AtXPB1, the XPB/RAD25 homologue gene from *Arabidopsis thaliana*, in DNA repair and plant development. *Plant J.*, 28(4):385-95

Culligan, K., Tissier, A. & Britt, A. (2004). ATR regulates a G2-phase cell-cycle checkpoint in *Arabidopsis thaliana*. *Plant Cell*, 16(5):1091-104

Curtis, M.J. & Hays, J.B. (2007). Tolerance of dividing cells to replication stress in UVB-irradiated *Arabidopsis* roots: requirements for DNA translesion polymerases eta and zeta. *DNA Repair (Amst).*, 6(9):1341-58

Danon, A., Rotari, V.I., Gordon, A., Mailhac, N. & Gallois, P. (2004). Ultraviolet-C overexposure induces programmed cell death in *Arabidopsis*, which is mediated by caspase-like activities and which can be suppressed by caspase inhibitors, p35 and Defender against Apoptotic Death. *J Biol Chem.*, 279(1):779-87

Deisenhofer, J. (2000). DNA photolyases and cryptochromes. *Mutat Res.*, 460(3-4):143-9

Draper, C.K. & Hays, J.B. (2000). Replication of chloroplast, mitochondrial and nuclear DNA during growth of unirradiated and UVB-irradiated *Arabidopsis* leaves. *Plant J.*, 23(2):255-65

Dubest, S., Gallego, M.E. & White, C.I. (2002). Role of the AtRad1p endonuclease in homologous recombination in plants. *EMBO Rep.*, 3(11):1049-54

Dubest, S., Gallego, M.E. & White, C.I. (2004). Roles of the AtErcc1 protein in recombination. *Plant J.*, 39(3):334-42

Farmer, L.M., Book, A.J., Lee, K.H., Lin, Y.L., Fu, H. & Vierstra, R.D. (2010). The RAD23 family provides an essential connection between the 26S proteasome and ubiquitylated proteins in *Arabidopsis*. *Plant Cell*, 22(1):124-42

Fidantsef, A.L., Mitchell, D.L. & Britt, A.B. (2000). The *Arabidopsis UVH1* gene is a homolog of the yeast repair endonuclease RAD1. *Plant Physiol.*, 124(2):579-86

Fitch, M.E., Nakajima, S., Yasui, A. & Ford, J.M. (2003). In vivo recruitment of XPC to UV-induced cyclobutane pyrimidine dimers by the DDB2 gene product. *J Biol Chem.*, 278(47):46906-10

Fousteri, M., Vermeulen, W., van Zeeland, A.A. & Mullenders, L.H. (2006). Cockayne syndrome A and B proteins differentially regulate recruitment of chromatin remodeling and repair factors to stalled RNA polymerase II in vivo. *Mol Cell*, 23(4):471-82

Fousteri, M. & Mullenders, L.H. (2008). Transcription-coupled nucleotide excision repair in mammalian cells: molecular mechanisms and biological effects. *Cell Res.*, 18(1):73-84

Frit, P., Bergmann, E. & Egly, J.M. (1999). Transcription factor IIH: a key player in the cellular response to DNA damage. *Biochimie*, 81(1-2):27-38

Frohnmeyer, H. & Staiger, D. (2003). Ultraviolet-B Radiation-Mediated Responses in Plants. Balancing Damage and Protection. *Plant Physiol.*, 133(4):1420–1428

Furukawa, T., Kimura, S., Ishibashi, T., Mori, Y., Hashimoto, J. & Sakaguchi, K. (2003a). OsSEND-1: a new RAD2 nuclease family member in higher plants. *Plant Mol Biol.*, 51(1):59-70

Furukawa, T., Ishibashi, T., Kimura, S., Tanaka, H., Hashimoto, J. & Sakaguchi, K. (2003b). Characterization of all the subunits of replication factor C from a higher plant, rice (Oryza sativa L.), and their relation to development. *Plant Mol Biol.*, 53(1-2):15-25

Furukawa, T., Curtis, M.J., Tominey, C.M., Duong, Y.H., Wilcox, B.W., Aggoune, D., Hays, J.B. & Britt, A.B. (2010). A shared DNA-damage-response pathway for induction of stem-cell death by UVB and by gamma irradiation. *DNA Repair (Amst).*, 9(9):940-8

Gallego, F., Fleck, O., Li, A., Wyrzykowska, J. & Tinland, B. (2000). AtRAD1, a plant homologue of human and yeast nucleotide excision repair endonucleases, is involved in dark repair of UV damages and recombination. *Plant J.*, 21(6):507-18

Gao, C., Xing, D., Li, L. & Zhang, L. (2008). Implication of reactive oxygen species and mitochondrial dysfunction in the early stages of plant programmed cell death induced by ultraviolet-C overexposure. *Planta*, 227(4):755-67

Garcia-Diaz, M. & Bebenek, K. (2007). Multiple functions of DNA polymerases. *CRC Crit Rev Plant Sci.*, 26(2):105-122

García-Ortiz, M.V., Roldán-Arjona, T. & Ariza, R.R. (2007). The noncatalytic C-terminus of AtPOLK Y-family DNA polymerase affects synthesis fidelity, mismatch extension and translesion replication. *FEBS J.*, 274(13):3340-50

Gillet, L.C.J. & Scharer, O.D. (2006). Molecular mechanisms of mammalian global genome nucleotide excision repair. *Chem. Rev.*, 106(2):253-276

Grasser, M., Kane, C.M., Merkle, T., Melzer, M., Emmersen, J. & Grasser, K.D. (2009). Transcript elongation factor TFIIS is involved in *Arabidopsis* seed dormancy. *J Mol Biol.*, 386(3):598-611

Groisman, R., Polanowska, J., Kuraoka, I., Sawada, J., Saijo, M., Drapkin, R., Kissilev, A.F., Tanaka, K. & Nakatani, Y. (2003). The ubiquitin ligase activity in the DDB2 and CSA complexes is differentially regulated by the COP9 signalosome in response to DNA damage. *Cell*, 113(3): 357-367

Groisman, R., Kuraoka, I., Chevallier, O., Gaye, N., Magnaldo, T., Tanaka, K., Kisselev, A.F., Harel-Bellan, A. & Nakatani, Y. (2006). CSA-dependent degradation of CSB by the ubiquitin-proteasome pathway establishes a link between complementation factors of the Cockayne syndrome. *Genes Dev.*, 20(11):1429-34

Guerrero-Santoro, J., Kapetanaki, M.G., Hsieh, C.L., Gorbachinsky, I., Levine, A.S. & Rapić-Otrin, V. (2008). The cullin 4B-based UV-damaged DNA-binding protein ligase binds to UV-damaged chromatin and ubiquitinates histone H2A. *Cancer Res.*, 68(13):5014-22

Gulbis, J.M., Kelman, Z., Hurwitz, J., O'Donnell, M. & Kuriyan, J. (1996). Structure of the C-terminal region of p21(WAF1/CIP1) complexed with human PCNA. *Cell*, 87(2):297-306

Hada, M., Hino, K., Buchholz, G., Goss, J., Wellmann, E. & Shin, M. (2000). Assay of DNA photolyase activity in spinach leaves in relation to cell compartmentation-evidence for lack of DNA photolyase in chloroplasts. *Biosci Biotechnol Biochem.*, 64:1288–1291

Hanawalt, P.C. & Spivak, G. (2008). Transcription-coupled DNA repair: two decades of progress and surprises. *Nat Rev Mol Cell Biol.*, 9(12):958-70

He, R., Drury, G.E., Rotari, V.I., Gordon, A., Willer, M., Farzaneh, T., Woltering, E.J. & Gallois, P. (2008). Metacaspase-8 modulates programmed cell death induced by ultraviolet light and H2O2 in *Arabidopsis*. *J Biol Chem.*, 283(2):774-83

He, Z., Henricksen, L.A., Wold, M.S. & Ingles, C.J. (1995). RPA involvement in the damage-recognition and incision steps of nucleotide excision repair. *Nature*, 374: 566–569

Hefner, E., Preuss, S.B. & Britt, A.B. (2003). *Arabidopsis* mutants sensitive to gamma radiation include the homologue of the human repair gene ERCC1. *J Exp Bot.*, 54(383):669-80

Hey, T., Lipps, G., Sugasawa, K., Iwai, S., Hanaoka, F. & Krauss, G. (2002). The XPC-HR23B complex displays high affinity and specificity for damaged DNA in a true-equilibrium fluorescence assay. *Biochemistry*, 41(21): 6583–6587

Hidema, J., Kumagai, T. & Sutherland, B.M. (2000). UV radiation-sensitive norin 1 rice contains defective cyclobutane pyrimidine dimer photolyase. *Plant Cell*, 12(9):1569-78

Hidema, J., Taguchi, T., Ono, T., Teranishi, M., Yamamoto, K. & Kumagai, T. (2007). Increase in CPD photolyase activity functions effectively to prevent growth inhibition caused by UVB radiation. *Plant J.*, 50(1):70-9

Higa, L.A., Wu, M., Ye, T., Kobayashi, R., Sun, H. & Zhang, H. (2006). CUL4-DDB1 ubiquitin ligase interacts with multiple WD40-repeat proteins and regulates histone methylation. *Nat Cell Biol.*, 8(11):1277-83

Hirouchi, T., Nakajima, S., Najrana, T., Tanaka, M., Matsunaga, T., Hidema, J., Teranishi, M., Fujino, T., Kumagai, T. & Yamamoto, K. (2003). A gene for a Class II DNA photolyase from *Oryza sativa*: cloning of the cDNA by dilution-amplification. *Mol Genet Genomics*, 269(4):508-16

Hoeijmakers, J.H. (2001). Genome maintenance mechanisms for preventing cancer. *Nature*, 411: 135-141

Hoffman, P.D., Curtis, M.J., Iwai, S. & Hays, J.B. (2008). Biochemical evolution of DNA polymerase eta: properties of plant, human, and yeast proteins. *Biochemistry*, 47(16):4583-96

Holmberg, C., Fleck, O., Hansen, H.A., Liu, C., Slaaby, R., Carr, A.M. & Nielsen, O. (2005). Ddb1 controls genome stability and meiosis in fission yeast. *Genes Dev.*,19:853–862

Hua, Z. & Vierstra, R.D. (2011). The Cullin-RING Ubiquitin-Protein Ligases. *Annu Rev Plant Biol.*, 62:299-334

Ishibashi, T., Kimura, S., Furukawa, T., Hatanaka, M., Hashimoto, J. & Sakaguchi, K. (2001). Two types of replication protein A 70 kDa subunit in rice, *Oryza sativa*: molecular cloning, characterization, and cellular & tissue distribution. *Gene*, 272(1-2):335-43

Ishibashi, T., Kimura, S., Yamamoto, T., Furukawa, T., Takata, K., Uchiyama, Y., Hashimoto, J. & Sakaguchi, K. (2003). Rice UV-damaged DNA binding protein homologues are most abundant in proliferating tissues. *Gene*, 308:79-87

Ishibashi, T., Koga, A., Yamamoto, T., Uchiyama, Y., Mori, Y., Hashimoto, J., Kimura, S. & Sakaguchi, K. (2005). Two types of replication protein A in seed plants. *FEBS J.*, 272(13):3270-81

Ishibashi, T., Kimura, S. & Sakaguchi, K. (2006). A higher plant has three different types of RPA heterotrimeric complex. *J Biochem.*, 139(1):99-104

Jansan, M.A.K., Hectors, K., O'Brien, N.M., Guisez, Y. & Potters, G. (2008). Plant stress and human health: Do human consumers benefit from UV-B acclimated crops? *Plant Science*, 175:449–458

Jenkins, G.I. (2009). Signal transduction in responses to UV-B radiation. *Annu Rev Plant Biol.*, 60:407-31

Jenkins, M.E., Suzuki, T.C. & Mount, D.W. (1997). Evidence that heat and ultraviolet radiation activate a common stress-response program in plants that is altered in the *uvh6* mutant of *Arabidopsis thaliana*. *Plant Physiol.*, 115(4):1351-8

Kaiser, G., Kleiner, O., Beisswenger, C. & Batschauer, A. (2009). Increased DNA repair in *Arabidopsis* plants overexpressing CPD photolyase. *Planta*, 230(3):505-15

Kapetanaki, M.G., Guerrero-Santoro, J., Bisi, D.C., Hsieh, C.L., Rapić-Otrin, V. & Levine, A.S. (2006). The DDB1-CUL4ADDB2 ubiquitin ligase is deficient in xeroderma pigmentosum group E and targets histone H2A at UV-damaged DNA sites. *Proc Natl Acad Sci U S A.*, 103(8):2588-93

Kim, S.H. & Michael, W.M. (2008). Regulated proteolysis of DNA polymerase eta during the DNA-damage response in *C. elegans*. *Mol Cell*, 32(6):757-66

Kimura, S., Tahira, Y., Ishibashi, T., Mori, Y., Mori, T., Hashimoto, J. & Sakaguchi, K. (2004). DNA repair in higher plants; photoreactivation is the major DNA repair pathway in non-proliferating cells while excision repair (nucleotide excision repair and base excision repair) is active in proliferating cells. *Nucleic Acids Res.*, 32(9):2760-7

Kimura, S. & Sakaguchi, K. (2006). DNA repair in plants. *Chem Rev.*, 106(2):753-66

Koga, A., Ishibashi, T., Kimura, S., Uchiyama, Y. & Sakaguchi, K. (2006). Characterization of T-DNA insertion mutants and RNAi silenced plants of *Arabidopsis thaliana* UV-damaged DNA binding protein 2 (AtUV-DDB2). *Plant Mol Biol.*, 61(1-2):227-40

Kraft, E., Stone, S.L., Ma, L., Su, N., Gao, Y., Lau, O.S., Deng, X.W. & Callis, J. (2005). Genome analysis and functional characterization of the E2 and RING-type E3 ligase ubiquitination enzymes of *Arabidopsis*. *Plant Physiol.*, 139(4):1597-611

Kunz, B.A., Anderson, H.J., Osmond, M.J. & Vonarx, E.J. (2005). Components of nucleotide excision repair and DNA damage tolerance in *Arabidopsis thaliana*. *Environ Mol Mutagen.*, 45(2-3):115-27

Kunz, B.A., Cahill, D.M., Mohr, P.G., Osmond, M.J. & Vonarx, E.J. (2006). Plant responses to UV radiation and links to pathogen resistance. *Int Rev Cytol.*, 255:1-40

Kuraoka, I., Ito, S., Wada, T., Hayashida, M., Lee, L., Saijo, M., Nakatsu, Y., Matsumoto, M., Matsunaga, T., Handa, H., Qin, J., Nakatani, Y. & Tanaka, K. (2008). Isolation of

XAB2 complex involved in pre-mRNA splicing, transcription, and transcription-coupled repair. *J Biol Chem.*, 283(2):940-50

Lainé, J.P. & Egly, J.M. (2006). Initiation of DNA repair mediated by a stalled RNA polymerase IIO. *EMBO J.*, 25(2):387-97

Landry, L.G., Stapleton, A.E., Lim, J., Hoffman, P., Hays, J.B., Walbot, V. & Last, R.L. (1997). An *Arabidopsis* photolyase mutant is hypersensitive to ultraviolet-B radiation. *Proc Natl Acad Sci U S A.*, 94(1):328-32

Lee, J. & Zhou, P. (2007). DCAFs, the missing link of the CUL4-DDB1 ubiquitin ligase. *Mol Cell*, 26(6):775-80

Lee, J.H., Terzaghi, W., Gusmaroli, G., Charron, J.B., Yoon, H.J., Chen, H., He, Y.J., Xiong, Y. & Deng, X.W. (2008). Characterization of *Arabidopsis* and rice DWD proteins and their roles as substrate receptors for CUL4-RING E3 ubiquitin ligases. *Plant Cell*, 20(1):152-67

Liang, L., Flury, S., Kalck, V., Hohn, B. & Molinier, J. (2006). CENTRIN2 interacts with the *Arabidopsis* homolog of the human XPC protein (AtRAD4) and contributes to efficient synthesis-dependent repair of bulky DNA lesions. *Plant Mol Biol.*, 61(1-2):345-56

Liu, Z., Hossain, G.S., Islas-Osuna, M.A., Mitchell, D.L. & Mount, D.W. (2000). Repair of UV damage in plants by nucleotide excision repair: *Arabidopsis* UVH1 DNA repair gene is a homolog of *Saccharomyces cerevisiae* Rad1. *Plant J.*, 21(6):519-28

Liu, Z., Hall, J.D. & Mount, D.W. (2001). *Arabidopsis UVH3* gene is a homolog of the *Saccharomyces cerevisiae* RAD2 and human XPG DNA repair genes. *Plant J.*, 26(3):329-38

Liu, Z., Hong, S.W., Escobar, M., Vierling, E., Mitchell, D.L., Mount, D.W. & Hall, J.D. (2003). *Arabidopsis* UVH6, a homolog of human XPD and yeast RAD3 DNA repair genes, functions in DNA repair and is essential for plant growth. *Plant Physiol.*, 132(3):1405-14

Luijsterburg, M.S., Goedhart, J., Moser, J., Kool, H., Geverts, B., Houtsmuller, A.B., Mullenders, L.H., Vermeulen, W. & van Driel, R. (2007). Dynamic in vivo interaction of DDB2 E3 ubiquitin ligase with UV-damaged DNA is independent of damage-recognition protein XPC. *J Cell Sci.*, 120(15):2706-16

Mackerness, S. (2000). Plant responses to ultraviolet-B (UV-B:280–320 nm) stress: What are the key regulators? *Plant Growth Regul.*, 37:27-39

Marwedel, T., Ishibashi, T., Lorbiecke, R., Jacob, S., Sakaguchi, K. & Sauter, M. (2003). Plant-specific regulation of replication protein A2 (OsRPA2) from rice during the cell cycle and in response to ultraviolet light exposure. *Planta.*, 217(3):457-65

Mellon, I. (2005). Transcription-coupled repair: a complex affair. *Mutat Res.*, 577(1-2):155-61

Mocquet, V., Lainé, J.P., Riedl, T., Yajin, Z., Lee, M.Y. & Egly, J.M. (2008). Sequential recruitment of the repair factors during NER: the role of XPG in initiating the resynthesis step. *EMBO J.*, 27(1):155-67

Molinier, J., Ramos, C., Fritsch, O. & Hohn, B. (2004). CENTRIN2 modulates homologous recombination and nucleotide excision repair in *Arabidopsis*. *Plant Cell*, 16(6):1633-43

Molinier, J., Lechner, E., Dumbliauskas, E. & Genschik, P. (2008). Regulation and role of *Arabidopsis* CUL4-DDB1A-DDB2 in maintaining genome integrity upon UV stress. *PloS Genetics*, 4(6):e10000

Morgante, P.G., Berra, C.M., Nakabashi, M., Costa, R.M., Menck, C.F. & Van Sluys, M.A. (2005). Functional XPB/RAD25 redundancy in *Arabidopsis* genome: characterization of AtXPB2 and expression analysis. *Gene*, 344:93-103

Nakagawa, M., Takahashi, S., Tanaka, A., Narumi, I. & Sakamoto, A.N. (2011). Role of AtPol{zeta}, AtRev1, and AtPol{eta} in UV light-induced mutagenesis in *Arabidopsis*. *Plant Physiol.*, 155(1):414-20

Nakajima, S., Sugiyama, M., Iwai, S., Hitomi, K., Otoshi, E., Kim, S.T., Jiang, C.Z., Todo, T., Britt, A.B. & Yamamoto, K. (1998). Cloning and characterization of a gene (*UVR3*) required for photorepair of 6-4 photoproducts in *Arabidopsis thaliana*. *Nucleic Acids Res.*, 26(2):638-44

Nakatsu, Y., Asahina, H., Citterio, E., Rademakers, S., Vermeulen, W., Kamiuchi, S., Yeo, J.P., Khaw, M.C., Saijo, M., Kodo, N., Matsuda, T., Hoeijmakers, J.H. & Tanaka, K. (2000). XAB2, a novel tetratricopeptide repeat protein involved in transcription-coupled DNA repair and transcription. *J Biol Chem.*, 275(45):34931-7

Nishi, R., Okuda, Y., Watanabe, E., Mori, T., Iwai, S., Masutani, C., Sugasawa, K. & Hanaoka, F. (2005). Centrin2 stimulates nucleotide excision repair by interacting with xeroderma pigmentosum group C protein. *Mol Cell Biol.*, 25(13):5664-74

Oravecz, A., Baumann, A., Máté, Z., Brzezinska, A., Molinier, J., Oakeley, E.J., Adám, E., Schäfer, E., Nagy, F. & Ulm, R. (2006). CONSTITUTIVELY PHOTOMORPHOGENIC1 is required for the UV-B response in *Arabidopsis*. *Plant Cell*, 18(8):1975-90

Pandey, R., Müller, A., Napoli, C.A., Selinger, D.A., Pikaard, C.S., Richards, E.J., Bender, J., Mount, D.W. & Jorgensen, R.A. (2002). Analysis of histone acetyltransferase and histone deacetylase families of *Arabidopsis thaliana* suggests functional diversification of chromatin modification among multicellular eukaryotes. *Nucleic Acids Res.*, 30(23):5036-55

Pang, Q. & Hays, J.B. (1991). UV-B-Inducible and Temperature-Sensitive Photoreactivation of Cyclobutane Pyrimidine Dimers in *Arabidopsis thaliana*. *Plant Physiol.*, 95(2):536-43

Parry, G. & Estelle, M. (2004). Regulation of Cullin based ubiquitin ligases by the Nedd8/RUB ubiquitin like proteins. *Semin Cell Dev. Biol.*, 15: 221-229

Pepper, A., Delaney, T., Washburn, T., Poole, D. & Chory, J. (1994). DET1, a negative regulator of light-mediated development and gene expression in *Arabidopsis*, encodes a novel nuclear-localized protein. *Cell*, 78(1):109-16

Preuss, S.B. & Britt, A.B. (2003). A DNA-damage-induced cell cycle checkpoint in *Arabidopsis*. *Genetics*, 164(1):323-34

Rapić-Otrin, V., McLenigan, M.P., Bisi, D.C., Gonzalez, M. & Levine, A.S. (2002). Sequential binding of UV DNA damage binding factor and degradation of the p48 subunit as early events after UV irradiation. *Nucleic Acids Res.*, 30(11):2588-98

Ribeiro, D.T., Machado, C.R., Costa, R.M., Praekelt, U.M., Van Sluys, M.A. & Menck, C.F. (1998). Cloning of a cDNA from *Arabidopsis thaliana* homologous to the human XPB gene. *Gene*, 208(2):207-13

Riedl, T., Hanaoka, F. & Egly, J.M. (2003). The comings and goings of nucleotide excision repair factors on damaged DNA. *EMBO J.*, 22(19):5293-303

Ries, G., Heller, W., Puchta, H., Sandermann, H., Seidlitz, H.K. & Hohn, B. (2000). Elevated UV-B radiation reduces genome stability in plants. *Nature*, 406(6791):98-101

Roy, S., Choudhury, S.R., Singh, S.K. & Das, K.P. (2011). AtPolλ, A Homolog of Mammalian DNA Polymerase λ in *Arabidopsis thaliana*, is Involved in the Repair of UV-B Induced DNA Damage through the Dark Repair Pathway. *Plant Cell Physiol.*, 52(2): 448-467

Sakaguchi, K., Ishibashi, T., Uchiyama, Y. & Iwabata, K. (2009). The multi-replication protein A (RPA) system--a new perspective. *FEBS J.*, 276(4):943-63

Sakamoto, A., Lan, V.T., Hase, Y., Shikazono, N., Matsunaga, T. & Tanaka, A. (2003). Disruption of the *AtREV3* gene causes hypersensitivity to ultraviolet B light and gamma-rays in *Arabidopsis*: implication of the presence of a translesion synthesis mechanism in plants. *Plant Cell,* 15(9):2042-57

Sakamoto, A.N., Lan, V.T., Puripunyavanich, V., Hase, Y., Yokota, Y., Shikazono, N., Nakagawa, M., Narumi, I. & Tanaka, A. (2009). A UVB-hypersensitive mutant in *Arabidopsis thaliana* is defective in the DNA damage response. *Plant J.*, 60(3):509-17

Sancar, A. (2003). Structure and function of DNA photolyase and cryptochrome blue-light photoreceptors. *Chem Rev.*, 103(6):2203-37

Sancar, A. (2008). Structure and function of photolyase and in vivo enzymology: 50th anniversary. *J Biol Chem.*, 283(47):32153-7

Santiago, M.J., Alejandre-Durán, E. & Ruiz-Rubio, M. (2006). Analysis of UV-induced mutation spectra in *Escherichia coli* by DNA polymerase eta from *Arabidopsis thaliana. Mutat Res.*, 601(1-2):51-60

Santiago, M.J., Ruiz-Rubio, M., Dio, L.D., González-Reyes, J.A. & Alejandre-Durán, E. (2008a). Ubiquitous expression of two translesion synthesis DNA polymerase genes in *Arabidopsis*. *Planta,* 227(6):1269-77

Santiago, M.J., Alejandre-Durán, E., Muñoz-Serrano, A. & Ruiz-Rubio, M. (2008b). Two translesion synthesis DNA polymerase genes, *AtPOLH* and *AtREV1*, are involved in development and UV light resistance in *Arabidopsis*. *J Plant Physiol.*, 165(15):1582-91

Santiago, M.J., Alejandre-Durán, E. & Ruiz-Rubio, M. (2009). Alternative splicing of two translesion synthesis DNA polymerases from *Arabidopsis thaliana*. *Plant Science,* 176(4):591-596

Saxowsky, T.T. & Doetsch, P.W. (2006). RNA polymerase encounters with DNA damage: transcription-coupled repair or transcriptional mutagenesis? *Chem Rev.*, 106(2):474-88

Schroeder, D.F., Gahrtz, M., Maxwell, B.B., Cook, R.K., Kan, J.M., Alonso, J.M., Ecker, J.R. & Chory, J. (2002). De-etiolated1 and Damaged DNA Binding Protein 1 interact to regulate *Arabidopsis* photomorphogenesis. *Curr Biol.*, 12(17):1462-72

Schultz, T.F. & Quatrano R.S. (1997). Characterization and expression of a rice *RAD23* gene. *Plant Mol Biol.*, 34: 557-562

Schwechheimer, C. & Deng, X.W. (2001). COP9 signalosome revisited: a novel mediator of protein degradation. *Trends Cell Biol.*, 11(10):420-426

Scrima, A., Konícková, R., Czyzewski, B.K., Kawasaki, Y., Jeffrey, P.D., Groisman, R., Nakatani, Y., Iwai, S., Pavletich, N.P. & Thomä, N.H. (2008). Structural basis of UV DNA-damage recognition by the DDB1-DDB2 complex. *Cell,* 135(7):1213-23

Shaked, H., Avivi-Ragolsky, N. & Levy, A.A. (2006). Involvement of the *Arabidopsis* SWI2/SNF2 chromatin remodeling gene family in DNA damage response and recombination. *Genetics,* 173(2):985-94

Shultz, R.W., Tatineni, V.M., Hanley-Bowdoin, L. & Thompson, W.F. (2007). Genome-wide analysis of the core DNA replication machinery in the higher plants *Arabidopsis* and rice. *Plant Physiol.*, 144(4):1697-714

Singh, S.K., Roy, S., Choudhury, S.R. & Sengupta, D.N. (2010). DNA repair and recombination in higher plants: insights from comparative genomics of *Arabidopsis* and rice. *BMC Genomics*, 11:443

Soria, G. & Gottifredi, V. (2010). PCNA-coupled p21 degradation after DNA damage: The exception that confirms the rule? *DNA Repair (Amst)*, 9(4):358-64

Strzalka, W. & Ziemienowicz, A. (2011). Proliferating cell nuclear antigen (PCNA): a key factor in DNA replication and cell cycle regulation. *Ann Bot.* 107(7):1127-40

Sturm, A. & Leinhard, S. (1998). Two isoforms of plant RAD 23 complement a UV sensitive rad23 mutant in yeast. *Plant J.*, 13(6): 815-821

Sugasawa, K., Okuda, Y., Saijo, M., Nishi, R., Matsuda, N., Chu, G., Mori, T., Iwai, S., Tanaka, K., Tanaka, K. & Hanaoka, F. (2005). UV-induced ubiquitylation of XPC protein mediated by UV-DDB-ubiquitin ligase complex. *Cell*, 121(3):387-400

Svejstrup, J.Q. (2002). Mechanisms of Transcription coupled repair. *Nat Rev Mol Cell Biol.*, 3(1):21-29

Takahashi, M., Teranishi, M., Ishida, H., Kawasaki, J., Takeuchi, A., Yamaya, T., Watanabe, M., Makino, A. & Hidema, J. (2011). Cyclobutane pyrimidine dimer (CPD) photolyase repairs ultraviolet-B-induced CPDs in rice chloroplast and mitochondrial DNA. *Plant J.*, 66(3):433-42

Takahashi, S., Nakajima, N., Saji, H. & Kondo, N. (2002). Diurnal change of cucumber CPD photolyase gene (*CsPHR*) expression and its physiological role in growth under UV-B irradiation. *Plant Cell Physiol.*, 43(3):342-9

Takahashi, S., Sakamoto, A., Sato, S., Kato, T., Tabata, S. & Tanaka, A. (2005). Roles of *Arabidopsis* AtREV1 and AtREV7 in translesion synthesis. *Plant Physiol.*, 138(2):870-81

Takahashi, S., Sakamoto, A.N., Tanaka, A. & Shimizu, K. (2007). AtREV1, a Y-family DNA polymerase in *Arabidopsis*, has deoxynucleotidyl transferase activity in vitro. *Plant Physiol.*, 145(3):1052-60

Takashi, Y., Kobayashi, Y., Tanaka, K. & Tamura, K. (2009). *Arabidopsis* replication protein A 70a is required for DNA damage response and telomere length homeostasis. *Plant Cell Physiol.*, 50(11):1965-76

Tanaka, A., Sakamoto, A., Ishigaki, Y., Nikaido, O., Sun, G., Hase, Y., Shikazono, N., Tano, S. & Watanabe, H. (2002). An ultraviolet-B resistant mutant with enhanced DNA repair in *Arabidopsis*. *Plant Physiol*, 129(1):64–71

Tapias, A., Auriol, J., Forget, D., Enzlin, J.H., Schärer, O.D., Coin, F., Coulombe, B. & Egly, J.M. (2004). Ordered conformational changes in damaged DNA induced by nucleotide excision repair factors. *J Biol Chem.*, 279(18):19074-83

Terai, K., Abbas, T., Jazaeri, A.A. & Dutta, A. (2010). CRL4(Cdt2) E3 ubiquitin ligase monoubiquitinates PCNA to promote translesion DNA synthesis. *Mol Cell*, 37(1):143-9

Todo, T., Ryo, H., Yamamoto, K., Toh, H., Inui, T., Ayaki, H., Nomura, T. & Ikenaga, M. (1996). Similarity among the Drosophila (6-4)photolyase, a human photolyase homolog, and the DNA photolyase-blue-light photoreceptor family. *Science*, 272(5258):109-12

Tornaletti, S. (2009). DNA repair in mammalian cells: Transcription-coupled DNA repair: directing your effort where it's most needed. *Cell Mol Life Sci.*, 66(6):1010-20

Ueda, T., Sato, T., Hidema, J., Hirouchi, T., Yamamoto, K., Kumagai, T. & Yano, M. (2005). qUVR-10, a major quantitative trait locus for ultraviolet-B resistance in rice, encodes cyclobutane pyrimidine dimer photolyase. *Genetics,* 171(4):1941-50

Ulm, R., Baumann, A., Oravecz, A., Máté, Z., Adám, E., Oakeley, E.J., Schäfer, E. & Nagy, F. (2004). Genome-wide analysis of gene expression reveals function of the bZIP transcription factor HY5 in the UV-B response of *Arabidopsis*. *Proc Natl Acad Sci U S A.*, 101(5):1397-402

Vannier, J.B., Depeiges, A., White, C. & Gallego, M.E. (2009). ERCC1/XPF protects short telomeres from homologous recombination in *Arabidopsis thaliana*. *PLoS Genet.*, 5(2):e1000380

van den Boom, V., Citterio, E., Hoogstraten, D., Zotter, A., Egly, J.M., van Cappellen, W.A., Hoeijmakers, J.H., Houtsmuller, A.B. & Vermeulen, W. (2004). DNA damage stabilizes interaction of CSB with the transcription elongation machinery. *J Cell Biol.*, 166(1):27-36

Volker, M., Mone, M.J., Karmakar, P., van Hoffen, A., Schul, W., Vermeulen, W., Hoeijmakers, J.H., van Driel, R., van Zeeland, A.A. & Mullenders, L.H. (2001). Sequential assembly of the nucleotide excision repair factors in vivo. *Mol Cell,* 8(1):213–224

Vonarx, E.J., Howlett, N.G., Schiestl, R.H. & Kunz, B.A. (2002). Detection of *Arabidopsis thaliana* AtRAD1 cDNA variants and assessment of function by expression in a yeast rad1 mutant. *Gene,* 296(1-2):1-9

Vonarx, E.J., Tabone, E.K., Osmond, M.J., Anderson, H.J. & Kunz, B.A. (2006). *Arabidopsis* homologue of human transcription factor IIH/nucleotide excision repair factor p44 can function in transcription and DNA repair and interacts with AtXPD. *Plant J.*, 46(3):512-21

Wang, H., Zhai, L., Xu, J., Joo, H.Y., Jackson, S., Erdjument-Bromage, H., Tempst, P., Xiong, Y. & Zhang, Y. (2006). Histone H3 and H4 ubiquitylation by the CUL4-DDB-ROC1 ubiquitin ligase facilitates cellular response to DNA damage. *Mol Cell,* 22(3):383-94

Waters, L.S., Minesinger, B.K., Wiltrout, M.E., D'Souza, S., Woodruff, R.V. & Walker, G.C. (2009). Eukaryotic translesion polymerases and their roles and regulation in DNA damage tolerance. *Microbiol Mol Biol Rev.*, 73(1):134-54

Waterworth, W.M., Jiang, Q., West, C.E., Nikaido, M. & Bray, C.M. (2002). Characterization of *Arabidopsis* photolyase enzymes and analysis of their role in protection from ultraviolet-B radiation. *J Exp Bot.*, 53(371):1005-15

Weeda, G., Donker, I., De Wit, J., Morreau, H. Janssens, R., Vissers, C.J., Nigg, A., van Steeg, H., Bootsma, D. & Hoeijmakers, J.H. (1997). Disruption of mouse ERCC1 results in a novel repair syndrome with growth failure, nuclear abnormalities and senescence. *Curr Biol.*, 7(6): 427-39

Wold, M.S. (1997). Replication protein A: a heterotrimeric, single-stranded DNA-binding protein required for eukaryotic DNA metabolism. *Annu Rev Biochem.*, 66:61-92

Xu, H., Swoboda, I., Bhalla, P.L., Sijbers, A.M., Zhao, C., Ong, E.K., Hoeijmakers, J.H. & Singh, M.B. (1998). Plant homologue of human excision repair gene ERCC1 points to conservation of DNA repair mechanisms. *Plant J.*, 13(6):823-9

Yamamoto, A., Hirouchi, T., Mori, T., Teranishi, M., Hidema. J., Morioka, H., Kumagai, T. & Yamamoto, K. (2007). Biochemical and biological properties of DNA photolyases derived from utraviolet-sensitive rice cultivars. *Genes Genet Syst.*, 82(4):311-9

Yamamoto, A., Tanbir, N., Hirouchi, T., Teranishi, M., Hidema, J., Morioka, H. & Yamamoto, K. (2008). Temperature-sensitive photoreactivation of cyclobutane thymine dimer in soybean. *J Radiat Res (Tokyo)*, 49(2):189-96

Yasui, A., Eker, A.P., Yasuhira, S., Yajima, H., Kobayashi, T., Takao, M. & Oikawa, A. (1994). A new class of DNA photolyases present in various organisms including aplacental mammals. *EMBO J.*, 13(24):6143-51

Yoshihara, R., Imaki, T., Hori, M., Watanabe, C., Yamamoto, K. & Takimoto, K. (2005). CPD photolyase gene from *Spinacia oleracea*: repair of UV-damaged DNA and expression in plant organs. *J Radiat Res (Tokyo)*, 46(2):157-64

Yoshiyama, K., Conklin, P.A., Huefner, N.D. & Britt, A.B. (2009). Suppressor of gamma response 1 (SOG1) encodes a putative transcription factor governing multiple responses to DNA damage. *Proc Natl Acad Sci USA*, 106(31):12843-8

Yuzhakov, A., Kelman, Z., Hurwitz, J. & O'Donnell, M. (1999). Multiple competition reactions for RPA order the assembly of the DNA polymerase delta holoenzyme. *EMBO J.*, 18(21):6189-99

Zhang, C., Guo, H., Zhang, J., Guo, G., Schumaker, K.S. & Guo, Y. (2010). *Arabidopsis* cockayne syndrome A-like proteins 1A and 1B form a complex with CULLIN4 and damage DNA binding protein 1A and regulate the response to UV irradiation. *Plant Cell*, 22(7):2353-69

Zhang, L., Xu, Q., Xing, D., Gao, C. & Xiong, H. (2009). Real-time detection of caspase-3-like protease activation in vivo using fluorescence resonance energy transfer during plant programmed cell death induced by ultraviolet C overexposure. *Plant Physiol.*, 150(4):1773-83

# 5

# DNA Helix Destabilization by Alkylating Agents: From Covalent Bonding to DNA Repair

Gaëlle Lenglet, Sabine Depauw, Denise Mendy-Belaiche and Marie-Hélène David-Cordonnier

*INSERM, Jean-Pierre Aubert Research Center (JPARC), Team 4 Molecular and Cellular Targeting for Cancer Treatment and University of Lille-Grand Nord, Institut pour la Recherche sur le Cancer de Lille, Place de Verdun, Lille France*

## 1. Introduction

Preservation of the integrity of the DNA, carrier of heritage information, is crucial for cell survival. Altered genetic information could lead to major perturbations in cell organization, function and proliferation of cancer cells. Because cancer cells are highly proliferative with high number of replication, DNA was the first clinically used anti-cancer therapeutic target with the drugs directly (intercalators/alkylating drugs) or indirectly (micro-tubules, topoisomerases inhibitors, modifiers of histone acetylation...) targeting DNA. Despite the actual development of targeted chemotherapies (against membrane receptors, kinases, the proteasome,...), direct DNA targeting drugs still represent a major part of the actual anti-cancer pharmacopeia in terms of total prescriptions and efficacy. Compounds mainly bind DNA in three different ways: non-covalent (fitting in major or minor grooves), intercalation between two successive base pairs, or covalent bonding to a base, and generally lead to a stabilization of the DNA double helix. Only a few number from intercalating and alkylating families destabilizes the DNA helix. Cytotoxic effects of alkylating agents (used/developed for chemotherapy or from carcinogens) are strongly attenuated by the cellular DNA repair processes. Optimal use of DNA alkylating drugs in therapy requires a clear understanding of their DNA repair processes. Similarly, knowing how cells cope with the carcinogens-induced DNA damages is of major interest regarding health in our actual society, so prompt to use chemical compounds insufficiently studied for long term toxicities and sometimes eventually identified as carcinogens (food and industries). DNA repair processes infer with both those Yin and Yang aspects of alkylating compounds using different machineries: base excision repair (BER); nucleotide excision repair (NER: long/short-patch, transcription-coupled/global genome); mismatch repair (MMR); homologous recombination (HR) or non-homologous end-joining (NHEJ). Fanconi anemia (FA) repair acts as a coordinator of those repair pathways (Moldovan & D'Andrea, 2009). Since there are yet various complete reviews on DNA repair processes in the literature, the present review will focus on the repair process of DNA destabilizing compounds.

## 2. DNA destabilizing compounds

Stability of DNA double helix is mainly due to reversible non-covalent hydrogen bonds between Watson-Crick base-pairs. Local or global denaturation (melting or breathing) of the double-stranded DNA (dsDNA) helix is dispensable for different cellular processes: DNA replication, transcription and repair (Choi et al., 2004; Schneider et al., 2001). DNA melting is affected by sequence (AT- or GC-rich portions, some successive base pairs arrangements) and their specific tilt, roll, twist effects (Benham, 1996; Dornberger et al., 1999; Krueger et al., 2006), the formation of local hairpins, 3D structures at terminal regions of the DNA helix (Putnam et al., 1981) or internal portions of B- to Z-DNA transition (Harvey, 1983). Such locally opened sites are good substrates for, or are generated by, some cellular proteins: DNA helicases (Betterton & Julicher, 2005), single strand binding proteins (SSBP) such as replication protein A (RPA) (Wold, 1997), UP1 and myeloma helix-destabilizing protein (Herrick & Alberts, 1976; Planck & Wilson, 1980), GAPDH-related protein P8 (Karpel & Burchard, 1981), High Mobility Group (HMG) proteins (Butler et al., 1985), c-Abl kinase (David-Cordonnier et al., 1998, 1999), HIV-1 nucleocapsid protein (Narayanan et al., 2006), prion protein (Bera et al., 2007), NF-$\kappa$B transcription factor (Mura & McCammon, 2008) and UHRF-1 protein (Arita et al., 2008). Besides large DNA opening, small modifications such as base flipping locally perturb DNA stability (Hornby & Ford, 1998) during mismatches or repair proteins interaction from NER (Cao et al., 2004), BER (Bellamy et al., 2007; Tubbs et al., 2007) or DNA methylases/demethylases (Sundheim et al., 2008).
Besides naturally occurring DNA breathing, unzipping is induced by clinically used or potential anti-tumor compounds. The vast majority of DNA-interacting compounds stabilize the DNA double helix; only a very few of them displays the pecular ability to destabilize DNA helix. In this latter group, most belong to DNA intercalating or alkylating families.

### 2.1 DNA intercalators as helix destabilizing agents

#### 2.1.1 Mono-intercalators

Historically, the first DNA intercalating compound evidencing DNA destabilization properties was acridine orange (Figure 1), a well-known dsDNA intercalating compound and a strong single-stranded DNA (ssDNA) binder. It emitted green fluorescence emission from dsDNA binding and red luminescence from ssDNA interaction. Acridine orange enhances the global helix stability but exerts local denaturation of DNA (Kapuscinski & Darzynkiewicz, 1983; 1984; Darzynkiewicz et al, 1983). Ellipticine and adriamycin (Figure 1) also induce local unzipping of the DNA and bind ssDNA (Zunino et al., 1972), in contrast with ethidium bromide (BET), highly specific to dsDNA and stabilizing DNA. Intercalation of acridine orange, ellipticine and adriamycin progressively unzip the DNA helix preferentially in heterochromatin, ribosomes and polysomes (Darzynkiewicz et al., 1983).

#### 2.1.2 Bis-intercalators

Bisacridine A (BisA) (Figure 1) is a DNA unwinding bis-intercalator deriving from acridine orange by cyclization of two acridine planar chromophores using polyammonium bridges. Initially designed to interact with ss- rather than ds-DNA (Teulade-Fichou et al., 1995), BisA shifts duplexes DNA toward hairpins and destabilizes dsDNA (Slama-Schwok et al., 1997).

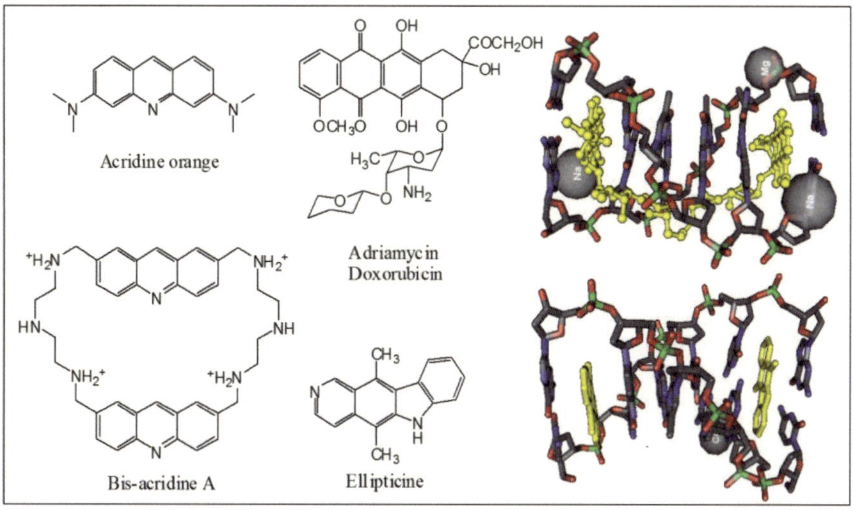


Fig. 1. DNA intercalators that destabilize the DNA helix: structures and 3D orientation of morpholino-doxorubicin (Top, [mmdbId:52942]) or ellipticine (Bottom, [mmdbId:52189]).

### 2.2 DNA alkylators as helix destabilizing agents

Some DNA alkylating drugs could also locally destabilize DNA double helix. Some of those are used/developed as anticancer drugs such as cisplatin and metal-derivatives, or more recently the benzoacronycine derivative S23906-1. They contrast with most DNA alkylating agents used or not in chemotherapy that stabilize DNA helix (for instance mitomycin C, dinuclear platinum, nitrogen mustards or ecteinascidine 743) (Basu et al., 1993; David-Cordonnier et al., 2005; Fridman et al., 2003; Kasparkova et al., 1999). Electrophilic alkylating drugs react at nucleophilic positions of G-C or A-T bp with preferential targets: $N^7$ position of dG or dA and $O^6$ position of dG in the major groove, $N^3$ positions of dG or dA and exocyclic $NH_2$ group on $C^2$ of dG (also called $N^2$) in the minor groove (Figure 2).

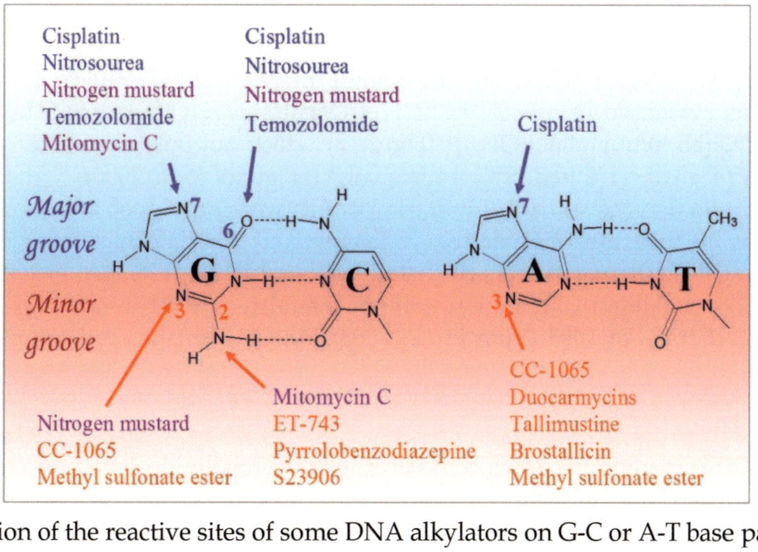


Fig. 2. Position of the reactive sites of some DNA alkylators on G-C or A-T base pairs.

### 2.2.1 Cisplatin and other transition-metal antitumor agents as DNA destabilizing drugs

Fortuitously discovered in 1965, cisplatin (or *cis*-diaminedichloridoplatinum(II) is used in clinic since 1978 and is still frequently administrated in combinatory chemotherapies as one of the most effective anticancer drugs against solid tumors (Figure 3). Cisplatin forms inter- and intra-strand crosslinks as well as monovalent adducts. Those lesions occur primarily though covalent bonding to the $N^7$ atom of guanines. The most common lesions are intra-strand crosslink at the 5′-GG (65%) or 5′-AG (25%) dinucleotides and inter-strand crosslinks (5-8%). This latter lesion is more frequent using transplatin (12%), *trans*-$PtCl_2(NH_3)$(quinoline) and *trans*-$PtCl_2(NH_3)$(thiazole) derivatives (up to 30%) (Figure 3). Cisplatin-induced intra-strand crosslinks at GpG base-pairs result in a strong DNA helix bending toward the major groove with an angle of 55-78° associated with DNA distortion, resulting in a destabilization of the Watson-Crick base pairing and local denaturation of the DNA helix (bending at 45° and unwinding by 79+/.4°) (Bellon, 1991; Malinge et al., 1994; Todd & Lippard, 2010). In platinated-GpG intra-strand crosslinks, the distortion varies and depends on the sequence context, with up to a 7 bp distortion for 1,3-intrastrand crosslinks within a TGTGT sequence (Kasparkova et al., 2008a). Such destabilization was found to be enthalpic, but not entropic, in origin. Similarly, when occurring at 5′-TGGT site, cisplatin adducts decrease the melting temperature of the DNA by more than 10°C which is much higher than that induced on 5′-CGGT and 5′-AGGC sequences (~6°C) (Malina et al., 2007). Such effects are not observed with transplatin which does not change the transition entropy or enthalpy and, consequently, does not destabilize the DNA helix (Kasparkova et al., 2008a). Third-generation platinum antitumor derivative oxaliplatin (Figure 3) induces greater DNA bending, unwinding and helix destabilization than cisplatin, whereas JM118 (Figure 3) induces DNA destabilization profiles similar to that of cisplatin (Kostrhunova et al., 2010). JM118 is the major metabolite of satraplatin (JM216), the first orally administered platinum drug that also evidenced promising therapeutic activities in prostate cancer. JM118 induces a DNA bending with an angle of 28° toward the major groove, an angle smaller than that obtained with cisplatin for the same sequence (34°) (Kostrhunova et al., 2010).
Besides the nature of the platinated drug, the surrounding DNA sequence is also of major importance for helix stability. Indeed, monofunctional platinum adducts at 5′-TGC triplet induces major DNA destabilization (Brabec et al., 1992) but none at 5′-AGT or 5′-TGA triplet (Schwartz et al., 1989). DNA is not the unique nucleic acid destabilized by platinated derivatives as evidenced using *cis*-$[PtCl(NH_3)_2(OH_2)]^+$, *cis*-$[PtCl(NH_3)(c\text{-}C_6H_{11}NH_2)(OH_2)]^+$ and *trans*-$[PtCl(NH_3)(\text{quinoline})(OH_2)]^+$ (Figure 3) which not only destabilize ds-DNA but also ds-RNA (ΔTm of -11°C and -5°C, respectively) (Hägerlöf et al., 2006).
Besides platinum derivatives, ruthenium compounds were developed as anti-cancer drugs. NAMI-A was the first ruthenium derivative that entered phase I clinical trials in 1999 as an anti-metastatic drug (Bergamo et al., 2002), followed by KP1019 (FFC14A) in 2003 (Hartinger et al., 2008). Two gallium compounds, gallium maltolate and KP46 (FFC11), also entered phase I clinical trials in 2003 (Lum et al., 2003). As for cisplatin, ruthenium derivatives evidenced DNA destabilization properties. This is particularly well described for Ru-CYM ([(η6-π-cymene)Ru(II)(en)-(Cl)]+ and Ru-BIP, Ru-DHA or Ru-THA as biphenyl, dihydroanthracene or tetrahydroanthracene derivatives, respectively (Figure 3). Such organometallic ruthenium(II) arene complexes were rationally designed for chemotherapy with the idea that changing platinum for ruthenium would provide additional coordination sites in the octahedral complexes to modify the oxidation rate and change ligand affinity

and binding kinetics (C.X. Zhang & Lippard, 2003). From this series, Ru-CYM presents the highest DNA helix destabilization activity, together with the smaller unwinding angle in supercoiled plasmid DNA (7° *vs.* 14° for Ru-BIP, Ru-DHA and Ru-THA), in correlation with its lack of intercalation and the formation of monoadducts at $N^7$-dG (Nováková et al., 2009). New Ru-derivatives monodentate-Ru(II) and $[Ru(terpy)(4,4'\text{-}(COLysCONH_2)_2bpy)Cl]^{3+}$ also destabilize DNA (Nováková et al., 2010; Triantafillidi et al., 2011). For gallium-complexed compounds, interaction of trivalent Ga-cations with calf-thymus DNA resulted in major helix destabilization with perturbations at A-T base pairs sites (R. Ahmad et al. 1996).

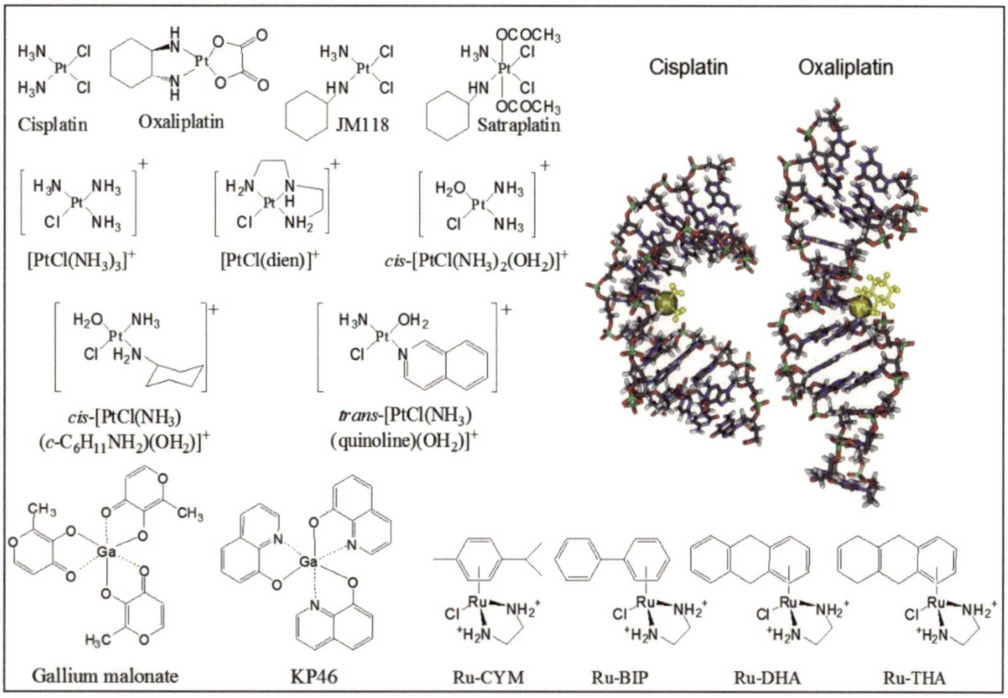


Fig. 3. Structure of cisplatin and other transition-metal agents as DNA destabilizing drugs and 3D orientation [mmdbId:47796] (cisplatin) and [mmdbId:69361] (oxaliplatin).

### 2.2.2 Carcinogens as DNA destabilizing agents

DNA interaction of carcinogen, adduct formation and their repair processes are widely studied using carcinogens from environmental and tobacco smoke. Some of them have the ability to destabilize the DNA helix: BPDE ((+/-)-*anti*-benzo[*a*]pyrene-7,8-dihydrodiol-9,10-epoxide) and 4-OHEN (4-hydroxyequilenin-O-quinone) (Figure 4).

The smoke carcinogen benzo[*a*]pyrene (BaP) is metabolized into several enantiomers of BPDE that covalently bond the exocyclic $NH_2$ group of guanines to form a bulky adduct in the minor groove of the DNA helix, resulting in its destabilization (Zou & Van Houten, 1999). Due to the orientation of the reactive epoxide group on asymmetric carbons, several enantiomers are produced. The most carcinogenic is 10S(+)-*trans-anti*-BPDE $N^2$-dG adduct followed by the stereo-isomeric 10R(+)-*cis-anti*-BPDE-$N^2$-dG adducts. Covalent bonding to DNA is associated with base-displaced intercalation where the bulky adduct prevents the hydrogen bonding of the amino group of guanine with the opposite cytosine. This results in a base-flipping where the (+)-*anti*-B[*a*]P-N$^2$-dG bulky adduct is located in the minor groove and the opposite cytosine is positioned in the major groove (Cosman et al., 1993). The precise orientation of this highly carcinogenic 10S(+)-*trans-anti*-B[*a*]P-N$^2$-dG adduct depends on the sequence surrounding the target guanine (Cai et al., 2010). DNA is untwisted at 5'-CGG*C sites where a large bend is induced in the DNA helix, but not at 5'-CG*GC sequences where, conversely, DNA helix is destabilized in its portion orientated 5' to the lesion (Rodríguez et al., 2007). Such differences result in different protein/DNA recognition and repair activities (see 3.4). Thermal destabilization was also observed using 14R(+)-*trans-anti*-DB[*a,l*]P-N$^2$-dG adduct (Zheng et al., 2010) or *14S*(-)-*trans-anti*-DB[*a,l*]P-N$^6$-dA adducts whereas *14R*(+) isomer stabilizes the ds-DNA (Cai et al., 2011).

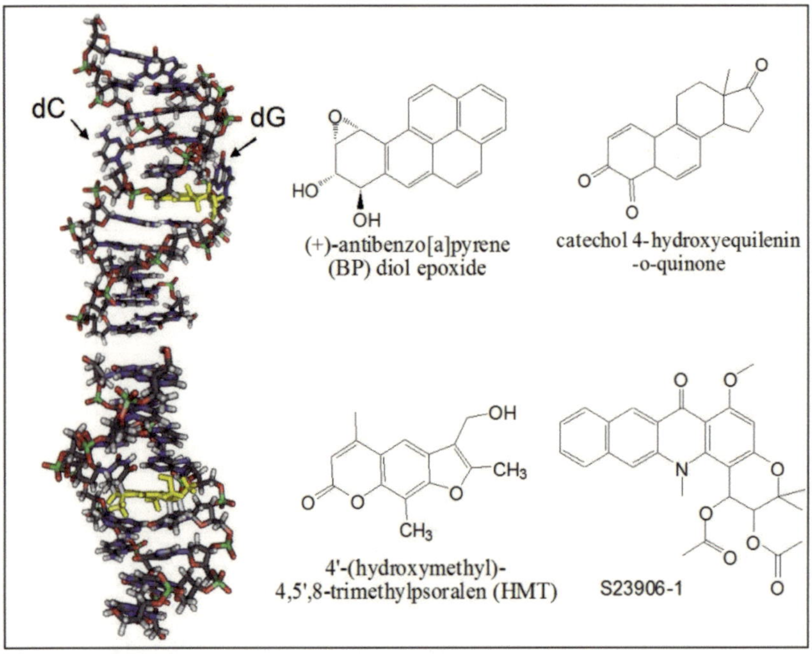


Fig. 4. 3D orientation of (+)-*anti*-BPDE [mmdbId:52106] and the psoralen derivative HMT [mmdbId:52343] and structure of some DNA alkylators that destabilize the DNA helix.

The hormone-derived genotoxic compound, 4-OHEN, derives from equilin and equilenin, two equine oestrogens present in hormone substitution therapies used to prevent the uncomfortable effects of menopauses but are also thought to increase breast cancer incidence in the population of hormonally-treated women (Rossouw et al., 2002). Its ortho-quinone form is cytotoxic and genotoxic (Pisha et al., 2001) through the formation of bulky DNA lesions at dA, dC and dG (but not at T residues) (Kolbanovskiy et al., 2005) which were detected in both cell culture and breast cancer biopsies from patients treated with hormone substitution therapies (Embrechts et al., 2003). 4-OHEN derived from the intermediate catechol 4-hydroxyequilenin which was generated from a rapid conversion of both equilin and equilenin in the organism to four stereo-isomers differently affecting the 3D-structure of the DNA helix (Ding et al., 2007). For adducts on cytosine, the *syn*- or *anti*-conformations of the bulky rings of 4-OHEN point along the major or the minor groove (Ding et al., 2005). Interestingly, alkylation at dA or dC residues is associated with a strong decrease in the melting temperature (Tm) of a 11-bp oligonucleotide, with the magnitude of the negative ΔTm values being lower when the adduct is located at 1 or 2-bp from the end of the 11-bp DNA (-6 to -9°C) then when it is located in its medium part (positions 4 to 8) with up to a -21 to -27°C decrease of Tm. Similarly, the stereoisomeric orientation of the 4-OHEN adduct affects the base-stacking, groove sizes and subsequent distortions and is also crucial for the extent of DNA destabilization (Kolbanovskiy et al., 2005).

### 2.2.3 Psoralen derivatives

Psoralen is a chemotherapeutic agent known to cause DNA inter-strand crosslinks (ICLs) upon absorption of two photons from UVA irradiation at 365 nm, preferentially at 5'-TA and to a lesser extend at 5'-AT dinucleotides. This activity was the basis for use of psoralen and UVA exposure (PUVA therapy) to treat cutaneous diseases like psoriasis, vitiligo, atopic dermatitis or cutaneous T cell lymphomas. However, such treatment increased the risk of squamous and basal cell carcinomas (Teicher, 1996). Psoralen-induced ICLs are classically used models for DNA repair of ICLs. The psoralen derivative 4'-(hydroxymethyl)-4,5',8-trimethylpsoralen (HMT) (Figure 4) evidenced DNA destabilization by mono-addition of a psoralen residue to both thymines (one on each strand) of 5'-GGGTACCC sequence.

### 2.2.4 Benzo-acronycine derivatives

Acronycine is a natural alkaloid extracted from the bark of an Australian ash scrub that presented interesting antitumor activities but was poorly soluble and, consequently, too toxic in first clinical trials. The discovery of an unstable acronycine epoxide opened the way to the rational drug design of S23906-1 (Figure 4), that appeared to be a highly active compound (Guilbaud et al., 2001) with an original mode of action (David-Cordonnier 2002; 2005; Depauw et al., 2009) and consequently entered phase I clinical trials in 2006. As for the clinically used drug Ecteinascidine 743 (ET-743, Trabectedin, Yondelis ™ from Pharmamar), S23906-1 alkylates the exocyclic $NH_2$ group of guanines in the minor groove. But, in contrast with ET-743, S23906-1 does not reinforce the stability of the ds-DNA helix but destabilizes it, generating portions of ss-DNA (David-Cordonnier et al., 2005; Depauw et al., 2009). Various spectral and biochemical approaches convinced with this conclusion. Indeed, classical DNA melting temperature studies evidenced a strong decrease of the Tm values upon alkylation with S23906-1 or other biologically active benzo-acronycine derivatives. Similarly, spectral analysis of the ratio of fluorescence properties of picogreen (a ds- and ss-DNA interacting dye) and BET (a ds-DNA specific dye) evidenced an increase of picogreen *vs.* BET fluorescence which enlightens the generation of single-stranded portions of the DNA upon S23906-1 alkylation. Biochemical approaches like digestion of the alkylated DNA by single-strand specific nuclease S1 and electrophoretic mobility shift assays (EMSAs) confirmed the opening of the DNA. The destabilization was relatively wide since mapping with nuclease S1 evidenced locally opened DNA portions within a 117 bp DNA fragment alkylated by S23906-1 whereas EMSAs, performed with oligonucleotides as long as 24 bp, evidenced fully single-stranded alkylated oligonucleotides in the presence of S23906-1 or derivatives (David-Cordonnier et al., 2005; Depauw et al., 2009).

## 3. Repair processes for DNA destabilizing lesions

DNA adducts are critical lesions for cell proliferation and survival. Single or multiple DNA repair machineries could be implicated in the removal of these damages, as for example

BER, GG-NER (global genome) or TC-NER (transcription-coupled), MMR, HR or NHEJ. Only few data are published about the consequences of non-covalent DNA destabilizing agents on protein/DNA binding from the repair machineries. These data on BisA function reported that insertion of BisA could flip the mispaired thymine to an extrahelical base subsequently inducing a sterical blockage of DNA glycosylases binding (David, 2003). The present section will therefore focus on alkylating compounds. As examples, we will shortly present the repair processes for the well-studied temolozomide-induced lesions in the major groove and for the DNA stabilizing drug ET-743, as an original minor groove alkylating agents that "poison" the NER machinery to exert its anti-tumor properties, before presenting the current knowledge on DNA repair of DNA destabilizing lesions.

### 3.1 Repair of temolozomide-induced DNA lesions

Temolozomide (TMZ, Temodar®, Figure 5) is a monofunctional alkylating agent chemically related to dacarbazine. It is active in vitro and in vivo against a wide variety of tumor type and particularly efficient in malignant glioma (Newlands et al., 1997). Contrasting with dacarbazine, TMZ does not require to be activated by enzymatic oxidation, but spontaneously hydrolyses to 5-(3-methyltriazen-l-yl)-imidazole-4-carboximide (MITC) at pH above 7. MITC is then broken down to (*i*) the reactive methyldiazonium cation which next loses the methyl group in the presence of DNA or proteins and (*ii*) the inactive 5-aminoimidazole-4-carboxyamide moiety (AIC) (**1**). TMZ treatment leads to different adducts on the double helix DNA: $N^3$-methyladenine, $N^7$-methylguanine and $O^6$-methylguanine

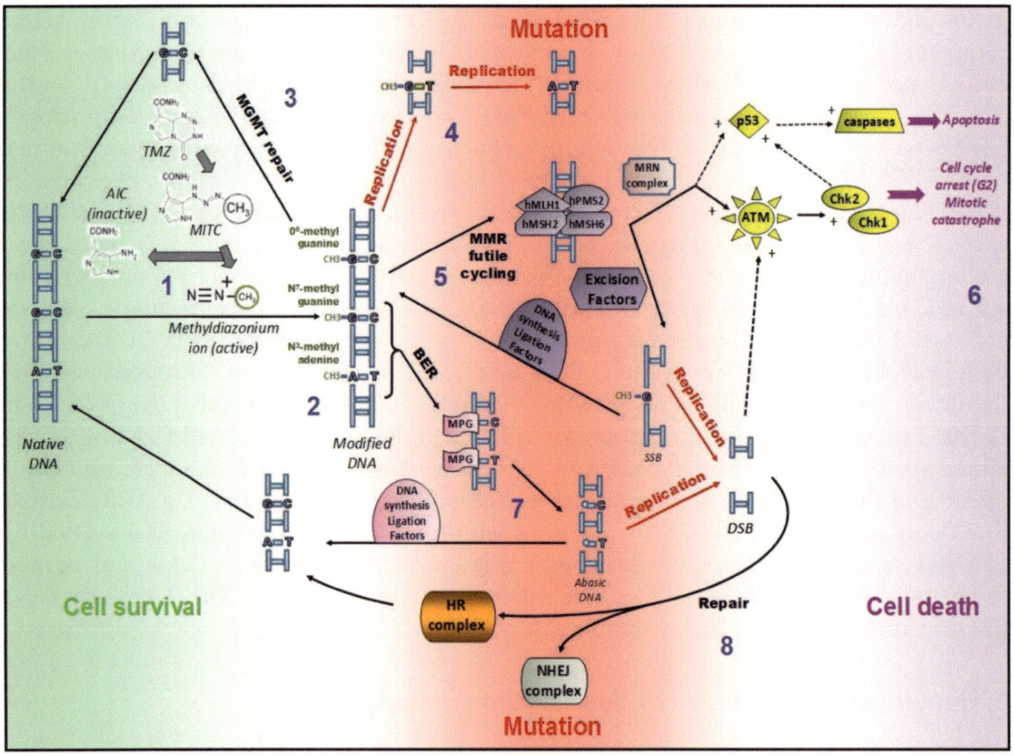


Fig. 5. DNA repair pathways for TMZ-induced damage.

(Newlands et al., 1997) and cell sensitivity to TMZ treatment depends on multiple DNA repair mechanisms (**2**). The major one is the recognition of methyl lesions from $O^6$ position of guanines by the $O^6$-methylguanine DNA methyltransferase (MGMT) protein which directly converts the methylated DNA to its normal, undamaged state (**3**). MGMT enzymatic activity is crucial for TMZ resistance in vivo suggesting that MGMT expression may predict the response of patients to TMZ treatment (Everhard et al., 2006; McCormack et al., 2009). However, other repair mechanisms are also implicated since some cell lines with low MGMT expression still evidence significant resistance to TMZ (Fukushima et al., 2009).

When $O^6$-methyguanine is not repaired by MGMT, it may lead to an $O^6$-methylguanine:thymine mismatch during DNA replication. The following DNA replication cycle can then pair thymine with adenine in place of the original guanine, thus leading to transition mutations (**4**). However, the cytotoxic property of TMZ is mostly linked to MMR pathway through $O^6$-methylguanine:thymine mismatch recognition and repair by this system (**5**). MMR is not involved in TMZ chemo-resistance but in TMZ cytotoxicity, associated with cell cycle blockade at G2 checkpoint (Caporali et al., 2004), activation of p53 and ATM, leading to cell death (**6**). The MRN (Mre11/Rad50/Nbs1) complex was evidenced as the earliest sensor of TMZ-induced damage (Mirzoeva et al., 2006). It undergoes a series of conformational changes that activates the protein sensor ATM (ataxia telangiectasia mutated) which, subsequently, activates Chk1 and Chk2 to block cell cycle. TMZ induces p53-mediated apoptosis in MMR-proficient but not in MMR-deficient cells (D'Atri et al., 1998). Thus, deficient MMR is another mechanism for resistance to TMZ (Cahill et al., 2007).

Besides MGMT and MMR, BER is also implicated in TMZ lesion repair. More than 80% of $N^7$-methylated purines are recognized and excised by the BER enzyme N-methylpurine DNA glycosylase (MPG) (Trivedi et al., 2008; J. Zhang et al., 2010) (**7**). As a consequence, disruption of BER system sensitizes MMR-deficient and proficient cells (Liu et al., 1999). The major MPG-dependent repair occurs via short-patch BER, a mechanism whereby only the damaged nucleotide is excised. So, BER pathway is another contributor of cell resistance to TMZ and its efficacy depends on specific BER gene expression and activity (Fishel et al., 2008). DNApol β or MPG-deficient cells are more sensitive than wild-type cells to TMZ-induced cell death, whereas MPG over-expression increases TMZ-induced cytotoxicity (Tang et al., 2011; Trivedi et al., 2008). Similarly, inhibition of poly(ADP-ribose) polymerase-1 partially restored sensitivity to TMZ (J. Zhang et al., 2010).

Both methylated DNA lesions can lead to SSBs in a DNA repair-dependent manner (BER, MMR). If unrepaired before replication, SSBs convert in DSBs, a more mutagenic and lethal lesion (Newlands et al., 1997). However, DSBs could be processed by the conservative HR pathway to give back undamaged double stand DNA or by NHEJ repair machinery potentially resulting in chromosomal rearrangements between chromatide or deleterious genomic rearrangements as other toxic lesions (**8**). Other inter-crossings between repair pathways are not presented in this scheme: a role of some MMR proteins in the NHEJ pathway to repair DSB during G1 phase of the cell cycle or in HR pathway through the regulation of the early G2 checkpoint and inhibition of DSB repair (Y. Zhang et al., 2009) as well as the implication of Fanconi anemia FANC-D1 (Kondo et al., 2011).

### 3.2 DNA repair process and implication in ET-743 expressing cytotoxicity

ET-743 is a tetrahydroisoquinoline alkaloid isolated from the tunicate *Ecteinascidia turbinata* which is approved as an orphan drug against advanced soft tissue sarcoma and, in

association with doxorubicine, in refractory cisplatin-sensitive ovarian cancers. This DNA minor groove binder (Pommier et al., 1996) bends DNA toward the major groove (Hurley & Zewail-Foote, 2001). ET-743 (Figure 6) is composed of three subunits: A and B are involved in DNA binding at specific sites (David-Cordonnier et al. 2005; García-Nieto et al., 2000; Pommier et al., 1996) and C protrudes out of the double helix thus facilitating the interaction of ET-743 with nuclear proteins such as transcription factors or DNA repair proteins (**1**). The formation of such protein/ET-743-DNA complex prevents the transcription of different genes (Friedman et al., 2002; Jin et al., 2000) and induces a rapid degradation of transcribing RNA polymerase II in TC-NER proficient, but not deficient, cells (Aune et al., 2008).
By contrast with other DNA damaging agents, NER-deficient cell lines are resistant to ET-743, and restoration of NER functions sensitizes cells to the drug. Indeed, the TC-NER complex is trapped during the repair process of ET-743-DNA damage (Damia et al., 2001; Takebayashi et al., 2001) through the formation of a stable XPG/DNA 'cytotoxic complex' (Herrero et al., 2006)(**2**). In a replication-independent manner, the MRN complex is recruited (**3**) and induces DSBs subsequently recognized by DNA-PK from the HR machinery. DNA-PK then phosphorylates H2AX and activates ATM (Damia et al., 2001) and Chk1 to bypass G2/M and S phases checkpoints and promote cell death (Herrero et al., 2006).
Protein recognition of ET-743-DNA adducts also induces the formation of DSBs through replication fork collapse (Soares et al., 2007; Takebayashi et al., 2001)(**4**), as well known for topoisomerase/drug/DNA poisoning complexes. Such DSBs are repaired by HR (acting mainly in G2-M phases) but not by NHEJ (Soares et al., 2007; Tavecchio et al., 2008)(**5**).

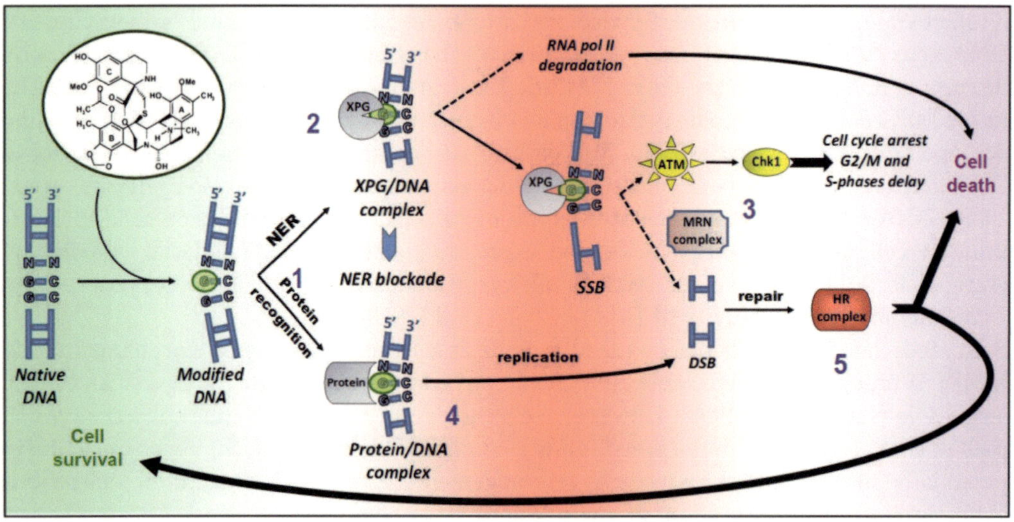


Fig. 6. DNA repair pathways for ET-743-induced DNA damage.

### 3.3 DNA repair for cisplatin and other transition-metal antitumor agents

Regarding DNA repair, local destabilization of the double helix, base-flipping, DNA bending and poor base-stacking following cisplatin alkylation are determinant for recognition of DNA lesions by repair proteins (C.G. Yang et al., 2009; W. Yang, 2006). Several repair machineries are implicated in metal-drug-induced DNA adduct recognition, removal and cytotoxicity (Basu & Krishnamurthy, 2010; S. Ahmad, 2010). First, NER is an important actor for the removal of both 5′-GG, 5′-AG and 5′-GNG cisplatin intra-strand crosslinks, with a preference for the latter site. The induced-kink, being greater for 5′-GNG than 5′-GG or 5′-AG alkylated sites, seems to be of major relevance for NER recognition (**1**, in Figure 7). Particularly, platinum adducts are recognized by the global genome-NER XPC/hHR23B "sensor complex" (Neher et al., 2010) and XPC expression or polymorphism predicts the response to cisplatin treatment in lung cancers (Lai et al., 2011; L.B. Zhu et al., 2010). Lesions induced by cisplatin, oxaliplatin and JM216 are similarly repaired whereas transplatin-induced lesions, which poorly affect 3D structure of DNA, are poorly repaired by NER.

MMR is also important to remove platinated lesions (**2**). Facilitated by cisplatin-induced kink, MSH2 binding is associated with a 60° angle generated through intercalation of its Phe39 at the lesion site. MSH2/MSH6 complex (Mut-Sα) recognizes cisplatin crosslinks (Castellano-Castillo et al., 2008; Fourrier et al., 2003) but not transplatin mono-adducts from $[Pt(dien)Cl]^+$. Translesion bypass is also implicated in cisplatin toxicity. Interestingly, oxaliplatin lesions are more bypassed by DNA polymerases than cisplatin, in relation with their difference in DNA bending/destabilization potencies. Mutants FANC-C and -D of Fanconi anemia pathway also sensitize cells to Pt-drug (Kachnic et al., 2010).

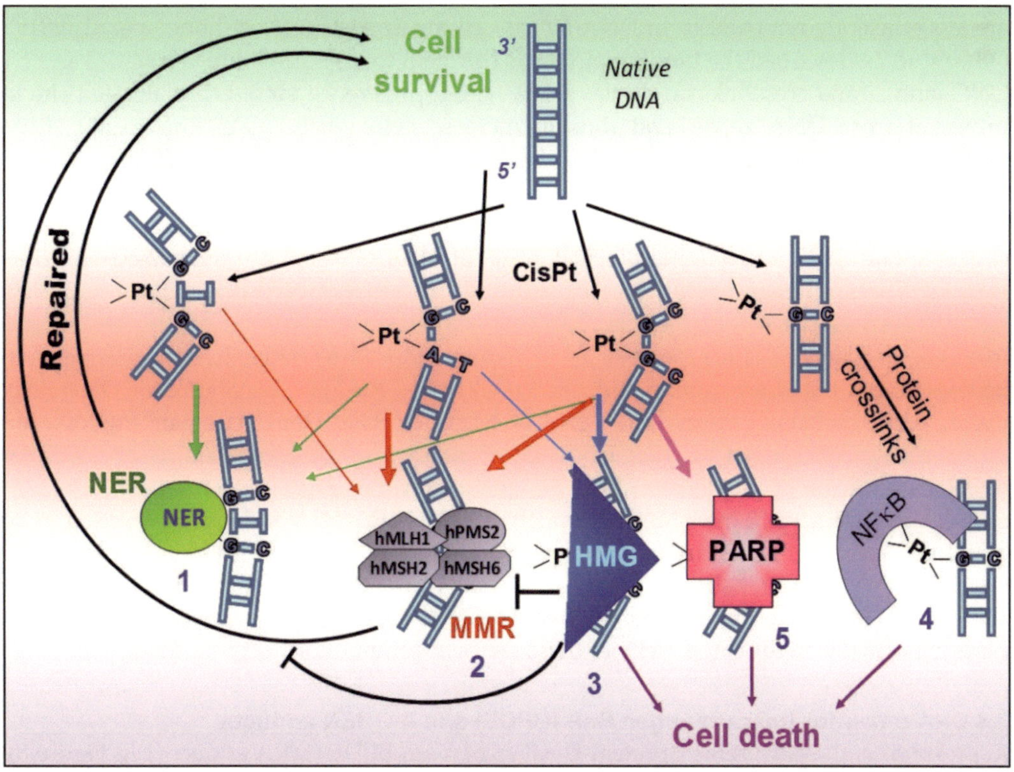


Fig. 7. DNA repair pathways for platinated DNA.

Of major concern, cisplatin adducts are also recognized by HMG proteins (**3**). Similarly to MutS complex recognition, the large induced bend is crucial for this recognition and fits perfectly with the L-shaped structure of HMG DNA binding domain (HMG-box) to reduce the "cost" of DNA bending for HMG-box (Privalov et al., 2009). Insertion of Phe37 between the two platinated guanines in 5'GG dinucleotide stabilizes the binding but is regulated in a redox manner. Indeed, the formation of a disulfure bond between the thiol groups of Cys22 and Cys44 on helix II and III, respectively, of HMG-box infers with the correct planar insertion of Phe37 between the two guanines at crosslink site (Park & Lippard, 2011). Binding of HMG-B1 (and HMG-B2) stabilizes the cisplatin-induced bent and supercoiling of the DNA helix, increases the sensitivity of the cells to cisplatin and shields the platinated adducts from repair by the human DNA excision machinery (J.C. Huang et al., 1994). As a consequence of the degree of kink of the DNA, HMG proteins poorly bind to oxaliplatin adducts which induce relatively small DNA-bending and DNA destabilization (Figure 3), and so poorly protects them from DNA repair (Kasparkova et al., 2008b). This difference correlates with the lower level of DNA lesions in oxaliplatin- versus cisplatin-treated cells. If HMG-B1 and -B2 binding participates in platinated-agent-induced cytotoxicity (Sharma et al., 2009), bent platinated-DNA is also a good substrate for transcription factors from HMG-box family such as SRY, LEF-1 and UBF-1, resulting in the transcriptional changes observed in treated cells (Chvalova et al., 2008; Treiber et al., 1994; Trimmer et al., 1998). For the repair of other platinum derivative-induced DNA damages, JM108 evidenced higher level of protein/DNA cross-links such as DNA-$Pt_{II}$-NF-κB cross-linked complexes (**4**). Those lesions are less efficiently removed from DNA by the cell repair system (Kostrhunova et al., 2010). Other studies described the binding of PARP-1 protein to cisplatin adduct at 5'-GG and 5'-GNG intra-strand crosslinks on duplex DNA with a preference for 5'-GG platinated site to protect it from DNA repair and thus to increase cytotoxicity (G.Y. Zhu et al., 2010), particularly in MSH3-deficient cells (Takahashi et al., 2011) (**5**). Such side effect of PARP-1 orientates current phase I/II clinical trials using PARP inhibitors (CEP-6800, AZD2281 or ABT-888) as sensitizing agents in combination with cisplatin and carboplatin. A recent paper suggests that PARP is a pharmacological target of platinum- and other metal-based drugs showing PARP inhibition using Pt- (cisplatin), Ru- (RAPTA-T, NAMI-A) or Au- (Auphen, Aubipy) derived drugs (Mendes et al., 2011).

In a general manner, NER process of DNA lesions induced by ruthenium-drug appears to be less efficient than for platinum adducts. Ru-CYM and Ru-THA destabilize the DNA helix via different enthalpic effects and differ in terms of their DNA base-pair intercalation propensities. Comparison of their DNA repair processes has been used as a model for understanding the link between DNA destabilization and repair. Interestingly, Ru-CYM adducts (that destabilize the DNA helix much more than Ru-THA adducts) are excised more efficiently than Ru-THA complex adducts. Such observation is in good agreement with lower binding of RPA helicase to Ru-THA- than to Ru-CYM- adducts (Nováková et al., 2005). Ru-THA is also more cytotoxic than Ru-CYM, suggesting that DNA destabilization plays a major role in the cytotoxicity of these series of compounds.

### 3.4 DNA repair for the carcinogen BaP (BPDE) and 4-OHEN adducts

In prokaryote, the NER sensor protein UvrB recognizes BPDE/DNA adduct (**1** in Figure 8). Lesion-induced local thermodynamic destabilization and associated nucleotide flipping facilitate this recognition (Jia et al., 2009) with excision efficiencies changing up to a factor of 3 with stereoisomery (i.e. (+) *vs.* (-), *cis- vs. trans-*orientation)(Zou & Van Houten, 1999).

By contrast, the BaP-induced lesions are recognized in eukaryotic higher cells by the NER machinery's "sensor" protein XPC, associated with HR23B to initiate DNA repair (**2**). Weaker recognition by XPC/HR23B complex of the (+)-*trans*-B[*a*]P-$N^2$-dG adduct, relatively to that of the other conformers, contributes to its higher mutagenic potential (Mocquet et al., 2007). Lesion recognition by XPC requires DNA bending facilitated by local conformational flexibility (Clement et al., 2010) and destabilization of the base-pairing (Brown et al., 2010). Such recognition is driven by Trp690 and Thp733 amino-acids identified as "aromatic sensors" (Maillard et al., 2007). Upon treatment with BaP, human bronchial epithelial 16HBE cells expressed higher levels of the heat shock protein 70 and the NER proteins XPA and XPG, both three proteins co-localizing in the nucleus, suggesting that Hsp70 is also implicated in the DNA repair response to BPDE-DNA adducts (J. Yang et al., 2009). The highly mutagenic (+)-(7R,8S,9S,10R)-7,8-dihydroxy-9,10-epoxy-7,8,9,10-tetrahydrobenzo[*a*]pyrene-DNA lesion leads to different repair processes depending on sequence context, associated with the destabilization potency. Indeed, for an identical BaP-DNA lesion leading to differently orientated bulky lesions, sequence-dependent effect was observed: DNA destabilized at 5′-CG*GC site is more rapidly excised in cell-free human HeLa extracts than DNA bent at 5′-CGG*C site (Rodríguez et al., 2007). As the DNA helix is readily opened upon alkylation, recognition of the lesion by repair protein (including induction of base flipping) is less energetic and, thus, is quicker for DNA already destabilized at 5′-CG*GC site than for duplex DNA bent at 5′-CGG*C site, clearly evidencing the importance of DNA sequence/global structure context for an efficient repair of BPDE-DNA adducts (Yuqin et al., 2009). Moreover, interesting data arise from comparison of the 3D conformation and the NER excision efficiencies for dA adducts formed using the bay region BPDE and the fjord region benzo[*c*]phenanthrene diol epoxide (B[*c*]PhDE) (M. Wu et al., 2002). The bay region of B[*a*]P is more extended, planar and rigid than the B[c]Ph fjord region, being twisted and curved. Consequently, B[*a*]P-dA adducts are associated with greater backbone distortion, unwinding, intercalation potency and

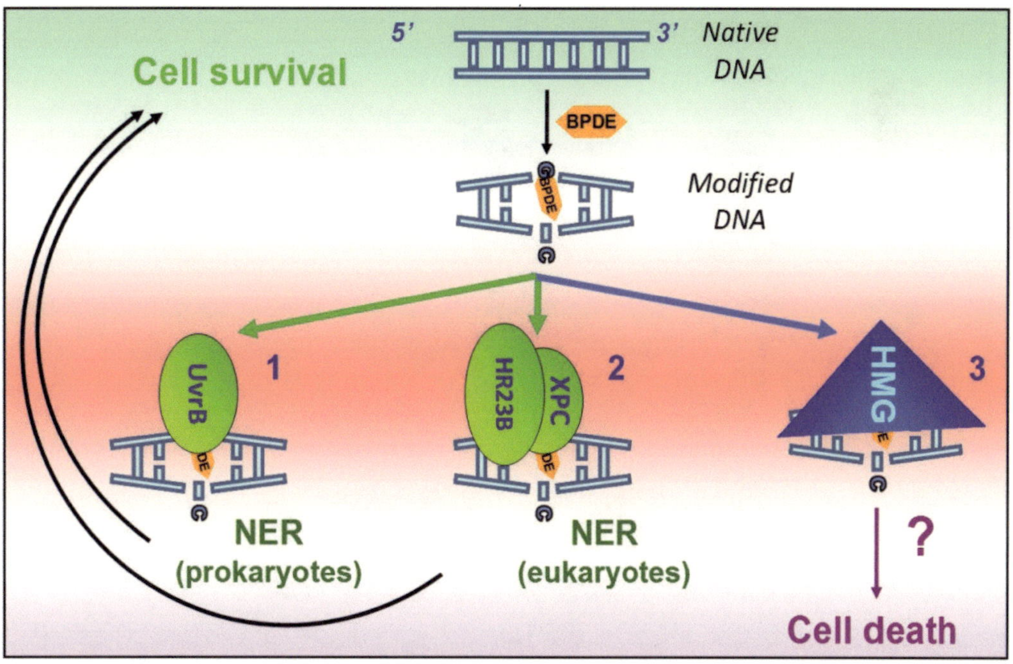


Fig. 8. DNA repair pathways for BPDE-induced DNA damage.

disturbed Watson-Crick hydrogen bonding than B[*c*]Ph-dA adducts, in correlation with stronger excision efficiency by NER machinery. The fjord region B[*c*]Ph-dA adducts being poorly excised lead to more tumorigenic activities. HMG-1 and -2 proteins are also implicated in bulky BPDE-adducts recognition (Lanuszewska & Widlak, 2000) but the consequences on repair or cell death are unknown (**3**). HMG binding might protects adduct recognition by repair proteins as for platinated DNA, but this needs further evaluation.

Excision of bulky 4-OHEN-DNA adducts by NER proteins also depends on both the nature of the alkylated base, its stereo-isomery and the sequence context. For instance, 4-OHEN-dC adducts are more efficiently excised from the DNA than the 4-OHEN-dA adducts (D. Chen et al., 2006). It was reported in male zebrafish that 17a-ethinylestradiol, as a source of 4-OHEN, induces a decrease in NER activity as part of a decrease of the expression level of some NER genes such as XPC, XPA, XPD and XPF, but not of HR23B (Notch et al., 2007).

### 3.5 DNA repair for psoralen-DNA adducts

DNA alkylation by psoralen can lead to inter-strand crosslinks (ICL) or mono-adducts (MA). Psoralen-ICLs (Figure 9) are eliminated during the replication process, associated with HR (**1**), MMR (**2**) and error-prone translesion DNA polymerases (Dronkert & Kanaar, 2001). NER proteins such as XPC/hHR23B complex and XPA/RPA complexes are also implicated in the repair of psoralen-ICL (Thoma et al., 2005) and could cooperate with MMR to excise the lesions (Zhao et al., 2009). By contrast, thymine-psoralen mono-adducts (**3**) are moderately excised from the DNA by the NER system (Vasquez et al., 2002), because of adduct recognition by HMG-B1 which recruits RPA helicase (**4**) (Lange et al., 2009) or by MMR

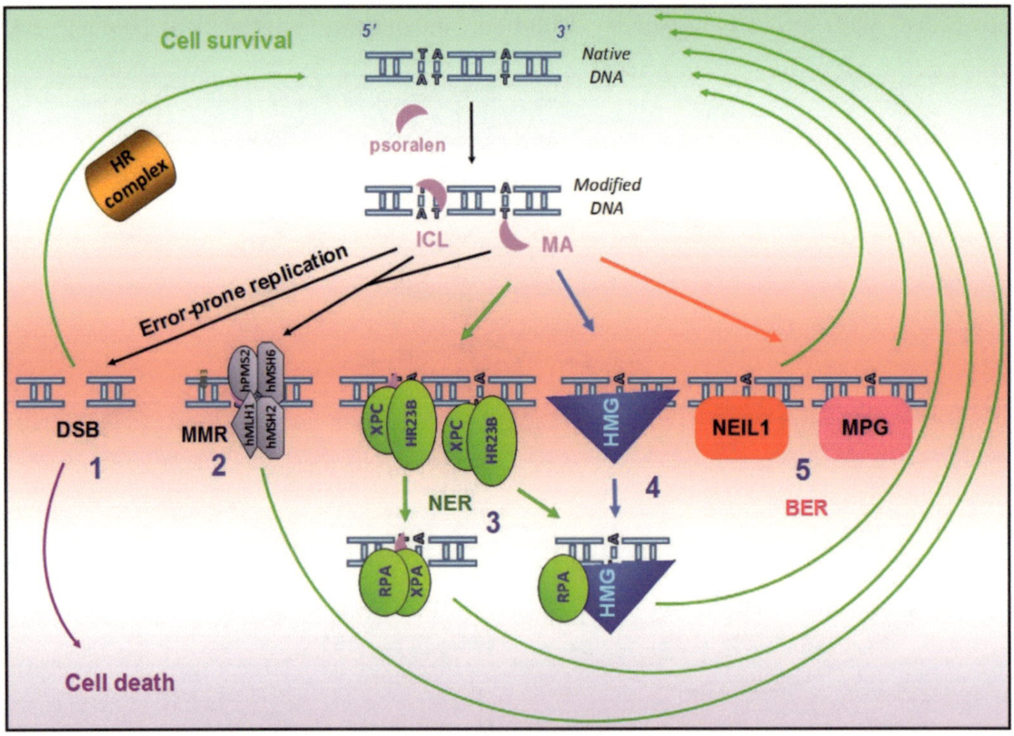


Fig. 9. DNA repair pathways for psoralen-induced DNA damage.

(Q. Wu et al., 2005; 2008). Psoralen monoadducts are good substrates for 3-Methyladenine DNA glycosylase (MPG) (Maor-Shoshani et al., 2008) and the human oxidative DNA glycosylase, NEIL1, which catalyses the β,δ-elimination at AP site, leaving a 3'-P termini at the resulting SSB (5) (Couvé-Privat et al., 2007). Fanconi anemia pathway was also implicated in the repair process, in link with NEIL1 stability and NER efficiency (Macé-Aimé et al., 2010).

### 3.6 DNA repair for benzoacronycine-DNA adducts

S23906-1 alkylates the DNA in the minor groove and induces a strong destabilization of the DNA helix. Two reactive acetate groups are positioned on asymmetric carbons leading to four pure enantiomers: 2 *cis* (1R;2R and 1S;2S) (the *cis*-racemate being S23906-1) and two *trans* (1R;2S and 1S;2R) isomers. Both pure enantiomers react with DNA and destabilize the DNA helix but at different extends. The most potent DNA destabilizing ones (1S;2S and 1S;2R) being those presenting the most active anti-tumour activities in animal models (Depauw et al., 2009). Therefore, the rate of DNA destabilization is different depending on the orientation of the core of the adducts regarding the opened drug/DNA structure, and correlates with different cellular and anti-tumour effects. Such strong destabilisation could affect single-stranded endonuclease and DNA repair activities. There is currently only partial knowledge on the repair of S23906-1 DNA adducts. The NER proteins XPC and CSB are involved in cell sensitivity to S23906-1, associated with both global genome repair and transcription-coupled NER (Rocca et al., 2010). ATR coordination, RPA recognition and Chk1 activation were also implicated in responses to S23906-1 DNA damages (Soares et al., 2011). Process of the lesions is associated with DSB as secondary DNA lesions important for cytotoxicity of S23906-1, associated with histone H2AX phosphorylation (Léonce et al., 2006). Of major interest, the most potent destabilizing isomer of S23906-1 was evidenced to be also the most cytotoxic on cellular models and the most efficient on xenografted animal models (Depauw et al., 2009). Current ongoing research is identifying proteins implicated in S23906-1/DNA adduct recognition and evaluating their impact on S23906-1 cytotoxic activity (personal communication). Locally destabilized DNA could favour the recognition of DNA lesion by "DNA repair sensors" thus increasing the efficiency/kinetic of the removal of the DNA lesion.

## 4. Conclusion

Destabilization of the DNA helix that is induced by drugs is an important aspect of the antitumor mechanism of action of this series of compounds besides they represent just few droplets in an ocean of DNA-interacting compounds that mainly stabilize the double helix. As evidenced here, stabilizing *vs.* destabilizing compounds differs in terms of molecular and cellular processes: DNA repair, transcription or replication. From the different series (platinum, ruthenium, BPDE, benzoacronycines), the level of DNA destabilization correlates with the efficiency of protein recognition and anti-tumor/cytotoxic activities. Therefore, we believe that it is important not to consider DNA destabilization as a unique process but in relation with potential associated bending of the DNA helix (as evidenced using oxaliplatin- and cisplatin-induced distortions or the different isomers of BPDE) and with the size of the locally destabilized DNA (for instance, portions of DNA opened by benzoacronycines are strongly sensitive to single-strand-specific nucleases). The most recent and ongoing studies on the importance of DNA destabilization on DNA repair processes and induced-cytotoxic activities illustrate the need for an accurate examination of precise mode of binding /bonding to DNA of potential anti-cancer drugs in terms of 3D structure/activity relationships and to clearly evaluate the cellular consequences (cytotoxicity, DNA repair processes).

## 5. Acknowledgment

We thank the Ligue Nationale Contre le Cancer (Comité du Nord) and the Institut pour la Recherche sur le Cancer de Lille (IRCL) for grants, as well as the Université de Lille 2, the Conseil Régional Nord/Pas-de-Calais and the IRCL for a PhD fellowship to Gaëlle Lenglet.

## 6. References

Ahmad, R.; Naoui, M.; Neault, J.F.; Diamantoglou, S. & Tajmir-Riahi, H.A. (1996). An FTIR spectroscopic study of calf-thymus DNA complexation with Al(III) and Ga(III) cations. *Journal of Biomolecular Structure & Dynamics*, Vol.13, No.5, (April 1996), pp. 795-802, ISSN 0739-1102

Ahmad, S. (2010). Platinum-DNA interactions and subsequent cellular processes controlling sensitivity to anticancer platinum complexes. *Chemistry & Biodiversity*, Vol.7, No.3, (March 2010), pp. 543-66, ISSN 1612-1880

Arita, K.; Ariyoshi, M.; Tochio, H.; Nakamura, Y. & Shirakawa, M. (2008). Recognition of hemi-methylated DNA by the SRA protein UHRF1 by a base-flipping mechanism. *Nature*, Vol.455, No.7214, (October 2008), pp. 818-21, ISSN 0028-0836

Aune, G.J.; Takagi, K.; Sordet, O.; Guirouilh-Barbat, J.; Antony, S.; Bohr, V.A. & Pommier, Y. (2008). Von Hippel-Lindau-coupled and transcription-coupled nucleotide excision repair-dependent degradation of RNA polymerase II in response to trabectedin. *Clinical Cancer Research*, Vol.14, No.20, (October 2008), pp. 6449-55, ISSN 1078-0432

Basu, A.K.; Hanrahan, C.J.; Malia, S.A.; Kumar, S.; Bizanek, R. & Tomasz, M. (1993). Effect of site-specifically located mitomycin C-DNA monoadducts on in vitro DNA synthesis by DNA polymerases. *Biochemistry*, Vol.32, No.18, (May 1993), pp. 4708-18, ISSN 0006-2960

Basu, A. & Krishnamurthy, S. (2010). Cellular responses to Cisplatin-induced DNA damage. *Journal of Nucleic Acids*, (August 2010), pp. 201367, ISSN 2036-7996

Bellamy, S.R.; Krusong, K. & Baldwin, G.S. (2007). A rapid reaction analysis of uracil DNA glycosylase indicates an active mechanism of base flipping. *Nucleic Acids Research*, Vol.35, No.5, (February 2007), pp. 1478-87, ISSN 0305-1048

Bellon, S.F.; Coleman, J.H. & Lippard, S.J. (1991). DNA unwinding produced by site-specific intrastrand cross-links of the antitumor drug *cis*-diamminedichloroplatinum(II). *Biochemistry*, Vol.30, No.32, (August 1991), pp. 8026-35, ISSN 0006-2960

Benham, C.J. (1996). Duplex destabilization in superhelical DNA is predicted to occur at specific transcriptional regulatory regions. *Journal of Molecular Biology*, Vol.255, No.3, (January 1996), pp. 425-34, ISSN 0022-2836

Bera, A.; Roche, A.C. & Nandi, P.K. (2007). Bending and unwinding of nucleic acid by prion protein. *Biochemistry*, Vol.46, No.5, (February 2007), pp. 1320-8, ISSN 0006-2960

Bergamo, A.; Gava, B.; Alessio, E.; Mestroni, G.; Serli, B.; Cocchietto, M.; Zorzet, S. & Sava, G. (2002). Ruthenium-based NAMI-A type complexes with in vivo selective metastasis reduction and in vitro invasion inhibition unrelated to cell cytotoxicity. *International Journal of Oncology*, Vol.21, No.6, (December 2002), pp. 1331-8, ISSN 1019-6439

Betterton, M.D. & Julicher, F. (2005). Opening of nucleic-acid double strands by helicases: active versus passive opening. *Physical Review E: Statistical, Nonlinear, and Soft Matter Physics*, Vol.71, No.1 Pt 1, (January 2005), pp. 011904, ISSN 1550-2376

Brabec, V.; Reedijk, J. & Leng M. (1992). Sequence-dependent distortions induced in DNA by monofunctional platinum(II) binding. *Biochemistry*, Vol.31, No.49, (December 1992), pp. 12397-402, ISSN 0006-2960

Brown, K.L.; Roginskaya, M.; Zou, Y.; Altamirano, A.; Basu, A.K. & Stone, M.P. (2010). Binding of the human nucleotide excision repair proteins XPA and XPC/HR23B to the 5R-thymine glycol lesion and structure of the *cis*-(*5R;6S*) thymine glycol epimer in the 5'-GTgG-3' sequence: destabilization of two base pairs at the lesion site. *Nucleic Acids Research*, Vol.38, No.2, (January 2010), pp. 428-40, ISSN 0305-1048

Butler, A.P.; Mardian, J.K. & Olins, D.E. (1985). Nonhistone chromosomal protein HMG 1 interactions with DNA. Fluorescence and thermal denaturation studies. *Journal of Biological Chemistry*, Vol.260, No.19, (September 1985), pp. 10613-20, ISSN 0021-9258

Cahill, D.P.; Levine, K.K.; Betensky, R.A.; Codd, P.J.; Romany, C.A.; Reavie, L.B.; Batchelor, T.T.; Futreal, P.A.; Stratton, M.R.; Curry, W.T.; Iafrate, A.J. & Louis, D.N. (2007). Loss of the mismatch repair protein MSH6 in human glioblastomas is associated with tumor progression during temozolomide treatment. *Clinical cancer research*, Vol.13, No.7, (April 2007), pp 2038-45, ISSN 2038-2045

Cai, Y; Patel, DJ; Broyde, S & Geacintov, NE. (2010). Base sequence context effects on nucleotide excision repair. *Journal of Nucleic Acids*. Pii.174252, (August 2010), ISSN 2036-7996

Cai, Y.; Ding, S.; Geacintov, N.E. & Broyde S. (2011). Intercalative conformations of the *14R* (+)- and *14S* (-)-*trans-anti*-DB[*a*;l]P-$N^6$-dA adducts: Molecular Modeling and MD Simulations. *Chemical Research in Toxicology*, In press, (February 2011), ISSN 0893-228X

Cao, C.; Jiang, Y.L., Stivers, J.T. & Song, F. (2004). Dynamic opening of DNA during the enzymatic search for a damaged base. *Nature Structural & Molecular Biology*, Vol.11, No.12, (December 2004), pp. 1230–36, ISSN 1545-9993

Caporali, S. ; Falcinelli, S.; Starace, G.; Russo, M.T.; Bonmassar, E.; Jiricny, J. & D'Atri, S. (2004). DNA damage induced by temozolomide signals to both ATM and ATR: role of the mismatch repair system. *Molecular Pharmacology*, Vol.66, (September 2004), pp 478 –91, ISSN 0026-895X

Castellano-Castillo, M.; Kostrhunova, H.; Marini, V.; Kasparkova, J.; Sadler, P.J; Malinge, J.M. & Brabec, V. (2008). Binding of mismatch repair protein MutS to mispaired DNA adducts of intercalating ruthenium(II) arene complexes. *Journal of Biological Inorganic Chemistry*, Vol.13, No.6, (August 2008), pp. 993-9, ISSN 0949-8257

Chen, D.; Kolbanovskiy, A.; Shastry, A.; Ding, S.; Broyde, S.; Bolton, J.L.; Van Houten, B. & Geacintov, N.E. (2006). Nucleotide excision repair of DNA adducts derived from the binding of the equine estrogen metabolite 4-OHEN to dC and dA adducts in vitro. *Proceedings of the 97th Annual Meeting of the American Association for Cancer Research, 2006 Apr 1-5, Washington, DC. Philadelphia (PA): AACR*, Vol.47, Abstract #5255.

Choi, C.H.; Kalosakas, G.; Rasmussen, K.O.; Hiromura, M.; Bishop, A.R. & Usheva, A. (2004). DNA dynamically directs its own transcription initiation. *Nucleic Acids Research*, Vol.32, No.4, (March 2004), pp. 1584-90, ISSN 0305-1048

Chvalova, K.; Sari, M.A. Bombard, S. & Kozelka, J. (2008). LEF-1 recognition of platinated GG sequences within double-stranded DNA. Influence of flanking bases. *Journal of Biological Inorganic Chemistry*, Vol.102, No.2, (February 2008), pp. 242-50, ISSN 0949-8257

Clement, F.C.; Camenisch, U.; Fei, J.; Kaczmarek, N.; Mathieu, N. & Naegeli, H. (2010). Dynamic two-stage mechanism of versatile DNA damage recognition by xeroderma pigmentosum group C protein. *Mutation Research*, Vol.685, No.1-2, (March 2010), pp. 21-8, ISSN 0027-5107

Cosman, M.; De los Santos, C.; Fiala, R.; Hingerty, B.E.; Ibanez, V.; Luna, E.; Harvey, R.; Geacintov, N.E.; Broyde, S. & Patel, D.J. (1993). Solution conformation of the (+)-*cis*-*anti*-[BP]dG adduct in a DNA duplex: intercalation of the covalently attached benzo[*a*]pyrenyl ring into the helix and displacement of the modified deoxyguanosine. *Biochemistry*, Vol.32, No.16, (April 1993), pp. 4145–55, ISSN 0006-2960

Couvé-Privat, S.; Macé, G.; Rosselli, F & Saparbaev, M.K. (2007). Psoralen-induced DNA adducts are substrates for the base excision repair pathway in human cells. *Nucleic Acids Research*, Vol.35, No. 18, (March 2009), pp. 5672–5682, ISSN 0305-1048

Damia, G.; Silvestri, S.; Carrassa, L.; Filiberti, L.; Faircloth, G.T.; Liberi, G.; Foiani, M. & D'Incalci, M. (2001). Unique pattern of ET-743 activity in different cellular systems with defined deficiencies in DNA-repair pathways. *International Journal of Cancer*, Vol.92, No.4, (May 2001), pp. 583-8, ISSN 1097-0215

Darzynkiewicz, Z.; Evenson, D.; Kapuscinski, J. & Melamed, M.R. (1983). Denaturation of RNA and DNA in situ induced by acridine orange. *Experimental Cell Research*, Vol.148, No.1, (October 1983), pp. 31-46, ISSN 0014-4827

D'Atri, S.; Tentori, L.; Lacal, P.M.; Graziani, G.; Pagani, E.; Benincasa, E.; Zambruno, G.; Bonmassar, E. & Jiricny, J. (1998). Involvement of the mismatch repair system in temozolomide-induced apoptosis. *Molecular Pharmacology*, Vol.54, No.2, (August 1998), pp. 334–341, ISSN 0026-895X

David-Cordonnier, M.-H.; Gajate, C.; Olmea, O.; Laine, W.; de la Iglesia-Vicente, J.; Perez, C.; Cuevas, C.; Otero, G.; Bailly, C. & Mollinedo F. (2005). DNA and non-DNA targets in the mechanism of action of the antitumor drug Yondelis™ (trabectedin, ET-743). *Chemistry and Biology*, Vol.12, No.11, (November 2005), pp. 1201-10, ISSN 1074-5521

David, A.; Bleimling, N.; Beuck, C.; Lehn, J.M.; Weinhold, E.; Teulade-Fichou, M.P. (2003). DNA mismatch-specific base flipping by a bisacridine macrocycle. *Chembiochem*, Vol.4, No.12, (December 2003), pp. 1326-31, ISSN 1439-4227

David-Cordonnier, M.-H.; Laine, W.; Lansiaux, A.; Kouach, M.; Briand, G.; Pierré, A.; Hickman, J.A. & Bailly, C. (2002). Alkylation of guanine in DNA by S23906-1, a novel potent antitumor compound derived from the plant alkaloid acronycine. *Biochemistry*, Vol.41, No. 31, (August 2002), pp. 9911-20, ISSN 0006-2960

David-Cordonnier, M.-H.; Laine, W.; Lansiaux, A.; Rosu, F.; Colson, P.; de Pauw, E.; Michel, S.; Tillequin, F.; Koch, M.; Hickman, J.A.; Pierré, A. & Bailly, C. (2005). Covalent binding of antitumor benzoacronycines to double-stranded DNA induces helix opening and the formation of single-stranded DNA: unique consequences of a novel DNA-bonding mechanism. *Molecular Cancer Therapeutics*, Vol.4, No.1, (January 2005), pp. 71-80, ISSN 1535-7163

David-Cordonnier, M.-H.; Payet, D.; D'Halluin, J.-C.; Waring, M.J.; Travers, A.A. & Bailly, C. (1999). The DNA-binding domain of human c-Abl tyrosine kinase promotes the interaction of a HMG chromosomal protein with DNA. *Nucleic Acids Research*, Vol.27, No.11, (June 1999), pp. 2265-70, ISSN 0305-1048

David-Cordonnier, M.-H.; Hamdane, M.; Bailly, C.; D'Halluin, J.-C. (1998). The DNA binding domain of the human c-Abl tyrosine kinase preferentially binds to DNA sequences containing an AAC-motif and to distorted DNA structures. *Biochemistry*, Vol.37, No.17, (April 1998), pp. 6065-76, ISSN 0006-2960

Depauw, S.; Gaslonde, T.; Léonce, S.; Kraus-Berthier, L.; Laine, W.; Lenglet, G.; Chiaroni, A.; Pfeiffer, B.; Bailly, C.; Michel, S.; Tillequin, F.; Pierré, A. & David-Cordonnier, M.-H. (2009). Influence of the stereoisomeric position of the reactive acetate groups of the benzo[*b*]acronycine derivative S23906-1 on its DNA alkylation, helix opening, cytotoxic and anti-tumor activities. *Molecular Pharmacoly*, Vol.76, No.6, (December 2009), pp. 1172-85, ISSN 0026-895X

Ding, S.; Shapiro, R.; Geacintov, N.E. & Broyde, S. (2005). Equilenin-derived DNA adducts to cytosine in DNA duplexes: structures and thermodynamics. *Biochemistry*, Vol.44, No.44, (November 2005), pp. 14565-76, ISSN 0006-2960

Ding, S.; Shapiro, R.; Geacintov, N.E. & Broyde, S. (2007). 4-hydroxyequilenin-adenine lesions in DNA duplexes: stereochemistry, damage site, and structure. *Biochemistry*, Vol.46, No.1, (January 2007), pp. 182-91, ISSN 0006-2960

Dornberger, U.; Leijon, M. & Fritzsche, H. (1999). High base pair opening rates in tracts of GC base pairs. *Journal of Biological Chemistry*, Vol.274, No.11, (March 1999), pp. 6957-62, ISSN 0021-9258

Dronkert, M.L. & Kanaar, R. (2001). Repair of DNA interstrand cross-links. *Mutation Research*, Vol.486, No.4, (September 2001), pp. 217–47, ISSN 0027-5107

Embrechts, J.; Lemiere, F.; Van Dongen, W.; Esmans, E.L.; Buytaert, P.; Van Marck, E.; Kockx, M. & Makar, A. (2003). Detection of estrogen DNA-adducts in human breast tumor tissue and healthy tissue by combined nano LC-nano ES tandem mass spectrometry. *Journal of the American Society of Mass Spectrometry*, Vol.14, No.5 (May 2003), pp. 482–91, ISSN

Everhard, S.; Kaloshi, G.; Crinière, E.; Benouaich-Amiel, A.; Lejeune, J.; Marie, Y.; Sanson, M.; Kujas, M.; Mokhtari, K.; Hoang-Xuan, K.; Delattre, J.Y. & Thillet, J. (2006). MGMT methylation: a marker of response to temozolomide in low-grade gliomas. *Annals of neurology* , Vol.60, No.6, (December 2006), pp 740-3, ISSN 0364-5134

Fishel, M.L.; He, Y.; Smith, M.L.; Kelley, M.R. (2008). Manipulation of base excision repair to sensitize ovarian cancer cells to alkylating agent temozolomide. *Molecular Pharmacology*, Vol.74, No.1, (July 2008), pp 173-83, ISSN 0026-895X

Fourrier, L.; Brooks, P. & Malinge, J.M. (2003). Binding discrimination of MutS to a set of lesions and compound lesions (base damage and mismatch) reveals its potential role as a cisplatin-damaged DNA sensing protein. *Journal of Biological Chemistry*, Vol.278, No.23, (June 2003), pp. 21267-75, ISSN 1044-0305

Fridman, A.S.; Brabec, V.; Haroutiunian, S.G.; Wartell, R.M. & Lando, D.Y. (2003). Melting of cross-linked DNA v. cross-linking effect caused by local stabilization of the double helix. *Journal of Biomolecular Structure & Dynamics*, Vol.20, No.4, (February 2003), pp. 533-45, ISSN 0739-1102

Friedman, D.; Hu, Z.; Kolb, E.A.; Gorfajn, B. & Scotto, K.W. (2002). Ecteinascidin-743 inhibits activated but not constitutive transcription. *Cancer Research*, Vol.62, No. 12, (June 2002), pp. 3377-81, ISSN 0008-5472

Fukushima, T.; Takeshima, H. & Kataoka, H. (2009). Anti-glioma Therapy with Temozolomide and Status of the DNA-Repair Gene MGMT. *Anticancer Research*, Vol.29, No.11, (November 2009), pp 4845-54, ISSN 0250-7005

García-Nieto, R.; Manzanares, I.; Cuevas, C. & Gago, F. (2000). Increased DNA binding specificity for antitumor ecteinascidin 743 through protein-DNA interactions? *Journal of Medicinal Chemistry*, Vol.43, No.23, (November 2000), pp. 4367-9, ISSN ISSN 0022-2623

Guilbaud, N.; Kraus-Berthier, L.; Meyer-Losic, F.; Malivet, V.; Chacun, C.; Jan, M.; Tillequin, F.; Koch, M.; Pfeiffer, B.; Atassi, G.; Hickman, J. & Pierré, A. (2001). Marked antitumor activity of a new potent acronycine derivative in orthotopic models of human solid tumors. *Clinical Cancer Research*, Vol.7, No.8, (August 2001), pp. 2573-80, ISSN 1078-0432

Hägerlöf, M.; Papsai, P.; Chow, C.S. & Elmroth, S.K. (2006). More pronounced salt dependence and higher reactivity for platination of the hairpin r(CGCGUUGUUCGCG) compared with d(CGCGTTGTTCGCG). *Journal of Biological Inorganic Chemistry*, Vol.11, No.8, (November 2006), pp. 974-90, ISSN 0949-8257

Hartinger, C.G.; Jakupec, M.A.; Zorbas-Seifried, S.; Groessl, M.; Egger, A.; Berger, W.; Zorbas, H.; Dyson, P.J. & Keppler, B.K. (2008). KP1019, a new redox-active anticancer agent--preclinical development and results of a clinical phase I study in tumor patients. *Chemistry and Biodiversity*, Vol.5, No.10, (October 2008), pp. 2140-55, ISSN 1612-1880

Harvey, S.C. (1983). DNA structural dynamics: longitudinal breathing as a possible mechanism for B↔Z transition. *Nucleic Acids Research*, Vol.11, No.14, (July 1983), pp. 4867-78, ISSN 0305-1048

Herrero, A.B.; Martín-Castellanos, C.; Marco, E.; Gago, F. & Moreno, S. (2006). Cross-talk between nucleotide excision and homologous recombination DNA repair pathways in the mechanism of action of antitumor trabectedin. *Cancer Research*, Vol.66, No.16, (August 2006), pp. 8155-62, ISSN 0008-5472

Herrick, G. & Alberts, B. (1976). Nucleic acid helix-coil transitions mediated by helix-unwinding proteins from calf thymus. *Journal of Biological Chemistry*, Vol.251, No.7, (April 1976), pp. 2133-41, ISSN 0021-9258

Hornby, D.P. & Ford, G.C. (1998). Protein-mediated base flipping. *Current Opinion in Biotechnology*, Vol.9, No.4, (August 1998), pp. 354-8, ISSN 0958-1669

Huang, J.C.; Zamble, D.B.; Reardon, J.T.; Lippard, S.J. & Sancar, A. (1994). HMG-domain proteins specifically inhibit the repair of the major DNA adduct of the anticancer drug cisplatin by human excision nuclease. *Proceedings of the National Academy of Sciences USA*, Vol.91, No.22, (October 1994), pp. 10394-8, ISSN 0027-8424

Hurley, L.H. & Zewail-Foote, M. (2001). The antitumor agent ecteinascidin 743: characterization of its covalent DNA adducts and chemical stability. *Advances in Experimental Medicine and Biology*, Vol.500, pp. 289-99, ISSN 0065-2598

Jia, L.; Kropachev, K.; Ding, S.; Van Houten, B.; Geacintov, N.E. & Broyde, S. (2009). Exploring damage recognition models in prokaryotic nucleotide excision repair with a benzo[*a*]pyrene-derived lesion in UvrB. *Biochemistry*, Vol.48, No.38, (September 2009), pp. 8948-57, ISSN 0006-2960

Jin, S.; Gorfajn, B.; Faircloth, G. & Scotto, K.W. (2000). Ecteinascidin 743; a transcription-targeted chemotherapeutic that inhibits MDR1 activation. *Proceedings of the National Academy of Sciences USA*, Vol.97, No.12, (June 2000), pp. 6775-9, ISSN 0027-8424

Kachnic, L.A.; Li. L; Fournier. L & Willers. H. (2010) Fanconi anemia pathway heterogeneity revealed by cisplatin and oxaliplatin treatments. *Cancer Letters*, Vol.292, No.1, (June 2010), pp. 73-9, ISSN 0304-3835

Kapuscinski, J. & Darzynkiewicz, Z. (1983). Increased accessibility of bases in DNA upon binding of acridine orange. *Nucleic Acids Research*, Vol.11, No.21, (November 1983), pp. 7555-68, ISSN 0305-1048

Kapuscinski, J. & Darzynkiewicz, Z. (1984). Denaturation of nucleic acids induced by intercalating agents. Biochemical and biophysical properties of acridine orange-DNA complexes. *Journal of Biomolecular Structure & Dynamics*, Vol.1, No.6, (June 1984), pp. 1485-99, ISSN 0739-1102

Karpel, R.L & Burchard, A.C. (1981). A basic isozyme of yeast glyceraldehyde-3-phosphate dehydrogenase with nucleic acid helix-destabilizing activity. *Biochimica and Biophysica Acta*, Vol.654, No.2, (July 1981), pp. 256-67, ISSN 0006-3002

Kaspárková, J.; Nováková, O.; Vrána, O.; Farrell, N. & Brabec, V. (1999). Effect of geometric isomerism in dinuclear platinum antitumor complexes on DNA interstrand cross-linking. *Biochemistry*, Vol.38, No.34, (August 1999), pp. 10997-1005, ISSN 0006-2960

Kasparkova, J.; Marini, V.; Bursova, V. & Brabec, V. (2008a). Biophysical studies on the stability of DNA intrastrand cross-links of transplatin. *Biophysical Journal*, Vol.95, No.9, (November 2008), pp. 4361-71, ISSN 0006-3495

Kasparkova, J.; Vojtiskova, M.; Natile, G. & Brabec, V. (2008b). Unique properties of DNA interstrand cross-links of antitumor oxaliplatin and the effect of chirality of the carrier ligand. *Chemistry*, Vol.14, No.4, (January 2008), pp. 1330-41, ISSN 1521-3765

Kolbanovskiy, A.; Kuzmin, V.; Shastry, A.; Kolbanovskaya, M.; Chen, D.; Chang, M.; Bolton, J.L. & Geacintov, N.E. (2005). Base selectivity and effects of sequence and DNA secondary structure on the formation of covalent adducts derived from the equine estrogen metabolite 4-hydroxyequilenin. *Chemical Research in Toxicology,* Vol.18, No.11, (November 2005), pp. 1737-47, ISSN 0893-228X

Kondo, N.; Takahashi, A.; Mori, E.; Noda, T.; Zdzienicka, M.Z.; Thompson, L.H.; Helleday, T.; Suzuki, M.; Kinashi, Y.; Masunaga, S.; Ono, K.; Hasegawa, M. & Ohnishi, T. (2011). FANCD1/BRCA2 plays predominant role in the repair of DNA damage induced by ACNU or TMZ. *PLoS One,* Vol.6, No5, (May 2011), e19659, ISSN 1932-6203

Kostrhunova, H.; Vrana, O.; Suchankova, T.; Gibson, D.; Kasparkova, J. & Brabec, V. (2010). Different features of the DNA binding mode of antitumor *cis*-amminedichlorido(cyclohexylamine)platinum(II) (JM118) and cisplatin in vitro. *Chemical Research in Toxicology,* Vol.23, No.11, (November 2010), pp. 1833–42, ISSN 0893-228X

Krueger, A.; Protozanova, E. & Frank-Kamenetskii, M.D. (2006). Sequence-dependent base pair opening in DNA double helix. *Biophysical Journal,* Vol.90, No.9, (May 2006), pp. 3091-9, ISSN 0006-3495

Lai, T.C.; Chow, K.C.; Fang, H.Y.; Cho, H.C.; Chen, C.Y.; Lin, T.Y.; Chiang, I.P. & Ho, S.P. (2011). Expression of xeroderma pigmentosum complementation group C protein predicts cisplatin resistance in lung adenocarcinoma patients. *Oncology Report,* Vol.25, No.5, (May 2011), pp. 1243-51, ISSN 1021-335X

Lange, S.S.; Reddy, M.C. & Vasquez K.M. (2009). Human HMGB1 directly facilitates interactions between nucleotide excision repair proteins on triplex-directed psoralen interstrand crosslinks. *DNA Repair (Amst),* Vol.8, No.7, (July 2009), pp. 865-72, ISSN 1568-7864

Lanuszewska, J. & Widlak, P. (2000). High mobility group 1 and 2 proteins bind preferentially to DNA that contains bulky adducts induced by benzo[*a*]pyrene diol epoxide and N-acetoxy-acetylaminofluorene. *Cancer Letters,* Vol.158, No.1, (September 2000), pp. 17–25, ISSN 0304-3835

Léonce, S.; Kraus-Berthier, L.; Golsteyn, R.; David-Cordonnier, M.-H.; Tardy, C.; Lansiaux, A.; Poindessous, V.; Larsen, A. K. & Pierré, A. (2006). Generation of replication-dependent double-strand breaks by the novel $N^2$-G-alkylator S23906-1. *Cancer Research,* Vol.66, No.14, (July 2006), pp. 7203-10, ISSN 0008-5472

Liu, L.; Taverna, P.; Whitacre CM, Chatterjee S. & Gerson S.L. (1999). Pharmacologic disruption of base excision repair sensitizes mismatch repair-deficient and -proficient colon cancer cells to methylating agents. *Clinical Cancer Research,* Vol.5, No.10, (October 1999), pp 2908-17, ISSN 1078-0432

Lum, B. L.; Srinivas, S.; Beck, J. T.; Vesole, D.; Largey, M.; Valone, F. H. & Sayre P. H. (2003). Phase I trial of oral gallium maltolate in refractory malignancies. 2003 ASCO Annual Meeting. *Proceedings - American Society of Clinical Oncology Program,* Vol.22, abstr 943, ISSN 1081-0641

Macé-Aimé, G.; Couvé, S.; Khassenov, B.; Rosselli, F. & Saparbaev, M.K. (2010). The Fanconi anemia pathway promotes DNA glycosylase-dependent excision of interstrand DNA crosslinks. *Environmental and Molecular Mutagenesis,* Vol.15, No.6, (July 2010), pp. 508-19, ISSN 0893-6692

Maillard, O.; Solyom, S. & Naegeli H. (2007). An aromatic sensor with aversion to damaged strands confers versatility to DNA repair. *PLoS Biology*, Vol.5, No.4, (April 2007), e79, ISSN 1544-9173

Malina, J.; Novakova, O.; Vojtiskova, M.; Natile, G. & Brabec, V. (2007). Conformation of DNA GG intrastrand cross-link of antitumor oxaliplatin and its enantiomeric analog. *Biophysical Journal*, Vol.93, No.11, (December 2007), pp. 3950-62, ISSN 0006-3495

Malinge, J.M.; Pérez, C. & Leng, M. (1994). Base sequence-independent distorsions induced by interstrand cross-links in *cis*-diamminedichloroplatinum (II)-modified DNA. *Nucleic Acids Research*, Vol.22, No.19, (September 1994), pp. 3834-9, ISSN 0305-1048

Maor-Shoshani, A.; Meira, L.B.; Yang, X. & Samson, L.D. (2008). 3-Methyladenine DNA glycosylase is important for cellular resistance to psoralen interstrand cross-links. *DNA Repair (Amst)*, Vol.7, No.8, (August 2008), pp. 1399-406, ISSN 1568-7864

McCormack; A.I.; McDonald, K.L.; Gill, A.J.; Clark, S.J.; Burt, M.G.; Campbell, K.A.; Braund, W.J.; Little, N.S.; Cook, R.J.; Grossman, A.B.; Robinson, B.G. & Clifton-Bligh, RJ. (2009). Low O6-methylguanine-DNA methyltransferase (MGMT) expression and response to temozolomide in aggressive pituitary tumours. *Clinical Endocrinology*, Vol.71, No.2, (August 2009), pp 226-33, ISSN 0300-0664

Mendes, F.; Groessl, M.; Nazarov, A.A.; Tsybin, Y.O.; Sava, G.; Santos, I.; Dyson, P.J. & Casini, A. (2011). Metal-Based Inhibition of Poly(ADP-ribose) Polymerase - The Guardian Angel of DNA. *Journal of Medicinal Chemistry*, Vol.54, No.7, (March 2011), pp. 2196–206, ISSN 0022-2623

Mirzoeva O.K.; Kawaguchi, T. & Pieper, R.O. (2006). The Mre11/Rad50/Nbs1 complex interacts with the mismatch repair system and contributes to temozolomide-induced G2 arrest and cytotoxicity. *Molecular Cancer Therapeutics*, Vol.5, No.11, (November 2006), pp. 2757-66, ISSN 1535-7163

Mocquet, V.; Kropachev, K.; Kolbanovskiy, M.; Kolbanovskiy, A.; Tapias, A.; Cai, Y.; Broyde, S.; Geacintov, N.E. & Egly, J.M. (2007). The human DNA repair factor XPC-HR23B distinguishes stereoisomeric benzo[*a*]pyrenyl-DNA lesions. *EMBO Journal*, Vol.26, No.12, (June 2007), pp. 2923-32, ISSN 0261-4189

Moldovan, G.L. & D'Andrea, A.D. (2009). How the fanconi anemia pathway guards the genome. *Annual Review of Genetic*, Vol.43, pp. 223-49, ISSN 0066-4197

Mura, C. & McCammon, J.A. (2008). Molecular dynamics of a kappaB DNA element: base flipping via cross-strand intercalative stacking in a microsecond-scale simulation. *Nucleic Acids Research*, Vol.36, No.15, (September 2008), pp. 4941-55, ISSN 0305-1048

Narayanan, N.; Gorelick, R.J & DeStefano, J.J. (2006). Structure/function mapping of amino acids in the N-terminal zinc finger of the human immunodeficiency virus type 1 nucleocapsid protein: residues responsible for nucleic acid helix destabilizing activity. *Biochemistry*, Vol.45, No.41, (October 2006), pp. 12617-28, ISSN 0006-2960

Neher, T.M.; Rechkunova, N.I.; Lavrik, O.I. & Turchi, J.J. (2010). Photo-cross-linking of XPC-Rad23B to cisplatin-damaged DNA reveals contacts with both strands of the DNA duplex and spans the DNA adduct. *Biochemistry*, Vol.49, No.4, (February 2010), pp. 669-78, ISSN 0006-2960

Newlands, E.S.; Stevens, M.F.G.; Wedge, S.R.; Wheelhouse, R.T. & Brock C. (1997). Temozolomide: a review of its discovery, chemical properties, pre-clinical development and clinical trials. *Cancer Treatment Reviews*, Vol.23, No.1, (January 1997), pp 35–61, ISSN 0305-7372

Notch, E.G. Miniutti, D.M. & Mayer, G.D. (2007). 17alpha-Ethinylestradiol decreases expression of multiple hepatic nucleotide excision repair genes in zebrafish (Danio rerio). *Aquatic Toxicology*, Vol.84, No.3, (October 2007), pp. 301-9, ISSN 0166-445X

Nováková, O.; Kasparkova, J.; Bursova, V.; Hofr, C.; Vojtiskova, M.; Chen, H.; Sadler, P.J. & Brabec, V. (2005). Conformation of DNA modified by monofunctional Ru(II) arene complexes: recognition by DNA binding proteins and repair. Relationship to cytotoxicity. *Chemistry & Biology*, Vol.12, No.1, (January 2005), pp. 121-9, ISSN 1074-5521

Nováková, O.; Nazarov, A.A.; Hartinger, C.G.; Keppler, B.K. & Brabec, V. (2009). DNA interactions of dinuclear RuII arene antitumor complexes in cell-free media. *Biochemical Pharmacology*, Vol.77, No.3, (February 2009), pp. 364-74, ISSN 0006-2952

Nováková, O.; Malina, J.; Suchankova, T.; Kasparkova, J.; Bugarcic, T.; Sadler, P.J. & Brabec, V. (2010). Energetics, conformation, and recognition of DNA duplexes modified by monodentate Ru(II) complexes containing terphenyl arenes. *Chemistry*, Vol.16, No.19, (May 2010), pp. 5744-54, ISSN 1521-3765

Park, S. & Lippard, S.J. (2011). Redox state-dependent interaction of HMGB1 and cisplatin-modified DNA. *Biochemistry*, Vol.50, No.13, (April 2011), pp. 2567-74, ISSN 0006-2960

Pisha, E.; Lui, X.; Constantinou, A. I. & Bolton, J. L. (2001). Evidence that a metabolite of equine estrogens, 4-hydroxyequilenin, induces cellular transformation in vitro. *Chemical Research in Toxicology*, Vol.14, No.1, (January 2001), pp. 82–90, ISSN 0893-228X

Planck, S.R. & Wilson, S.H. (1980). Studies on the structure of mouse helix-destabilizing protein-1. DNA binding and controlled proteolysis with trypsin. *Journal of Biological Chemistry*, Vol.255, No.23, (December 1980), pp. 11547-56, ISSN 0021-9258

Pommier, Y.; Kohlhagen, G.; Bailly, C.; Waring, M.J.; Mazumder, A. & Kohn, K.W. (1996). DNA sequence- and structure-selective alkylation of guanine $N^2$ in the DNA minor groove by ecteinascidin 743, a potent antitumor compound from the Caribbean tunicate Ecteinascidia turbinata. *Biochemistry*, Vol.35, No.41, (October 1996), pp. 13303-9, ISSN 0006-2960

Privalov, P.L.; Dragan, A.I. & Crane-Robinson, C. (2009). The cost of DNA bending. *Trends in Biochemical Sciences*, Vol.34, No.9, (September 2009), pp. 464-70, ISSN 0968-0004

Putnam, B.F.; Van Zandt, L.L.; Prohofsky, E.W. & Mei, W.N. (1981). Resonant and localized breathing modes in terminal regions of the DNA double helix. *Biophysical Journal*, Vol.35, No.2, (August 1981), pp. 271-87, ISSN 0006-3495

Rocca, C.J.; Poindessous, V.; Soares, D.G.; Ouadrani, K.E.; Sarasin, A.; Guérin, E.; de Gramont, A.; Henriques, J.A.; Escargueil, A.E. & Larsen, A.K. (2010). The NER proteins XPC and CSB, but not ERCC1, regulate the sensitivity to the novel DNA binder S23906: Implications for recognition and repair of antitumor alkylators. *Biochemical Pharmacology*, Vol.80, No.3, (August 2010), pp. 335-43, ISSN 0006-2952

Rodríguez, F.A.; Cai, Y.; Lin, C.; Tang, Y.; Kolbanovskiy, A.; Amin, S.; Patel, D.J.; Broyde, S. & Geacintov, N.E. (2007). Exocyclic amino groups of flanking guanines govern sequence-dependent adduct conformations and local structural distortions for minor groove-aligned benzo[*a*]pyrenyl-guanine lesions in a GG mutation hotspot context. *Nucleic Acids Research*, Vol.35, No.5, (March 2007), pp. 1555-68, ISSN 0305-1048

Rossouw, J.E.; Anderson, G.L.; Prentice, R.L.; LaCroix, A.Z.; Kooperberg, C.; Stefanick, M.L.; Jackson, R.D.; Beresford, S.A.; Howard, B.V.; Johnson, K.C.; Kotchen, J.M. & Ockene, J. (2002). Risks and benefits of estrogen plus progestin in healthy postmenopausal women: principal results From the Women's Health Initiative randomized controlled trial. *Journal of the American Medical Association*, Vol.288, No.3, (July 2002), pp. 321–33, ISSN 0002-9955

Schneider, T.D. (2001). Strong minor groove base conservation in sequence logos implies DNA distortion or base flipping during replication and transcription initiation. *Nucleic Acids Research*, Vol.29, No.23, (December 2001), pp. 4881-91, ISSN 0305-1048

Schwartz, A.; Marrot, L. & Leng, M. (1989). Conformation of DNA modified at a d(GG) or a d(AG) site by the antitumor drug *cis*-diamminedichloroplatinum(II). *Biochemistry*, Vol.28. No.20, (October 1989), pp. 7975-9, ISSN 0006-2960

Sharma, A.; Ramanjaneyulu, A.; Ray, R. & Rajeswari, M.R. (2009). Involvement of high mobility group B proteins in cisplatin-induced cytotoxicity in squamous cell carcinoma of skin. *DNA and Cell Biology*, Vol.28, No.7, (July 2009), pp. 311-8, ISSN 1044-5498

Slama-Schwok, A.; Peronnet, F.; Hantz-Brachete, E.; Taillandier, E.; Teulade-Fichou, M.P.; Vigneron, J.P.; Baudoin, O.; Best-Belpomme, M. & Lehn J.M. (1997). A macrocyclic bis-acridine shifts the equilibrium from duplexes towards DNA hairpins. *Nucleic Acids Research*, Vol.25, No.13, (July 1997), pp. 2574-81, ISSN 0305-1048

Soares, D.G.; Battistella, A.; Rocca, C.J.; Matuo, R.; Henriques, J.A.; Larsen, A.K. & Escargueil, A.E. (2011). Ataxia telangiectasia mutated- and Rad3-related kinase drives both the early and the late DNA-damage response to the monofunctional antitumour alkylator S23906. *Biochemical Journal*, Vol.47, No.1, (July 2011), pp. 63-73, ISSN 0264-6021

Soares, D.G.; Escargueil, A.E.; Poindessous, V.; Sarasin, A.; de Gramont, A.; Bonatto, D.; Henriques, J.A. & Larsen A.K. (2007). Replication and homologous recombination repair regulate DNA double-strand break formation by the antitumor alkylator ecteinascidin 743. *Proceedings of the National Academy of Sciences USA*, Vol.104, No32, (August 2007), pp. 13062-7; ISSN 0027-8424

Sundheim, O.; Talstad, V.A.; Vågbø, C.B.; Slupphaug, G. & Krokan, H.E. (2008). AlkB demethylases flip out in different ways. *DNA Repair (Amst)*, Vol.7, No. 11, (November 2008), pp. 1916-23, ISSN 1568-7864

Takahashi, M.; Koi, M.; Balaguer, F.; Boland, C.R. & Goel, A. (2011). MSH3 mediates sensitization of colorectal cancer cells to cisplatin, oxaliplatin and a poly(ADP-ribose) polymerase inhibitor. *Journal of Biological Chemistry*, Vol.286, No.14, (April 2011), pp. 12157-65, ISSN 0021-9258

Takebayashi, Y.; Pourquier, P.; Zimonjic, D.B.; Nakayama, K.; Emmert, S.; Ueda, T.; Urasaki, Y.; Kanzaki, A.; Akiyama, S.I.; Popescu, N.; Kraemer, K.H. & Pommier, Y. (2001). Antiproliferative activity of ecteinascidin 743 is dependent upon transcription-coupled nucleotide-excision repair. *Nature Medicine*, Vol.7,No.8, (August 2001), pp. 961-6, ISSN 1078-8956

Tang, J.B.; Svilar, D.; Trivedi, R.N.; Wang, X.H.; Goellner, E.M.; Moore, B.; Hamilton, R.L.; Banze, L.A.; Brown, A.R. & Sobol, R.W. (2011). N-methylpurine DNA glycosylase and DNA polymerase {beta} modulate BER inhibitor potentiation of glioma cells to temozolomide, *Neuro-Oncology*, (April 2011), online, ISSN 1522-8517

Tavecchio, M.; Simone, M.; Erba, E.; Chiolo, I.; Liberi, G.; Foiani, M.; D'Incalci, M. & Damia, G. (2008). Role of homologous recombination in trabectedin-induced DNA damage. *European Journal of Cancer*, Vol.44, No4, (March 2008), pp. 609-18, ISSN 1359-6349

Teicher, BA. (1996). Cancer therapeutics: Experimental and clinical agents. *Cancer Drug Discovery and Development*, Beverly A. Teicher Editor.

Teulade-Fichou, M.P; Vigneron, J.P & Lehn, J.M. (1995). Molecular recognition of nucleosides and nucleotides by a water soluble cyclo-bis-intercaland type receptor molecule based on acridine subunits. *Supramolecular Chemistry*, Vol.5, No.2, (February 1995), pp. 139-47, ISSN 1061-0278

Thoma, B.S.; Wakasugi, M.; Christensen, J.; Reddy, M.C. & Vasquez, K.M. (2005). Human XPC-hHR23B interacts with XPA-RPA in the recognition of triplex-directed psoralen DNA interstrand crosslinks. *Nucleic Acids Research*, Vol.33, No.9, (May 2005), pp. 2993-3001, ISSN 0305-1048

Todd, R.C. & Lippard S.J. (2010). Structure of duplex DNA containing the cisplatin 1,2-$\{Pt(NH_3)_2\}^{2+}$-d(GpG) cross-link at 1.77 A resolution. *Journal of Inorganic Biochemistry*, Vol.104, No.9, (September 2010), pp. 902-8, ISSN 0162-0134

Treiber, D.K; Zhai, X.; Jantzen, H.M. & Essigmann, J.M. (1994). Cisplatin-DNA adducts are molecular decoys for the ribosomal RNA transcription factor hUBF (human upstream binding factor). *Proceedings of the National Academy of Sciences USA*, Vol.91, No.12, (June 1994), pp. 5672-6, ISSN 0027-8424

Triantafillidi, K.; Karidi, K.; Novakova., O; Malina, J. & Garoufis, A. (2011). DNA binding selectivity of oligopyridine-ruthenium(II)-lysine conjugate. *Dalton Transactions*, Vol.40, No.2, (January 2011), pp. 472-83, ISSN 0022-4944

Trimmer, E.E.; Zamble, D.B.; Lippard, S.J. & Essigmann, J.M. (1998). Human testis-determining factor SRY binds to the major DNA adduct of cisplatin and a putative target sequence with comparable affinities. *Biochemistry*, Vol.37, No.1, (January 1998), pp. 352-362, ISSN 0006-2960

Trivedi, R.N.; Wang X.; Jelezcova, E.; Goellner, E.M.; Tang, J. & Sobol R.W. (2008). Human methyl purine DNA glycosylase and DNA polymerase β expression collectively predict sensitivity to Temozolomide. *Molecular Pharmacology*, Vol.74, No.2, (August 2008), pp 505–516, ISSN 0026-895X

Tubbs, J.L.; Pegg, A.E. & Tainer, J.A. (2007). DNA binding, nucleotide flipping, and the helix-turn-helix motif in base repair by O6-alkylguanine-DNA alkyltransferase and its implications for cancer chemotherapy. *DNA Repair (Amst)*, Vol.6, No8, (August 2007), pp. 1100-15, ISSN 1568-7864

Vasquez, K.M.; Christensen, J.; Li, L.; Finch, R.A. & Glazer, P.M. (2002). Human XPA and RPA DNA repair proteins participate in specific recognition of triplex-induced helical distortions. *Proceedings of the National Academy of Sciences USA*, Vol.99, No.9, (April 2002), pp. 5848–53, ISSN 0027-8424

Wold, M.S. (1997). Replication protein A: a heterotrimeric, single-stranded DNA-binding protein required for eukaryotic DNA metabolism. *Annual Review of Biochemistry*, Vol.66, (July 1997), pp. 61-92, ISSN 1545-4509

Wu, M.; Yan, S.; Patel, D.J.; Geacintov, N.E. & Broyde, S. (2002). Relating repair susceptibility of carcinogen-damaged DNA with structural distortion and thermodynamic stability. *Nucleic Acids Research*, Vol.30, No.15, (August 2002), pp. 3422-32, ISSN 0305-1048

Wu, Q.; Christensen, L.A.; Legerski, R.J. & Vasquez, K.M. (2005). Mismatch repair participates in error-free processing of DNA interstrand crosslinks in human cells. EMBO Reports, Vol.6, No.6, (June 2005), pp. 551–7, ISSN 1469-221X.

Wu, Q & Vasquez, K.M. (2008). Human MLH1 protein participates in genomic damage checkpoint signaling in response to DNA interstrand crosslinks, while MSH2 functions in DNA repair. PLoS Genetics, Vol.4, No.9 (September 2008), e1000189, ISSN 1553-7390

Yang, C.G.; Garcia, K. & He, C. (2009). Damage detection and base flipping in direct DNA alkylation repair. *Chembiochem*, Vol.10, No.3, (February 2009), pp. 417-423, ISSN 1439-4227

Yang, J.; Liu, X.; Niu, P.; Zou, Y. & Duan, Y. (2009). Correlations and co-localizations of Hsp70 with XPA, XPG in human bronchial epithelia cells exposed to benzo[*a*]pyrene. *Toxicology*, Vol. 265, No.1-2, (November 2009), pp. 10-4, ISSN 0300-483X

Yang, W. (2006). Poor base stacking at DNA lesions may initiate recognition by many repair proteins. *DNA Repair (Amst)*, Vol.5, No6, (June 2006), pp. 654-66, ISSN 1568-7864

Yuqin, C.; Dinshaw, J.P.; Nicholas, E.G. & Suse, B. (2009). Differential nucleotide excision repair susceptibility of bulky DNA adducts in different sequence contexts: Hierarchies of recognition signals. *Journal of Molecular Biology*, Vol.385, No.1, (January 2009), pp. 30-44, ISSN 0022-2836

Zhang, C.X. & Lippard, S.J. (2003). New metal complexes as potential therapeutics. *Current Opinion in Chemical Biology*, Vol.7, No.4, (August 2003), pp. 481-9, ISSN 1367-5931

Zhang, J.; Stevens, M.F.; Laughton, C.A.; Madhusudan, S. & Bradshaw, T.D. (2010). Acquired resistance to temozolomide in glioma cell lines: molecular mechanisms and potential translational applications. *Oncology*. Vol.78, No.2, (March 2010), pp 103-14, ISSN 0030-2414

Zhang, Y.; Rohde, L.H. & Wu, H. (2009). Involvement of nucleotide excision and mismatch repair mechanisms in double strand break repair. *Current Genomics*, Vol.10, No.4, (June 2009), pp 250–8, ISSN 1389-2029

Zhao, J.; Jain, A.; Iyer, R.R.; Modrich, P.L. & Vasquez, K.M. (2009). Mismatch repair and nucleotide excision repair proteins cooperate in the recognition of DNA interstrand crosslinks. *Nucleic Acids Research*, Vol.37, No.13, (July 2009), pp. 4420-9, ISSN 0305-1048

Zheng, H.; Cai, Y.; Ding, S.; Tang, Y.; Kropachev, K.; Zhou, Y.; Wang, L.; Wang, S.; Geacintov, N.E.; Zhang, Y. & Broyde, S. (2010). Base flipping free energy profiles for damaged and undamaged DNA. *Chemical Research in Toxicology*, Vol.23, No.12, (November 2010), pp. 1868–70, ISSN 0893-228X

Zhu, G.Y.; Chang, P. & Lippard, S.J. (2010). Recognition of Pplatinum- DNA damage by poly(ADP-ribose) polymerase-1. *Biochemistry*, Vol.49, No12, (November 2010), pp. 6177–83, ISSN 0006-2960

Zhu, L.B.; Xu, Q.; Hong, C.Y.; Yue, Z.; Zhang, Y.; Ye, H.N. & Yuan, Y. (2010). XPC gene intron 11 C/A polymorphism is a predictive biomarker for the sensitivity to NP chemotherapy in patients with non-small cell lung cancer. *Anticancer Drugs*, Vol.21, No.7, (August 2010), pp. 669-73, ISSN 0959-4973

Zou, Y. & Van Houten, B. (1999). Strand opening by the UvrA(2)B complex allows dynamic recognition of DNA damage. *EMBO Journal*, Vol.18, No.17, (September 1999), pp. 4889–901, ISSN 0261-4189

Zunino, F.; Gambetta, R.; Di Marco, A. & Zaccara, A. (1972). Interaction of daunomycin and its derivatives with DNA. *Biochimica and Biophysica Acta*, Vol.277, No.3, (September 1972), pp. 489-98, ISSN 0006-3002

# DNA Damage Caused by Polycyclic Aromatic Hydrocarbons: Mechanisms and Markers

Balam Muñoz and Arnulfo Albores
*Departamento de Toxicología,*
*Centro de Investigación y de Estudios Avanzados del I.P.N.*
*México*

## 1. Introduction

Polycyclic Aromatic Hydrocarbons (PAHs) are a group of chemicals that occur naturally in coal, crude oil and gasoline. Incomplete combustion of organic material results in emission of PAHs (ATSDR, 1996). These molecules consist of two or more aromatic rings fused in linear, angular or cluster arrangements (Fig. 1) and by definition are composed of hydrogen and carbon. PAHs containing up to six fused aromatic rings are often known as "small" PAHs while those containing more than six aromatic rings are called "large" PAHs. As pure chemicals, these compounds are colorless, white or pale yellow solids. Their physicochemical properties, vapor pressure and solubility vary according to their molecular weight. PAHs possess a highly characteristic UV absorbance spectra although some may be fluorescent (Fetzer & Biggs, 1994). PAHs are ubiquitous and persistent as a consequence of natural (forest fires and volcanic eruptions) and human activities (Jongeneelen, 2001). PAHs may distribute in water, soil and the atmosphere according to different weather and geographical factors. Although industrial activity such as coke manufacturing or asphalt production are major contributors to PAH emissions, incineration, power generation and several mobile sources also emit a considerable amount of PAHs. Significant sources of PAHs in surface waters include deposition of airborne PAHs, municipal wastewater discharge, urban storm-water runoff, and industrial waste. Food groups that tend to have the highest levels of PAHs include charcoal broiled or smoked meats, leafy vegetables, grains, and vegetable fats and oils (Yu, 2005). Therefore, workers of these industries and the general population are continually exposed to different concentrations of PAH mixtures. The Agency for Toxic Substances and Disease Registry (ATSDR) has grouped 17 PAHs according to their health effects (ATSDR, 1996). The United States Environmental Protection Agency (EPA) has designated 28 PAH compounds as priority pollutants (EPA, 2009) (Table 1). The International Agency for Research on Cancer (IARC) has classified some these compounds as carcinogenic (group 1) or likely carcinogenic (group 2A) to humans, for example benzo[*a*]pyrene and dibenz[*a,h*]anthracene, respectively (IARC, 2010). Finally, the National Institute of Standards and Technology has created a classification of PAHs according to their symbols, molecular formulas, class and notation among other properties (NIST, 2010).

The most common mechanism of carcinogenesis induced by PAHs is DNA damage through the formation of adducts. Alternatively, in the presence of reactive oxidative species, DNA damage can also result. In this chapter, we review the mechanisms of damage caused by exposure to PAHs, factors involved in repairing the damage, and the important role of biomarkers.

## 2. Metabolism of PAHs

Once PAHs enter the body they are metabolized in a number of organs (including liver, kidney, lungs), excreted in bile, urine or breast milk and stored to a limited degree in adipose tissue. The principal routes of exposure are: inhalation, ingestion, and dermal contact. The lipophilicity of PAHs enables them to readily penetrate cellular membranes (Yu, 2005). Subsequent metabolism renders them more water-soluble making them easier for the body to remove. However, PAHs can also be converted to more toxic or carcinogenic metabolites.

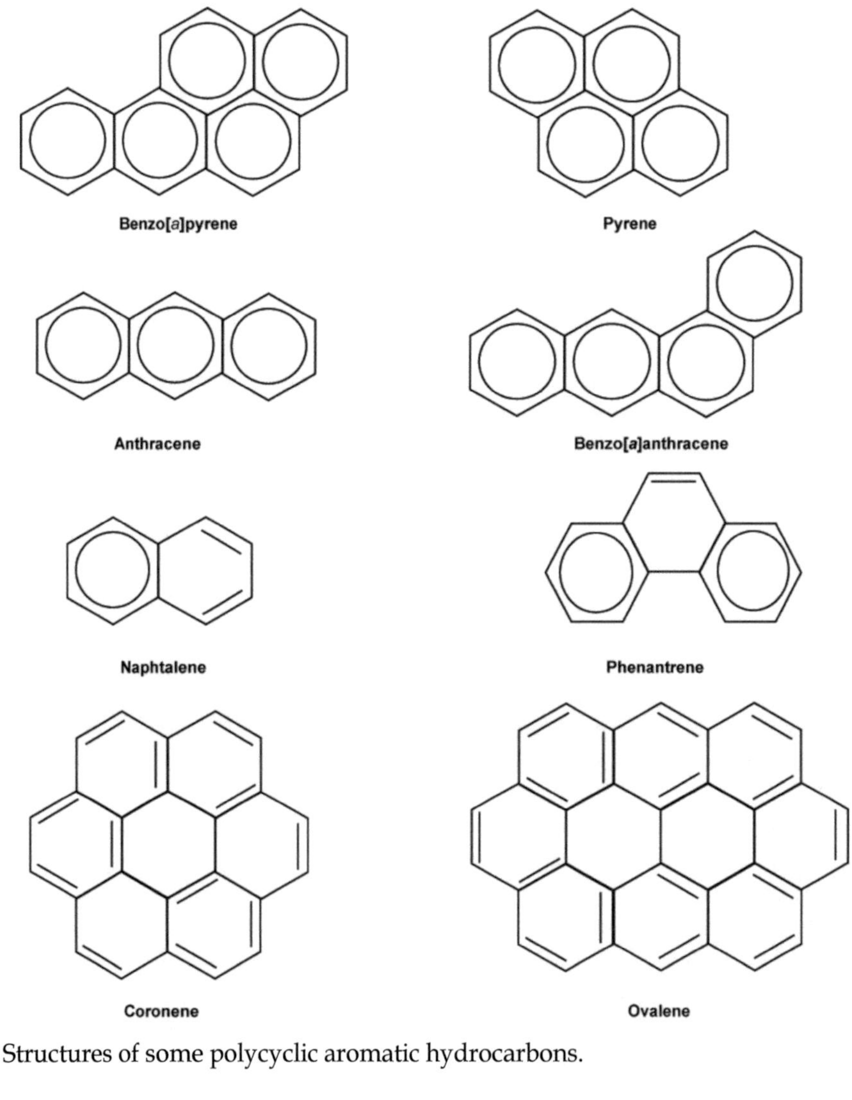


Fig. 1. Structures of some polycyclic aromatic hydrocarbons.

| Name | CAS[1] | Name | CAS |
|---|---|---|---|
| Acenaphthene | 83-32-9 | Dibenz(a,j)acridine, | 224-42-0 |
| Acenaphtylene | 208-96-8 | Dibenzo(a,h)anthracene | 53-70-3 |
| Benzo(a)anthracene | 56-55-3 | Dibenzo(a,e)fluoranthene | 5385-75-1 |
| Benzo(a)phenanthrene (chrysene) | 218-01-9 | Dibenzo(a,e)pyrene | 192-65-4 |
| Benzo(a)pyrene | 50-32-8 | Dibenzo(a,h)pyrene | 189-64-0 |
| Benzo(b)fluoranthene | 205-99-2 | Dibenzo(a,l)pyrene | 191-30-0 |
| Benzo(j)fluoranthene | 205-82-3 | 7H-Dibenzo(c,g)carbazole | 194-59-2 |
| Benzo(k)fluoranthene | 207-08-9 | 7,12-Dimethylbenz(a)anthracene | 57-97-6 |
| Benzo(g,h,i)perylene | 191-24-2 | Fluorene | 86-73-7 |
| Benzo(j,k)fluorene (fluoranthene) | 206-44-0 | Indeno(1,2,3-cd)pyrene | 193-39-5 |
| Benzo(r,s,t)pentaphene | 189-55-9 | 3-Methylcholanthrene | 56-49-5 |
| Dibenz(a,h)acridine | 226-36-8 | 5-Methylchrysene | 3697-24-3 |
| Phenanthrene | 85-01-8 | Pyrene | 129-00-0 |
| 1-Nitropyrene | 5222-43-0 | Anthracene | 120-12-7 |

Table 1. US EPA priority polycyclic aromatic hydrocarbons.

After exposure, these molecules induce expression of phase I and II metabolizing enzymes (Shimada, 2006) including aldo-ketone reductases, cytochrome P-450s, catechol-O-methyltransferase, epoxide hydrolase, peroxidases, glutathione S-transferases, N-acetyltransferases, sulfotransferases, and other enzymes catalyzing conjugation reactions (Williams & Phillips, 2000).

### 2.1 Phase I metabolism of PAHs

There are three main pathways for activation of PAHs: the formation of a PAH radical cation in a metabolic oxidation process involving cytochrome P450 peroxidase, the formation of PAH-o-quinones by dihydrodiol dehydrogenase-catalyzed oxidation and finally the creation of dihydrodiol epoxides, catalyzed by cytochrome P450 enzymes (Guengerich, 2000). The most common mechanism of metabolic activation of PAHs, such as benzo[a]pyrene (B[a]P), is via the formation of bay-region dihydrodiol epoxides e.g. benzo[a]pyrene-7,8-dihydrodiol-9,10-epoxide (BPDE), via CYP450 and epoxide hydrolase (EH) (Fig. 2). The most important enzymes in the metabolism of PAHs are CYPs 1A1, 1A2, 1B1 and 3A4. CYP1A1 is highly inducible by PAHs such as B[a]P and some polyhalogenated hydrocarbons. Recombinant human CYP1A1 metabolizes compounds such as B[a]P, 2-acetylaminofluorene and 7,8-diol,7-12-dimethylbenz[a]anthracene (Kim, et al., 1998). CYP1A2 and CYP1B2 are also inducible by the exposure to PAHs. In fact, these enzymes share the same mechanism with which PAH molecules interact with, the aryl hydrocarbon receptor (AhR). The AhR is present in the cytoplasm as a complex with other proteins such as heat shock protein 90 (Hsp90), p23 and AhR-interacting protein. After forming a complex with PAHs, the Hsp90 is released and the AhR-PAH complex translocates to the nucleus (Fig 3). Here, it creates a heterodimer with a ARNT (Ah Receptor Nuclear Translocator) and

[1] CAS (Chemical Abstracts Service) registry number

afterwards binds to DNA via the xenobiotic response element (XRE) situated in the promoter region of CYP1A and CYP1B genes (Shimada, et al., 2002)). CYP3A4 and CYP3A5 are known to activate PAHs present in cigarette smoke, such that increased protein levels and activity of these enzymes in cells exposed to smoke have been detected (Piipari, et al., 2000)). Furthermore, genetic variants of CYPs are associated with risk of carcinogenesis. Some polymorphisms of CYP1A1 are associated with adduct formation and mutagenesis in several populations and species (Ichiba, et al., 1994, Rojas, et al., 2000, Shields, et al., 1992). This fact is related to the metabolizing rate and the subsequent repair mechanism associated with DNA damage. Polycyclic aromatic hydrocarbons are activated by a pathway that involves both CYP enzymes and epoxide hydrolase.

Other phase I enzymes related to PAHs metabolism are the aldo-keto reductases. These enzymes oxidize polycyclic aromatic (PAH) trans-dihydrodiols to reactive and redox-active o-quinones *in vitro* (Quinn & Penning, 2006). Specifically, AKR1A1, and members of the AKR1C dihydrodiol/hydroxysteroid dehydrogenase subfamily, AKR1C1-AKR1C4 are involved in metabolic activation of PAH trans-dihydrodiol. Production of o-quinone metabolites by these enzymes has been shown *in vitro* and in cell lines to amplify ROS and oxidative damage to DNA bases to form the highly mutagenic lesion 8-oxo-dGuo and render damaged and carcinogenic DNA (Quinn, et al., 2008).

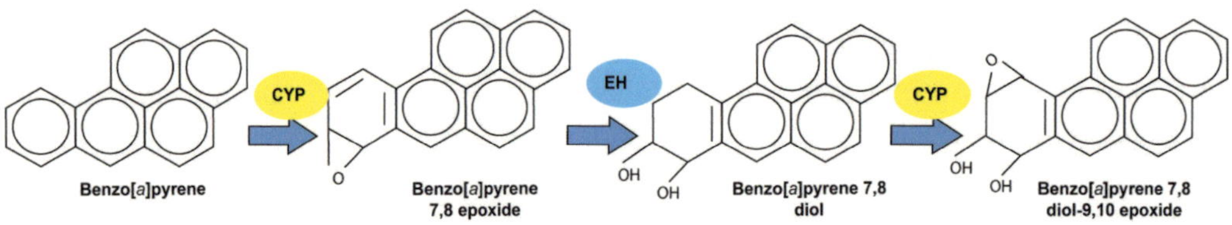


Fig. 2. Mechanism of activation of BaP by cytochrome P450 (CYP) and epoxide hydrolase (EH).

### 2.2 Phase II metabolism of PAHs

Phase II metabolism includes conjugation of metabolites from phase I with small molecules catalyzed by specific enzymes such as sulfotransferases (SULTs), UDP-glucuronyl transferases (UGTs) or glutathione S-transferases (GSTs). SULTs have been shown to activate some metabolites of PAHs such as 7,12-dimethylbenz[a]anthracene and its methyl-hydroxylated derivatives, in different tissues (Chou, et al., 1998). Polymorphisms of SULT1A1 have been associated with PAH-DNA adduct levels (Tang, et al., 2003). Glucuronidation is also a main pathway for PAH detoxification metabolism. Like sulfation, glucuronidation produces polar conjugates that are readily excreted. Oxygenated benzo[*a*]pyrene derivatives are common substrates of UDP-glucuronyltransferase (Bansal, et al., 1981), the resulting metabolite, 1-hydroxypyrene glucuronide, and the parental 1-hydroxypyrene are used as biomarkers of PAH exposure (Strickland, et al., 1994). Finally, GSTs are also involved in conjugation of PAH derivatives. The importance of this activity has been demonstrated *in vitro* using the corresponding diol epoxides of dibenzo[*a,l*]pyrene and benzo[*a*]pyrene as substrates for these enzymes (Sundberg, et al., 2002). Activity of GSTs is related to their glutathione redox status and genotoxic damage, at least in placenta tissue, therefore this status can be used as biomarker of PAH exposure (Obolenskaya, et al., 2010). On the other hand, polymorphisms of phase II metabolism are associated with carcinogenesis and with DNA damage. For instance, there is an important association between GSTM1 gene polymorphism and the DNA adduct levels (Binkova, et al., 2007). GSTs are also important for quenching and detoxifying ROS and their derivatives (Bonner, et al., 2005).

## 3. Mechanisms of damage

PAHs undergo metabolic activation to diol-epoxides as we discussed before, which bind covalently to DNA. Afterwards, they form adducts or induce oxidative stress that provokes mutations. If DNA repair mechanisms are afflicted by the adduct formation rate the result is an accumulation of mutations in DNA that may induce carcinogenesis. Several studies indicate that the number of adducts formed is related to the degree of PAH exposure. However, is also important to consider the effect of life stage of the organism at exposure to PAHs (Bolognesi, et al., 1991), as well as concentration and genetic profiles of PAHs, among other factors. PAH exposure induces several molecular and cellular responses that modify the endogenous environment. Exposure to PAHs induces genes involved in apoptosis, cell cycle control and DNA repair (Castorena-Torres, et al., 2008).

### 3.1 Adduct formation

When PAHs are metabolized reactive diol epoxide enantiomers are generated. These enantiomers form DNA adducts with different structures, motifs and biological activities. DNA adducts of diverse conformations are excised by DNA repair enzymes at different rates. PAH diol epoxides (PAHDEs) bind covalently to exocyclic amino groups of guanine and adenine, forming stable adducts within DNA (Lin, et al., 2001). Futhermore, there are correlations between DNA adduct levels and mutagenesis. The structure of some PAHDEs forms a region called "Fjord", which some studies indicate is a region that is highly involved with high tumorigenicity. These molecules are mostly non-planar, reactive, and bind preferentially to adenine nucleotides. On the other hand, PAHDES with a "bay" region are planar, less reactive and bind to guanine nucleotides (Fig. 4). Geacintov and colleagues (1997) have described several structural motifs by nuclear magnetic resonance analysis. These structural types are divided into: (a) minor groove, when the PAH is partially accessible to the solvent; (b) classical intercalation, when the PAH is protected from the environment and forms a "sandwich structure" and (c) base-displaced intercalation, when PAHs substitute the healthy base (Buterin, et al., 2000, Geacintov, et al., 1997).
Molecular studies have revealed that adducts in DNA block polymerase replication activity, contributing to increased DNA damage by reducing repair activity (Hsu, et al., 2005). An example of adduct formation between adenine or guanine and benzopyrene diol epoxide (BPDE) is shown in Figure 5. Interestingly, some compounds present in food are capable of preventing adducts such as ellagic acid (EA) by the formation of adducts previous to DNA binding (Lagerqvist, et al., 2011). The presence of adducts have been evaluated in marine and aquatic species as an indicator of environmental occurrence of PAHs. Some studies have revealed, by X-ray crystallography, structures of PAH-adducted oligonucleotides bound to bacterial DNA polymerases (Hsu, et al., 2005, Ling, et al., 2004).

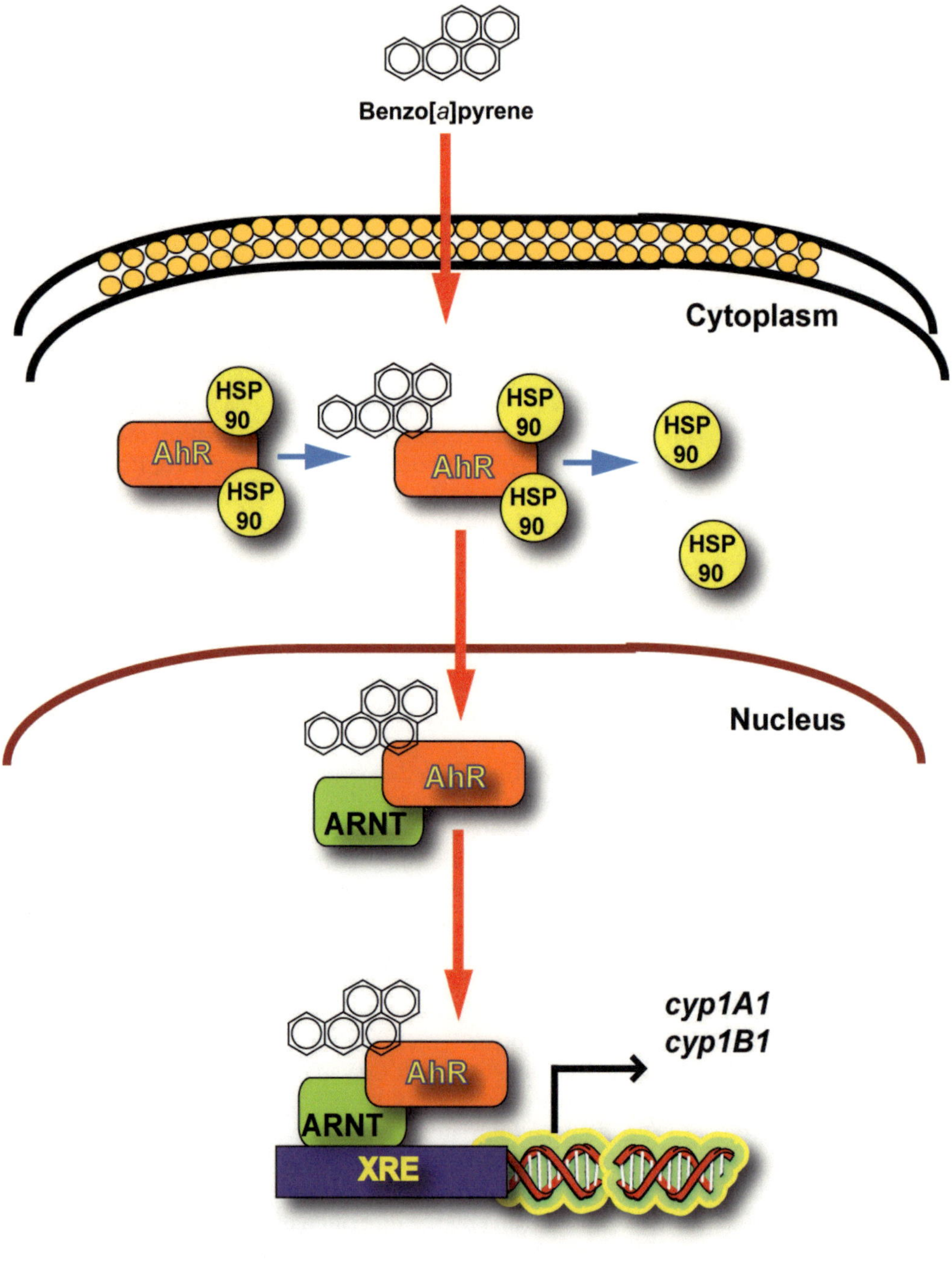


Fig. 3. Aryl hydrocarbon receptor (AhR) pathway activated by BaP induces expression of *cyp1A1* and *cyp1B1*.

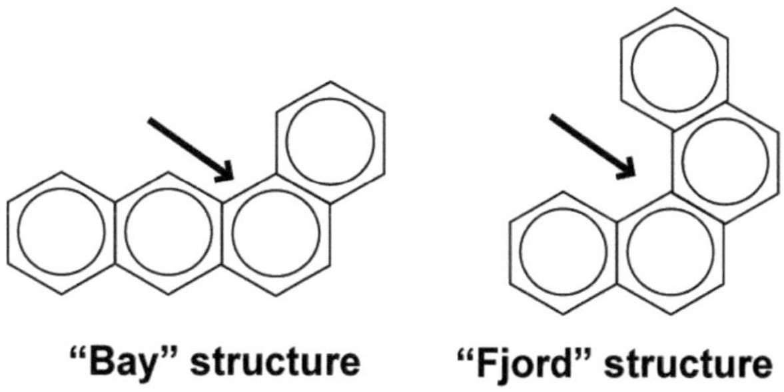


Fig. 4. Difference between bay and fjord regions in two PAH conformations.

### 3.2 Oxidative stress

It has been reported that BaP derivatives have the capacity to enter redox cycles and induce the production of reactive oxygen species (ROS), thereby causing oxidative stress (An, et al., 2011). BaP radical-cations are precursors for 6-OH-BaP. Auto-oxidation of this derivative may result in the formation of BaP quinones such as 6, 12-, 1,6- and 3,6-BaP dione (Briede, et al., 2004). These metabolites can undergo redox-cycling to their corresponding BaP diols and produce superoxide reactive oxygen species which are then converted to hydroxyl radicals by the Haber-Weiss reaction (Lesko & Lorentzen, 1985). Free radicals react with guanine and cause DNA damage, including the production of 7-hydro-8-oxo-20-deoxyguanosine (8-oxo-dG) (Chatgilialoglu & O'Neill, 2001). The OGG1 gene codes for a DNA glycosylase involved in base excision repair of 8-oxo-dG that arises from ROS. When this system fails there is an increase in mutation rate (Bonner, et al., 2005). Balance between generation of ROS species and scavenging of these molecules is fundamental in repairing DNA damage. If the rate of ROS generation is greater than their removal it is likely that more DNA damage will result. PAHs may absorb light energy in UVR (280–400 nm) region and may induce DNA damage by production of ROS. For example, chrysene, induces apoptosis and DNA damage in human keratinocytes by generating ROS in response to UVB radiation (Ali, et al., 2011).

### 3.3 Mutations

The failure of repair mechanisms and constant exposure to PAHs induce mutagenesis in cells. These mutations are present in multiple genes including those that participate in cell survival. In particular, p53 mutations are associated with risk of carcinogenesis in PAH-exposed individuals. Since the p53 protein is a transcription factor that regulates cell proliferation, differentiation, apoptosis, and DNA repair, mutations induced in this important protein could lead to severe damage in cells and genes. Some studies have associated p53 mutations to PAH exposure (Mordukhovich, et al., 2010, Yoon, et al., 2003). Another common target of mutagenesis is the ras gene (Ross & Nesnow, 1999). A study by Gray et al. (2001) revealed that exposure to BaP in mice increases mutation of the K-ras gene.

### 3.4 Carcinogenesis

Forming adducts in DNA repair-related genes is not the only mechanism by which PAHs induce carcinogenesis. An additional danger amounts from their resemblance to steroid hormones allowing PAHs the ability to activate estrogen receptors and metabolism. The ability of several PAHs to displace natural estrogens and occupy ER binding sites, at least to some extent, implies a potential mechanism of action in endocrine tissues that is ER-mediated (Santodonato, 1997). Nevertheless, the most important mechanism of carcinogenesis is a deficient DNA repair system in key genes involved in cell cycle control. Since chronic exposure to PAHs is related to a high rate of mutagenesis it is probable that damage to DNA is cumulative. Several studies have associated chronic occupational PAH exposure to multiple types of cancer including cancer of the bladder, lung, kidney, liver, and breast (Boffetta, et al., 1997, Dickey, et al., 1997, Karami, et al., 2011, Shen, et al., 2003).

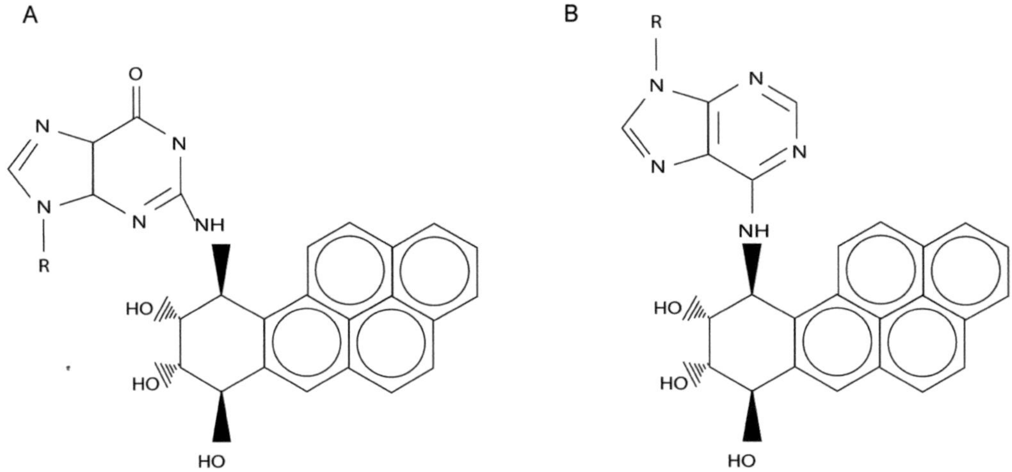


Fig. 5. Structures and interaction of two common adducts: (A) BPDE-dG adduct and (B) BPDE-dA adduct.

## 4. Mechanisms of repair

Several molecular processes exist in cells that repair damage caused from PAH exposure, adduct formation, and ROS production. If the damage is repaired by these mechanisms no further consequences should result. However, if the lesions escape repair and survive to the next round of DNA replication faulty translesion bypass can occur causing mutagenesis and carcinogenesis. The most common mechanisms of repair used by cells exposed to PAHs are: nucleotide excision repair (NER), base excision repair (BER), non-homologous end joining (NHEJ) of DNA double-strand breaks (DSBs), homologous recombinational repair (HRR) and transcription coupled repair (TCR). On the other hand, some studies indicate that DNA damage induced by PAHs is preferentially repaired by NER or BER (Braithwaite, et al., 1998), and to a lesser extent by HRR (Meschini, et al., 2010).

### 4.1 Nucleotide excision repair (NER)

In this process, cells recognize damaged DNA regions based on their abnormal structure or chemistry, then excise and replace them. This pathway is complex, requiring more than 20 different proteins. NER is considered the main pathway for removal of bulky DNA adducts (Braithwaite, et al., 1998). There are two distinct forms of NER: GG-NER (Global Genomic-NER) and TC-NER (Transcription Coupled-NER). The first corrects damage in transcriptionally silent areas of the genome, while the second repairs lesions on the actively transcribed strand of the DNA. In GG-NER, the XPC (Xeroderma Pigmentosum Complementation Group-C)/hHR23B (Rad23 homolog B) protein complex is responsible for the initial detection of damaged DNA. On the other hand, TC-NER does not require XPC, however the stalled RNA Polymerase complex is displaced in order to allow the NER proteins to access the damaged DNA. After this process, TC-NER and GG- NER proceed in identical ways. XPA and RPA (Replication Protein-A) then bind at the location of injury and further aid in damage detection. Subsequently, the XPB and XPD helicases unwind the DNA duplex in the surrounding area of the lesion. The endonucleases XPG and ERCC1 (Excision Repair Cross-Complementing group-1)/XPF then cleave one strand of the DNA at positions 3' and 5' to the damage, respectively, generating a 30 base oligonucleotide containing the lesion. This oligonucleotide is displaced, permitting gap repair synthesis (performed by DNA Pol Delta/Epsilon, and other accessory proteins). Finally, DNA ligase seals the nick in the repaired strand (Fig. 6). Several studies demonstrate that certain polymorphisms in NER genes alter the efficiency of DNA repair (Shen, et al., 2006, Vodicka, et al., 2004). Four polymorphisms, XPA -4G/A (rs1800975), ERCC1 C8092A (rs3212986), XPD Lys751Gln (rs1052559), and XPF Ser835Ser (rs1799801), are associated with a reduced capacity for DNA repair and an increased susceptibility to various cancers (Hu, et al., 2004, Monzo, et al., 2007). However, a recent study reports that significant opportunities exist for an interaction between the XPA-4 G/A polymorphism and PAH exposure on sperm DNA damage (Gu, et al., 2010). Although some PAHs lack "bay" and/or "fjord" regions, such as anthracene for example, this molecule also induces DNA damage, activating repair mechanisms, and has in fact has been shown to induce NER and MMR pathways (Desler, et al., 2009).These findings provide support for the importance of NER pathway in DNA damage induced by PAHs.

### 4.2 Base excision repair (BER)

BER involves the combined activity of some specific proteins that recognize and excise DNA damage, replacing the damaged moiety with normal nucleotides. PAH adducts are repaired by this mechanism. BER consists of three important steps: first, removal of the incorrect base by an appropriate DNA N-glycosylase to create an AP site (apurinic/apyrimidinic site); second, cutting off the damaged DNA strand by AP endonuclease upstream of the AP site, therefore creating a 3'-OH terminus adjacent to the AP site and finally, extension of the 3'-OH terminus by DNA polymerase, accompanied by excision of the AP site. Several enzymes are required to complete these three steps. In humans, there are at least six different glycosylases that bind specifically to a target base and hydrolyze the N-glycosylic bond generating the AP or abasic site. Next, the AP site is processed by the APE1 system (AP Endonuclease-1, or HAP1/REF1/APEX), which cuts the phosphodiester backbone adjacent to the 5' end of the AP site, resulting in a 3' hydroxyl group and a transient 5′ dRP (abasic deoxyribose phosphate). The removal of the dRP is accomplished by DNA Pol Beta (polymerase beta) activity, which adds one nucleotide to the 3′ end of the nick and removes the dRP moiety through the action of an AP lyase (Bennett, et al., 1997). DNA Pol Beta also interacts with XRCC1. DNA Pol Beta is therefore crucial for the inclusion of different components of BER at sites of DNA damage and promoting repair efficiency (Fig. 6). The BER pathway deals with smaller damage to individual bases, such as oxidation, methylation, depurination, and deamination. If the adducts are left unrepaired, they may cause permanent mutations (Boysen & Hecht, 2003). If these mutations are situated at critical sites, including tumor suppressor genes, DNA repair-related genes or oncogenes, they may lead to cellular transformation and the development of tumors. A recent study demonstrates that BER plays an important role in DNA repair in cells exposed to PAHs. Chinese hamster ovary cells (CHO) deficient in the BER pathway were found to be more sensitive to damage induced by DBPDE, as measured by frequency of chromosomal aberrations (Meschini, et al., 2010). Polymorphisms in proteins of the BER pathway are associated with an increase in DNA damage. One of these proteins, XRCC1, was discovered to have four functional polymorphisms: T-77C, Arg194Trp, Arg280His and Arg399Gln, associated with alteration in repair capacity of DNA damage induced by PAH adducts (Ji, et al., 2010).

### 4.3 Homologous recombination (HR)

Homologous recombination (HR) is a DNA metabolic process found in all forms of life that provides high-fidelity, template-dependent repair or tolerance of complex DNA damage including DNA gaps, DNA double-stranded breaks (DSBs), and DNA interstrand crosslinks (ICLs). The primary function of HR is to search for homology and DNA strand invasion through the Rad51-ssDNA presynaptic filament by positioning the invading 3'-end on a template duplex DNA to initiate repair synthesis. This mechanism participates in DNA repair induced by three specific PAHs: 1-nitrosopyrene (1-NOP), N-acetoxy-2-acetylaminofluorene (N-AcO-AAF), and 4-nitroquinoline 1-oxide (4-NQO). These PAHs were compared for their ability to cause intrachromosomal homologous recombination between two identical genes stably integrated into a genome of a mouse cell. In each case a dose-dependent increase in recombination frequency with differences in the efficiency of each compound was observed (Bhattacharyya, et al., 1989). Polymorphisms in the proteins related to the HR seem to be associated with a protective effect against PAH exposure.

One of these proteins, XRCC3, participates in homologous recombination repair of DNA double strand breaks and cross-links. This factor is a member of a family of Rad-51-related proteins. According to Shen, et al. (2003), it plays a protective role against bladder cancer for the XRCC3 codon 241 polymorphism, a higher risk in smokers. Considering that tobacco smoke has a high concentration of PAHs, this finding suggests that HR is related to some extent in the repair of damaged DNA induced by PAH exposure. Moreover, in an *in vitro* study using CHO cells deficient in the HR pathway, these cells were more sensitive to PAH exposure suggesting that this mechanism plays an important role in DNA repair (Meschini, et al., 2010).

### 4.4 Translesion synthesis (TLS)

To avoid cell death that may occur as a result of arrested DNA replication at unrepaired lesions cells have a mechanism, referred to as translesion synthesis (TLS), which allows them to overcome replication blockage from DNA damage. Once the lesion is generated in the DNA, the replication machine stalls, followed by either lesion repair or bypass by specialized polymerases (DNA polymerase IV or V, from the Y Polymerase family). Polymerase switching is mediated by, among other factors, the protein PCNA. TLS polymerases often have low fidelity; however, they are highly efficient, inserting the correct nucleotides at specific sites of damage. This process has been studied using the TLS performed by *Sulfolobus solfataricus* DNA polymerase Dpo4. The analysis of an oligonucleotide primer-extended and its dA−PAH adducts, using a liquid chromatography (LC)−mass spectrometry (MS)/MS, revealed this process in-depth including other proteins that may be involved (Zang, et al., 2006). The structure and nature, among other properties, of TLS polymerases is related to their fidelity and efficiency (Rechkoblit, et al., 2002). For a complete review of this process and the role of PAH adducts we recommend a review of Eoff et al. (2010).

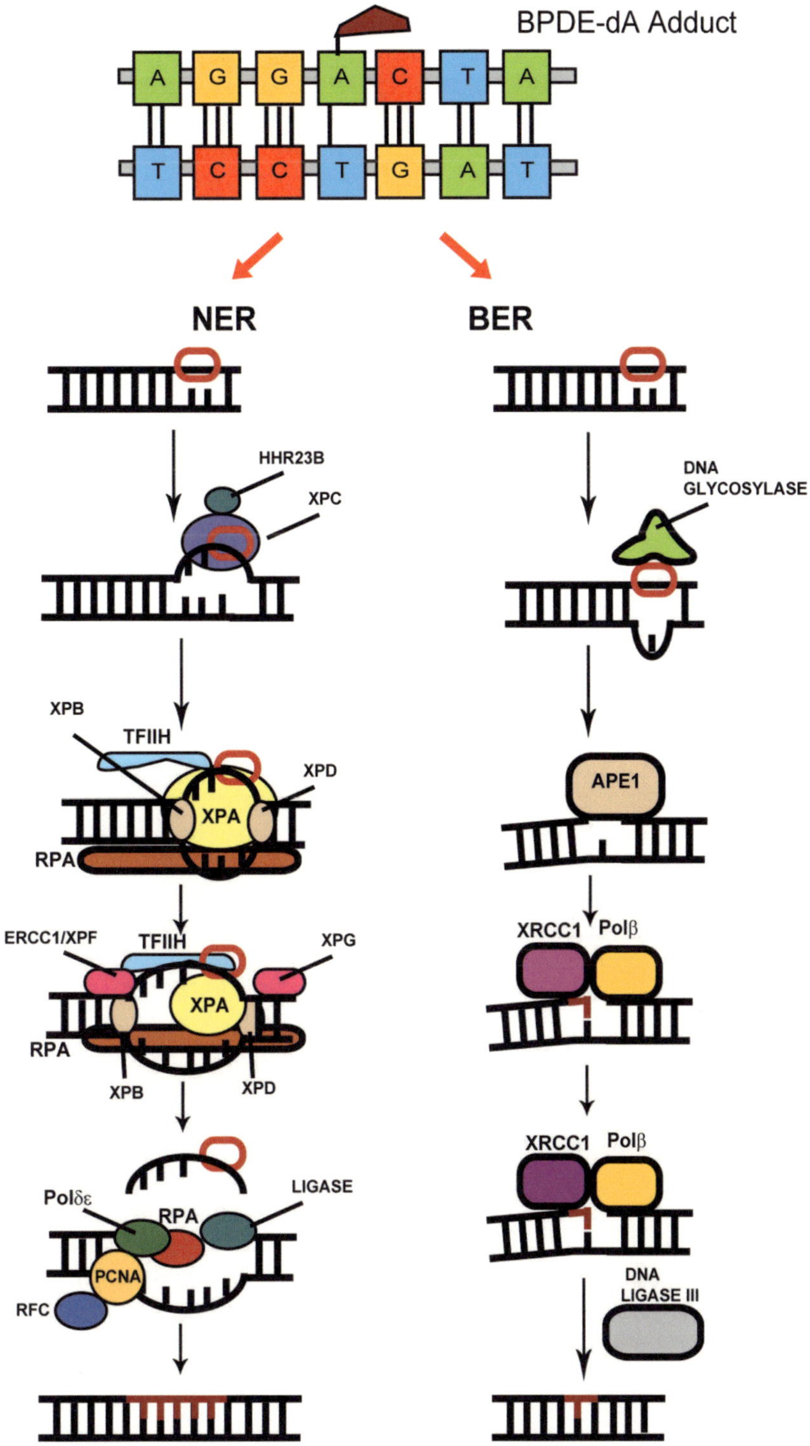


Fig. 6. Common mechanisms of DNA repair from PAH exposure and adduct formation: nucleotide excision repair (NER) and base excision repair (BER).

### 4.5 Mismatch repair (MMR)

The MMR system is responsible for the post-replicative repair of mismatches and small single stranded DNA loops, and is essential to the prevention of recombination between homologous DNA sequences. Although MMR repair in eukaryotic cells is not fully understood, studies of this mechanism in bacteria have contributed considerably to our understanding of this pathway. MMR is dependent on three highly conserved proteins: MutS, MutL, and MutH. In eukaryotes, homologous proteins as PCNA, RPA, HMGB1, RFC, and ligase I participate and coordinate the MMR process. Eukaryotic cells that are deficient in MMR have a 10-1,000-fold increase in mutation rates (Kunkel & Erie, 2005). In another study, MMR deficient mice showed an increase in PAH-induced lymphoma compared to controls (Zienolddiny, et al., 2006). MMR corrects strand-specific base mispairs and small loop structures. Furthermore, this mechanism recognizes smaller base analoges as mispairs that are participating in oxidative DNA damage repair. Cells deficient in the hMLH1 protein (essential for MMR initiation) have a reduced repair activity when exposed to anthracene (Desler, et al., 2009). This result indicates that MMR has a probable role in DNA repair response resulting from PAH exposure.

### 4.6 Other repair mechanisms

Further studies are necessary to confirm two other possible mechanisms involved in DNA repair following PAH exposure: non-homologous end joining (NHEJ) and transcription coupled repair (TCR). NHEJ appears to participate in DNA repair after PAH exposure. A recent report described that the V3-3 CHO cell line (NHEJ-deficient), showed a statistically significant dose-dependent enhancement during induced sister chromatid exchanges under PAH exposure. This result indicates that this process is important in DNA repair (Meschini, et al., 2010).

Some adducts perform alterations to the transcription process. The current model for TCR is dependent on the stalling of RNA pol II. Some PAHs such as BPDE and B[c]PhDE produce adducts repaired by TCR, while other studies indicate that PAHs such as B[g]Ch-DE and DB[a,l]P-DE also produce adducts. The efficiency and rate for repairing DNA depends of intrinsic adduct properties (Zhong, et al., 2010). For a complete review of this process we suggest consulting Scicchitano (2005).

## 5. Methods for detection of DNA damage

DNA damage associated with PAH exposure is mainly assessed by measuring the number of adducts formed. Several methods, such as $^{32}$P-postlabelling or immunochemical analysis with specific antibodies, have been applied extensively. However, the arrival of new molecular techniques and innovations in previously well-established biochemical methods, have increased the possibility of the early detection of DNA damage. Polymorphisms and gene expression analysis are helping to determine susceptibility of individuals and populations. Use of mass spectrometry and high performance liquid chromatography (HPLC) with increased sensitivity is another common tool to evaluate and quantify adduct formation. A brief description of the available methods to detect DNA damage is listed in Table 2.

On the other hand, some studies have proposed using molecules included in natural compounds to reduce DNA damage induced by PAHs (Chan, et al., 2003). Green tea consumption may reduce the risk of lung cancer by several hypothesized mechanisms including scavenging oxidative radicals (Bonner, et al., 2005). In previous studies, the role of green tea polyphenols has been associated with protective effects against tumor induction in mice to which PAHs were topically applied (Wang, et al., 1989). Resveratrol (Leung, et al., 2009) and Genistain (Leung, et al., 2009) reduced DNA oxidative damage and adduct formation induced by 7,12-dimethylbenz[*a*]anthracene in MCF-10A cells.

| **Strategies for detection of PAH exposure** | **Target molecule or experimental technique** | **Advantages** | **Disadvantages** | **Examples** |
|---|---|---|---|---|
| **Metabolites detection and quantitation** | Metabolites as a result of exposure detected by chromatography | Sensitive methods and multiple biological sources | Unstable metabolites | 1-hydroxypyrene |
| **Adduct detection** | Radiolabeled compounds | High sensitive to stable adducts | It may not be possible to detect unstable adducts | DNA adducts |
| | Mass spectrometry | High sensitivity and selectivity | Suitable just for isotopes | |
| | $^{32}$P-Postlabeling assay | High sensitivity to low concentrations, detection of different structures | Interference due endogen adducts | |
| | Immunoassays | Very high sensitivity | Hard to obtain and validate antibodies | |
| **Primary compound detection** | PAH molecules | Indicators of exposure | Some compounds are volatile | Pyrene |
| **Polymorphism analysis** | Genotyping | Susceptibility markers | Few studies on populations | CYP1A1 polymorphisms |
| **Gene expression** | Molecular biology methods | Changes in gene expression of some genes are related with PAH exposure | Expensive and highly skilled techniques | CYP1B1 expression |

Table 2. Methods to detect DNA damage caused by PAH exposure.

These studies offer novel alternatives for the prevention of further DNA damage caused by PAH exposure. Additionally, mechanisms of damage and repair are revealed through understanding the interactions and pathways involved when these molecules come into contact.

Both methods of detection and prevention of DNA damage are candidates for becoming new molecular alternatives for therapy and diagnosis of PAH-exposed individuals, and new tools in environmental biomonitoring.

## 6. Conclusions

Worldwide, the population is, to some extent, exposed to PAHs. Of primary concern are the carcinogenic, teratogenic and mutagenic properties exhibited by some PAHs. The occurrence of cancer and other diseases associated with PAH exposure has increased in recent decades. As we discussed in this chapter, the major mechanisms of carcinogenesis induced by these compounds are the interaction of PAHs with DNA to form adducts and the generation of reactive oxygen species. Both activities result in DNA damage and mutagenesis in important sites of the genome. Maintenance of genome integrity is critically dependent on efficient repair of DNA lesions by specific DNA repair mechanisms. In addition, the metabolism of PAHs is related with the ability of cells to prevent damage. Polymorphisms in DNA repair or xenobiotic metabolism-related genes are therefore associated with PAH-induced carcinogenesis. For this reason, understanding the metabolic pathways, biochemical transformations and interactions of PAHs with DNA will help to develop better strategies for risk analysis in exposed individuals. Some studies have shown that several natural compounds could help to reduce DNA damage caused by PAH exposure.

These findings offer the possibility for the development of novel drugs that help in the treatment of diseases related to PAH exposure. The analysis of specific polymorphisms of DNA repair genes will help to determine susceptibility in defined populations and the development of new biomarkers and diagnostic tools. Moreover, the study of DNA damage induced by these compounds has included other environmentally important species, such as fish, shrimp and worms. These studies are important in the development of biomarkers for biomonitoring and environmental assessment.

## 7. Acknowledgments

This work was supported by CONACyT Mexico (60463) to AA and CONACyT (104316) to BM.

## 8. References

Ali, D., Verma, A., Mujtaba, F., Dwivedi, A., Hans, R. K.& Ray, R. S. (2011). UVB-induced apoptosis and DNA damaging potential of chrysene via reactive oxygen species in human keratinocytes. Toxicol Lett, Vol. 204, No.2-3, (Jul 28), pp. 199-207, 1879-3169 (Electronic) 0378-4274 (Linking)

An, J., Yin, L., Shang, Y., Zhong, Y., Zhang, X., Wu, M., Yu, Z., Sheng, G., Fu, J. & Huang, Y. (2011). The combined effects of BDE47 and BaP on oxidatively generated DNA damage in L02 cells and the possible molecular mechanism. *Mutation Research/Genetic Toxicology and Environmental Mutagenesis,* Vol. In Press, Corrected Proof, pp.

ATSDR. (1996). ToxFAQs™ for Polycyclic Aromatic Hydrocarbons (PAHs), In: Agency for Toxic Substances and Disease Registry, 16.01.2011, Available from http://www.atsdr.cdc.gov/toxfaqs/tf.asp?id=121&tid=25

Bansal, S. K., Zaleski, J.& Gessner, T. (1981). Glucuronidation of oxygenated benzo(a)pyrene derivatives by UDP-glucuronyltransferase of nuclear envelope. *Biochemical and Biophysical Research Communications,* Vol. 98, No.1, pp. 131-139,

Bennett, R. A., Wilson, D. M., 3rd, Wong, D. & Demple, B. (1997). Interaction of human apurinic endonuclease and DNA polymerase beta in the base excision repair pathway. *Proceedings of the National Academy of Sciences of the U S A,* Vol. 94, No.14, (Jul 8), pp. 7166-7169, 0027-8424 (Print) 0027-8424 (Linking)

Bhattacharyya, N. P., Maher, V. M.& McCormick, J. J. (1989). Ability of structurally related polycyclic aromatic carcinogens to induce homologous recombination between duplicated chromosomal sequences in mouse L cells. *Mutation Research/Fundamental and Molecular Mechanisms of Mutagenesis*, Vol. 211, No.2, pp. 205-214,

Binkova, B., Chvatalova, I., Lnenickova, Z., Milcova, A., Tulupova, E., Farmer, P. B.& Sram, R. J. (2007). PAH-DNA adducts in environmentally exposed population in relation to metabolic and DNA repair gene polymorphisms. *Mutation Research/Fundamental and Molecular Mechanisms of Mutagenesis*, Vol. 620, No.1-2, pp. 49-61,

Boffetta, P., Jourenkova, N.& Gustavsson, P. (1997). Cancer risk from occupational and environmental exposure to polycyclic aromatic hydrocarbons. *Cancer Causes Control*, Vol. 8, No.3, (May), pp. 444-472, 0957-5243 (Print) 0957-5243 (Linking)

Bolognesi, C., Parrini, M., Aiello, C.& Rossi, L. (1991). DNA damage induced by 7,12-dimethylbenz[a]anthracene in the liver and the mammary gland of rats exposed to polycyclic aromatic hydrocarbon enzyme inducers during perinatal life. *Mutagenesis*, Vol. 6, No.2, (Mar), pp. 113-116, 0267-8357 (Print) 0267-8357 (Linking)

Bonner, M. R., Rothman, N., Mumford, J. L., He, X., Shen, M., Welch, R., Yeager, M., Chanock, S., Caporaso, N.& Lan, Q. (2005). Green tea consumption, genetic susceptibility, PAH-rich smoky coal, and the risk of lung cancer. Mutat Res, Vol. 582, No.1-2, (Apr 4), pp. 53-60, 0027-5107 (Print) 0027-5107 (Linking)

Boysen, G.& Hecht, S. S. (2003). Analysis of DNA and protein adducts of benzo[a]pyrene in human tissues using structure-specific methods. *Mutation Research/Reviews in Mutation Research*, Vol. 543, No.1, pp. 17-30,

Braithwaite, E., Wu, X.& Wang, Z. (1998). Repair of DNA lesions induced by polycyclic aromatic hydrocarbons in human cell-free extracts: involvement of two excision repair mechanisms in vitro. *Carcinogenesis*, Vol. 19, No.7, (Jul), pp. 1239-1246, 0143-3334 (Print) 0143-3334 (Linking)

Briede, J. J., Godschalk, R. W., Emans, M. T., De Kok, T. M., Van Agen, E., Van Maanen, J., Van Schooten, F. J.& Kleinjans, J. C. (2004). In vitro and in vivo studies on oxygen free radical and DNA adduct formation in rat lung and liver during benzo[a]pyrene metabolism. *Free Radicals Research*, Vol. 38, No.9, (Sep), pp. 995-1002, 1071-5762 (Print)1029-2470 (Linking)

Buterin, T., Hess, M. T., Luneva, N., Geacintov, N. E., Amin, S., Kroth, H., Seidel, A.& Naegeli, H. (2000). Unrepaired fjord region polycyclic aromatic hydrocarbon-DNA adducts in ras codon 61 mutational hot spots. *Cancer Research*, Vol. 60, No.7, (Apr 1), pp. 1849-1856, 0008-5472 (Print) 0008-5472 (Linking)

Castorena-Torres, F., Bermudez de Leon, M., Cisneros, B., Zapata-Perez, O., Salinas, J. E.& Albores, A. (2008). Changes in gene expression induced by polycyclic aromatic hydrocarbons in the human cell lines HepG2 and A549. *Toxicology In Vitro*, Vol. 22, No.2, (Mar), pp. 411-421, 0887-2333 (Print)

Chan, H. Y., Wang, H., Tsang, D. S., Chen, Z. Y.& Leung, L. K. (2003). Screening of chemopreventive tea polyphenols against PAH genotoxicity in breast cancer cells by a XRE-luciferase reporter construct. *Nutrition and Cancer*, Vol. 46, No.1, pp. 93-100, 0163-5581 (Print) 0163-5581 (Linking)

Chatgilialoglu, C.& O'Neill, P. (2001). Free radicals associated with DNA damage. *Experimental Gerontology*, Vol. 36, No.9, (Sep), pp. 1459-1471, 0531-5565 (Print) 0531-5565 (Linking)

Chou, H. C., Ozawa, S., Fu, P. P., Lang, N. P.& Kadlubar, F. F. (1998). Metabolic activation of methyl-hydroxylated derivatives of 7,12-dimethylbenz[a]anthracene by human liver dehydroepiandrosterone-steroid sulfotransferase. *Carcinogenesis*, Vol. 19, No.6, (Jun), pp. 1071-1076, 0143-3334 (Print) 0143-3334 (Linking)

Desler, C., Johannessen, C.& Rasmussen, L. J. (2009). Repair of DNA damage induced by anthanthrene, a polycyclic aromatic hydrocarbon (PAH) without bay or fjord regions. *Chemico-Biological Interactions*, Vol. 177, No.3, (Feb 12), pp. 212-217, 1872-7786 (Electronic) 0009-2797 (Linking)

Dickey, C., Santella, R. M., Hattis, D., Tang, D., Hsu, Y., Cooper, T., Young, T. L.& Perera, F. P. (1997). Variability in PAH-DNA adduct measurements in peripheral mononuclear cells: implications for quantitative cancer risk assessment. *Risk Analysis*, Vol. 17, No.5, (Oct), pp. 649-656, 0272-4332 (Print) 0272-4332 (Linking)

Eoff, R. L., Egli, M.& Guengerich, P. (2010).Impact of Chemical Adducts on Translesion Synthesis in Replicative and Bypass DNA Polymerases From Structure to Function. In: *The Chemical Biology of DNA damage* Wiley-VCH Verlag GmbH & Co. KGaA, 9783527630110,

EPA. (2009). List of Priority Chemicals, In: United States Environmental Protection Agency Web Site, 03.02.2011, Available from http://www.epa.gov/osw/hazard/wastemin/priority.htm

Fetzer, J. C.& Biggs, W. R. (1994). A Review of the Large Polycyclic Aromatic Hydrocarbons. *Polycyclic aromatic compounds*, Vol. 4, No.1, pp. 3 - 17, 1040-6638 March 18, 2011

Geacintov, N. E., Cosman, M., Hingerty, B. E., Amin, S., Broyde, S.& Patel, D. J. (1997). NMR Solution Structures of Stereoisomeric Covalent Polycyclic Aromatic Carcinogen-DNA Adducts: Principles, Patterns, and Diversity. *Chemical Research in Toxicology*, Vol. 10, No.2, pp. 111-146,

Gray, D. L., Warshawsky, D., Xue, W., Nines, R., Wang, Y., Yao, R.& Stoner, G. D. (2001). The effects of a binary mixture of benzo(a)pyrene and 7H-dibenzo(c,g)carbazole on lung tumors and K-ras oncogene mutations in strain A/J mice. *Experimental Lung Research*, Vol. 27, No.3, (Apr-May), pp. 245-253, 0190-2148 (Print) 0190-2148 (Linking)

Gu, A., Ji, G., Zhu, P., Zhou, Y., Fu, G., Xia, Y., Song, L., Wang, S. & Wang, X. (2010). Nucleotide excision repair polymorphisms, polycyclic aromatic hydrocarbon exposure, and their effects on sperm deoxyribonucleic acid damage and male factor infertility. *Fertility and Sterility*, Vol. 94, No.7, pp. 2620-2625.e2625,

Guengerich, F. P. (2000). Metabolism of chemical carcinogens. *Carcinogenesis*, Vol. 21, No.3, (Mar), pp. 345-351, 0143-3334 (Print) 0143-3334 (Linking)

Hsu, G. W., Huang, X., Luneva, N. P., Geacintov, N. E.& Beese, L. S. (2005). Structure of a high fidelity DNA polymerase bound to a benzo[a]pyrene adduct that blocks replication. *Journal of Biological Chemistry*, Vol. 280, No.5, (Feb 4), pp. 3764-3770, 0021-9258 (Print) 0021-9258 (Linking)

Hu, J. J., Hall, M. C., Grossman, L., Hedayati, M., McCullough, D. L., Lohman, K.& Case, L. D. (2004). Deficient nucleotide excision repair capacity enhances human prostate cancer risk. Cancer Res, Vol. 64, No.3, (Feb 1), pp. 1197-1201, 0008-5472 (Print) 0008-5472 (Linking)

IARC. (2010). IARC monographs on the evaluation of carcinogenic risks to humans., In: International Agency for Research in Cancer Web site, 22.02.2011, Available from http://monographs.iarc.fr/ENG/Classification/index.php

Ichiba, M., Hagmar, L., Rannug, A., Hogstedt, B., Alexandrie, A. K., Carstensen, U.& Hemminki, K. (1994). Aromatic DNA adducts, micronuclei and genetic polymorphism for CYP1A1 and GST1 in chimney sweeps. *Carcinogenesis*, Vol. 15, No.7, (Jul), pp. 1347-1352, 0143-3334 (Print) 0143-3334 (Linking)

Ji, G., Gu, A., Zhou, Y., Shi, X., Xia, Y., Long, Y., Song, L., Wang, S.& Wang, X. (2010). Interactions between Exposure to Environmental Polycyclic Aromatic Hydrocarbons and DNA Repair Gene Polymorphisms on Bulky DNA Adducts in Human Sperm. *PLoS ONE*, Vol. 5, No.10, pp. e13145,

Jongeneelen, F. J. (2001). Benchmark guideline for urinary 1-hydroxypyrene as biomarker of occupational exposure to polycyclic aromatic hydrocarbons. *Annals of Occupationa Hygiene*, Vol. 45, No.1, (Jan), pp. 3-13, 0003-4878 (Print) 0003-4878 (Linking)

Karami, S., Boffetta, P., Brennan, P., Stewart, P. A., Zaridze, D., Matveev, V., Janout, V., Kollarova, H., Bencko, V., Navratilova, M., Szeszenia-Dabrowska, N., Mates, D., Gromiec, J. P., Sobotka, R., Chow, W.-H., Rothman, N.& Moore, L. E. (2011). Renal Cancer Risk and Occupational Exposure to Polycyclic Aromatic Hydrocarbons and Plastics. *Journal of Occupational & Environmental Medicine*, Vol. 53, No.2, pp. 218-223 1076-2752

Kim, J. H., Stansbury, K. H., Walker, N. J., Trush, M. A., Strickland, P. T.& Sutter, T. R. (1998). Metabolism of benzo[a]pyrene and benzo[a]pyrene-7,8-diol by human cytochrome P450 1B1. *Carcinogenesis*, Vol. 19, No.10, (Oct), pp. 1847-1853, 0143-3334 (Print) 0143-3334 (Linking)

Kunkel, T. A.& Erie, D. A. (2005). DNA mismatch repair. *Annual Review of Biochemistry*, Vol. 74, pp. 681-710, 0066-4154 (Print) 0066-4154 (Linking)

Lagerqvist, A., Hakansson, D., Frank, H., Seidel, A.& Jenssen, D. (2011). Structural requirements for mutation formation from polycyclic aromatic hydrocarbon dihydrodiol epoxides in their interaction with food chemopreventive compounds. *Food and Chemical Toxicology*, Vol. 49, No.4, (Apr), pp. 879-886, 1873-6351 (Electronic) 0278-6915 (Linking)

Leung, H. Y., Yung, L. H., Poon, C. H., Shi, G., Lu, A. L.& Leung, L. K. (2009). Genistein protects against polycyclic aromatic hydrocarbon-induced oxidative DNA damage in non-cancerous breast cells MCF-10A. *British Journal of Nutrition*, Vol. 101, No.2, (Jan), pp. 257-262, 1475-2662 (Electronic) 0007-1145 (Linking)

Leung, H. Y., Yung, L. H., Shi, G., Lu, A. L.& Leung, L. K. (2009). The red wine polyphenol resveratrol reduces polycyclic aromatic hydrocarbon-induced DNA damage in MCF-10A cells. *British Journal of Nutrition*, Vol. 102, No.10, (Nov), pp. 1462-1468, 1475-2662 (Electronic) 0007-1145 (Linking)

Lin, C. H., Huang, X., Kolbanovskii, A., Hingerty, B. E., Amin, S., Broyde, S., Geacintov, N. E.& Patel, D. J. (2001). Molecular topology of polycyclic aromatic carcinogens determines DNA adduct conformation: a link to tumorigenic activity. Journal of Molecular Biology, Vol. 306, No.5, pp. 1059-1080,

Ling, H., Sayer, J. M., Plosky, B. S., Yagi, H., Boudsocq, F., Woodgate, R., Jerina, D. M.& Yang, W. (2004). Crystal structure of a benzo[a]pyrene diol epoxide adduct in a ternary complex with a DNA polymerase. *Proceedings of the National Academy of Sciences of the U S A*, Vol. 101, No.8, (Feb 24), pp. 2265-2269, 0027-8424 (Print) 0027-8424 (Linking)

Meschini, R., Berni, A., Marotta, E., Filippi, S., Fiore, M., Mancinelli, P., Natarajan, A. T.& Palitti, F. (2010). DNA repair mechanisms involved in the removal of DBPDE-induced lesions leading to chromosomal alterations in CHO cells. *Cytogenetics and Genome Research*, Vol. 128, No.1-3, pp. 124-130, 1424-859X (Electronic) 1424-8581 (Linking)

Monzo, M., Moreno, I., Navarro, A., Ibeas, R., Artells, R., Gel, B., Martinez, F., Moreno, J., Hernandez, R.& Navarro-Vigo, M. (2007). Single nucleotide polymorphisms in nucleotide excision repair genes XPA, XPD, XPG and ERCC1 in advanced colorectal cancer patients treated with first-line oxaliplatin/fluoropyrimidine. *Oncology*, Vol. 72, No.5-6, pp. 364-370, 1423-0232 (Electronic) 0030-2414 (Linking)

Mordukhovich, I., Rossner, P., Jr., Terry, M. B., Santella, R., Zhang, Y. J., Hibshoosh, H., Memeo, L., Mansukhani, M., Long, C. M., Garbowski, G., Agrawal, M., Gaudet, M. M., Steck, S. E., Sagiv, S. K., Eng, S. M., Teitelbaum, S. L., Neugut, A. I., Conway-Dorsey, K.& Gammon, M. D. (2010). Associations between polycyclic aromatic hydrocarbon-related exposures and p53 mutations in breast tumors. *Environmental Health Perspectives*, Vol. 118, No.4, (Apr), pp. 511-518, 1552-9924 (Electronic) 0091-6765 (Linking)

NIST. (2010). NIST chemical kinetics model database., In: National Institute of Standards and Tecnonology database, 03.03.2011, Available from http://kinetics.nist.gov/CKMech/SpeciesSearch.jsp#Help PAH Class

Obolenskaya, M. Y., Teplyuk, N. M., Divi, R. L., Poirier, M. C., Filimonova, N. B., Zadrozna, M.& Pasanen, M. J. (2010). Human placental glutathione S-transferase activity and polycyclic aromatic hydrocarbon DNA adducts as biomarkers for environmental oxidative stress in placentas from pregnant women living in radioactivity- and chemically-polluted regions. *Toxicology Letters*, Vol. 196, No.2, pp. 80-86,

Piipari, R., Savela, K., Nurminen, T., Hukkanen, J., Raunio, H., Hakkola, J., Mantyla, T., Beaune, P., Edwards, R. J., Boobis, A. R.& Anttila, S. (2000). Expression of CYP1A1, CYP1B1 and CYP3A, and polycyclic aromatic hydrocarbon-DNA adduct formation in bronchoalveolar macrophages of smokers and non-smokers. *International Journal of Cancer*, Vol. 86, No.5, (Jun 1), pp. 610-616, 0020-7136 (Print) 0020-7136 (Linking)

Quinn, A. M., Harvey, R. G.& Penning, T. M. (2008). Oxidation of PAH trans-Dihydrodiols by Human Aldo-Keto Reductase AKR1B10. *Chemical Research in Toxicology*, Vol. 21, No.11, pp. 2207-2215,

Quinn, A. M.& Penning, T. M. (2006). Oxidation of PAH trans-dihydrodiols by human aldo-keto reductase (AKR) 1B isoforms: A new AKR subfamily implicated in PAH activation. *Proceedings of Frontiers in Cancer Prevention Research Conference*, Boston, MA, USA, April 1, 2006

Rechkoblit, O., Zhang, Y., Guo, D., Wang, Z., Amin, S., Krzeminsky, J., Louneva, N.& Geacintov, N. E. (2002). trans-Lesion synthesis past bulky benzo[a]pyrene diol epoxide N2-dG and N6-dA lesions catalyzed by DNA bypass polymerases. *Journal of Biological Chemistry*, Vol. 277, No.34, (Aug 23), pp. 30488-30494, 0021-9258 (Print) 0021-9258 (Linking)

Rojas, M., Cascorbi, I., Alexandrov, K., Kriek, E., Auburtin, G., Mayer, L., Kopp-Schneider, A., Roots, I.& Bartsch, H. (2000). Modulation of benzo[a]pyrene diolepoxide-DNA adduct levels in human white blood cells by CYP1A1, GSTM1 and GSTT1 polymorphism. *Carcinogenesis*, Vol. 21, No.1, (Jan), pp. 35-41, 0143-3334 (Print) 0143-3334 (Linking)

Ross, J. A.& Nesnow, S. (1999). Polycyclic aromatic hydrocarbons: correlations between DNA adducts and ras oncogene mutations. *Mutation Research*, Vol. 424, No.1-2, (Mar 8), pp. 155-166, 0027-5107 (Print) 0027-5107 (Linking)

Santodonato, J. (1997). Review of the estrogenic and antiestrogenic activity of polycyclic aromatic hydrocarbons: relationship to carcinogenicity. *Chemosphere*, Vol. 34, No.4, (Feb), pp. 835-848, 0045-6535 (Print) 0045-6535 (Linking)

Scicchitano, D. A. (2005). Transcription past DNA adducts derived from polycyclic aromatic hydrocarbons. *Mutation Research*, Vol. 577, No.1-2, (Sep 4), pp. 146-154, 0027-5107 (Print) 0027-5107 (Linking)

Shen, J., Desai, M., Agrawal, M., Kennedy, D. O., Senie, R. T., Santella, R. M. & Terry, M. B. (2006). Polymorphisms in nucleotide excision repair genes and DNA repair capacity phenotype in sisters discordant for breast cancer. *Cancer Epidemiology, Biomarkers & Prevention*, Vol. 15, No.9, (Sep), pp. 1614-1619, 1055-9965 (Print) 1055-9965 (Linking)

Shields, P. G., Sugimura, H., Caporaso, N. E., Petruzzelli, S. F., Bowman, E. D., Trump, B. F., Weston, A. & Harris, C. C. (1992). Polycyclic aromatic hydrocarbon-DNA adducts and the CYP1A1 restriction fragment length polymorphism. Environ Health Perspect, Vol. 98, (Nov), pp. 191-194, 0091-6765 (Print) 0091-6765 (Linking)

Shimada, T. (2006). Xenobiotic-metabolizing enzymes involved in activation and detoxification of carcinogenic polycyclic aromatic hydrocarbons. *Drug Metabolic Pharmacokinetics*, Vol. 21, No.4, (Aug), pp. 257-276, 1347-4367 (Print) 1347-4367 (Linking)

Strickland, P. T., Kang, D., Bowman, E. D., Fitzwilliam, A., Downing, T. E., Rothman, N., Groopman, J. D. & Weston, A. (1994). Identification of 1-hydroxypyrene glucuronide as a major pyrene metabolite in human urine by synchronous fluorescence spectroscopy and gas chromatography-mass spectrometry. *Carcinogenesis*, Vol. 15, No.3, (Mar), pp. 483-487, 0143-3334 (Print) 0143-3334 (Linking)

Sundberg, K., Dreij, K., Seidel, A. & Jernström, B. (2002). Glutathione Conjugation and DNA Adduct Formation of Dibenzo[a,l]pyrene and Benzo[a]pyrene Diol Epoxides in V79 Cells Stably Expressing Different Human Glutathione Transferases. *Chemical Research in Toxicology*, Vol. 15, No.2, pp. 170-179,

Tang, D., Rundle, A., Mooney, L., Cho, S., Schnabel, F., Estabrook, A., Kelly, A., Levine, R., Hibshoosh, H.& Perera, F. (2003). Sulfotransferase 1A1 (SULT1A1) Polymorphism, PAH-DNA Adduct Levels in Breast Tissue and Breast Cancer Risk in a Case-Control Study. *Breast Cancer Research and Treatment*, Vol. 78, No.2, pp. 217-222,

Vodicka, P., Kumar, R., Stetina, R., Sanyal, S., Soucek, P., Haufroid, V., Dusinska, M., Kuricova, M., Zamecnikova, M., Musak, L., Buchancova, J., Norppa, H., Hirvonen, A., Vodickova, L., Naccarati, A., Matousu, Z.& Hemminki, K. (2004). Genetic polymorphisms in DNA repair genes and possible links with DNA repair rates, chromosomal aberrations and single-strand breaks in DNA. *Carcinogenesis*, Vol. 25, No.5, (May), pp. 757-763, 0143-3334 (Print) 0143-3334 (Linking)

Wang, Z. Y., Khan, W. A., Bickers, D. R.& Mukhtar, H. (1989). Protection against polycyclic aromatic hydrocarbon-induced skin tumor initiation in mice by green tea polyphenols. Carcinogenesis, Vol. 10, No.2, (Feb), pp. 411-415, 0143-3334 (Print) 0143-3334 (Linking)

Williams, J. A.& Phillips, D. H. (2000). Mammary expression of xenobiotic metabolizing enzymes and their potential role in breast cancer. *Cancer Research*, Vol. 60, No.17, (Sep 1), pp. 4667-4677, 0008-5472 (Print) 0008-5472 (Linking)

Yoon, J. H., Lee, C. S.& Pfeifer, G. P. (2003). Simulated sunlight and benzo[a]pyrene diol epoxide induced mutagenesis in the human p53 gene evaluated by the yeast functional assay: lack of correspondence to tumor mutation spectra. *Carcinogenesis*, Vol. 24, No.1, (Jan), pp. 113-119, 0143-3334 (Print) 0143-3334 (Linking)

Yu, M.-H. (2005).Environmental toxicology: biological and health effects of pollutants (2nd), CRC Press, 156670670X (alk. paper), Boca Raton

Zang, H., Chowdhury, G., Angel, K. C., Harris, T. M.& Guengerich, F. P. (2006). Translesion synthesis across polycyclic aromatic hydrocarbon diol epoxide adducts of deoxyadenosine by Sulfolobus solfataricus DNA polymerase Dpo4. *Chemical Research in Toxicology*, Vol. 19, No.6, (Jun), pp. 859-867, 0893-228X (Print) 0893-228X (Linking)

Zhong, Q., Amin, S., Lazarus, P.& Spratt, T. E. (2010). Differential repair of polycyclic aromatic hydrocarbon DNA adducts from an actively transcribed gene. *DNA Repair (Amsterdam)*, Vol. 9, No.9, (Sep 4), pp. 1011-1016, 1568-7856 (Electronic) 1568-7856 (Linking)

Zienolddiny, S., Ryberg, D., Svendsrud, D. H., Eilertsen, E., Skaug, V., Hewer, A., Phillips, D. H., te Riele, H.& Haugen, A. (2006). Msh2 deficiency increases susceptibility to benzo[a]pyrene-induced lymphomagenesis. *International Journal of Cancer*, Vol. 118, No.11, (Jun 1), pp. 2899-2902, 0020-7136 (Print) 0020-7136 (Linking)

7

# DNA Repair: Lessons from the Evolution of Ionizing-Radiation-Resistant Prokaryotes – Fact and Theory

Haïtham Sghaier
*Research Unit UR04CNSTN01 "Medical and Agricultural Applications of Nuclear Techniques", National Center for Nuclear Sciences and Technology (CNSTN), Sidi Thabet Technopark, Sidi Thabet, Tunisia*

## 1. Introduction

At the outset, I believe that the concept of ionizing-radiation (IR) resistance needs to be clarified in a tangible manner for readers of this chapter. I propose the following general definition adopted in a previous paper (Sghaier et al., 2008): An ionizing-radiation-resistant prokaryotes (IRRP) is any vegetative prokaryote that can thrive after exposure to high, acute IR (generally, with a $D_{10}$ value - the dose necessary to effect a 90% reduction in Colony Forming Units - greater than 1 kGy) using efficient physiological, genetic and proteic protection and repair mechanisms to fully amend its DNA DSBs. IR resistance has been observed in a broad range of prokaryotic groups (Kopylov et al., 1993), including hyperthermophilic Archaea (*P. abyssi, P. furiosus, Thermococcus marinus, Thermococcus radiotolerans* and *Thermococcus gammatolerans*) (DiRuggiero et al., 1997; Jolivet et al., 2003a; Jolivet et al., 2003b; Jolivet et al., 2004), halophilic Archaea (*Halobacterium* sp.) (Kottemann et al., 2005), the *Deinococcus-Thermus* group (many *Deinococcus* sp. and *Truepera radiovictrix*) (Albuquerque et al., 2005), Actinobacteria (*Rubrobacter radiotolerans, Rubrobacter xylanophilus* and *Kineococcus radiotolerans*) (Yoshinaka et al., 1973; Ferreira et al., 1999; Phillips et al., 2002; Chen et al., 2004), Proteobacteria (*Methylobacterium radiotolerans* and *Acinetobacter radioresistens*) (Ito and Iizuka, 1971; Nishimura et al., 1994), Cyanobacteria (*Chroococcidiopsis* sp.) (Billi et al., 2000), and Sphingobacteria (*Hymenobacter actinosclerus*) (Collins et al., 2000). However, with the exception of *Deinococcus* and *Pyrococcus*, very little information is available regarding the mechanisms of IR resistance and comparative genomics in the above-mentioned prokaryotes. *D. radiodurans* is the current gold-medallist of IR resistance among prokaryotes with a completely sequenced genome (Liolios et al., 2006; Liolios et al., 2010), and can amend more than 100 DSBs per chromosome, induced by IR, without loss of viability (Moseley, 1983; White et al., 1999). After breaking of its 3.2 Mb genome into 20–30 kb pieces by a high dose of IR, *D. radiodurans* fascinatingly reassembles its genome such that 3 hr later fully restructured nonrearranged chromosomes are present (Galhardo and Rosenberg, 2009). Nine interrelated explanations for the extreme IR resistance of *D. radiodurans* have been proposed: (i) the binding of IrrI (DR0171) to genomic repeat sequences that might prevent exhaustive chromosomal degradation after IR exposure - *irr* for IR resistance - (Udupa et al., 1994), (ii) the

RecA(DR2340)-promoted DNA strand exchangeby quite efficient pathways (Kim and Cox, 2002; Sghaier et al., 2010), (iii) the unusual genomic toroidal morphology (Levin-Zaidman et al., 2003) commented in an another paper (Battista et al., 2003), (iv) the prompt PprI/IrrE(DR0167)-induced DNA repair in response to IR stress - *pprI* for inducer of pleiotropic proteins promoting DNA repair - (Earl et al., 2002; Hua et al., 2003; Lu et al., 2009), (v) the critical role played by PprA (DRA0346) in a presumed IR-induced DNA end-joining repair mechanism - PprA for pleiotropic protein promoting DNA repair A - (Narumi et al., 2004), (vi) the divergent evolutionary route of adaptation to IR resistance in comparison to IR-sensitive prokaryotes (IRSP) (Omelchenko et al., 2005; Makarova et al., 2007; Sghaier et al., 2008) including the acquisition of a putative radiation/desiccation response motif (RDRM) and regulon (RDR) (Makarova et al., 2007; Makarova and Daly, 2011), (vii) the stabilization by "holding proteins" of base pairing between closely opposed strand breaks (Cox and Battista, 2005), (viii) the extended synthesis-dependent strand annealing (ESDSA) process, which involves PolA-accomplished DNA synthesis (completed by crossovers achieved by RecA) (Zahradka et al., 2006), with the participation of Pol III and RadA (Galhardo and Rosenberg, 2009; Slade et al., 2009), and (ix) the protein-centered view of IR toxicity (Daly et al., 2007; Daly, 2010; Daly et al., 2010) based on the Mn(II)-facilitated recovery from IR injury (Daly et al., 2004). Yet, why *D. radiodurans* is an extremely IR-resistant bacterium whereas *Escherichia coli* is not is still an open question. For instance, previous literature (Daly et al., 2004; Daly et al., 2007; Daly, 2010; Daly et al., 2010) have suggested that protein protection from damage by oxidation and IR is what makes *D. radiodurans* IR-resistant compared to IRSP including *E. coli*. If so, it raises the question of whether *E. coli* might be able to amend a genome fragmented by restriction enzymes even though it can not amend severe damage induced by IR (Slade et al., 2009), unless it is mutated (Harris et al., 2009).

Interestingly, *D. radiodurans* and *P. furiosus* are able to efficiently repair DSBs in a similar manner (DiRuggiero et al., 1997). In addition, *D. radiodurans* and *P. abyssi* respond in a similar fashion to DNA damage caused by IR (Jolivet et al., 2003b). DNA replication in *D. radiodurans* is known to cease following irradiation (Dean et al., 1966; Moseley and Copland, 1976), which is comparable to the efficient strategy utilized by *P. abyssi* in response to DNA damage that includes an uncoupling of DNA repair and DNA synthesis (Jolivet et al., 2003b). Another shared feature in irradiated *D. radiodurans* and *P. abyssi* is the transport of damaged DNA that should prevent the accumulation of genetic mistakes (Jolivet et al., 2003b). Further study will be necessary to discover mechanistic commonalities among IRRP.

Presently, one of the most significant conclusions that investigators drew by comparing IRRP with IRSP was that the most resistant cells accumulated about 300 times more Mn and about three times less Fe than the most sensitive cells which contributes to protecting their enzymes and the repair functions they catalyze (Daly et al., 2004; Daly et al., 2007; Daly, 2010; Daly et al., 2010). Interestingly, a recent survey of an Fe-rich site in Tunisia (Tamra mine in Nefza) showed relatively high concentrations of Fe (~9.9%) and Mn (~2242 ppm) with a high environmental radioactivity level (~1.5 microsieverts/hour (μSv/h)) nearby the site. In the United States of America (USA), the Ocean Drilling Program, under contract with the National Science Foundation, has recently surveyed environments representative of a broad range of subsurface conditions found in marine sediments (D'Hondt et al., 2004). Among the most striking features of deeply buried sediments (20-100 meters below the sea floor (mbsf)) are Mn-rich sites with high natural γ-radiation levels (see Figure F14 in http://www-odp.tamu.edu/publications/prelim/201_prel/201PREL.PDF and http://www.ldeo.columbia.edu/BRG/ODP/ODP/LEG_SUMM/201/leg201.html#fig4) (Daly MJ, personal communication, 2006). In this context, anaerobic and hyperthermophilic *Deinococcus* sp. have been isolated from the subsurfaces of hydrothermal vents at depths of 64.8 to 128.9 mbsf, where temperatures range from 76 to 91.4°C (Kimura et al., 2003). This finding supports the possibility of the coexistence within the same ecological niche of *Deinococcus* species and other anaerobic hyperthermophilic archaea.

16 rDNA-based phylogenies place *Deinococcus* very close to hyperthermophiles and the root of the phylogenetic tree, with organisms exhibiting IR resistance forming a scattered group (Woese, 1987; Cox and Battista, 2005). In this context, Cavalier-Smith employed aspects of palaeontology, sequence trees, and the methods of transition analysis and congruence testing to demonstrate that the last universal common ancestor (LUCA) lies within eubacteria; specifically, among negibacteria of the superphylum Eobacteria (Hadobacteria and Chlorobacteria) (Cavalier-Smith, 2006). Several important characters indicate that Hadobacteria, including the genus *Deinococcus*, are more primitive than other phyla, with the exception of Chlorobacteria (Cavalier-Smith, 2006). As far as the dispersed phylogenetic clades of IRRP are concerned, the idea of Cox and Battista (Cox and Battista, 2005) concerning convergent evolution remains possible, but it needs further explanation as to how IR-resistant lineages became similar to each other. An immediate question is whether horizontal gene transfer was involved in the convergent evolution of some pivotal genes essential for IR resistance in IRRP. If so, several different evolutionary scenarios are possible: either the genetic gain consisted of a few relatively large DNA fragments, or the genetic gain included individual genes one-by-one. Additionally, the theory of convergent evolution requires that IRRP responded in a similar fashion to DNA damage caused by IR (DSBs) through adaptation to identical environments under the same driving forces. More interestingly, Cox and Battista raised the possibility that IR resistance could be a vestige of DNA repair systems that were present in ancestral species, and has been retained in those organisms that continue to require this phenotype (Cox and Battista, 2005). Their explanation asserts that most descendents "lost" the ancestor's ability to cope with DNA damage and predicts that the molecular mechanisms of IR resistance should be similar among IR-resistant species. Given new insights from pertinent organisms, novel comparative analytical tools, and extensive phylogenetic endeavours, it should soon be possible to test current and future hypotheses concerning the origin of IRRP (see (Omelchenko et al., 2005; Makarova et al., 2007; Sghaier et al., 2007; Makarova and Daly, 2011) and references therein).

Presently, besides many genome projects of IRRP in progress (*e.g. Acinetobacter radioresistens*), many completely sequenced IR-resistant genomes are available on public genome databases (*e.g. Deinococcus proteolyticus* MRP (Liolios et al., 2010)) or were published very recently (*e.g. Deinococcus maricopensis* DSM21211 (Pukall et al., 2011)). However, completely sequenced IR-resistant genomes (Liolios et al., 2010), with published information regarding their IR resistance, are relatively limited in number and restricted in genera: *Deinococcus deserti* VCD115 (de Groot et al., 2005; de Groot et al., 2009; Baudet et al., 2010), *Deinococcus geothermalis* DSM 11300 (Makarova et al., 2007), *D. radiodurans* $R_1$ (White et al., 1999), two species of *Halobacterium* (*H. salinarum* R1 (Pfeiffer et al., 2008) and *Halobacterium* sp. NRC-1 (Ng et al., 2000)) (Ng et al., 2008), *Kineococcus radiotolerans* SRS30216 (Bagwell et al., 2008), *Rubrobacter xylanophilus* DSM 9941, *Methylobacterium radiotolerans* JCM 2831 (Liolios et al., 2010), three species of *Pyrococcus* (*P. abyssi* GE5 (Cohen et al., 2003), *P. furiosus* DSM 3638 (Maeder et al., 1999), and *P. horikoshii* OT3 (Kawarabayasi et al., 1998)), *Thermococcus gammatolerans* EJ3

(Jolivet et al., 2003a; Liolios et al., 2010), and *Truepera radiovictrix* DSM 17093 (Ivanova et al., 2011). In concordance with previous literature (Koonin, 2003), genes shared by the above-mentioned members of prokaryotic IR-resistant taxa based on TaxPlot available through the NCBI database (Sayers et al., 2011) suggest that the hypothesis of a common ancestor is quantitatively tenable. Qualitatively (Ouzounis et al., 2006), and in contrast to other phenotypes such as those characterized by (hyper)thermophily or pathogenecity, IR resistance does not have characteristic large genetic traits (mutagenesis cassettes, genomic islets (< 10 kilobase pairs (kb)) or fitness islands (> 10 kb), *etc.*) that are either correlated to IR resistance, specific to IRRP, or absent in IRSP. Hallmark genes correlated to IR resistance could be classified into four major evolutionary families on the basis of their mode of contribution to DNA repair (directly through interactions with DNA or indirectly by interactions without DNA) and their prokaryotic distribution:

- Family 1: Composed of genes assuming fundamental and direct functions related to DNA replication and repair (*e.g. polA*, *recA*) (Kim and Cox, 2002; Zahradka et al., 2006). Members of this family, or their orthologs, are present in all previously studied IRRP (Ouzounis et al., 2006; Sghaier et al., 2008). For instance, RecA protein is quintessential for the fidelity of repair of IR-induced DNA breaks and, consequently, for genome stability in *D. radiodurans* (Repar et al., 2010). In addition, the RecA mutant is among the most IR-sensitive mutants found in *D. radiodurans* (Moseley and Copland, 1975).
- Family 2: Containing genes that contribute directly to IR resistance (*e.g.* DNA nonhomologous end-joining complex) (Weller et al., 2002). Genes of this family are present in several IR-resistant lineages (Aravind and Koonin, 2001).
- Family 3: Comprising genes that contribute indirectly to IR resistance (*e.g.* superoxide dismutase, catalase) (Markillie et al., 1999). These genes are shared by some IRRP (Klotz and Loewen, 2003).
- Family 4: Containing genus- or species-specific genes that contribute directly or indirectly to IR resistance (*e.g. pprI* and *pprA* in *Deinococcus*) (Hua et al., 2003; Narumi et al., 2004). Interestingly, genes of this family enhance DNA repair abilities (Narumi et al., 2004) and regulation mechanisms through check points (Hua et al., 2003).

Previous work by Zahradka *et al.* revealed the relevant two-stage DNA repair process involving PolA and RecA DNA repair enzymes during recovery of *D. radiodurans* from IR (Zahradka et al., 2006). Moreover, the key steps and enzymes involved in ESDSA were identified (Galhardo and Rosenberg, 2009; Slade et al., 2009). Particularly, *polA* and *recA* homologs, belonging to Family 1 (see above), are found among all IRRP. Therefore, the proposal of an ancestral ESDSA repair process (Zahradka et al., 2006) is plausible from a comparative genomics perspective. Since ancestral proteins are reconstructable (Thornton, 2004), the above data suggest that ESDSA might shed light through complementation assays on the IR sensitivity or IR resistance of any node in a phylogenetic tree of PolA or RecA. For instance, a resurrected ancestral PolA protein might be used to complement IR-sensitive cells that are deficient in PolA and for which the wild-type is IR-resistant. The PolA-RecA-mediated repair process possesses the following important characteristics:

1. Functionally, its proteins (PolA and RecA) are important for IR resistance (DiRuggiero et al., 1997; Cox and Battista, 2005; Zahradka et al., 2006; Galhardo and Rosenberg, 2009; Slade et al., 2009; Repar et al., 2010).
2. Phylogenetically, it is a ubiquitous repair mechanism, and it is traced back to LUCA (DiRuggiero et al., 1999; Koonin, 2003; Ouzounis et al., 2006).

3. Evolutionarily, its informational proteins have not been subject to lateral gene transfer (Jain et al., 1999; Koonin, 2003; Ouzounis et al., 2006; Cohen et al., 2011).

The first stage of the two-stage DNA repair process involves a PolA-dependent ESDSA mechanism (Zahradka et al., 2006). This stage mainly requires a functional PolA enzyme and at least two genome copies that are broken at different positions. Knowing that IR-sensitive *D. radiodurans polA* mutants are fully complemented by expression of the *polA* gene from the relatively IR-sensitive *E. coli* (Gutman et al., 1994), and that many IRSP are polyploid (Daly and Minton, 1995), it is legitimate to propose that the first stage of the two-stage DNA repair process could be functional in IRSP. However, the possibility that some deinococcal hypothetical protein(s) or orphan(s) facilitates DNA synthesis by 'any' functional PolA must be seriously considered. This preparation of chromosomal fragments by hypothetical protein(s), albeit not demonstrated, might explain the delay of 1.5 hours in DNA synthesis in the wild-type (Zahradka et al., 2006) and is consistent with the presence of many species-specific proteins in *D. radiodurans*.

The second stage of the two-stage DNA repair process involves RecA-dependent crossovers in *D. radiodurans* (Zahradka et al., 2006), belonging to Mn-accumulating bacteria (Daly et al., 2004). In general, (1) ionic strength affects RecA binding preferential affinity to DNA in relation to single-stranded DNA or double-stranded DNA (Cazenave et al., 1983), and (2) Mn ions have possible effects on DNA structure (stabilization of the helix, neutralization of the negative charge of the phosphate backbone, prevention of DNA renaturation, *etc.*) (Polyanichko et al., 2004). Thus, it is legitimate at this point to assume that the *in vivo* affinity for DNA of 'any' RecA within *D. radiodurans* will differ from its *in vivo* affinity for DNA within an IR-sensitive cell like *E. coli*. Until more research is done, investigators presently agree that repair of DNA DSBs mediated by *recA*-like genes is an extremely active and distinct repair mechanism in *Deinococcus* and *Pyrococcus* (DiRuggiero et al., 1997; Kim and Cox, 2002; Zahradka et al., 2006; Sghaier et al., 2010).

Experimental support for the theory of an ancestral ESDSA repair process is needed. Having been discovered in *D. radiodurans* (Zahradka et al., 2006), an essential attribute of ESDSA is that its presence should also be testable experimentally in IR-resistant archaea.

A consideration of the evolution of IRRP in terms of phenotypic consequences representing genetic change would provide answers on how these organisms evolved. For example, comparative genomic surveys revealed that the radiation-desiccation resistance phenotype of *D. radiodurans* might have gradually evolved via cross-species gene transfer (Omelchenko et al., 2005). One aspect of this theory does seem correct: in contrast to *Pyrococcus*, *Deinococcus* clearly escaped with other Terrabacteria from a state of genetic shrinkage to "genetic gamble" in response to stress during land colonization (Battistuzzi et al., 2004). In this context, the "desiccation adaptation hypothesis" (Mattimore and Battista, 1996) suggests that the IR resistance of *D. radiodurans* is a consequence of its adaptation to desiccation. However, there is no genome-wide data or any experimental data to suggest that desiccation tolerance is antecedent to IR resistance. If this hypothesis is wrong, evolution of IRRP can be misinterpreted profoundly in numerous ways. Briefly, the data presented by Mattimore and Battista (Mattimore and Battista, 1996) only implied a strong positive correlation between these two phenotypes. In fact, a co-author of the "desiccation adaptation hypothesis" showed that inactivation of DRB0118, a constitutively expressed protein, greatly sensitizes *D. radiodurans* to desiccation, but not to IR (Battista et al., 2001). In addition, the ill-founded "desiccation adaptation hypothesis" (Mattimore and Battista, 1996) fails to explain the extreme IR resistance observed in several members of the domain

Archaea (*e.g. Pyrococcus, Thermococcus*). A recent *in vitro* investigation (Beblo et al., 2011) led to a definitive refutation of the "desiccation adaptation hypothesis" (Mattimore and Battista, 1996) and to an implicit vindication of the "radiation adaptation hypothesis" (Sghaier et al., 2007). In brief, it was demonstrated that desiccation-tolerant as well as desiccation-intolerant (hyper-) thermophilic archaea survived comparably high doses of IR (Beblo et al., 2011). In so far as other mechanisms of IR resistance are concerned, it is not surprising that the *Deinococcus* lineage does not share with *Pyrococcus* its five transcripts (DR0423, *ddrA*; DR0070, *ddrB*; DR0003, *ddrC*; DR0326, *ddrD*; DRA0346, *pprA*), most likely evolving in response to IR and desiccation (Tanaka et al., 2004). This network of five transcripts is *Deinococcus* lineage-specific. Similarly, a putative DNA-repair gene cluster of five conserved hypothetical genes in *P. furiosus* (PF0639, PF0640, PF0641, PF0642, PF0643), specifically induced by exposure to IR and probably involved in translesion synthesis, seems to be unique to thermophilic archaea and bacteria (Williams et al., 2007). Does this mean that this putative cluster is important for thermophily? The answer is probably no. One could highlight the fact that the mechanism that protects the DNA against thermal degradation does not prevent the formation of DNA breaks during irradiation (Gerard et al., 2001).

A corollary to all these analyses is the notion that there is a multiplicity of evolutionary and functional processes associated with IR resistance (Omelchenko et al., 2005; Makarova et al., 2007; Sghaier et al., 2007; Daly, 2010; Makarova and Daly, 2011; Slade and Radman, 2011). However, this integrative appraisal does not exclude the possibility of common processes among IRRP. Future analyses might consider more experimental and genomic data from a variety of IRRP in order to determine whether they possess a set of genes that would refute either the concept of convergent evolution or the idea of a common ancestor.

## 2. Acknowledgements

This work was performed under the auspices of the Tunisian National Center for Nuclear Sciences and Technology (CNSTN). Special thanks to Dr. Issay Narumi from Japan Atomic Energy Agency (JAEA) for previous discussions that improved an initial draft.

## 3. References

Albuquerque, L., Simoes, C., Nobre, M.F., Pino, N.M., Battista, J.R., Silva, M.T. et al. (2005) *Truepera radiovictrix* gen. nov., sp. nov., a new radiation resistant species and the proposal of *Trueperaceae* fam. nov. *FEMS Microbiol Lett* 247: 161-169.

Aravind, L., and Koonin, E.V. (2001) Prokaryotic homologs of the eukaryotic DNA-end-binding protein Ku, novel domains in the Ku protein and prediction of a prokaryotic double-strand break repair system. *Genome Res* 11: 1365-1374.

Bagwell, C.E., Bhat, S., Hawkins, G.M., Smith, B.W., Biswas, T., Hoover, T.R. et al. (2008) Survival in nuclear waste, extreme resistance, and potential applications gleaned from the genome sequence of *Kineococcus radiotolerans* SRS30216. *PLoS One* 3: e3878.

Battista, J.R., Park, M.J., and McLemore, A.E. (2001) Inactivation of two homologues of proteins presumed to be involved in the desiccation tolerance of plants sensitizes *Deinococcus radiodurans* R1 to desiccation. *Cryobiology* 43: 133-139.

Battista, J.R., Cox, M.M., Daly, M.J., Narumi, I., Radman, M., and Sommer, S. (2003) The structure of *D. radiodurans*. *Science* 302: 567-568; author reply 567-568.

Battistuzzi, F.U., Feijao, A., and Hedges, S.B. (2004) A genomic timescale of prokaryote evolution: insights into the origin of methanogenesis, phototrophy, and the colonization of land. *BMC Evol Biol* 4: 44.

Baudet, M., Ortet, P., Gaillard, J.C., Fernandez, B., Guerin, P., Enjalbal, C. et al. (2010) Proteomics-based refinement of *Deinococcus deserti* genome annotation reveals an unwonted use of non-canonical translation initiation codons. *Mol Cell Proteomics* 9: 415-426.

Beblo K, Douki T, Schmalz G, Rachel R, Wirth R, Huber H, Reitz G, Rettberg P. (2011) Survival of thermophilic and hyperthermophilic microorganisms after exposure to UV-C, ionizing radiation and desiccation. *Arch Microbiol* [Epub ahead of print]

Billi, D., Friedmann, E.I., Hofer, K.G., Caiola, M.G., and Ocampo-Friedmann, R. (2000) Ionizing-radiation resistance in the desiccation-tolerant cyanobacterium *Chroococcidiopsis*. *Appl Environ Microbiol* 66: 1489-1492.

Cavalier-Smith, T. (2006) Rooting the tree of life by transition analyses. *Biol Direct* 1: 19.

Cazenave, C., Toulme, J.J., and Helene, C. (1983) Binding of RecA protein to single-stranded nucleic acids: spectroscopic studies using fluorescent polynucleotides. *EMBO J* 2: 2247-2251.

Chen, M.Y., Wu, S.H., Lin, G.H., Lu, C.P., Lin, Y.T., Chang, W.C., and Tsay, S.S. (2004) Rubrobacter taiwanensis sp. nov., a novel thermophilic, radiation-resistant species isolated from hot springs. *Int J Syst Evol Microbiol* 54: 1849-1855.

Cohen, G.N., Barbe, V., Flament, D., Galperin, M., Heilig, R., Lecompte, O. et al. (2003) An integrated analysis of the genome of the hyperthermophilic archaeon *Pyrococcus abyssi*. *Mol Microbiol* 47: 1495-1512.

Cohen, O., Gophna, U., and Pupko, T. (2011) The complexity hypothesis revisited: connectivity rather than function constitutes a barrier to horizontal gene transfer. *Mol Biol Evol* 28: 1481-1489.

Collins, M.D., Hutson, R.A., Grant, I.R., and Patterson, M.F. (2000) Phylogenetic characterization of a novel radiation-resistant bacterium from irradiated pork: description of *Hymenobacter actinosclerus* sp. nov. *Int J Syst Evol Microbiol* 50 Pt 2: 731-734.

Cox, M.M., and Battista, J.R. (2005) *Deinococcus radiodurans* - the consummate survivor. *Nat Rev Microbiol* 3: 882-892.

D'Hondt, S., Jorgensen, B.B., Miller, D.J., Batzke, A., Blake, R., Cragg, B.A. et al. (2004) Distributions of microbial activities in deep subseafloor sediments. *Science* 306: 2216-2221.

Daly, M.J. (2010) *Deinococcus radiodurans*: Revising the Molecular Basis for Radiation Effects on Cells. In *Extremophiles Handbook*. Horikoshi, K. (ed): Springer Japan KK, pp. 1-16.

Daly, M.J., and Minton, K.W. (1995) Interchromosomal recombination in the extremely radioresistant bacterium *Deinococcus radiodurans*. *J Bacteriol* 177: 5495-5505.

Daly, M.J., Gaidamakova, E.K., Matrosova, V.Y., Kiang, J.G., Fukumoto, R., Lee, D.Y. et al. (2010) Small-molecule antioxidant proteome-shields in *Deinococcus radiodurans*. *PLoS One* 5: e12570.

Daly, M.J., Gaidamakova, E.K., Matrosova, V.Y., Vasilenko, A., Zhai, M., Leapman, R.D. et al. (2007) Protein oxidation implicated as the primary determinant of bacterial radioresistance. *PLoS Biol* 5: e92.

Daly, M.J., Gaidamakova, E.K., Matrosova, V.Y., Vasilenko, A., Zhai, M., Venkateswaran, A. et al. (2004) Accumulation of Mn(II) in *Deinococcus radiodurans* facilitates gamma-radiation resistance. *Science* 306: 1025-1028.

de Groot, A., Chapon, V., Servant, P., Christen, R., Saux, M.F., Sommer, S., and Heulin, T. (2005) *Deinococcus deserti* sp. nov., a gamma-radiation-tolerant bacterium isolated from the Sahara Desert. *Int J Syst Evol Microbiol* 55: 2441-2446.

de Groot, A., Dulermo, R., Ortet, P., Blanchard, L., Guerin, P., Fernandez, B. et al. (2009) Alliance of proteomics and genomics to unravel the specificities of Sahara bacterium *Deinococcus deserti*. *PLoS Genet* 5: e1000434.

Dean, C.J., Feldschreiber, P., and Lett, J.T. (1966) Repair of x-ray damage to the deoxyribonucleic acid in *Micrococcus radiodurans*. *Nature* 209: 49-52.

DiRuggiero, J., Brown, J.R., Bogert, A.P., and Robb, F.T. (1999) DNA repair systems in archaea: mementos from the last universal common ancestor? *J Mol Evol* 49: 474-484.

DiRuggiero, J., Santangelo, N., Nackerdien, Z., Ravel, J., and Robb, F.T. (1997) Repair of extensive ionizing-radiation DNA damage at 95 degrees C in the hyperthermophilic archaeon *Pyrococcus furiosus*. *J Bacteriol* 179: 4643-4645.

Earl, A.M., Mohundro, M.M., Mian, I.S., and Battista, J.R. (2002) The IrrE protein of *Deinococcus radiodurans* R1 is a novel regulator of *recA* expression. *J Bacteriol* 184: 6216-6224.

Ferreira, A.C., Nobre, M.F., Moore, E., Rainey, F.A., Battista, J.R., and da Costa, M.S. (1999) Characterization and radiation resistance of new isolates of *Rubrobacter radiotolerans* and *Rubrobacter xylanophilus*. *Extremophiles* 3: 235-238.

Galhardo, R.S., and Rosenberg, S.M. (2009) Extreme genome repair. *Cell* 136: 998-1000.

Gerard, E., Jolivet, E., Prieur, D., and Forterre, P. (2001) DNA protection mechanisms are not involved in the radioresistance of the hyperthermophilic archaea *Pyrococcus abyssi* and *P. furiosus*. *Mol Genet Genomics* 266: 72-78.

Gutman, P.D., Fuchs, P., and Minton, K.W. (1994) Restoration of the DNA damage resistance of *Deinococcus radiodurans* DNA polymerase mutants by *Escherichia coli* DNA polymerase I and Klenow fragment. *Mutat Res* 314: 87-97.

Harris, D.R., Pollock, S.V., Wood, E.A., Goiffon, R.J., Klingele, A.J., Cabot, E.L. et al. (2009) Directed evolution of ionizing radiation resistance in *Escherichia coli*. *J Bacteriol* 191: 5240-5252.

Hua, Y., Narumi, I., Gao, G., Tian, B., Satoh, K., Kitayama, S., and Shen, B. (2003) PprI: a general switch responsible for extreme radioresistance of *Deinococcus radiodurans*. *Biochem Biophys Res Commun* 306: 354-360.

Ito, H., and Iizuka, H. (1971) Taxonomic studies on a radio-resistant *Pseudomonas*. Part XII. Studies on the microorganisms of cereal grain. *Agric Biol Chem* 35: 1566-1571.

Ivanova, N., Rohde, C., Munk, C., Nolan, M., Lucas, S., Del Rio, T.G. et al. (2011) Complete genome sequence of *Truepera radiovictrix* type strain (RQ-24). *Stand Genomic Sci* 4: 91-99.

Jain, R., Rivera, M.C., and Lake, J.A. (1999) Horizontal gene transfer among genomes: the complexity hypothesis. *Proc Natl Acad Sci U S A* 96: 3801-3806.

Jolivet, E., L'Haridon, S., Corre, E., Forterre, P., and Prieur, D. (2003a) *Thermococcus gammatolerans* sp. nov., a hyperthermophilic archaeon from a deep-sea hydrothermal vent that resists ionizing radiation. *Int J Syst Evol Microbiol* 53: 847-851.

Jolivet, E., Corre, E., L'Haridon, S., Forterre, P., and Prieur, D. (2004) *Thermococcus marinus* sp. nov. and *Thermococcus radiotolerans* sp. nov., two hyperthermophilic archaea from deep-sea hydrothermal vents that resist ionizing radiation. *Extremophiles* 8: 219-227.

Jolivet, E., Matsunaga, F., Ishino, Y., Forterre, P., Prieur, D., and Myllykallio, H. (2003b) Physiological responses of the hyperthermophilic archaeon "*Pyrococcus abyssi*" to DNA damage caused by ionizing radiation. *J Bacteriol* 185: 3958-3961.

Kawarabayasi, Y., Sawada, M., Horikawa, H., Haikawa, Y., Hino, Y., Yamamoto, S. et al. (1998) Complete sequence and gene organization of the genome of a hyper-thermophilic archaebacterium, *Pyrococcus horikoshii* OT3. *DNA Res* 5: 55-76.

Kim, J.I., and Cox, M.M. (2002) The RecA proteins of *Deinococcus radiodurans* and *Escherichia coli* promote DNA strand exchange via inverse pathways. *Proc Natl Acad Sci U S A* 99: 7917-7921.

Kimura, H., Asada, R., Masta, A., and Naganuma, T. (2003) Distribution of microorganisms in the subsurface of the manus basin hydrothermal vent field in Papua New Guinea. *Appl Environ Microbiol* 69: 644-648.

Klotz, M.G., and Loewen, P.C. (2003) The molecular evolution of catalatic hydroperoxidases: evidence for multiple lateral transfer of genes between prokaryota and from bacteria into eukaryota. *Mol Biol Evol* 20: 1098-1112.

Koonin, E.V. (2003) Comparative genomics, minimal gene-sets and the last universal common ancestor. *Nat Rev Microbiol* 1: 127-136.

Kopylov, V.M., Bonch-Osmolovskaya, E.A., Svetlichnyi, V.A., Miroshnicheko, M.L., and Skobin, V.S. (1993) Gamma-irradiation resistance and UV sensitivity of extremely thermophilic archaebacteria and eubacteria. *Mikrobiologiya* 62: 90-95.

Kottemann, M., Kish, A., Iloanusi, C., Bjork, S., and DiRuggiero, J. (2005) Physiological responses of the halophilic archaeon *Halobacterium* sp. strain NRC1 to desiccation and gamma irradiation. *Extremophiles* 9: 219-227.

Levin-Zaidman, S., Englander, J., Shimoni, E., Sharma, A.K., Minton, K.W., and Minsky, A. (2003) Ringlike structure of the *Deinococcus radiodurans* genome: a key to radioresistance? *Science* 299: 254-256.

Liolios, K., Tavernarakis, N., Hugenholtz, P., and Kyrpides, N.C. (2006) The Genomes On Line Database (GOLD) v.2: a monitor of genome projects worldwide. *Nucleic Acids Res* 34: D332-334.

Liolios, K., Chen, I.M., Mavromatis, K., Tavernarakis, N., Hugenholtz, P., Markowitz, V.M., and Kyrpides, N.C. (2010) The Genomes On Line Database (GOLD) in 2009: status of genomic and metagenomic projects and their associated metadata. *Nucleic Acids Res* 38: D346-354.

Lu, H., Gao, G., Xu, G., Fan, L., Yin, L., Shen, B., and Hua, Y. (2009) *Deinococcus radiodurans* PprI switches on DNA damage response and cellular survival networks after radiation damage. *Mol Cell Proteomics* 8: 481-494.

Maeder, D.L., Weiss, R.B., Dunn, D.M., Cherry, J.L., Gonzalez, J.M., DiRuggiero, J., and Robb, F.T. (1999) Divergence of the hyperthermophilic archaea *Pyrococcus furiosus* and *P. horikoshii* inferred from complete genomic sequences. *Genetics* 152: 1299-1305.

Makarova, K.S., and Daly, M.J. (2011) Comparative Genomics of Stress Response Systems in *Deinococcus* Bacteria. In *Bacterial Stress Responses*. Storz, G., and Hengge, R. (eds). Washington, DC: ASM Press, pp. 445-457.

Makarova, K.S., Omelchenko, M.V., Gaidamakova, E.K., Matrosova, V.Y., Vasilenko, A., Zhai, M. et al. (2007) *Deinococcus geothermalis*: the pool of extreme radiation resistance genes shrinks. *PLoS One* 2: e955.

Markillie, L.M., Varnum, S.M., Hradecky, P., and Wong, K.K. (1999) Targeted mutagenesis by duplication insertion in the radioresistant bacterium *Deinococcus radiodurans*: radiation sensitivities of catalase (*katA*) and superoxide dismutase (*sodA*) mutants. *J Bacteriol* 181: 666-669.

Mattimore, V., and Battista, J.R. (1996) Radioresistance of *Deinococcus radiodurans*: functions necessary to survive ionizing radiation are also necessary to survive prolonged desiccation. *J Bacteriol* 178: 633-637.

Moseley, B.E., and Copland, H.J. (1975) Isolation and properties of a recombination-deficient mutant of *Micrococcus radiodurans*. *J Bacteriol* 121: 422-428.

Moseley, B.E., and Copland, H.J. (1976) The rate of recombination repair and its relationship to the radiation-induced delay in DNA synthesis in *Micrococcus radiodurans*. *J Gen Microbiol* 93: 251-258.

Moseley, B.E.B. (1983) Photobiology and radiobiology of *Micrococcus* (*Deinococcus*) *radiodurans*. *Photochem Photobiol Rev* 7: 223-274.

Narumi, I., Satoh, K., Cui, S., Funayama, T., Kitayama, S., and Watanabe, H. (2004) PprA: a novel protein from *Deinococcus radiodurans* that stimulates DNA ligation. *Mol Microbiol* 54: 278-285.

Ng, W.V., Berquist, B.R., Coker, J.A., Capes, M., Wu, T.H., DasSarma, P., and DasSarma, S. (2008) Genome sequences of *Halobacterium* species. *Genomics* 91: 548-552; author reply 553-544.

Ng, W.V., Kennedy, S.P., Mahairas, G.G., Berquist, B., Pan, M., Shukla, H.D. et al. (2000) Genome sequence of *Halobacterium* species NRC-1. *Proc Natl Acad Sci U S A* 97: 12176-12181.

Nishimura, Y., Uchida, K., Tanaka, K., Ino, T., and Ito, H. (1994) Radiation sensitivities of *Acinetobacter* strains isolated from clinical sources. *J Basic Microbiol* 34: 357-360.

Omelchenko, M.V., Wolf, Y.I., Gaidamakova, E.K., Matrosova, V.Y., Vasilenko, A., Zhai, M. et al. (2005) Comparative genomics of *Thermus thermophilus* and *Deinococcus radiodurans*: divergent routes of adaptation to thermophily and radiation resistance. *BMC Evol Biol* 5: 57.

Ouzounis, C.A., Kunin, V., Darzentas, N., and Goldovsky, L. (2006) A minimal estimate for the gene content of the last universal common ancestor--exobiology from a terrestrial perspective. *Res Microbiol* 157: 57-68.

Pfeiffer, F., Schuster, S.C., Broicher, A., Falb, M., Palm, P., Rodewald, K. et al. (2008) Evolution in the laboratory: the genome of *Halobacterium salinarum* strain R1 compared to that of strain NRC-1. *Genomics* 91: 335-346.

Phillips, R.W., Wiegel, J., Berry, C.J., Fliermans, C., Peacock, A.D., White, D.C., and Shimkets, L.J. (2002) *Kineococcus radiotolerans* sp. nov., a radiation-resistant, gram-positive bacterium. *Int J Syst Evol Microbiol* 52: 933-938.

Polyanichko, A.M., Andrushchenko, V.V., Chikhirzhina, E.V., Vorob'ev, V.I., and Wieser, H. (2004) The effect of manganese(II) on DNA structure: electronic and vibrational circular dichroism studies. *Nucleic Acids Res* 32: 989-996.

Pukall R, Zeytun A, Lucas S, Lapidus A, Hammon N, Deshpande S, Nolan M, Cheng JF, Pitluck S, Liolios K, Pagani I, Mikhailova N, Ivanova N, Mavromatis K, Pati A, Tapia R, Han C, Goodwin L, Chen A, Palaniappan K, Land M, Hauser L, Chang YJ, Jeffries CD, Brambilla EM, Rohde M, Göker M, Detter JC, Woyke T, Bristow J, Eisen JA, Markowitz V, Hugenholtz P, Kyrpides NC, Klenk HP. (2011) Complete genome sequence of *Deinococcus maricopensis* type strain (LB-34). *Stand Genomic Sci* 4(2):163-172.

Repar, J., Cvjetan, S., Slade, D., Radman, M., Zahradka, D., and Zahradka, K. (2010) RecA protein assures fidelity of DNA repair and genome stability in *Deinococcus radiodurans*. *DNA Repair (Amst)* 9: 1151-1161.

Sayers, E.W., Barrett, T., Benson, D.A., Bolton, E., Bryant, S.H., Canese, K. et al. (2011) Database resources of the National Center for Biotechnology Information. *Nucleic Acids Res* 39: D38-51.

Sghaier, H., Ghedira, K., Benkahla, A., and Barkallah, I. (2008) Basal DNA repair machinery is subject to positive selection in ionizing-radiation-resistant bacteria. *BMC Genomics* 9: 297.

Sghaier, H., Satoh, K., Ohba, H., and Narumi, I. (2010) Assessing the role of RecA protein in the radioresistant bacterium *Deinococcus geothermalis*. *African Journal of Biochemistry Research* 4: 111-118.

Sghaier, H., Narumi, I., Satoh, K., Ohba, H., and Mitomo, H. (2007) Problems with the current deinococcal hypothesis: an alternative theory. *Theory Biosci* 126: 43-45.

Slade, D., and Radman, M. (2011) Oxidative stress resistance in *Deinococcus radiodurans*. *Microbiol Mol Biol Rev* 75: 133-191.

Slade, D., Lindner, A.B., Paul, G., and Radman, M. (2009) Recombination and replication in DNA repair of heavily irradiated *Deinococcus radiodurans*. *Cell* 136: 1044-1055.

Tanaka, M., Earl, A.M., Howell, H.A., Park, M.J., Eisen, J.A., Peterson, S.N., and Battista, J.R. (2004) Analysis of *Deinococcus radiodurans*'s transcriptional response to ionizing radiation and desiccation reveals novel proteins that contribute to extreme radioresistance. *Genetics* 168: 21-33.

Thornton, J.W. (2004) Resurrecting ancient genes: experimental analysis of extinct molecules. *Nat Rev Genet* 5: 366-375.

Udupa, K.S., O'Cain, P.A., Mattimore, V., and Battista, J.R. (1994) Novel ionizing radiation-sensitive mutants of *Deinococcus radiodurans*. *J Bacteriol* 176: 7439-7446.

Weller, G.R., Kysela, B., Roy, R., Tonkin, L.M., Scanlan, E., Della, M. et al. (2002) Identification of a DNA nonhomologous end-joining complex in bacteria. *Science* 297: 1686-1689.

White, O., Eisen, J.A., Heidelberg, J.F., Hickey, E.K., Peterson, J.D., Dodson, R.J. et al. (1999) Genome sequence of the radioresistant bacterium *Deinococcus radiodurans* R1. *Science* 286: 1571-1577.

Williams, E., Lowe, T.M., Savas, J., and DiRuggiero, J. (2007) Microarray analysis of the hyperthermophilic archaeon *Pyrococcus furiosus* exposed to gamma irradiation. *Extremophiles* 11: 19-29.

Woese, C.R. (1987) Bacterial evolution. *Microbiol Rev* 51: 221-271.

Yoshinaka, T., Yano, K., and Yamaguchi, H. (1973) Isolation of highly radioresistant bacterium, *Arthrobacter radiotolerans* nov. sp. *Agric Biol Chem* 37: 2269-2275.

Zahradka, K., Slade, D., Bailone, A., Sommer, S., Averbeck, D., Petranovic, M. et al. (2006) Reassembly of shattered chromosomes in *Deinococcus radiodurans*. *Nature* 443: 569-573.

# 8

# Involvement of Non-Homologous End-Joining in Radiation-Induced Genomic Instability

Keiji Suzuki, Motohiro Yamauchi, Masatoshi Suzuki, Yasuyoshi Oka and Shunichi Yamashita
*Nagasaki University Graduate School of Biomedical Sciences, Atomic Bomb Disease Institute, Department of Radiation Medical Sciences, Japan*

## 1. Introduction

DNA double-strand breaks are the most detrimental form of DNA damage induced by either endogenous and exogenous sources. DNA double-strand breaks are generated in response to ionizing radiation, radiomimic drugs, and topoisomerase inhibitors. They also created during V(D)J and class switch recombination in lymphocytes, meiotic recombination in germ cells, and by retroviral integrations (Downs et al., 2007, Polo and Jackson, 2011). Since DNA double-strand breaks discontinue chromosome structure, they may result in cell death that are associated with radiosensitivity, immunodeficiency, neurodegeneration, and developmental defects (Jackson and Bartek, 2009, Mahaney et al., 2009, O'Driscoll and Jeggo, 2006, Weterings and Chen, 2007, Wyman and Kanaar, 2006). Thus, cells have evolved sophisticated mechanisms, by which DNA double-strand breaks are repaired. Two major pathways to repair DNA double-strand breaks are non-homologous end-joining and homologous and homologous recombination (Hartlerode and Scully, 2009, Mahaney et al., 2009, Weterings and Chen, 2007, Wyman and Kanaar, 2006). While rejoining of DNA breaks are indispensable for the survival of cells, DNA repair, by itself, may threaten the stability of the genome. (Burma et al., 2006, Pastink et al., 2001, Sonoda et al., 2006, van Gent et al., 2001). In particular, non-homologous end-joining, which is the primary DNA repair pathway functions in G1 phase, is error-prone (Hartlerode and Scully, 2009, Lieber, 2010). It causes loss or rearrangement of the genetic information through mis-rejoining of DNA double strand breaks. Processing of DNA broken ends by exonucleases and endonucleases also provide another chance to alter DNA sequences. Consequently, surviving cells can avoid lethal effects of DNA double-strand breaks but it results in a loss of heterozygosity as well as gross genome rearrangements that are associated with cancer predisposition. Although most genome rearrangements have been thought to be generated directly by the initial radiation exposure (Leonhardt et al., 1999), recent findings have demonstrated that the integrity of the genome is also endangered eventually, if the cells were survived exposure to DNA damaging agents. In this chapter, the results showing that delayed DNA double-strand breaks are induced several generations after the initial insult in the progenies of surviving cells are presented, and a role of non-homologous end-joining on delayed manifestation of radiation effects and the integrity of the genome in the cells surviving radiation exposure will be discussed.

## 2. Radiation-induced genomic instability

It has been well established that ionizing radiation induces delayed effects in the progeny of surviving cells (Little, 2003, Lorimore et al., 2003, Morgan et al., 1996, Suzuki et al., 2003). This phenomenon is now called radiation-induced genomic instability, which is manifested as the delayed expression of various radiation effects, such as delayed reproductive death, delayed chromosomal instability, and delayed mutagenesis (Figure 1). Radiation-induced genomic instability has been commonly observed in many cell culture systems as well as in various animals (Lorimore et al., 2003, Morgan, 2003). In addition, there are a series of studies showing that radiation-induced genomic instability is attributed to transgenerational effects in mice using hypervariable minisatellite sequences, which have been renamed as expanded simple tandem repeats (Niwa, 2006). Radiation-induced genomic instability results in accumulating gene mutations and chromosomal rearrangements in addition to the direct genome damage caused by the primary radiation exposure. Therefore, it has been thought to play a pivotal role in accelerating the process of radiation-induced carcinogenesis (Huang et al., 2003, Kadhim et al., 1992, Niwa, 2003, Suzuki, 1997).

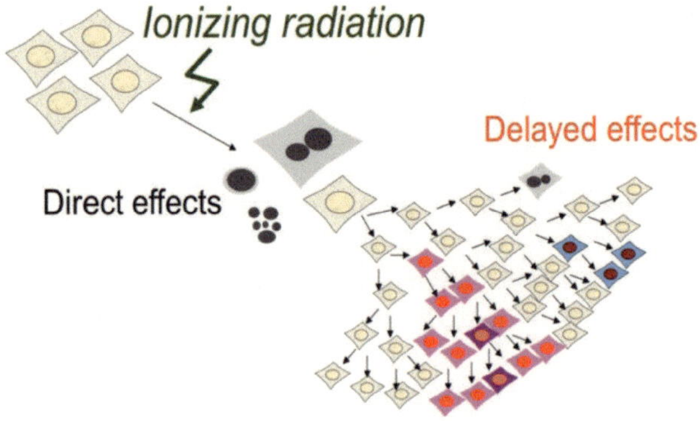


Fig. 1. Radiation-induced genomic instability.

Because radiation-induced genomic instability is induced in a certain fraction of the progenies originated from a single survived cell, not a single gene mutation but some epigenetic changes could be involved in the initiation of radiation-induced genomic instability (Wright, 2010). Persistently elevated levels of oxidative stress was found is association with radiation-induced genomic instability (Azzam et al., 2003, Kim et al., 2006a, Limoli et al., 2003). Further association was confirmed in studies where chronic hydrogen peroxide treatment initiated instability. Administration of free-radical scavengers, antioxidant treatment, and reducing oxygen tension each reduced delayed chromosomal instability, suggesting a role of oxidative stress in perpetuating genomic instability (Roy et al., 2000). Moreover, unstable clones showed mitochondrial dysfunction, which might explain elevated levels of oxidative stress (Kim et al., 2006b). An inflammatory response has also been proposed to be involved in radiation-induced genomic instability particularly in bone marrow (Wright, 2010). Furthermore, possible involvement of bystander effects has also been discussed. Bystander effects are responses observed in unirradiated cells as a result of receiving signals from irradiated cells (Mothersill and Seymour, 2004, Prise and O'Sullivan, 2009). A variety of responses have been described including DNA damage induction, chromosomal instability, and cell death. As bystander effects have been observed in coculture of irradiated and unirradiated cells, and after the transfer of medium from irradiated cells to unirradiated cells, secreted factor(s) may be involved in transducing the bystander signals (Sowa and Morgan, 2004). It has been hypothesized that increased secretion of transforming growth factor beta results in stimulation of production of reactive oxygen species through a membrane NADPH oxidase. In fact, previous study demonstrated that transforming growth factor beta increased oxidative stress through decreased activity of mitochondrial complex IV (Kim et al., 2006b).

Although oxidative stress is surely involved in perpetuation of radiation-induced genomic instability (Azzam et al., 2003, Coates et al., 2008, Miller et al., 2008, Kim et al., 2006a, Limoli et al., 2003, Wright, 2007), alternative mechanisms could be associated with manifestation of radiation-induced genomic instability in non-hematopoietic cells. We have shown that delayed unscheduled induction of DNA double strand breaks is involved in the manifestation of delayed phenotypes (Suzuki et al., 2003). In fact, our study indicated that increased phosphorylated histone H2AX foci, which correspond to DNA double-strand breaks, were frequently detected in the progeny of normal human diploid cells surviving X-rays. Moreover, delayed reactivation of p53 in response to DNA damage was manifested in the surviving clones. Delayed induction of DNA double strand breaks was also confirmed by delayed induction of chromosomal aberrations (Toyokuni et al., 2009). Thus, it is evidenced that induction of DNA double strand breaks is induced indirectly in surviving cells from exposure to radiation, indicating that DNA repair pathways could play roles in amending delayed DNA double-strand breaks in surviving cells.

Previously, Chang and Little reported that radiation-induced genomic instability was absent in xrs5 cells, which are NHEJ-deficient Chinese hamster cells defective in Ku80 protein (Chang and Little, 1992a). Interestingly, delayed reproductive death was not observed in these cells, even though they harbor sufficient amount of DNA double-strand breaks. Since the mechanism of delayed reproductive death has not been fully described yet, we have hypothesized that defective NHEJ in xrs5 cells decreases the chance of mis-rejoining of the broken ends, which result in the formation of dicentric chromosomes involved in division halt. To test this possibility we examined delayed chromosomal instability in two NHEJ-defective cells, xrs-5 and xrs-6 cells, and compared the frequency with the wild-type CHO cells. Furthermore, delayed induction of dicentric chromosomes was examined in cells defective in the catalytic subunit of DNA-dependent protein kinase (DNA-PKcs).

## 3. Non-homologous end-joining and its mutants

Non-homologous end-joining is one of the two major pathways involved in amending DNA double-strand breaks in multicellular eukaryotes. It primarily plays a critical role during G0-, G1- and early S-phase of cell cycle (Lieber 2010, Polo and Jackson, 2011). Non-homologous end-joining is initiated by binding a heterodimeric protein complex consists of Ku80 and Ku70 to both ends of DNA double-strand breaks (Jackson and Bartek, 2009, Mahaney et al., 2009, O'Driscoll and Jeggo, 2006, Weterings and Chen, 2007, Wyman and Kanaar, 2006). Then, DNA-PKcs, a catalytic subunit of DNA-dependent protein kinase, is recruited to Ku-DNA complex, which results in activation of the protein kinase activity of DNA-PKcs and tethering two broken DNA ends. DNA-PKcs phosphorylates a number of proteins, including Ku80, Ku70, XRCC4, Artemis, DNA ligase IV and DNA-PKcs itself (Mahaney et al., 2009, Weterings and Chen, 2007). Autophosphorylation alters the conformation of DNA-PKcs, allowing the recruitment of DNA end-processing enzymes, such as MRE11 and Artemis (Huertas, 2010). MRE11 exhibits a 3' to 5' exonuclease activity and plays a critical role in homologous recombination, but its function in non-homologous end-joining is still to be determined. On the other hand, Artemis shows a 5' to 3' exonuclease activity, and it is suggested to be involved in a subset of DNA double-strand breaks. In fact, cells defective in both nucleases do not show significant radiation sensitivity. Processing of broken ends might create DNA single-strand breaks, which are amended by the DNA polymerase X family, such as polymerase mu and polymerase lambda, and terminal deoxyribonucleotidyltransferase. DNA double-strand breaks are finally rejoined by a complex composed of DNA ligase IV, XRCC4, and XLF.

Until now, several mutants defective in DNA double-strand break repair have been cloned (Jeggo, 1998). They are highly sensitive to radiation and show chromosome instability in response to DNA damaging agents. As shown in Table 1, at least four independent groups were identified. XR-1 mutant belong to X-ray repair complementing defective repair in Chinese hamster cells 4 (XRCC4) group holds mutations in the XRCC4 gene. Both xrs-5 and xrs-6 cells are the members of the XRCC5 group, and they show profound defect in the Ku80 function (Singleton et al., 1997). In xrs-5 cells, the expression of the Ku80 gene is significantly compromised. In xrs-6 cells, a 13-base pair insertion causes a truncation of KU80 protein, which accelerates degradation of KU80 protein. The responsible gene for the XRCC7 group is the DNA-PKcs (Zdzienicka, 1999). Both scid and V-3 mutants harbor premature termination of the protein in the C-terminus. In irs-20 a mutation that causes substitution of the amino acid located in the C-terminal region.

| Mutants | Complementation group | Gene |
|---|---|---|
| XR-1 | XRCC4 | *XRCC4* |
| xrs-5, xrs-6 | XRCC5 | *Ku80* |
| - | XRCC6 | *Ku70* |
| scid, V3 | XRCC7 | *DNA-PKcs* |

Table 1. Rodent cell mutants with defective non-homologous end-joining repair.

Radiation sensitivity of these mutants was determined by colony formation assay. A single cell is able to form a cluster of progenitor cells, namely, a colony, when it is incubated for 10 days or more. After X-irradiation, numbers of colonies are decreased in a dose dependent manner. Consequently, cell survival can be calculated by dividing the number of colonies after X-irradiation by the number of colonies formed by the control cells. As shown in Figure 2, both xrs-5 (closed diamond), xrs-6 (closed triangle), and scid (closed square) cells show significant reduction of cell survival as compared to CHO cells (open circle). These cells lose the shoulder of the survival curve observed in CHO cells, indicating that they lose DNA repair capacity. To compliment the defect in xrs5 cells, the human Ku86 gene was introduced by electroporation, and as a result, radiation sensitivity was significantly recovered (open diamond), confirming that a single gene mutation causes profound DNA repair defect.

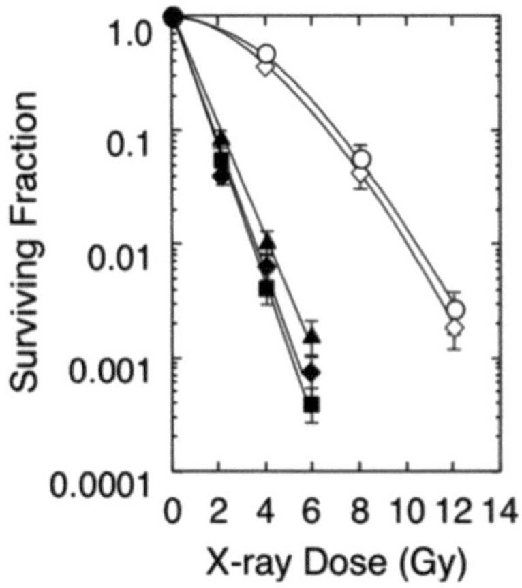


Fig. 2. Survival curves of CHO cells and Ku80-deficient cells.

These cells were irradiated with X-rays from an X-ray generator at 150 kVp and 5 mA with a 0.1-mm copper. The dose rate was 0.44 Gy/min. Dose rates were determined with an ionization chamber.

## 4. Induction of delayed phenotypes in DNA repair-deficient cells

### 4.1 Methods for detection of delayed phenotypes

Since radiation-induced genomic instability is manifested as the expression of delayed effects in the progeny of surviving cells, most of the study isolated colonies formed by the cells surviving X-irradiation. The primary colonies were cloned 10 days after irradiation. The cells obtained from each colony have already passed 15 to 20 population doublings. Then, the primary clones were subjected to the secondary colony formation. After 10 day, the secondary clones were isolated, and the cells were at 30 to 35 population doubling levels after irradiation. Delayed reproductive death was examined by colony-forming ability. Colonies derived from the surviving cells often contain giant cells, which occupied an area in the colony several times greater than the rest of the cells. Colonies containing at least one giant cell were judged as giant cell-positive colony. Delayed chromosomal bridges were detected between two dividing daughter nuclei in the anaphase cells in the surviving colonies. Delayed chromosomal aberrations were examined in metaphase cells derived from the primary and the secondary clones. Both chromatid- and chromosome-type aberrations were analyzed, and total 200 metaphases were counted per each sample.

Delayed induction of DNA double strand breaks was determined by 53BP1 foci by immunofluorescence. 53BP1 is a protein, which was originally discovered as a p53-binding protein. Lately, it turns to be clear that 53BP1 is a critical component of DNA damage signalling pathway (Polo and Jackson, 2011). ATM-dependent DNA damage checkpoint plays a central role in protecting integrity of the genome (Kastan and Bartek, 2004, Lavin, 2008, Shiloh and Kastan, 2001, Shiloh, 2003). ATM, which forms dimer or oligomer in the control cells, dissociates into monomer through autophosphorylation at serine 1981 in response to ionizing radiation (Bakkenist and Kastan, 2003). Activated ATM transduces DNA damage signal through phosphorylation of down-stream factors, including histone H2AX, MDC1 and 53BP1 (Ciccia and Elledge, 2010, Kastan and Lim, 2000)(Figure 3), and DNA damage signal is amplified through the formation of ionizing radiation-induced foci

(Bonner et al., 2008). Activated ATM also phosphorylates p53 and CHK2/Cds1, which result in an induction of apoptosis as well as cell cycle arrest. Furthermore, ATM phosphorylates MRE11, NBS1, and Artemis, by which DNA repair ability may be regulated. Previously, it was demonstrated that the number of DNA double-strand breaks and the number of foci are well correlated, and since then, ionizing radiation-induced foci have been treated as a trustable marker for DNA double-strand breaks (Bonner et al., 2008). Foci of phosphorylated histone H2AX at serine 139 were the first ones to be used as DNA damage marker (Paull et al., 2000). Subsequently, foci of phosphorylated ATM at serine 1981 were demonstrated to illustrate low level of DNA double-strand breaks (Suzuki et al., 2006). Compared to these foci, 53BP1 foci create larger discrete foci, which can be detected even in tissue specimens (Nakashima et al., 2008). Thus, 53BP1 foci have been treated as DNA damage marker.

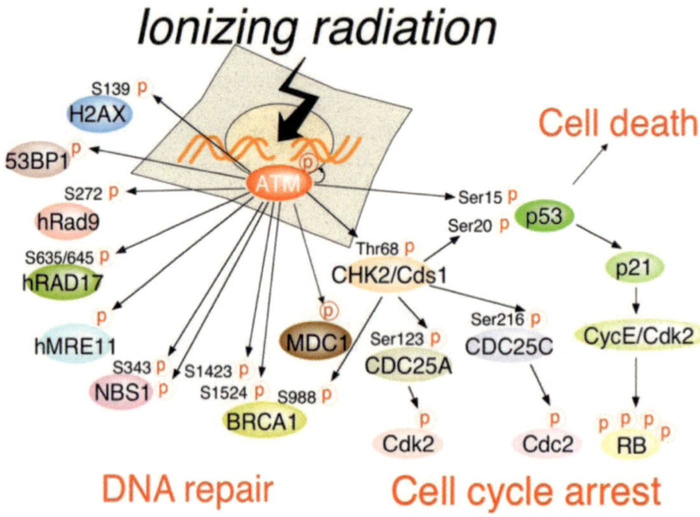


Fig. 3. ATM-dependent DNA damage checkpoint signalling.

53BP1 foci were detected by a specific antibody against the human 53BP1 protein. The primary antibody was visualized by Alexa594-labelled anti-rabbit IgG antibody. The nuclei were counterstained with DAPI. The samples were examined with an Olympus fluorescence microscope. Digital images were captured by a cooled CCD camera, and the images were analyzed by image analysis software.

### 4.2 Manifestation of delayed phenotypes

Radiation-induced genomic instability needs to be examined at the same survival levels, so that 8 Gy and 10 Gy of X-rays were irradiated to CHO, while 2 and 4 Gy of X-rays were exposed to xrs-5 and xrs-6 cells, respectively. The primary clones were isolated, and they were subjected to the secondary colony formation. As shown in Figure 4, colony-forming ability is significantly reduced in CHO cells derived from surviving clones compared with those derived from the control clones. In contrast, no such difference is observed in both xrs-5 and xrs-6 cells, indicating that delayed reproductive death was completely absent in both xrs-5 and xrs-6 cells. In CHO cells, the frequency of giant cells and chromosomal bridges is also increased only in surviving clones, whereas, delayed induction of these phenotypes was completely abrogated in xrs-5 and xrs-6 cells (Figures 5 and 6).

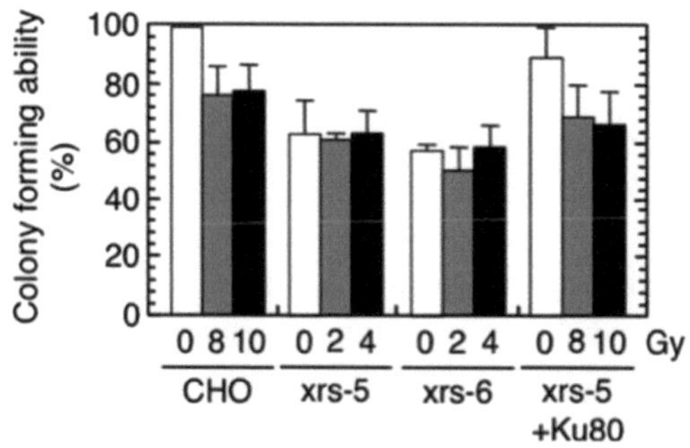


Fig. 4. Delayed reproductive death at 30-35 population doublings post-irradiation.

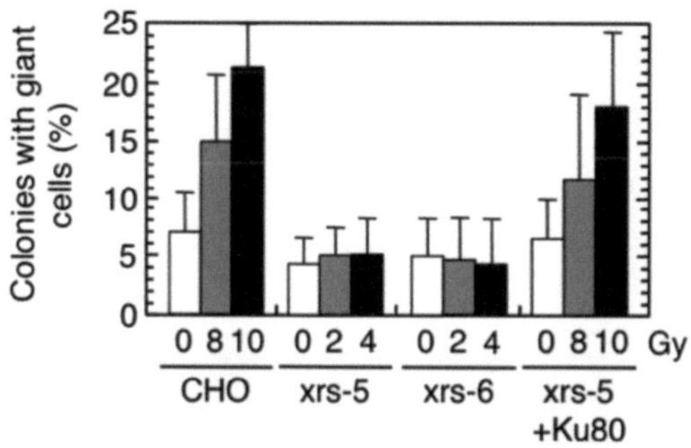


Fig. 5. Delayed giant cell formation at 30-35 population doublings post-irradiation.

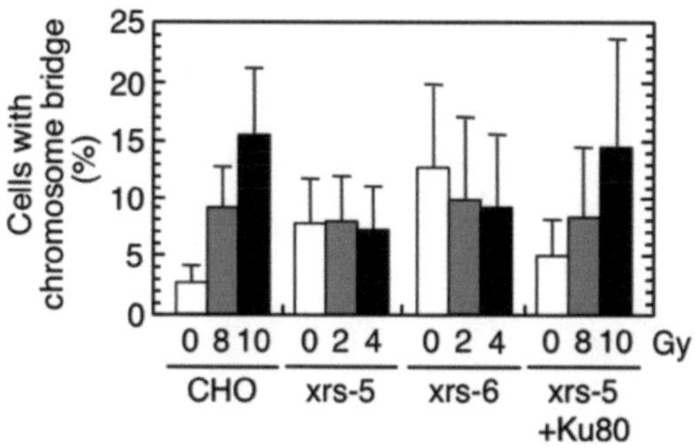


Fig. 6. Delayed chromosome bridge (right) at 30-35 population doublings post-irradiation.

In order to confirm that defective induction of these delayed phenotypes are caused by the simple Ku80-deficiency, the human Ku86 gene was introduced into xrs-5 cells. Expression of human KU80 protein was confirmed by western blotting, and sufficient amount of KU80 protein was detected in the complimented cells. Accordingly, it was confirmed that complementation of the defective Ku80 function in xrs-5 cells simultaneously restored delayed reproductive death, giant cell formation and delayed chromosomal bridge formation to the levels observed in CHO cells. Thus, the results clearly indicated that Ku80-dependent rejoining is involved in the manifestation of delayed phenotypes in the progenies of X-ray-surviving cells.

### 4.3 Delayed induction of DNA double-strand breaks

It is possible that delayed phenotypes are caused by delayed DNA double strand breaks and Ku80-dependent mis-rejoining. Delayed induction of DNA double strand breaks were examined by 53BP1 foci in cells at 30-35 PDL post-irradiation (Figure 7). Since the primary antibody against 53BP1 is visualized by the secondary antibody labeled with Alexa594, 53BP1 foci are detected as discrete large red dots within the blue nuclei. Upon X-irradiation, the foci of DNA damage checkpoint factors become detectable within a few minutes after exposure. At 1 to 2 hours after X-irradiation, the initial foci are detectable in all exposed cells. Many small foci, most of which diameter distributed between 0.4 and 1.0 micrometer, were observed. The number of foci is decreased thereafter, indicating DNA repair. While the number of the initial foci reduced significantly during the first 6 to 10 hours, some fraction of the initial foci is remained as residual foci. Diameter of these residual foci increased time-dependently, and they are quite large in size after 24 hours (Yamauchi et al., 2008). The number of foci shows no significant change thereafter, however, the cells with large residual foci are diluted out, when the foci-negative cells dominate the population. Thus, the background foci is rarely detectable even in the cells surviving 10 Gy of X-rays. While the frequency of 53BP1 foci per cell in the control CHO cells was approximately 0.14 ± 0.07, it was increased to 0.41 ± 0.19 in 10 Gy-surviving cells. The frequency of 53BP1 foci in the unirradiated xrs5 cells were relatively higher (0.18 ± 0.08) compared to the CHO cells, and it was about 0.51 ± 0.27 in 4 Gy-surviving cells.

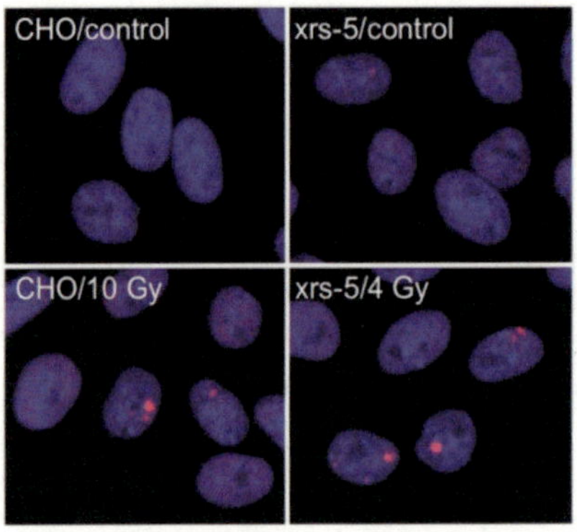


Fig. 7. Delayed induction of 53BP1 foci in CHO and xrs-5 cells at 30-35 population doublings post-irradiation.

Previously, a few studies including ours have suggested that delayed DNA double strand breaks are induced several generations after the initial insult (Barber et al., 2006, Huang et al., 2007, Suzuki et al., 2003), which has been proven by examining the delayed induction of foci of DNA damage checkpoint factors, such as phosphorylated histone H2AX. While phosphorylated histone H2AX foci are frequently used as biochemical markers for DNA double strand breaks, the foci of other DNA damage checkpoint factors, such as phosphorylated ATM foci and 53BP1 foci, are colocalized with phosphorylated histone H2AX foci, and they could also be used as alternative markers for DNA damage. In the present study, we demonstrated that the frequency of 53BP1 foci was higher in the progenies of surviving cells compared to unirradiated cells. Thus, it is confirmed that delayed induction of DNA double strand breaks in the progeny of surviving cells associated with pleiotropic manifestation of radiation-induced genomic instability.

### 4.4 Mis-rejoining of delayed DNA double-strand breaks

Although the number of spontaneous foci per cell in the foci-positive cells is 1, we found multiple numbers of foci in not a small numbers of surviving cells. Therefore, it is possible that mis-rejoining of delayed DNA double-strand breaks results in delayed chromosomal instability. We tested this possibility by examining delayed induction of dicentric chromosomes at 30-35 PDL post irradiation (Figure 8).

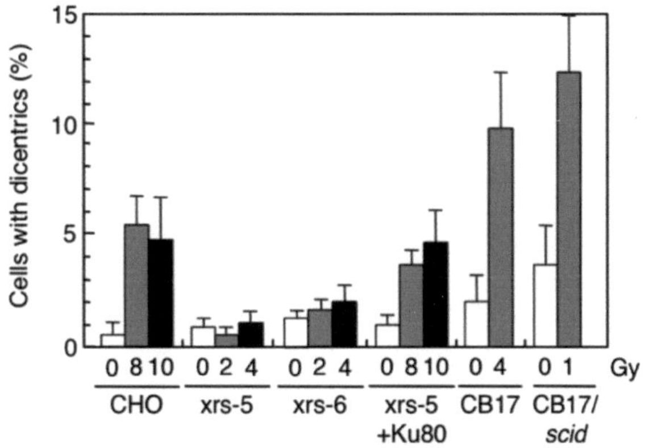


Fig. 8. Delayed chromosomal instability at 30-35 population doublings post-irradiation.

We found that delayed formation of dicentric chromosomes was significantly increased in CHO cells. Whereas, it is absent in xrs5 and xrs6 cells, while the control levels of dicentric chromosome were comparable among those cells. To confirm whether defective induction of dicentric chromosomes is related to Ku80-deficiency, delayed chromosomal instability was examined in the complimented xrs5 cells. We observed that delayed induction of dicentric chromosomes was increased to the level observed in CHO cells. Delayed chromosomal instability was also examined in cells derived from DNA-PKcs-defective *scid* mouse (Figure 8). Cells were irradiated with equivalent 10% survival doses and delayed induction of dicentric chromosomes was analyzed 30-35 PDL post-irradiation. The frequency of dicentric chromosomes in the unirradiated *scid* was higher than that in the wild-type cells, and increased dicentric frequencies in surviving cells were observed.

## 5. Role of non-homologous end-joining on radiation-induced genomic instability

Radiation-induced genomic instability has been reported commonly in various cell systems including human and rodent cells (Little, 2003, Lorimore et al., 2003, Morgan et al., 1996, Suzuki et al., 2003). However, Chang and Little demonstrated that delayed reproductive death, one characteristic manifestation of radiation-induced genomic instability, was not observed in Ku80-deficient xrs5 cells (Chang and Little, 1992a). The authors suggested that the cellular processing of DNA double strand breaks during repair must play a role in delayed reproductive death. In fact, our current study confirmed their results and found that not only delayed cell death but also delayed induction of giant cells and chromosome bridge were absent in xrs-5 cells (Figures 5 and 6). Furthermore, other Ku80-deficient cell line, xrs6, also revealed deficiency in the induction of those delayed phenotypes. Thus, it becomes clear that Ku80-dependent non-homologous end-joining is involved in the manifestation of radiation-induced genomic instability. Then the question should be about the mechanism. One possible explanation of the defective induction of some delayed phenotypes is that error-free DNA repair, such as homologous recombination, reduced the incidence of transmissible damage in the absence of error-prone non-homologous end-joining repair. If so, delayed induction of DNA double strand breaks should be lower in Ku80-defective cells than the control CHO cells. Therefore, we checked whether delayed DNA damage was less frequent in xrs5 cells. The results clearly indicated that it was not the case. Thus, even without Ku80-dependent repair, genomic instability by itself could be induced in the progenies of surviving cells. The second possibility is that defective DNA repair in xrs5 cells decreased the chance of mis-rejoining of the broken ends that occurred many generations after the initial insult. In fact, delayed induction of chromosome bridges between two daughter cells was significantly reduce in xrs-5 and xrs-6 cells (Figure 6). Furthermore, delayed induction of dicentric chromosomes was completely absent in both xrs-5 and xrs-6 cells (Figure 8). Although several studies have reported that chromosome breakages are more frequent in Ku80-deficient cells (Darroudi and Natarajan, 1987, Kemp and Jeggo, 1986), the frequency of dicentric chromosome was relatively low considering the frequency of chromosome breaks. These results support our conclusion that the formation of dicentric chromosome caused by delayed DNA damage was compromised in Ku80-deficient cells. Although a back-up non-homologous end-joining may undertake mis-rejoining of broken ends in the absence of Ku80-dependent DNA repair (Iliakis et al., 2004), it is highly likely that a major pathway of illegitimate rejoining the DNA breaks is Ku80-dependent process (Liang et al., 1996). We also confirmed that radiation-induced genomic instability was manifested in cells derived from DNA-PKcs-defective *Scid* mouse. Moreover, delayed dicentric formation was normally detected in *Scid* cells. Therefore, DNA-PK-independent rejoining, which was suggested previously (Gao et al., 1998), is involved in delayed dicentric formation. Recently, it has been postulated that XRCC4/DNA Ligase IV-dependent but DNA-PKcs-independent rejoining needs Ku80/70 complex. Thus, it is highly possible that Ku80-dependent mis-rejoining is involved in delayed generation of dicentric chromosomes, by which chromosome bridges is generated. Such mis-rejoining inhibits segregation of two daughter cells, which results in delayed induction of giant cells as well as delayed reproductive death.

It has been well described that genomic instability, which is known as gross chromosomal rearrangement, is commonly observed in yeast. Gross chromosomal rearrangements manifest as translocations, chromosomal deletions, and inversions, indicating that they could be means to accelerate multiple genetic alterations associated with carcinogenesis (Kolodner et al., 2002). Although multiple pathways cooperate to suppress gross chromosomal rearrangement, homologous recombination plays a pivotal role in avoiding gross chromosomal rearrangement (Myung et al., 2001). Moreover, the restrained recruitment of homologous recombination proteins has been reported to promote gross chromosomal rearrangement. Thus, non-homologous end-joining has little effect on gross chromosomal rearrangement in yeast.

It should be very interesting to know the consequence of cells harboring mis-rejoined chromosomes. Previously, it was reported that ionizing radiation induced genomic instability in the progeny of surviving CHO cells, which resulted in a heritable mutator phenotypes. For example, mutation frequency at the hypoxanthine-guanine phosphoribosyltransferase locus in surviving clones was persistently higher than the unirradiated progenies (Lim et al., 2000). It was expected that such mis-rejoining caused large deletions at the gene locus, however, multiplex polymerase chain reaction analysis revealed that point mutations are the predominant type of genetic alterations in the mutants (Chang and Little, 1992b). Because cells with micronuclei were frequently observed among the surviving cells, persistent break induction, which may not be involved in delayed cell death under the p53-dysfunctional condition (Tzang et al., 1999), may be resulted from mis-rejoined chromosomes. In fact, previous study demonstrated that delayed chromosomal instability was mediated by bridge-breakage-fusion cycle, which could also be involved in the perpetuation of radiation-induced genomic instability. It has been proved that ionizing radiation induces delayed genomic instability, which accumulates genetic alterations including gene mutations, loss of heterozygosity, and chromosome rearrangements, concurrently with delayed reproductive death. As Ku80-deficiency compromised delayed cell death through the formation of dicentric chromosomes, it is likely that such cells with defective DNA repair capacity are more susceptible to carcinogenesis induced by DNA damaging agents.

## 6. Molecular nature of radiation signature involved in radiation-induced genomic instability

Radiation-induced genomic instability is transmitted through many generations after the initial X-irradiation, indicating that there should be some mechanism(s), by which the initial radiation insults are memorized (Suzuki, 1997). As delayed DNA double-strand breaks are identified in surviving cells, persistent DNA damage is one candidate for radiation signature. In fact, a recent study has proved that DNA double-strand breaks induced by very low dose of X-rays remain unrepaired for many days in confluent cells (Rothkamm and Lobrich, 2003). Furthermore, if persistent DNA is radiation signature, radiation-induced genomic instability is more prevailing in xrs-5 and xrs-6 cells compared with CHO cells. But, we observed radiation-induced genomic instability at similar level between these cells (Suzuki et al., 2009). Thus, these results exclude the possibility that radiation signature is DNA double-strand breaks *per se*. Previously, we compared delayed aberrations of X chromosome with or without large deletion at the hypoxanthine-quanine-phosphorybosyltransferase gene, which is located at Xq26.1 (Toyokuni et al., 2009, Suzuki et al., 2003). Because cells defective in the gene were able to grow in the presence of 6-thioguanine, we cloned 6-thioguanine resistant clones after 3 Gy of X-rays, and examine gene deletion. We found some of the resistant clones had large deletions expanding over several megabases. Interestingly, these clones with large deletions showed higher probability to induce delayed chromosomal instability. Thus, altered higher-order chromatin structure could be a candidate for radiation signature. It is possible that such altered higher-order chromatin structure results in replication stress, which causes DNA double-strand breaks.

## 7. Conclusion

Ionizing radiation induces delayed destabilization of the genome in the progenies of surviving cells. This phenomenon, which is called radiation-induced genomic instability, is manifested by delayed induction of radiation effects, such as cell death, chromosome aberration, and mutation in the progeny of cells surviving radiation exposure. Previously, it was reported that delayed cell death was absent in Ku80-deficient cells. We have proved that this is because delayed induction of dicentric chromosomes is significantly compromised in those cells. In fact, reintroduction of the human Ku86 gene complimented the defective DNA repair and recovered delayed induction of dicentric chromosomes and delayed cell death. Thus, our current study demonstrated that DNA repair pathway is an important determinant of cellular response to ionizing radiation not only in the immediate response but also in cells surviving radiation exposure. Survived cells induced DNA double strand breaks many generations after the initial insult. Although the mechanism of delayed DNA damage induction has to be determined, delayed dicentric formation indicated that delayed DNA damage was induced in G1 phase. Such delayed DNA damage could be repaired by NHEJ repair, but it also provided a chance to engender mis-rejoining. These results should bring a new insight into how DNA repair protects the integrity of the genome from the insults of DNA damaging agents.

## 8. Acknowledgements

This work was supported in part by grants for scientific research and by Nagasaki University Global COE program from the Ministry of Education, Culture, Sports, Science, and Technology, Japan. The authors greatly appreciated Dr. Penny A. Jeggo for providing the plasmid containing the human Ku86 gene.

## 9. References

Azzam, E.I.; de Toledo, S.M. & Little, J.B. (2003). Oxidative metabolism, gap junctions and the ionizing radiation-induced bystander effect. *Oncogene*, Vol.22, No.45, (October 2003), pp. 7050-7057, ISSN 0950-9232

Bakkenist, C.J. & Kastan M.B. (2003). DNA damage activates ATM through intermolecular autophosphorylation and dimer dissociation. *Nature*, Vol.421, No.6922, (January 2003), pp. 499-506, ISSN 0028-0836

Barber, R.C.; Hickenbotham, P., Hatch, T., Kelly, D., Topchiy, N., Almeida, G.M., Jones, G.D., Johnson, G.E., Parry, J.M., Rothkamm, K. & Dubrova, Y.E. (2006). Radiation-induced transgenerational alterations in genome stability and DNA damage. *Oncogene*, Vol.25, No. 56, (November 2006), pp. 7336-7342, ISSN 0950-9232

Bonner, W.M.; Redon, C.E., Dickey, J.S., Nakamura, A.J., Sedelnikova, O.A., Solier, S. & Pommier, Y. (2008). GammaH2AX and cancer. *Nature Review of Cancer*, Vol. 8, No.12, (December 2008), pp. 957-967, ISSN 1474-175X

Burma, S.; Chen, B.P. & Chen, D.J. (2006). Role of non-homologous end joining (NHEJ) in maintaining genomic integrity. *DNA Repair*, Vol.5, No.9-10, (September 2006), pp. 1042-1048, ISSN 1568-7864

Chang, W.P. & Little, J.B. (1992a). Evidence that DNA double-strand breaks initiate the phenotype of delayed reproductive death in Chinese hamster ovary cells. *Radiation Research*, Vol.131, No.1, (July 1992), pp. 53-59, ISSN 0033-7587

Chang, W.P. & Little, J.B. (1992b). Persistent elevated frequency of spontaneous mutations in progeny of CHO clones surviving X-irradiation: association with delayed reproductive death phenotypes. *Mutation Research*, Vol.270, No.2, (November 1992), pp. 191-199, ISSN 0027-5107

Ciccia, A. & Elledge, S.J. (2010). The DNA damage response: making it safe to play with knives. *Molecular Cell*, Vol.28, No.2, (October 2007), pp. 739-745, ISSN 1097-2765

Coates, P.J.; Rundle, J.K., Lorimore, S.A. & Wright, E.G. (2008). Indirect macrophage responses to ionizing radiation: implications for genotype-dependent bystander signaling. *Cancer Research*, Vol.68, No.2 ,(January 2008), pp. 450-456, ISSN 0008-5472

Darroudi, F. & Natarajan, A.T. (1987). Cytogenetical characterization of Chinese hamster ovary X-ray-sensitive mutant cells xrs 5 and xrs 6. I. Induction of chromosomal aberrations by X-irradiation and its modulation with 3-aminobenzamide and caffeine. *Mutation Research*, Vol.177, No.1, (March 1987), pp. 133-148, ISSN 0027-5107

Downs, J.A.; Nussenzweig, M.C. & Nussenzweig, A. (2007). Chromatin dynamics and the preservation of genetic information. *Nature*, Vol.447, No.7147, (June 2007), pp. 951-958, ISSN 0028-0836

Gao, Y.; Chaudhuri, J., Zhu, C., Davidson, L., Weaver, D.T. & Alt, F.W. (1998). A targeted DNA-PKcs-null mutation reveals DNA-PK-independent functions for KU in V(D)J recombination. *Immunity*, Vol.9, No.3, (September 1998), pp. 367-376, ISSN 1074-7613

Hartlerode, A.J. & Scully, R. (2009). Mechanisms of double-strand break repair in somatic mammalian cells. *The Biochemical Journal*, Vol.423, (September 2009), pp. 157-168, ISSN 0264-6021

Huang, L.; Snyder, A.R. & Morgan, W.F. (2003). Radiation-induced genomic instability and its implications for radiation carcinogenesis. *Oncogene*, Vol.22, No.45, (October 2003), pp. 5848-5854, ISSN 0950-9232

Huang, L.; Kim, P.M., Nickoloff, J.A. & Morgan, W.F. (2007). Targeted and nontargeted effects of low-dose ionizing radiation on delayed genomic instability in human cells. *Cancer Research*, Vol.67, No.3, (February 2007), pp. 1099-1104, ISSN 0008-5472

Huertas, P. (2010). DNA resection in eukaryotes: deciding how to fix the break. *Nature Structual and Molecular Biology*, Vol.17, No. 1, (January 2010), pp. 11-16, ISSN 1545-9993

Iliakis, G.; Wang, H., Perrault, A.R., Boecker, W., Rosidi, B., Windhofer, F., Wu, W., Guan, J., Terzoudi, G. & Pantelias, G. (2004). Mechanisms of DNA double strand break repair and chromosome aberration formation. *Cytogenetic Genome Research*, Vol.104, No.1-4, (November 2004), pp. 14-20, ISSN 1424-8581

Jackson S.P. & Bartek, J. (2009). The DNA-damage response in human biology and diseases. *Nature*, Vo.461, No.7267, (October 2009), pp. 1071-1078, ISSN 0028-0836

Jeggo, P.A. (1998). Identification of genes involved in repair of DNA double-strand breaks in mammalian cells. *Radiation Research*, Vol.150, No.5, (November 1998), pp. 80-91, ISSN 0033-7587

Kadhim, M.A.; MacDonald, D.A., Goodhead, D.T., Lorimore, S.A., Marsden, S.J. & Wright, E.G. (1992). Transmission of chromosomal instability after plutonium alpha-particle irradiation. *Nature*, Vol.355, No.6362, (February 1992), pp. 738-740, ISSN 0028-0836

Kastan, M.B. & Lim, D.S. (2000). The many substrates and functions of ATM. *Nature Reviews. Molecular and Cellular Biology*, Vol.1, No.3, (December 2000), pp. 179-186, ISSN 1471-0072

Kastan, M.B. & Bartek, J. (2004). Cell-cycle checkpoints and cancer. *Nature*, Vol.432, No.7015, (November 2004), pp. 316-323, ISSN 0028-0836

Kemp, L.M. & Jeggo, P.A. (1986). Radiation-induced chromosome damage in X-ray-sensitive mutants (xrs) of the Chinese hamster ovary cell line. *Mutation Research*, Vol.166, No.3, (November 1986), pp. 255-263, ISSN 0027-5107

Kim, G.J.; Chandrasekaran, K. & Morgan, W.F. (2006a). Mitochondrial dysfunction, persistently elevated levels of reactive oxygen species and radiation-induced genomic instability: a review. *Mutagenesis*, Vol.21, No.6, (October 2006), pp. 361-368, ISSN 0267-8357

Kim, G.J.; Fiskum, G.M. & Morgan, W.F. (2006b). A role for mitochondrial dysfunction in perpetuating radiation-induced genomic instability. *Cancer Research*, Vol.66, No.21, (November 2006), pp. 10377-10383, ISSN 0008-5472

Kolodner, R.D.; Putnam, C.D., Myung, K. (2002) Maintenance of genome stability in *Saccharomyces cerevisiae*. *Science*, Vol.297, (July 2002), pp. 552-557, ISSN 0193-4511

Lavin, M.F. (2008). Ataxia-telangiectasia: from a rare disorder to a paradigm for cell signalling and cancer. *Nature Reviews. Molecular and Cellular Biology*, Vol.9, No.10, (October 2008), pp. 759-769, ISSN 1471-0072

Leonhardt, E.A.; Trinh, M., Chu, K. & Dewey, W.C. (1999). Evidence that most radiation-induced HPRT mutants are generated directly by the initial radiation exposure. *Mutation Research*, Vol.426, No.1, (May 1999), pp. 23-30, ISSN 0027-5107

Liang, F.; Romanienko, P.J., Weaver, D.T., Jeggo, P.A. & Jasin, M. (1996). Chromosomal double-strand break repair in ku80-deficient cells. *Proceedings of the National Academy of Science USA*, Vol.93, No.17, (August 1996), pp. 8929-8933, ISSN 0027-8424

Lieber, M.R. (2010). The mehanism of Double-strand DNA break repair by the nonhomologous DNA end-joining pathway. *Annual review of Biochemistry*, Vol.79, No.1, (July 2010), pp. 181-211, ISSN 0066-4154

Lim, D.S.; Vogel, H., Willefrod, D.M., Sands, A.T., Platt, K.A. & Hasty, P. (2000). Analysis of ku80-mutant mice and cells with deficient levels of p53. *Molecular and Cellular Biology*, Vol.20, No.11, (June 2000), pp. 3772-3780, ISSN 0270-7306

Limoli, C.L.; Giedzinski, E., Morgan, W.F., Swarts, S.G., Jones, G.D. & Hyun, W. (2003). Persistent oxidative stress in chromosomally unstable clones. *Cancer Research*, Vol.63, No.12, (June 2003), pp. 3107-3111, ISSN 0008-5472

Little, J.B. (2003). Genomic instability and bystander effects: a historical perspective. *Oncogene*, No.22, Vol.45, (October 2003), pp. 6978-6987, ISSN 0950-9232

Lorimore, S.A.; Coates, P.J. & Wright, E.G. (2003). Radiation-induced genomic instability and bystander effects: inter-related nontargeted effects of exposure to ionizing radiation. *Oncogene*, Vol.22, No.45 (October 2003), pp. 7058-7069, ISSN 0950-9232

Rothkamm, K. & Löbrich, M. (2003). Evidence for a lack of DNA double-strand break repair in human cells exposed to very low x-ray doses. *Proceedings of the National Academy of Science U S A*, Vol.100, No. 9, (April 2003), pp. 5057-5062, ISSN 0027-8424

Mahaney, B.L.; Meek, K. & Lees-Miller, S.P. (2009). Repair of ionizing radiation-induced DNA double-strand breaks by non-homologous end-joining. *The Biochemical Journal*, Vol.417, No.3, (February 2009), pp. 639-650, ISSN 0264-6021

Miller, J.H.; Jin, S., Morgan, W.F., Yang, A., Wan, Y., Aypar, U., Peters, J.S. & Springer, D.L. (2008). Profiling mitochondrial proteins in radiation-induced genome-unstable cell lines with persistent oxidative stress by mass spectrometry, *Radiation Research*, Vol.169, No.6, (June 2008), pp. 700-706, ISSN 0033-7587

Morgan, W.F.; Day, J.P., Kaplan, M.I., McGhee, E.M. & Limoli, C.L. (1996). Genomic instability induced by ionizing radiation. *Radiation Research*, Vol.146, No.3, (September 1996), pp. 247-258, ISSN 0033-7587

Morgan W.F. (2003). Non-targeted and delayed effects of exposure to ionizing radiation: I. Radiation-induced genomic instability and bystander effects in vitro. *Radiation Research*, Vol.159, No.5, (May 2003), pp. 567-580, ISSN 0033-7587

Mothersill, C. & Seymour, C. (2004). Radiation-induced bystander effects--implications for cancer. *Nature Review of Cancer*, Vol.4, No.2, (February 2004), pp. 158-164, ISSN 1474-175X

Myung, K.; Chen, C., Kolodner, R.D. (2001) Multiple pathways cooperate in the suppression of genomic instability in *Saccharomyces cerevisiae*. *Nature*, Vol.411, No.6841, (June 2001), pp. 1073-1076, ISSN 0028-0836

Nakashima, M.; Suzuki, K., Meirmanov, S., Naruke, Y., Matsuu-Matsuyama, M., Shichijo, K., Saenko, V., Kondo, H., Hayashi, T., Ito, M., Yamashita, S. & Sekine, I. (2008). Foci formation of p53-binding protein 1 in thyroid tumors: activation of genomic instability during thyroid carcinogenesis. *International Journal of Cancer*, Vol.122, No.5, (March 2008), pp. 1082-1088, ISSN 0828-6924

Niwa, O. (2003). Induced genomic instability in irradiated germ cells and in the offspring; reconciling discrepancies among the human and animal studies. *Oncogene*, Vol.22, No.45, (October 2003), pp. 7078-7086, ISSN 0950-9232

Niwa, O. (2006). Radiation induced dynamic mutations and transgenerational effects. *Journal of Radiation Research*, Vol.47, No.1, (January 2006), pp. 25-30, ISSN 0449-3060

O'Driscoll, M. & Jeggo, P.A. (2006). The role of double-strand break repair - insights from human genetics. *Nature Review of Genetics*, Vol.7, No.1, (January 2006), pp. 45-54, ISSN 1471-0056

Pastink, A.; Eeken, J.C. & Lohman, P.H. (2001). Genomic integrity and the repair of double-strand breaks. *Mutation Research*, Vol.480-481, (September 2001), pp. 37-50, ISSN 0027-5107

Paull, T.T.; Rogakou. E.P., Yamazaki, V., Kirchgessner, C.U., Gellert, M. & Bonner WM. (2000). A critical role for histone H2AX in recruitment of repair factors to nuclear foci after DNA damage. *Current Biology*, Vol.10, No. 15, (July 2000), pp. 886-895, ISSN 0960-9822

Polo, S.E. & Jackson, S.P. (2011). Dynamics of DNA damage response proteins at DNA breaks: a focus on protein modifications. *Genes and Development*, Vol.25, No. 5, (March 2011), pp. 409-433, ISSN 0890-9369

Prise, K. & O'Sullivan, J.M. (2009). Radiation-induced bystander signalling in cancer therapy. *Nature Review of Cancer*, Vol.9, No.5, (May 2009), pp. 351-360, ISSN 1474-175X

Roy, K.; Kodama, S., Suzuki, K., Fukase, K. & Watanabe, M. (2000). Hypoxia relieves X-ray-induced delayed effects in normal human embryo cells. *Radiation Research*, Vol.154, No.6, (December 2000), pp. 659-666, ISSN 0033-7587

Shiloh, Y. & Kastan, M.B. (2001). ATM: genome stability, neuronal development, an cancer cross paths. *Advances in Cancer Research*, Vol.83, (January 2001), pp. 209-254, ISSN 0065-230X

Shiloh, Y. (2003). ATM and related protein kinases: safeguarding genome integrity. *Nature Review of Cancer*, Vol.3, No.3, (March 2003), pp. 155-168, ISSN 1474-175X

Singleton, B.K.; Priestley, A., Steingrimsdottir, H., Gell, D., Blunt, T., Jackson, S.P., Lehmann, A.R. & Jeggo, P.A. (1997). Molecular and biochemical characterization of xrs mutants defective in Ku80. *Molecular and Cellular Biology*, Vol.17, No.3, (March 1997), pp. 1264-1273, ISSN 0270-7360

Sonoda, E.; Hochegger, H., Saberi, A., Taniguchi, Y. & Takeda, S. (2006). Differential usage of non-homologous end-joining and homologous recombination in double strand break repair. *DNA Repair*, Vol.5, No.9-10, (September 2006), pp. 1021-2129, ISSN 1568-7864

Sowa Resat, M.B. & Morgan, W.F. (2004). Radiation-induced genomic instability: a role for secreted soluble factors in communicating the radiation response to non-irradiated cells. *Journal of Cell Biochemistry*, Vol.92, No.5, (August 2004), pp. 1013-1019, ISSN 0730-2312

Suzuki, K. (1997). Multistep nature of X-ray-induced neoplastic transformation in mammalian cells: genetic alteration and instability. Journal of Radiation Research, Vol.38, No.1, (March 1997), pp. 55-63, ISSN0449-3060

Suzuki, K.; Ojima, M., Kodama, S. & Watanabe, M. (2003). Radiation-induced DNA damage and delayed induced genomic instability. *Oncogene*, Vol.22, No.45, (October 2003), pp. 6988-6993 ISSN 0950-9232

Suzuki, K.; Yokoyama, S., Waseda, S., Kodama, S. & Watanabe, M. (2003). Delayed reactivation of p53 in the progeny of cells surviving ionizing radiation. *Cancer Research*, Vol.63, No.5, (March 2003), pp. 936-941, ISSN 0008-5472

Suzuki, K.; Okada, H., Yamauchi, M., Oka, Y., Kodama, S. & Watanabe, M. (2006). Qualitative and quantitative analysis of phosphorylated ATM foci induced by low-dose ionizing radiation. *Radiation Research*, Vol.165, No. 5, (May 2006), pp. 499-504, ISSN 0033-7587

Suzuki, K.; Kodama, S. & Watanabe, M. (2009). Role of Ku80-dependent end-joining in delayed genomic instability in mammalian cells surviving ionizing radiation. *Mutation Research*, Vol.683, No.1-2, (January 2009), pp. 29-34, ISSN 0027-5107

Toyokuni, H.; Maruo, A., Suzuki, K. & Watanabe, M. (2009). The contribution of radiation-induced large deletion of the genome to chromosomal instability. *Radiation Research*, Vol.171, No.2, (February 2009), pp. 198-203, ISSN 0033-7587

Tzang, B.S.; Lai, Y.C., Hsu, M., Chang, H.W., Chang, C.C., Huang, P.C. & Liu, Y.C. (1999). Function and sequence analysis of tumor suppressor gene p53 of CHO.K1 cells.*DNA and Cell Biology*, Vol.18, No.4, (April 1999), pp. 315-321, ISSN 1044-5498

van Gent, D.C.; Hoeijmakers, J.H. & Kanaar, R. (2001). Chromosomal stability and the DNA double-stranded break connection. *Nature Review of Genetics*, Vol.2, No.3, (March 2001), pp. 196-206, ISSN 1471-0056

Weterings, E. & Chen, D.J. (2007). DNA-dependent protein kinase in nonhomologous end joining: a lock with multiple keys? The *Journal of Cell Biology*, Vol.179, No. 2, (October 2007), pp. 183-186, ISSN 0021-9525

Wright, E.G. (2007). Microenvironment and genetic factors in haemopoietic radiation responses. *International Journal of Radiation Biology*, Vol.83, No.11-12, (November-December 2007), pp. 813-818, ISSN 0955-3002

Wright, E.G. (2010). Manifestations and mechanisms of non-targeted effects of ionizing radiation. *Mutation Research*, Vol.687, No.1-2, (May 2010), pp. 28-33, ISSN 0027-5107

Wynman, C. & Kannar, R. (2006). DNA double strand break repair: all's well that ends well. *Annual Review of Genetics*, Vol.40, No.1, (December 2006), pp. 363-383, ISSN 0066-4197

Yamauchi, M.; Oka, Y., Yamamoto, M., Niimura, K., Uchida, M., Kodama, S., Watanabe, M., Sekine, I., Yamashita, S. & Suzuki, K. (2008). Growth of persistent foci of DNA damage checkpoint factors is essential for amplification of G1 checkpoint signaling. *DNA Repair*, Vol.7, No.3, (March 2008), pp. 405-17, ISSN 1568-7864

Zdzienicka, M.Z. (1999). Mammalian X-ray-sensitive mutants which are defective in non-homologous (illegitimate) DNA double-strand break repair. *Biochimie*, Vol.81, No.1-2, (January-February 1999), pp. 107-116, ISSN 0300-9084

# Part 2

## Mechanistic Insights

# 9

# Role of RPA Proteins in Radiation Repair and Recovery

Patrick E. Gygli, J. Scott Lockhart and Linda C. DeVeaux
*Idaho State University,*
*USA*

## 1. Introduction

Repair of radiation-induced DNA damage requires a complex series of protein interactions. Single-stranded DNA (ssDNA) binding proteins (RPA/SSB) have long been known to play a passive, protective role in DNA replication and repair, by coating ssDNA. Recent evidence, however, suggests a much more active function for these ubiquitous proteins. In this review, we provide a summary of the background of ssDNA binding proteins, and incorporate recent experimental observations into current models of dynamic interactions between these proteins and cellular DNA repair enzymes. These results point to a highly choreographed, interactive mechanism, with RPA/SSB at the center of the coordination.

## 2. Structure

There are two primary classes of ssDNA binding proteins, which share secondary and tertiary structural features, but are distinct in their quaternary structures. The eukaryotic Replication Protein A class (RPAs) consists of heterotrimeric proteins while the bacterial class (SSBs) consists of a range of homo-multimers. Members of the archaeal domain may possess either the RPA or SSB types, or combinations unique to this domain, illustrated in Figure 1 (Kerr, et al., 2003; Lin, et al., 2008; Richard, et al., 2009; Shereda, et al., 2008; Wold, 1997).
SSBs/RPAs are primarily identified by the presence of a structurally conserved oligonucleotide/oligosaccharide binding motif (OB-fold) (Kerr, et al., 2003; Richard, et al., 2009; Shereda, et al., 2008; Theobald, et al., 2003; Wold, 1997). The canonical OB-fold consists of five structurally conserved β-strands, forming two β-sheets, and their inter-spaced variable loops, which form a tertiary flattened β-barrel. The non-specific binding of ssDNA occurs on the surface of the β-barrel in a cleft between the variable loops. The binding of nucleotides is mediated through stacking interactions with aromatic residues and packing interactions with hydrophobic residues. Binding to the phosphodiester backbone also occurs through electrostatic interactions. The OB-folds have a binding polarity that specifies the orientation on the bound ssDNA (Shereda, et al., 2008; Theobald, et al., 2003).
The majority of bacterial and mitochondrial SSBs function as homotetramers, with a single OB-fold per monomer and thus four OB-folds per complex. For members of the *Deinococcus/Thermus* branch, the SSB functions as a homodimer and maintains the theme of four OB-folds per complex by having two non-identical OB-folds per monomer (Bernstein, et al., 2004; Eggington, et al., 2004; Filipkowski, et al., 2006; Filipkowski & Kur, 2007;

Shereda, et al., 2008). These SSB complexes occlude up to 65 and 35 nucleotides of ssDNA, respectively (Filipkowski & Kur, 2007; Meyer & Laine, 1990; Shereda, et al., 2008). Other, less common SSB configurations have also been identified, including an alternative homopentameric Deinococcal SSB (Norais, et al., 2009; Sugiman-Marangos & Junop, 2010). In general, the N-terminal region of the SSB contains the oligomerization domain while the C-terminal region is implicated in heterologous protein interactions (Shereda, et al., 2008).

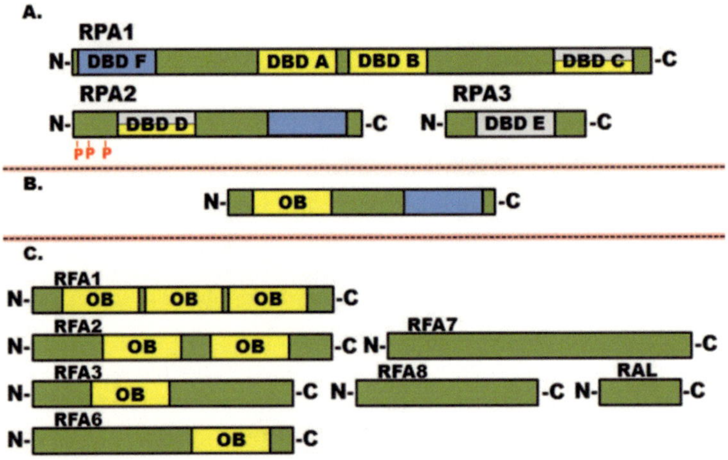


Fig. 1. RPA and SSB structures from eukaryotes, bacteria, and archaea. (A) The canonical eukaryotic RPA comprises three protein subunits, each containing OB-folds designated DBD A-F. Yellow OB-folds are DNA interacting domains, blue domains are involved in heterologous protein interactions, and gray domains are involved in maintenance of RPA structure. The N-terminus of RPA2 is the primary phosphorylation domain, denoted by red Ps. (B) The canonical bacterial SSB functions as a homotetramer and contains a single OB-fold (yellow) and a C-terminal heterologous protein interacting domain (blue) per monomer. (C) Archaeal RPAs are diverse and display characteristics of both eukaryotic RPA and bacterial SSB. Examples from *H. salinarum* are shown. RFA6 resembles bacterial SSB, whereas RFA1 is uniquely archaeal. The genes encoding RFA2 and RFA7, which are found in an operon, likely function as a multimeric protein, as do RFA3, RFA8, and RAL.

The eukaryotic RPA is a heterotrimer composed of a large RPA1 (~72 kDa), medium RPA2 (~32 kDa), and small RPA3 (~14 kDa) subunit. RPA1 and RPA2 tend to be conserved subunits with a variable RPA3, though considerable variation can occur throughout domains (Lin, et al., 2008; Wold, 1997). RPA1 contains four OB-folds referred to as DNA binding domains (DBD). DBD A and B are centrally located, DBD C is in the C-terminal region, and DBD F is in the N-terminal region. RPA2 contains a single centrally located OB-fold, DBD D, and RPA3 a single centrally located OB-fold, DBD E (Binz, et al., 2004; Oakley, et al., 2009; Pretto, et al., 2010). ssDNA binding occurs primarily through interaction with DBD A-D, which together are capable of occluding approximately 30 nucleotides (Blackwell & Borowiec, 1994; Iftode, et al., 1999; C. Kim, et al., 1992; Theobald, et al., 2003). A binding polarity of the complex is achieved through decreased ssDNA affinity from DBD A to D (Oakley, et al., 2009; Pretto, et al., 2010). The N-terminal domain of RPA1 is implicated in heterologous protein interactions and regulation, particularly through DBD F, while the C-terminal domain is involved in heterotrimer structure interactions (Broderick, et al., 2010;

Fanning, et al., 2006; Oakley, et al., 2009; Wold, 1997). The N-terminus of RPA2 contains a regulatory phosphorylation domain that affects interactions of RPA with other proteins, as well as its DNA binding kinetics (Machwe, et al., 2011; Nuss, et al., 2005; Oakley, et al., 2009; Patrick, et al., 2005; Vassin, et al., 2009). The C-terminal region of RPA2 is also involved in heterologous protein interactions and regulation. RPA3 consists almost entirely of DBD E and is thought to be involved primarily in heterotrimer formation, but potential roles in heterologous protein interactions have been identified (Cavero, et al., 2010; Wold, 1997).

## 3. Multiplicity of homologs

The highly conserved nature of the OB-fold has allowed identification of potential RPA/SSB homologs in the ever-expanding genome sequence database. To our knowledge, there have been no reports of genomes lacking an RPA/SSB homolog, with the possible exception of the crenarchaea *Pyrobaculum aerophilum* and *Aeropyrum pernix* (Luo, et al., 2007).

There are numerous excellent and extensive reviews covering the history, genetics and biochemical characterization of *E. coli* SSB and its encoding gene (Lohman & Ferrari, 1994; Meyer & Laine, 1990; Shereda, et al., 2008). The single gene, *ssb*, is located adjacent to, but divergently transcribed from, the *uvrA* gene (Brandsma, et al., 1985). In *Bacillus subtilis*, there are two SSB genes, *ssb* and *ywpH* (Lindner, et al., 2004). Although the amino acid sequences of the two proteins are similar, YwpH lacks the C-terminal region found in both the *E. coli* and *B. subtilis* SSBs. *B. subtilis ssb* is essential, but unlike in *E. coli*, is found between ribosomal protein genes. Of 87 bacterial genomes analyzed, all contained at least one SSB gene (Lindner, et al., 2004). Based on gene organization, four groupings were proposed: Group I organisms display *B. subtilis*-type gene organization and more than one SSB. Group II organisms contain only one gene for SSB. *E. coli* represents the type organism for Group III bacteria, where the single *ssb* gene is divergently transcribed from the adjacent *uvrA* gene. Group IV consists of organisms whose SSB organization does not resemble either *B. subtilis* or *E. coli*. *Thermotoga maritima* and *T. neopolitana* likely fall into Group IV, whereas *Thermoanaerobacter tengcongensis* is in Group I (Olszewski, et al., 2010; Olszewski, et al., 2008).

Recently, a novel homopentameric SSB, DdrB, was identified in *Deinococcus radiodurans*, which may challenge previous notions regarding canonical SSB structure (Norais, et al., 2009; Sugiman-Marangos & Junop, 2010). Restricted to the Deinococcal lineage, it may represent an adaptation related to the unusually high DNA repair capacity of this organism. However, it should be kept in mind that other SSB proteins that deviate from the traditional consensus may yet be identified (Norais, et al., 2009; G. Xu, et al., 2010).

Three separate genes encode the canonical eukaryotic RPA, which is the subject of several recent review articles (Binz, et al., 2004; Broderick, et al., 2010; Richard, et al., 2009; Wold, 1997). However, in higher plants each subunit of RPA may be represented by multiple genes whose proteins function in distinct processes (Sakaguchi, et al., 2009).

Both *Saccharomyces cerevisiae* and *Schizosaccharomyces pombe* contain a single gene for each of the three RPA subunits. All three are essential in *S. cerevisiae*, but RPA3 appears to be non-essential in *S. pombe* (Brill & Stillman, 1991; Cavero, et al., 2010; Dickson, et al., 2009; Maniar, et al., 1997). Given that RPA3 is the most variable, and the essential role that the intact protein plays in replication, an additional RPA3 gene may yet be identified that carries out this role in *S. pombe*. In addition to heterotrimeric RPA, a protein complex, Stn1/Ten1, resembling an RPA2/RPA3 dimer has been found to be necessary for telomere maintenance and protection in *S. cerevisiae, S. pombe* and *Candida albicans* (Sun, et al., 2009). Together with Cdc13, the Stn1/Ten1 complex may represent a highly conserved telomere binding RPA.

Mammals are thought to have only one nuclear RPA protein, which functions in both replication and repair (Fanning, et al., 2006; Iftode, et al., 1999; Wold, 1997). However, an alternative RPA2 homolog (RPA4) found only in mammals has been identified (Keshav, et al., 1995). RPA4 binds with the single RPA1 and RPA3 subunits to form an alternative RPA that does not interact with DNA polymerase α, and consequently, does not support replication (Haring, et al., 2010; Mason, et al., 2009; Mason, et al., 2010). Rather, its role is restricted to repair, particularly in quiescent cells. A mitochondrial SSB has also been identified in many eukaryotes, which has sequence and structural similarities to *E. coli* SSB (Curth, et al., 1994). In addition, two human proteins, hSSB1 and hSSB2, which structurally resemble bacterial SSB, have been reported. hSSB1 has been characterized, and appears not to be involved in replication, but is required for genome stability and DNA repair processes (Richard, Cubeddu, et al., 2011; Richard, Savage, et al., 2011).

Although much less is known about RPA genes in plants, the recent sequencing of higher plant genomes has revealed a large diversity of homologs (Sakaguchi, et al., 2009). Rice contains three genes each for RPA1 and RPA2, but only a single gene for RPA3 (Ishibashi, et al., 2006; Shultz, et al., 2007). Each RPA1 associates with a particular RPA2, and RPA3 is common among the different complexes. One complex is unique to chloroplasts, whereas the other two are nuclear. Like rice, *Arabidopsis* contains multiple homologs for the RPA1 and RPA2 subunits, but also has two RPA3 genes (Shultz, et al., 2007). In both plants, one of the large subunits has been shown to be non-essential for vegetative growth, but is required for meiosis, demonstrating specialization of function among the multiple species of protein (Chang, et al., 2009; Osman, et al., 2009). This homolog is involved in response to DNA damage as well as maintenance of telomeres (Takashi, et al., 2009). The degree of similarity among the multiple homologs suggests that they arose through duplication of ancestral genes after the establishment of the plant lineage.

By far the most diversity in RPA/SSB homologs is found in the archaea. Although many hypothetical RPA proteins have been identified in the numerous genomes analyzed, there is no quaternary structure that is common to all. In the crenarchaea, the RPA from *Sulfolobus solfataricus* is encoded by a single gene and exists as a monomer or a homotetramer (Haseltine & Kowalczykowski, 2002; Kerr, et al., 2001; Kerr, et al., 2003; Wadsworth & White, 2001). The different quaternary structures confer distinct binding capabilities (Rolfsmeier & Haseltine, 2010). Despite the similarity to bacterial SSB, and the ability of the gene to complement the lethality of an *E. coli ssb* mutation, the DNA-binding domain of this protein more closely resembles those of eukaryotic RPA1 (Haseltine & Kowalczykowski, 2002; Kerr, et al., 2003). Although the genomes of two related crenarchaea, *P. aerophilum* and *A. pernix*, have been reported to contain no obvious RPA or SSB homolog (Luo, et al., 2007), a previous study found a *Sulfolobus*-like SSB in *A. pernix* (Haseltine & Kowalczykowski, 2002). Given the recent identification of a novel SSB in *D. radiodurans*, and the fundamental role that ssDNA binding proteins play in replication and repair, it is likely that a protein carrying out these essential functions will be found in all organisms.

RPAs in euryarchaea present a multitude of OB-fold conformations that presumably provide unique functions (Lin, et al., 2005; Robbins, et al., 2005). Genomes of several euryarchaea, including *Thermoplasma acidophilum, Archaeoglobus fulgidus, Ferroplasma acidarmanus,* and *Halobacterium salinarum*, contain genes with similar organization to the crenarchaeal SSB/RPA gene, with one OB-fold; however, in each case, there is also at least one additional homolog that shows different domain structure, as seen in Figure 1 (Komori & Ishino, 2001; Pugh, et al., 2008; Robbins, et al., 2005). Other euryarchaea, such as *Methanococcus jannaschii, Methanobacter thermoautotrophicus*, and the Methanosarcinae, have proteins with four OB-folds, which may act as monomers, or in a complex with an adjacently encoded RPA2 homolog (Chedin, et al., 1998; Kelly, et al., 1998; Komori & Ishino, 2001; Lin, et al., 2008; Robbins, et al., 2004). In addition, *M. jannaschii* contains a two-OB-fold homolog which appears to function as a homotrimer (Robbins, et al., 2005). The *Pyrococcus furiosis* RPA more closely resembles eukaryotic RPA, with three distinct subunits that function as a heterotrimer and whose genes compose an operon (Komori & Ishino, 2001). In *H. salinarum*, Rfa3, Rfa8, and Ral, and Rfa2 and Rfa7 resemble the *P. furiosis* RPA with respect to operon structure and sequence homology to eukaryotic RPA (Figure 1). Rfa6 resembles the crenarchaeal SSB/RPA in gene and OB-fold structure, while Rfa1 appears more uniquely archaeal, with three OB-folds (DeVeaux, et al., 2007; Robbins, et al., 2005). The roles of the RPA-like homologs in *H. salinarum* will be discussed further below.

## 4. Characterized mutations of RPA and SSB

*E. coli* SSB mutants were first isolated in a screen for DNA replication mutants (Meyer & Laine, 1990). Although the two best-characterized of these temperature-sensitive (ts) mutations, *ssb-1* and *ssb-113*, fail to grow at 42° C due to inability of the labile SSB to participate in DNA replication, *ssb-1* mutants have essentially normal phenotypes at the permissive temperature. The mutation (H55Y) resides in the OB-fold and affects the ability of the protein to form homotetramers (Shereda, et al., 2008). In contrast, even at the permissive growth temperature, *ssb-113* mutants are severely compromised in their ability to survive numerous DNA damaging agents, and display recombination deficiencies (Chase, et al., 1984). The extremely pleiotropic phenotype conferred by the amino acid change (P176S of 177) in *ssb-113* suggests that the protein interaction capabilities of the C-terminal region are necessary for more than just replication. A protein lacking only 10 amino acids from the C-terminus is non-functional (Curth, et al., 1996). Indeed, mutation of the terminal phenylalanine is lethal, and disrupts protein-protein interactions (Genschel, et al., 2000). These phenotypes provided support not only for the commonality of protein function in recombination, repair, and replication, but also early evidence that these roles were separable within an individual protein. In contrast, a *B. subtilis* mutant in which SSB lacks the C-terminal 35 amino acids, involved in interaction with the helicase PriA, is viable, demonstrating that this conserved region is not essential in all bacteria (Lecointe, et al., 2007). In the budding yeast *S. cerevisiae*, all three subunits of RPA are essential (Brill & Stillman, 1991; Maniar, et al., 1997). Like *E. coli ssb-113* mutants, ts-mutants of RPA1 are profoundly UV- and ionizing radiation (IR)-sensitive at the permissive temperature (Parker, et al., 1997). Several ts-mutants display a mutator phenotype, which is likely related to defects in replication rather than repair (Chen, et al., 1998). Small insertions in either the RPA1 DNA-binding domain or the N-terminal protein-interaction domain result in a marked decrease in survival after UV exposure; however, only the latter is defective in the cell-cycle response to such damage. In addition, only the DNA-binding mutant is defective in repair of UV-induced lesions (Longhese, et al., 1996; Teng, et al., 1998). The N-terminal domain is required for interactions with the clamp loader. This binding is abolished in the *rfa1-t11* mutation, which contains a single change (K45E) (H. S. Kim & Brill, 2001; Majka, et al., 2006; Umezu, et al., 1998). This same allele is deficient in many pathways requiring interactions with DNA processing proteins, including repair of DNA breaks incurred during meiotic recombination, and interaction with Rad51 and its mediator Rad52 (Soustelle, et al., 2002; Sugiyama & Kantake, 2009). Deletion of either the N-terminal 20 amino acids or any deletion at the C-terminus is lethal (Philipova, et al., 1996). In the fission yeast *S. pombe*, as in *S. cerevisiae*, mutations in the large subunit gene confer sensitivity to DNA damaging agents such as UV; in addition, these mutations confer a deficiency in telomere maintenance that is seen in *S. cerevisiae* only in combination with a Ku mutation (Ono, et al., 2003).

In *S. cerevisiae*, mutations in RPA2 also confer sensitivity to various DNA-damaging agents and display defects in replication fidelity (Maniar, et al., 1997; Santocanale, et al., 1995). Ts-mutants arrest in S phase at the nonpermissive temperature. Although the protein is essential, the DNA-binding domain is not; only the central protein-interaction domain is required (Dickson, et al., 2009; Philipova, et al., 1996). Temperature-sensitive mutations in RPA3 confer a replication defect in *S. cerevisiae*. Whereas replication ceases immediately in ts-mutants of RPA2, RPA3 mutations allow one round of replication before cessation (Maniar, et al., 1997). As in RPA1, deletions of the RPA3 N-terminus are viable, but C-terminal deletions are not tolerated (Philipova, et al., 1996). Interestingly, RPA3 is not essential in *S. pombe*, and is dispensible in meiosis (Cavero, et al., 2010). However, cells containing a gene deletion show marked sensitivity to DNA damaging agents, particularly those interfering with replication, but not to IR. This suggests that RPA3 in *S. pombe* is involved in repair of replication damage, but not homologous recombination. It is possible that an additional RPA3 homolog will be discovered in *S. pombe* that carries out the essential role in replication performed by a single RPA3 in other organisms.

In human cells, depletion of RPA results not only in increased spontaneous DNA damage and decreased cell viability, but also in asynchrony, arrest at the G1/S boundary, a slowing of progression through S phase, and arrest at the G2/M checkpoint (Dodson, et al., 2004; Haring, et al., 2008). The G2/M arrest was found to be the result of constitutive activation of ATM (ataxia telangiectasia mutated) kinase resulting from lack of RPA. Cells harboring mutations in DBD A, B or C are able to replicate DNA, and traverse S phase, but arrest at the G2/M checkpoint. In contrast to yeast, the N-terminal 168 amino acids of RPA1 are not essential for replication or cell-cycle progression. RPA1 mutants defective in ssDNA binding are still able to support replication; however, some mutants with very modest defects in DNA binding are severely compromised in cell-cycle progression (Haring, et al., 2008). One mutation, L221P, in which a highly conserved leucine in DBD A is changed to proline, has been characterized in yeast (Chen & Kolodner, 1999; Chen, et al., 1998), in mice (Wang, et al., 2005), and in humans (Hass, et al., 2010), and has been shown to promote chromosomal instability. This mutation is lethal in mice; heterozygosity leads to shortened life spans and increased cancer incidence. The conservation of this residue and the drastic phenotype associated with its replacement indicates a critical role of this DNA binding domain in the fundamental role of RPA in replication. A mutation changing another conserved residue in the same domain, D227Y, causes telomere shortening in human cancer cells (Kobayashi, et al., 2010), as does the analogous change in yeast (Ono, et al., 2003). Much less is known about mutations of the two smaller subunits in mammalian systems. However, as in yeast, human RPA2 is required for replication, and the only essential region is the central protein-interacting domain (Fanning, et al., 2006; Haring, et al., 2010).

Higher plants contain multiple homologs of at least the large and medium subunits. In rice, one homolog of RPA1 is not essential during vegetative growth, but mutants are sterile, indicating a meiotic defect (Chang, et al., 2009). Also, mutants are sensitive to DNA-damaging agents, indicating a role in repair but not replication. Likewise, in *Arabidopsis thaliana*, deletion of one RPA1 homolog results in meiotic defects; although DNA breaks appear to be repaired normally, there is a deficiency in meiotic crossover (Osman, et al., 2009). During vegetative growth, plants containing this mutation are sensitive to DNA-damaging agents (Takashi, et al., 2009). The presence of multiple homologs, some of which are not essential and appear not to be involved with replication, suggests that RPAs in plants have duplicated and diverged, resulting in specialization and separation of function.

## 5. Interactive roles of RPA and SSB in DNA metabolism

While RPAs and SSBs are indispensible for normal replication, they are also central to nearly all DNA repair pathways. The overarching theme for RPA/SSB in these repair pathways is their function as directors of key enzymatic proteins without themselves being enzymatic. The following sections will pertain to the canonical RPA and SSB unless otherwise noted.

### 5.1 Interactive role of RPA and SSB in the unstressed cell cycle

RPA plays a critical role in replication of DNA and was first identified as a factor for replication of the Simian Virus 40 (SV40). Several reviews provide great detail about the role of RPA in replication; however, most current work examines its function in DNA repair (Fanning, et al., 2006; Iftode, et al., 1999; Wold, 1997). Nevertheless, it is important to understand the role of RPA in normal DNA replication as the switch between its replication role and its repair role is of great interest.

During replication, RPA functions to protect ssDNA and direct the assembly of the replication machinery. In SV40 replication, RPA interacts with T-antigen to facilitate unwinding of the replication origin, through ssDNA stabilization as well as DNA-duplex melting (Georgaki & Hubscher, 1993; Georgaki, et al., 1992; Iftode, et al., 1999; Wold, 1997). Interestingly, nearly all RPAs and SSBs are able to replace human RPA in this role, indicating that stability of the ssDNA intermediate is critical for progression of replication (Wold, 1997). In addition, RPA and SSB serve to direct the formation of the replication complex through direct protein-protein interactions (Binz, et al., 2006; Naue, et al., 2011; Shereda, et al., 2008; Witte, et al., 2003; Wold, 1997; Yuzhakov, Kelman, Hurwitz, et al., 1999).

RPA spatially and temporally directs the addition of key proteins of the replication complex at the site of replication. Temporal control is obtained through competitive binding of the replication components to RPA. Initially, the primase complex is directed to the ssDNA template. Following primer synthesis, Replication Factor C (RFC) binds RPA and loads the replicative clamp PCNA. DNA polymerase $\delta$ then binds RPA and is loaded at the DNA-primer junction, allowing DNA replication to begin (Yuzhakov, et al., 1999). These protein-protein interactions are RPA-specific; SSB cannot substitute, underscoring the important dual role of RPA in both ssDNA binding and protein interactions (Wold, 1997).

Though RPA and SSB cannot always substitute for each other, they play similar roles in the systems in which they reside. Like RPA, SSB serves not only to stabilize ssDNA but also to direct assembly of the replication complex proteins. Through interactions with the C-terminus of SSB, the primase is loaded and retained at the priming site. This interaction may be facilitated through further interactions of SSB with DnaB. This binding is disrupted by the $\chi$ subunit of the replicative DNA polymerase III through a multi-step handoff mechanism (Sharma, et al., 2009; Shereda, et al., 2008; Witte, et al., 2003; Yuzhakov, Kelman, & O'Donnell, 1999). Loss of these protein-protein interactions results in cellular demise.

Integral to the role of RPA in DNA replication is its cell-cycle dependent phosphorylation/dephosphorylation (Figure 2). Specifically, RPA2 is phosphorylated at two consensus sites for Cdc2/Cdk2, resulting in three forms of RPA: unphosphorylated, and two distinct phosphorylated forms (Iftode, et al., 1999; J. S. Liu, et al., 2006; Oakley, et al., 2003; Patrick, et al., 2005; Wold, 1997; Zernik-Kobak, et al., 1997). The majority of RPA is unphosphorylated during G1 phase, and is phosphorylated at either S23 or S29 of RPA2 at the G1/S phase boundary, which is maintained through S phase and into G2 (Anantha, et al., 2007; Oakley, et al., 2003; Stephan, et al., 2009). Near the G2/M phase boundary, a mitotic phosphorylation form becomes abundant (Oakley, et al., 2003; Zernik-Kobak, et al., 1997). This is presumably due to further phosphorylation of RPA2 at the remaining Cdc2/Cdk2 consensus site, which may regulate the ability of RPA to interact with and bind other proteins, thereby modulating its functional role through the cell-cycle (Oakley, et al., 2003; Stephan, et al., 2009). However, the effects of S phase phosphorylation of RPA have not yet been determined, as its ability to support replication and repair are unchanged (Henricksen, et al., 1996; Oakley, et al., 2003; Pan, et al., 1995). In contrast, M phase phosphorylation of RPA abrogates binding to DNA polymerase α, as well as to the checkpoint proteins ATM and DNA-PK (DNA-dependent protein kinase). In addition, its ability to bind duplex DNA is significantly reduced. These modifications may serve to switch RPA away from its replicative role after S phase (Oakley, et al., 2003; Stephan, et al., 2009). It has also been demonstrated that SSB is phosphorylated on tyrosine residues, but the consequences of this phosphorylation remain to be elucidated (Mijakovic, et al., 2006). As such, phosphorylation will be discussed only in relation to RPA for the remainder of this review. Nevertheless, it is reasonable to hypothesize that phosphorylation of SSB plays a similar regulatory role.

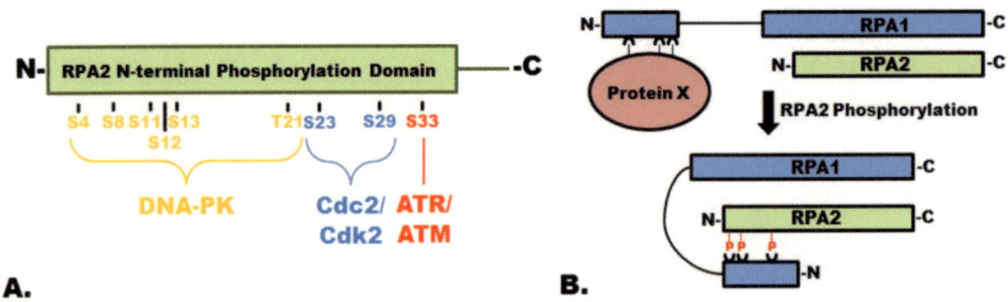


Fig. 2. (A) Phosphorylation sites on the N-terminus of RPA2. DNA-PK, Cdc2/Cdk2 and ATR/ATM phosphorylate different sites, which depends on the type of damage and point in the cell-cycle. (B) Proposed mechanism for phosphoregulation of RPA1 N-terminal heterologous protein interactions. Upon phosphorylation of RPA2, the basic N-terminus of RPA1 binds phosphorylated RPA2 and abrogates heterologous protein binding. Protein X represents any of a number of RPA1-interacting proteins.

### 5.2 Interactive role of RPA and SSB in NER, BER and MMR

Cellular DNA is under a constant barrage of damaging agents, which may cause crosslinking, base modification or base loss. In general, these types of damage may be repaired by excising the offending lesion and re-synthesizing DNA. RPA and SSB play critical roles in the coordination of these processes. Base excision repair (BER) processes remove damaged bases, forming apurinic/apyrimidinic sites, which are removed and replaced with undamaged DNA (Krokan, et al., 2000). RPA physically interacts with and regulates multiple BER glycosylases, including NEIL1 and Ung2, to facilitate correct repair of lesions, in part by inhibiting excisions on ssDNA and promoting incisions on duplex DNA (Mer, et al., 2000; Theriot, et al., 2010). Similarly, SSB interacts with the glycosylase UDG, stimulating or inhibiting its excision activity, depending on the DNA structure at the lesion (Kumar & Varshney, 1997). Nucleotide excision repair (NER) processes remove helix-distorting lesions by excising a patch of DNA, followed by re-synthesis. In this case, RPA physically interacts with the NER mediator XPA to direct incision to the damaged strand, and to help prevent excessive incision events, which could lead to further degradation of the genome (Krasikova, et al., 2010; Overmeer, et al., 2011; Saijo, et al., 2011). In mismatch repair (MMR), RPA and SSB interact with the exonuclease EXO1 to stimulate excision processes, as well as ensure correct excision termination (Genschel & Modrich, 2009; Lu & Keck, 2008).

### 5.3 Interactive role of RPA and SSB in the recovery of stalled replication forks

An advancing replication fork must traverse a myriad of DNA lesions through a normal replicative cycle, and the abundance of these lesions increases dramatically under DNA-damaging conditions. Depletion of the nucleotide pool or a single-strand lesion blocks progression of the polymerase complex, while the replicative helicase uncouples from the replisome and continues to unwind template DNA. Such uncoupling results in long segments of ssDNA to which RPA or SSB may bind and actively participate in restart of the stalled fork (Atkinson & McGlynn, 2009; Byun, et al., 2005; McInerney & O'Donnell, 2007; Pages & Fuchs, 2003). Additionally, lesions such as inter-strand crosslinks or covalently linked proteins block advancement of the entire replisome. Such stalls may be repaired and restarted through a fork regression pathway. Several competing fork regression models exist, but all of them require protein elements that closely function and interact with RPA and SSB (Atkinson & McGlynn, 2009; Dronkert & Kanaar, 2001; Machwe, et al., 2011; Shereda, et al., 2007; Shereda, et al., 2008; Sowd, et al., 2009; Sugiyama & Kantake, 2009; Suhasini, et al., 2009; Woodman, et al., 2010; Yuan, et al., 2009; Yusufzai, et al., 2009).

When the replicative helicase is uncoupled from the replisome, large tracts of ssDNA are formed. In eukaryotes this lengthy ssDNA is rapidly coated with RPA, which serves as a signal of replication stress to activate the S phase checkpoint kinase ATR (ATM and Rad3-related), a member of the phosphatidylinositol 3-kinase-like kinase (PIKK) family (Byun, et al., 2005; J. S. Liu, et al., 2006; Zou & Elledge, 2003). In bacteria, the ssDNA is similarly coated with SSB, but a strict cell-cycle control response is absent. ATR is found in a complex with its activator ATRIP (ATR interacting protein) and recruitment of ATR/ATRIP to sites of replication stress is mediated by direct interaction between the N-terminus of RPA1 (DBD F) and ATRIP. This interaction is sufficient for localization of ATR/ATRIP to the stalled replication fork, but activation of ATR requires further protein interactions, also mediated by RPA (X. Xu, et al., 2008; Zou & Elledge, 2003). The Rad17 complex, which comprises Rad17 and RFC subunits 2-5, loads the Rad9-Rad1-Hus1 (9-1-1) DNA damage checkpoint clamp at damage sites. To facilitate loading of the 9-1-1 complex, the Rad17 complex is recruited to damage sites in an RPA-dependent manner (Majka, et al., 2006; Zou, et al., 2003). Rad9 of the 9-1-1 complex binds topoisomerase 2 binding protein 1 (TopBP1), another factor for ATR activation. Simultaneously, Rad9 binds the N-terminus of RPA1 which correctly orients TopBP1 for activation of ATR. Rad9 and ATRIP compete for binding of the N-terminus of RPA1, but each must be bound for efficient activation of ATR. This suggests a model in which two adjacent RPAs are required to be bound to ssDNA at a damage site (X. Xu, et al., 2008). This model is further supported by studies describing a ssDNA length-dependent activation of ATR via RPA (J. S. Liu, et al., 2006; Zou & Elledge, 2003).

Activated ATR initiates the intra-S phase checkpoint signal cascade resulting in cell-cycle arrest, stabilization of replication forks, and initiation of damage repair through phosphorylation of effector molecules, including the checkpoint kinase Chk1 (Cimprich & Cortez, 2008; Kastan & Bartek, 2004; Yang, et al., 2003). Activation also leads ATR to phosphorylate S33, a PIKK consensus site, of the RPA2 subunit of ssDNA-bound RPA, which stimulates the Cdc2/Cdk2 kinases to phosphorylate their consensus sites on RPA2 if not already phosphorylated. This, in turn, stimulates phosphorylation of T21 by DNA-PK, which leads to further phosphorylation of RPA2 at residues S4, S8, S11, S12, and S13 by DNA-PK (Anantha, et al., 2007; Vassin, et al., 2009; Zernik-Kobak, et al., 1997). Such hyperphosphorylation of RPA is the major switch from its role in normal uninterrupted replication to an activator and director of DNA damage repair.

Hyperphosphorylation inhibits replicative functions of RPA while stimulating repair and fork stabilization, likely by modifying its protein interaction and duplex DNA binding and destabilizing capabilities. In a rather elegant regulatory mechanism, the phosphorylated RPA2 competitively binds the basic N-terminal region of RPA1, displacing proteins from one of the primary binding surfaces and modulating its interaction capability (Figure 2) (Oakley, et al., 2009). Competitive binding and conformational changes such as this may be responsible for many of the protein interactions that are altered upon phosphorylation of RPA2. Hyperphosphorylation abolishes interaction of RPA with DNA polymerase α, as well as decreases its duplex unwinding ability, which is critical for replication (Oakley, et al., 2003; Patrick, et al., 2005; Wold, 1997). Additionally, in an SV40 *in vitro* system, hyperphosphorylation of RPA leads to a 50% reduction in replication, which can be rescued by unphosphorylated RPA (Patrick, et al., 2005). Hyperphosphorylation, coupled with other aspects of the intra-S phase checkpoint, effectively halts chromosomal replication. However, other RPA-dependent processes, such as damage-dependent DNA synthesis, are unchanged or stimulated. Hyperphosphorylated RPA stimulates *in vivo* synthesis of DNA on RPA-coated ssDNA via a currently unidentified repair polymerase, minimizing ssDNA accumulation during replication stress (Vassin, et al., 2009). Additionally, essential interactions between RPA and NER proteins are unaffected by hyperphosphorylation of RPA (see above) (Oakley, et al., 2003; Patrick, et al., 2005). Many of these repair proteins are capable of interacting with the unphosphorylated C-terminus of RPA2 rather than the N-terminus of RPA1, which may explain the separation of functions between unphosphorylated and hyperphosphorylated RPA (Ali, et al., 2010; Saijo, et al., 2011). Regardless of the mechanism, this demonstrates the versatility of RPA in DNA metabolism.

The previous discussion has focused on a restart and repair pathway for replication fork stalls in which the replicative helicase uncouples from the replisome. A replisome may also encounter double-strand lesions, such as interstrand crosslinks, that prevent progression of the entire complex. These lesions, as well as some ssDNA lesions, result in stalled forks that may be repaired and restarted though fork regression. Among the most important proteins in fork regression are repair helicases including those in the RecQ, RecG, HARP, and FANC families. These helicases may perform the complex winding and unwinding of nascent and template strands necessary to form a Holliday junction-like structure referred to as a "chicken foot." Additionally, proteins of the Fanconi anemia pathway may be important for

RPA focus formation in regression of forks stalled by interstrand crosslinks (Huang, et al., 2010). For a review of fork regression models, see Atkinson and McGlynn, 2009.

Many studies support the hypothesis that RPA directs activity of helicases in fork regression. In eukaryotes, RPA interacts with the RecQ-like helicases WRN and BLM, which have been implicated in the regression of stalled replication forks *in vitro*. RecQ helicases are important for maintenance of chromosome stability; it is therefore not unexpected that they would be involved in fork regression. The interaction of RPA with these proteins may also recruit them to stalled forks; regardless, it stimulates their helicase activity (Brosh, et al., 2000; Brosh, et al., 1999; Doherty, et al., 2005; Machwe, et al., 2011; Machwe, et al., 2006; Machwe, et al., 2007; Ralf, et al., 2006). RPA also recruits the annealing helicase HARP to stalled forks through direct interaction. HARP has been implicated in stabilization and restart of stalled replication forks and may be well suited to assisting fork regression in which complementary DNA strands must be annealed to form stable structures (Ciccia, et al., 2009; Yuan, et al., 2009; Yusufzai, et al., 2009). Thus, the RecQ-like helicases may work with the HARP helicases in the regression of stalled forks. In addition to the human RecQ-like helicases, the archaeal RecQ-like helicase Hel308 is also recruited by RPA and is capable of fork regression *in vitro* (Li, et al., 2008; Woodman, et al., 2010). Additionally, the FANCM protein, which is involved in fork regression, interacts with RPA at stalled forks to promote formation of RPA foci (Banerjee, et al., 2008; Huang, et al., 2010).

In bacterial fork regression, similar interactions between SSB and helicases have been observed. SSB binds RecQ through its C-terminus *in vitro* and stimulates RecQ helicase activity (Lecointe, et al., 2007; Shereda, et al., 2007; Shereda, et al., 2008). RecG helicase not only interacts with SSB through the C-terminus but is stabilized by this interaction and supports fork regression (Buss, et al., 2008; Lecointe, et al., 2007; Shereda, et al., 2008). The replication restart helicase PriA also interacts with SSB, which would complete the fork regression process and initiate restart of replication (Cadman & McGlynn, 2004; Kozlov, et al., 2010; Lecointe, et al., 2007; Shereda, et al., 2008). In addition to helicases, SSB interacts with and actively directs the activity of several recombination proteins necessary for the repair of regressed forks before they may be restarted. These processes are essential to other aspects of DNA repair as well, including double-strand break (DSB) repair, discussed below.

### 5.4 Interactive role of RPA and SSB in DNA double-strand break repair

The types of DNA damage discussed previously may be repaired directly through NER or in response to replication fork stall. A far more grave form of DNA damage is the DSB, arising from either exogenous or endogenous stresses. A well-known exogenous physical stress that causes DSBs is IR, which is the major reason that it is so detrimental to living systems. A variety of chemical agents, such as bleomycin, phleomycin, and mitomycin C, also act by inducing DSBs. Additionally, a stalled replication fork that is unrepaired may collapse into a special type of DSB with a single double-strand end (Allen, et al., 2011). Regardless, these DSBs are all repaired via similar pathways, which rely on RPA and SSB.

Until recently, models of eukaryotic DSB repair indicated that the conserved DNA repair protein complex MRN (Mre11-Rad50-Nbs1) was the first responder and signaler at the site of a DSB. However, recent evidence implicates the novel ssDNA binding protein hSSB1 as the DSB-recognition protein in humans. At the site of damage this protein may bind short ssDNA overhangs and provide protection from incorrect end-processing by nucleases. Additionally, hSSB1 is found complexed with MRN independent of damage, through an interaction between the C-terminal tail of hSSB1 and the N-terminal region of Nbs1. This direct interaction, along with the ssDNA-bound hSSB1, stimulates the recruitment of the MRN complex to DSB sites. RPA cannot replace hSSB1 in this function (Richard, Cubeddu, et al., 2011; Richard, Savage, et al., 2011). hSSB1 may also have duplex melting capabilities similar to that seen in other SSBs, which would further help to provide a substrate for MRN binding (Cubeddu & White, 2005; Eggington, et al., 2006; Richard, Cubeddu, et al., 2011).

Once recruited to a DSB, the MRN complex tethers the broken DNA ends; its endonuclease activity is stimulated through hSSB1 association. MRN then activates the ATM kinase, which in turn initiates a phosphorylation signal cascade similar to ATR. Among the many phosphorylation targets of ATM are the cell-cycle checkpoint kinase Chk2, histone variant H2AX, and hSSB1 (Czornak, et al., 2008; Richard, et al., 2008; Richard, Cubeddu, et al., 2011; Richard, Savage, et al., 2011; Williams, et al., 2010). Phosphorylation of Chk2 results in cell-cycle arrest, while phosphorylated H2AX serves as a local binding point for repair proteins (Kastan & Bartek, 2004; J. E. Kim, et al., 2006). hSSB1 phosphorylation has unknown consequences, but it is likely to alter its repair role in a manner similar to the phospho-regulation of RPA (Richard, et al., 2008; Richard, Savage, et al., 2011). The nuclease activity of MRN results in limited end-resection at the DSB providing a substrate to which RPA may then bind (Richard, Cubeddu, et al., 2011; Richard, Savage, et al., 2011). ssDNA-bound RPA activates the ATR response and may also be phosphorylated by either activated ATM or ATR, switching it to a repair-process director (Jazayeri, et al., 2006; Oakley, et al., 2001).

In both eukaryotic and bacterial systems, DSB repair and fork regression may proceed via homologous recombination when a homologous template is present. Not surprisingly, RPA and SSB play central roles in this process as well. The RPA or SSB coating ssDNA at the site of damage is replaced with recombinase Rad51 or RecA, respectively, through direct interaction with mediators of homologous recombination. Specifically, the replacement of RPA by Rad51 is facilitated by interactions between the N-terminus of RPA1 and the homologous recombination mediator Rad52 (Plate, et al., 2008; Sugiyama & Kantake, 2009). Akin to requirements for ATR activation, multiple RPAs are necessary to promote this exchange. Similarly, bacterial SSB interacts through its C-terminal tail with the recombination mediator RecO to facilitate loading of RecA onto ssDNA by RecFOR (Costes, et al., 2010; Inoue, et al., 2011). Another interesting interaction of SSB is its apparent competition with the RecA inhibitor RecX for the common ssDNA ligand. By outcompeting RecX for access to ssDNA, SSB prevents RecX from inhibiting RecA loading onto the ssDNA (Baitin, et al., 2008). Interactions between archaeal SSB and a RadA-mediator Rad55 have also been demonstrated *in vitro*. This interaction promotes loading of RadA onto ssDNA suggesting a similar function to that seen in eukaryotes and bacteria (Sheng, et al., 2008).

## 6. Transcriptional regulation

The post-translational modifications of RPA/SSB provide virtually instantaneous response to conditions within the cell. Less well-documented, but potentially as important to survival, is transcriptional regulation of the genes in response to more global DNA damage. There is evidence of such regulation in all three domains of life. In general, where damage-induced transcriptional regulation has been reported, the organism contains multiple homologs, and the damage-regulated RPA is generally not required for replication.

In bacteria, the well-studied *E. coli ssb* gene contains multiple promoters, one of which has been shown to be damage-inducible (Brandsma, et al., 1985). Despite this, the level of *E. coli*

SSB protein does not appear to respond to DNA damage, suggesting that any regulation on this promoter is compensated by opposite regulation on the others (Meyer & Laine, 1990). One of the two homologs in *B. subtilis* functions in natural competence, whereas the gene for the replication SSB is not damage-inducible (Lindner, et al., 2004). The promoters for both the canonical SSB and the newly identified DdrB in *D. radiodurans* contain a recognizable "radiation-desiccation response motif"; both genes are up-regulated in response to IR, but *ssb* is not induced by desiccation or UV (Ujaoney, et al., 2010). The SSB protein is present in *D. radiodurans* at ten-fold higher levels than in *E. coli*, and, unlike in *E. coli*, levels increase 4-fold after irradiation (Bernstein, et al., 2004; Y. Liu, et al., 2003). In contrast, the transcript for the *ddrB* gene is normally almost absent, but is induced 40-fold within minutes after exposure to IR (Tanaka, et al., 2004). The IR-sensitivity, and viability, of *ddrB* knockouts underscores its specific role in DNA repair, and not replication.

In yeast and humans, the presence of a single RPA makes transcriptional regulation in response to damage less likely. In yeast, expression of RPA is cell-cycle dependent, with maximal expression prior to S phase (Brill & Stillman, 1991). Human RPA levels remain constant throughout the cell cycle (Wold, 1997). However, the alternative RPA2 subunit, RPA4, is more highly expressed in quiescent cells, and, since it competes with RPA2 for binding to RPA1 and RPA3, must be down-regulated in dividing cells (Haring, et al., 2010). This long-term regulation, however, is presumably not readily reversible, and is not a damage response. Interestingly, RPA1 and RPA2 levels are higher in colon cancer cells but it is not clear how this increase is achieved (Givalos, et al., 2007). Plants have multiple homologs, which are differentially expressed in tissues. There is evidence for regulation of certain homologs in response to DNA damage, as well as in response to certain hormones (Marwedel, et al., 2003; Sakaguchi, et al., 2009).

The single crenarchaeal RPA homolog would not be expected to be transcriptionally regulated to any significant extent, given its essential role in replication. In the euryarchaea, however, where multiple homologs are common, regulation has been reported. The transcriptome of *H. salinarum* during recovery from exposure to IR or UV has been analyzed and only one of the five RPA homologs showed any any increase in expression (Baliga, et al., 2004; Kottemann, et al., 2005; McCready, et al., 2005). This homolog, encoded by the *rfa3* operon, is one of two eukaryotic-like RPAs present in *H. salinarum*. Constitutive up-regulation of this operon was found as the only transcriptomic difference among multiple radiation-resistant mutants of *H. salinarum* (DeVeaux, et al., 2007). This homolog is significantly up-regulated following IR-treatment of wild type *H. salinarum*, but not in the radiation-resistant mutants, presumably because the protein is being constitutively expressed at the induced level. In addition, both wild-type and mutant strains show induced expression of the second RPA-like homolog, encoded by the *rfa2* operon. Neither of the crenarchaeal nor the euryarchaeal-like SSB/RPA homologs shows significant transcriptional differences after irradiation (Gygli and DeVeaux, unpublished observations). These results suggest that the eukaryotic RPA-like homologs present in this organism may be more directly involved in repair of radiation damage.

## 7. Conclusion

The highly conserved and essential nature of the RPA/SSB family underscores the fundamental role that these proteins play in basic DNA metabolic processes. The interactions that these proteins are involved in illustrate an intricate network and temporal sequence of events that are only beginning to be understood. The multiplicity of homologs present in some lineages suggests that ancestral duplications have resulted in specialization of function. These organisms provide models for study of individual activities, such as DNA repair, which are not essential for viability.

## 8. Acknowledgment

We thank all of the researchers whose hard work provided us with material for this review. We thank Dr. Dring Crowell and the members of the DeVeaux lab for support and helpful comments. The following agencies provided support for P.E.G. and J.S.L.: The Henry M. Jackson Foundation, NASA ISGC, and The United States Department of Defense.

## 9. References

Ali, S. I., Shin, J. S., Bae, S. H., et al. (2010). Replication Protein A 32 interacts through a similar binding interface with TIPIN, XPA, and UNG2. *Int J Biochem Cell Biol*, Vol. 42, No. 7 (pp. 1210-1215), 1878-5875 (Electronic) 1357-2725 (Linking)

Allen, C., Ashley, A. K., Hromas, R., et al. (2011). More forks on the road to replication stress recovery. *J Mol Cell Biol*, Vol. 3, No. 1 (pp. 4-12), 1759-4685 (Electronic)

Anantha, R. W., Vassin, V. M., & Borowiec, J. A. (2007). Sequential and synergistic modification of human RPA stimulates chromosomal DNA repair. *J Biol Chem*, Vol. 282, No. 49 (pp. 35910-35923), 0021-9258 (Print) 0021-9258 (Linking)

Atkinson, J., & McGlynn, P. (2009). Replication fork reversal and the maintenance of genome stability. *Nucleic Acids Res*, Vol. 37, No. 11 (pp. 3475-3492), 1362-4962 (Electronic) 0305-1048 (Linking)

Baitin, D. M., Gruenig, M. C., & Cox, M. M. (2008). SSB antagonizes RecX-RecA interaction. *J Biol Chem*, Vol. 283, No. 21 (pp. 14198-14204), 0021-9258 (Print) 0021-9258 (Linking)

Baliga, N. S., Bjork, S. J., Bonneau, R., et al. (2004). Systems level insights into the stress response to UV radiation in the halophilic archaeon *Halobacterium* NRC-1. *Genome Res*, Vol. 14, No. 6 (pp. 1025-1035), 1088-9051 (Print) 1088-9051 (Linking)

Banerjee, S., Smith, S., Oum, J. H., et al. (2008). Mph1p promotes gross chromosomal rearrangement through partial inhibition of homologous recombination. *J Cell Biol*, Vol. 181, No. 7 (pp. 1083-1093), 1540-8140 (Electronic) 0021-9525 (Linking)

Bernstein, D. A., Eggington, J. M., Killoran, M. P., et al. (2004). Crystal structure of the *Deinococcus radiodurans* single-stranded DNA-binding protein suggests a mechanism for coping with DNA damage. *Proc Natl Acad Sci U S A*, Vol. 101, No. 23 (pp. 8575-8580), 0027-8424 (Print) 0027-8424 (Linking)

Binz, S. K., Dickson, A. M., Haring, S. J., et al. (2006). Functional assays for Replication Protein A (RPA). *Methods Enzymol*, Vol. 409, (pp. 11-38), 0076-6879 (Print) 0076-6879 (Linking)

Binz, S. K., Sheehan, A. M., & Wold, M. S. (2004). Replication Protein A phosphorylation and the cellular response to DNA damage. *DNA Repair (Amst)*, Vol. 3, No. 8-9 (pp. 1015-1024), 1568-7864 (Print) 1568-7856 (Linking)

Blackwell, L. J., & Borowiec, J. A. (1994). Human Replication Protein A binds single-stranded DNA in two distinct complexes. *Mol Cell Biol*, Vol. 14, No. 6 (pp. 3993-4001), 0270-7306 (Print) 0270-7306 (Linking)

Brandsma, J. A., Bosch, D., de Ruyter, M., et al. (1985). Analysis of the regulatory region of the *ssb* gene of *Escherichia coli*. *Nucleic Acids Res*, Vol. 13, No. 14 (pp. 5095-5109), 0305-1048 (Print) 0305-1048 (Linking)

Brill, S. J., & Stillman, B. (1991). Replication factor-A from *Saccharomyces cerevisiae* is encoded by three essential genes coordinately expressed at S phase. *Genes Dev*, Vol. 5, No. 9 (pp. 1589-1600), 0890-9369 (Print) 0890-9369 (Linking)

Broderick, S., Rehmet, K., Concannon, C., et al. (2010). Eukaryotic single-stranded DNA binding proteins: central factors in genome stability. *Subcell Biochem*, Vol. 50, (pp. 143-163), 0306-0225 (Print) 0306-0225 (Linking)

Brosh, R. M., Jr., Li, J. L., Kenny, M. K., et al. (2000). Replication Protein A physically interacts with the Bloom's syndrome protein and stimulates its helicase activity. *J Biol Chem*, Vol. 275, No. 31 (pp. 23500-23508), 0021-9258 (Print) 0021-9258 (Linking)

Brosh, R. M., Jr., Orren, D. K., Nehlin, J. O., et al. (1999). Functional and physical interaction between WRN helicase and human Replication Protein A. *J Biol Chem*, Vol. 274, No. 26 (pp. 18341-18350), 0021-9258 (Print) 0021-9258 (Linking)

Buss, J. A., Kimura, Y., & Bianco, P. R. (2008). RecG interacts directly with SSB: implications for stalled replication fork regression. *Nucleic Acids Res*, Vol. 36, No. 22 (pp. 7029-7042), 1362-4962 (Electronic) 0305-1048 (Linking)

Byun, T. S., Pacek, M., Yee, M. C., et al. (2005). Functional uncoupling of MCM helicase and DNA polymerase activities activates the ATR-dependent checkpoint. *Genes Dev*, Vol. 19, No. 9 (pp. 1040-1052), 0890-9369 (Print) 0890-9369 (Linking)

Cadman, C. J., & McGlynn, P. (2004). PriA helicase and SSB interact physically and functionally. *Nucleic Acids Res*, Vol. 32, No. 21 (pp. 6378-6387), 1362-4962 (Electronic) 0305-1048 (Linking)

Cavero, S., Limbo, O., & Russell, P. (2010). Critical functions of Rpa3/Ssb3 in S-phase DNA damage responses in fission yeast. *PLoS Genet*, Vol. 6, No. 9, 1553-7404 (Electronic) 1553-7390 (Linking)

Chang, Y., Gong, L., Yuan, W., et al. (2009). Replication Protein A (RPA1a) is required for meiotic and somatic DNA repair but is dispensable for DNA replication and homologous recombination in rice. *Plant Physiol*, Vol. 151, No. 4 (pp. 2162-2173), 1532-2548 (Electronic) 0032-0889 (Linking)

Chase, J. W., L'Italien, J. J., Murphy, J. B., et al. (1984). Characterization of the *Escherichia coli* SSB-113 mutant single-stranded DNA-binding protein. Cloning of the gene, DNA and protein sequence analysis, high pressure liquid chromatography peptide mapping, and DNA-binding studies. *J Biol Chem*, Vol. 259, No. 2 (pp. 805-814), 0021-9258 (Print) 0021-9258 (Linking)

Chedin, F., Seitz, E. M., & Kowalczykowski, S. C. (1998). Novel homologs of Replication Protein A in archaea: implications for the evolution of ssDNA-binding proteins. *Trends Biochem Sci*, Vol. 23, No. 8 (pp. 273-277), 0968-0004 (Print) 0968-0004 (Linking)

Chen, C., & Kolodner, R. D. (1999). Gross chromosomal rearrangements in *Saccharomyces cerevisiae* replication and recombination defective mutants. *Nat Genet*, Vol. 23, No. 1 (pp. 81-85), 1061-4036 (Print) 1061-4036 (Linking)

Chen, C., Umezu, K., & Kolodner, R. D. (1998). Chromosomal rearrangements occur in *S. cerevisiae rfa1* mutator mutants due to mutagenic lesions processed by double-strand-break repair. *Mol Cell*, Vol. 2, No. 1 (pp. 9-22), 1097-2765 (Print) 1097-2765 (Linking)

Ciccia, A., Bredemeyer, A. L., Sowa, M. E., et al. (2009). The SIOD disorder protein SMARCAL1 is an RPA-interacting protein involved in replication fork restart. *Genes Dev*, Vol. 23, No. 20 (pp. 2415-2425), 1549-5477 (Electronic) 0890-9369 (Linking)

Cimprich, K. A., & Cortez, D. (2008). ATR: an essential regulator of genome integrity. *Nat Rev Mol Cell Biol*, Vol. 9, No. 8 (pp. 616-627), 1471-0080 (Electronic) 1471-0072 (Linking)

Costes, A., Lecointe, F., McGovern, S., et al. (2010). The C-terminal domain of the bacterial SSB protein acts as a DNA maintenance hub at active chromosome replication forks. *PLoS Genet*, Vol. 6, No. 12 (pp. e1001238), 1553-7404 (Electronic) 1553-7390 (Linking)

Cubeddu, L., & White, M. F. (2005). DNA damage detection by an archaeal single-stranded DNA-binding protein. *J Mol Biol*, Vol. 353, No. 3 (pp. 507-516), 0022-2836 (Print) 0022-2836 (Linking)

Curth, U., Genschel, J., Urbanke, C., et al. (1996). *In vitro* and *in vivo* function of the C-terminus of *Escherichia coli* single-stranded DNA binding protein. *Nucleic Acids Res*, Vol. 24, No. 14 (pp. 2706-2711), 0305-1048 (Print) 0305-1048 (Linking)

Curth, U., Urbanke, C., Greipel, J., et al. (1994). Single-stranded-DNA-binding proteins from human mitochondria and *Escherichia coli* have analogous physicochemical properties. *Eur J Biochem*, Vol. 221, No. 1 (pp. 435-443), 0014-2956 (Print) 0014-2956 (Linking)

Czornak, K., Chughtai, S., & Chrzanowska, K. H. (2008). Mystery of DNA repair: the role of the MRN complex and ATM kinase in DNA damage repair. *J Appl Genet*, Vol. 49, No. 4 (pp. 383-396), 1234-1983 (Print) 1234-1283 (Linking)

DeVeaux, L. C., Muller, J. A., Smith, J., et al. (2007). Extremely Radiation-Resistant Mutants of a Halophilic Archaeon with Increased Single-Stranded DNA-Binding Protein (RPA) Gene Expression. *Radiat Res*, Vol. 168, No. 4 (pp. 507-514), 0033-7587 (Print) 0033-7587 (Linking)

Dickson, A. M., Krasikova, Y., Pestryakov, P., et al. (2009). Essential functions of the 32 kDa subunit of yeast Replication Protein A. *Nucleic Acids Res*, Vol. 37, No. 7 (pp. 2313-2326), 1362-4962 (Electronic) 0305-1048 (Linking)

Dodson, G. E., Shi, Y., & Tibbetts, R. S. (2004). DNA replication defects, spontaneous DNA damage, and ATM-dependent checkpoint activation in Replication Protein A-deficient cells. *J Biol Chem*, Vol. 279, No. 32 (pp. 34010-34014), 0021-9258 (Print) 0021-9258 (Linking)

Doherty, K. M., Sommers, J. A., Gray, M. D., et al. (2005). Physical and functional mapping of the Replication Protein A interaction domain of the Werner and Bloom syndrome helicases. *J Biol Chem*, Vol. 280, No. 33 (pp. 29494-29505), 0021-9258 (Print) 0021-9258 (Linking)

Dronkert, M. L., & Kanaar, R. (2001). Repair of DNA interstrand cross-links. *Mutat Res*, Vol. 486, No. 4 (pp. 217-247), 0027-5107 (Print) 0027-5107 (Linking)

Eggington, J. M., Haruta, N., Wood, E. A., et al. (2004). The single-stranded DNA-binding protein of *Deinococcus radiodurans*. *BMC Microbiol*, Vol. 4, (pp. 2), 1471-2180 (Electronic) 1471-2180 (Linking)

Eggington, J. M., Kozlov, A. G., Cox, M. M., et al. (2006). Polar destabilization of DNA duplexes with single-stranded overhangs by the *Deinococcus radiodurans* SSB protein. *Biochemistry*, Vol. 45, No. 48 (pp. 14490-14502), 0006-2960 (Print) 0006-2960 (Linking)

Fanning, E., Klimovich, V., & Nager, A. R. (2006). A dynamic model for Replication Protein A (RPA) function in DNA processing pathways. *Nucleic Acids Res*, Vol. 34, No. 15 (pp. 4126-4137), 1362-4962 (Electronic) 0305-1048 (Linking)

Filipkowski, P., Duraj-Thatte, A., & Kur, J. (2006). Novel thermostable single-stranded DNA-binding protein (SSB) from *Deinococcus geothermalis*. *Arch Microbiol*, Vol. 186, No. 2 (pp. 129-137), 0302-8933 (Print) 0302-8933 (Linking)

Filipkowski, P., & Kur, J. (2007). Identification and properties of the *Deinococcus grandis* and *Deinococcus proteolyticus* single-stranded DNA binding proteins (SSB). *Acta Biochim Pol*, Vol. 54, No. 1 (pp. 79-87), 0001-527X (Print) 0001-527X (Linking)

Genschel, J., Curth, U., & Urbanke, C. (2000). Interaction of *E. coli* single-stranded DNA binding protein (SSB) with exonuclease I. The carboxy-terminus of SSB is the recognition site for the nuclease. *Biol Chem*, Vol. 381, No. 3 (pp. 183-192), 1431-6730 (Print) 1431-6730 (Linking)

Genschel, J., & Modrich, P. (2009). Functions of MutLα, Replication Protein A (RPA), and HMGB1 in 5'-directed mismatch repair. *J Biol Chem*, Vol. 284, No. 32 (pp. 21536-21544), 0021-9258 (Print) 0021-9258 (Linking)

Georgaki, A., & Hubscher, U. (1993). DNA unwinding by Replication Protein A is a property of the 70 kDa subunit and is facilitated by phosphorylation of the 32 kDa subunit. *Nucleic Acids Res*, Vol. 21, No. 16 (pp. 3659-3665), 0305-1048 (Print) 0305-1048 (Linking)

Georgaki, A., Strack, B., Podust, V., et al. (1992). DNA unwinding activity of Replication Protein A. *FEBS Lett*, Vol. 308, No. 3 (pp. 240-244), 0014-5793 (Print) 0014-5793 (Linking)

Givalos, N., Gakiopoulou, H., Skliri, M., et al. (2007). Replication Protein A is an independent prognostic indicator with potential therapeutic implications in colon cancer. *Mod Pathol*, Vol. 20, No. 2 (pp. 159-166), 0893-3952 (Print) 0893-3952 (Linking)

Haring, S. J., Humphreys, T. D., & Wold, M. S. (2010). A naturally occurring human RPA subunit homolog does not support DNA replication or cell-cycle progression. *Nucleic Acids Res*, Vol. 38, No. 3 (pp. 846-858), 1362-4962 (Electronic) 0305-1048 (Linking)

Haring, S. J., Mason, A. C., Binz, S. K., et al. (2008). Cellular functions of human RPA1. Multiple roles of domains in replication, repair, and checkpoints. *J Biol Chem*, Vol. 283, No. 27 (pp. 19095-19111), 0021-9258 (Print) 0021-9258 (Linking)

Haseltine, C. A., & Kowalczykowski, S. C. (2002). A distinctive single-strand DNA-binding protein from the Archaeon *Sulfolobus solfataricus*. *Mol Microbiol*, Vol. 43, No. 6 (pp. 1505-1515), 0950-382X (Print) 0950-382X (Linking)

Hass, C. S., Gakhar, L., & Wold, M. S. (2010). Functional characterization of a cancer causing mutation in human Replication Protein A. *Mol Cancer Res*, Vol. 8, No. 7 (pp. 1017-1026), 1557-3125 (Electronic) 1541-7786 (Linking)

Henricksen, L. A., Carter, T., Dutta, A., et al. (1996). Phosphorylation of human Replication Protein A by the DNA-dependent protein kinase is involved in the modulation of

DNA replication. *Nucleic Acids Res*, Vol. 24, No. 15 (pp. 3107-3112), 0305-1048 (Print) 0305-1048 (Linking)

Huang, M., Kim, J. M., Shiotani, B., et al. (2010). The FANCM/FAAP24 complex is required for the DNA interstrand crosslink-induced checkpoint response. *Mol Cell*, Vol. 39, No. 2 (pp. 259-268), 1097-4164 (Electronic) 1097-2765 (Linking)

Iftode, C., Daniely, Y., & Borowiec, J. A. (1999). Replication Protein A (RPA): the eukaryotic SSB. *Crit Rev Biochem Mol Biol*, Vol. 34, No. 3 (pp. 141-180), 1040-9238 (Print) 1040-9238 (Linking)

Inoue, J., Nagae, T., Mishima, M., et al. (2011). A Mechanism for Single-stranded DNA-binding Protein (SSB) Displacement from Single-stranded DNA upon SSB-RecO Interaction. *J Biol Chem*, Vol. 286, No. 8 (pp. 6720-6732), 1083-351X (Electronic) 0021-9258 (Linking)

Ishibashi, T., Kimura, S., & Sakaguchi, K. (2006). A higher plant has three different types of RPA heterotrimeric complex. *J Biochem*, Vol. 139, No. 1 (pp. 99-104), 0021-924X (Print) 0021-924X (Linking)

Jazayeri, A., Falck, J., Lukas, C., et al. (2006). ATM- and cell cycle-dependent regulation of ATR in response to DNA double-strand breaks. *Nat Cell Biol*, Vol. 8, No. 1 (pp. 37-45), 1465-7392 (Print) 1465-7392 (Linking)

Kastan, M. B., & Bartek, J. (2004). Cell-cycle checkpoints and cancer. *Nature*, Vol. 432, No. 7015 (pp. 316-323), 1476-4687 (Electronic) 0028-0836 (Linking)

Kelly, T. J., Simancek, P., & Brush, G. S. (1998). Identification and characterization of a single-stranded DNA-binding protein from the archaeon *Methanococcus jannaschii*. *Proc Natl Acad Sci U S A*, Vol. 95, No. 25 (pp. 14634-14639), 0027-8424 (Print) 0027-8424 (Linking)

Kerr, I. D., Wadsworth, R. I., Blankenfeldt, W., et al. (2001). Overexpression, purification, crystallization and data collection of a single-stranded DNA-binding protein from *Sulfolobus solfataricus*. *Acta Crystallogr D Biol Crystallogr*, Vol. 57, No. Pt 9 (pp. 1290-1292), 0907-4449 (Print) 0907-4449 (Linking)

Kerr, I. D., Wadsworth, R. I., Cubeddu, L., et al. (2003). Insights into ssDNA recognition by the OB fold from a structural and thermodynamic study of *Sulfolobus* SSB protein. *EMBO J*, Vol. 22, No. 11 (pp. 2561-2570), 0261-4189 (Print) 0261-4189 (Linking)

Keshav, K. F., Chen, C., & Dutta, A. (1995). Rpa4, a homolog of the 34-kilodalton subunit of the Replication Protein A complex. *Mol Cell Biol*, Vol. 15, No. 6 (pp. 3119-3128), 0270-7306 (Print) 0270-7306 (Linking)

Kim, C., Snyder, R. O., & Wold, M. S. (1992). Binding properties of Replication Protein A from human and yeast cells. *Mol Cell Biol*, Vol. 12, No. 7 (pp. 3050-3059), 0270-7306 (Print) 0270-7306 (Linking)

Kim, H. S., & Brill, S. J. (2001). Rfc4 interacts with Rpa1 and is required for both DNA replication and DNA damage checkpoints in *Saccharomyces cerevisiae*. *Mol Cell Biol*, Vol. 21, No. 11 (pp. 3725-3737), 0270-7306 (Print) 0270-7306 (Linking)

Kim, J. E., Minter-Dykhouse, K., & Chen, J. (2006). Signaling networks controlled by the MRN complex and MDC1 during early DNA damage responses. *Mol Carcinog*, Vol. 45, No. 6 (pp. 403-408), 0899-1987 (Print) 0899-1987 (Linking)

Kobayashi, Y., Sato, K., Kibe, T., et al. (2010). Expression of mutant RPA in human cancer cells causes telomere shortening. *Biosci Biotechnol Biochem*, Vol. 74, No. 2 (pp. 382-385), 1347-6947 (Electronic) 0916-8451 (Linking)

Komori, K., & Ishino, Y. (2001). Replication Protein A in *Pyrococcus furiosus* is involved in homologous DNA recombination. *J Biol Chem,* Vol. 276, No. 28 (pp. 25654-25660), 0021-9258 (Print) 0021-9258 (Linking)

Kottemann, M., Kish, A., Iloanusi, C., et al. (2005). Physiological responses of the halophilic archaeon *Halobacterium* sp. strain NRC1 to desiccation and gamma irradiation. *Extremophiles,* Vol. 9, No. 3 (pp. 219-227), 1431-0651 (Print) 1431-0651 (Linking)

Kozlov, A. G., Jezewska, M. J., Bujalowski, W., et al. (2010). Binding specificity of *Escherichia coli* single-stranded DNA binding protein for the chi subunit of DNA pol III holoenzyme and PriA helicase. *Biochemistry,* Vol. 49, No. 17 (pp. 3555-3566), 1520-4995 (Electronic) 0006-2960 (Linking)

Krasikova, Y. S., Rechkunova, N. I., Maltseva, E. A., et al. (2010). Localization of xeroderma pigmentosum group A protein and Replication Protein A on damaged DNA in nucleotide excision repair. *Nucleic Acids Res,* Vol. 38, No. 22 (pp. 8083-8094), 1362-4962 (Electronic) 0305-1048 (Linking)

Krokan, H. E., Nilsen, H., Skorpen, F., et al. (2000). Base excision repair of DNA in mammalian cells. *FEBS Lett,* Vol. 476, No. 1-2 (pp. 73-77), 0014-5793 (Print) 0014-5793 (Linking)

Kumar, N. V., & Varshney, U. (1997). Contrasting effects of single stranded DNA binding protein on the activity of uracil DNA glycosylase from *Escherichia coli* towards different DNA substrates. *Nucleic Acids Res,* Vol. 25, No. 12 (pp. 2336-2343), 0305-1048 (Print) 0305-1048 (Linking)

Lecointe, F., Serena, C., Velten, M., et al. (2007). Anticipating chromosomal replication fork arrest: SSB targets repair DNA helicases to active forks. *EMBO J,* Vol. 26, No. 19 (pp. 4239-4251), 0261-4189 (Print) 0261-4189 (Linking)

Li, Z., Lu, S., Hou, G., et al. (2008). Hjm/Hel308A DNA helicase from *Sulfolobus tokodaii* promotes replication fork regression and interacts with Hjc endonuclease *in vitro. J Bacteriol,* Vol. 190, No. 8 (pp. 3006-3017), 1098-5530 (Electronic) 0021-9193 (Linking)

Lin, Y., Lin, L. J., Sriratana, P., et al. (2008). Engineering of functional Replication Protein A homologs based on insights into the evolution of oligonucleotide/oligosaccharide-binding folds. *J Bacteriol,* Vol. 190, No. 17 (pp. 5766-5780), 1098-5530 (Electronic) 0021-9193 (Linking)

Lin, Y., Robbins, J. B., Nyannor, E. K., et al. (2005). A CCCH zinc finger conserved in a Replication Protein A homolog found in diverse Euryarchaeotes. *J Bacteriol,* Vol. 187, No. 23 (pp. 7881-7889), 0021-9193 (Print) 0021-9193 (Linking)

Lindner, C., Nijland, R., van Hartskamp, M., et al. (2004). Differential expression of two paralogous genes of *Bacillus subtilis* encoding single-stranded DNA binding protein. *J Bacteriol,* Vol. 186, No. 4 (pp. 1097-1105), 0021-9193 (Print) 0021-9193 (Linking)

Liu, J. S., Kuo, S. R., & Melendy, T. (2006). Phosphorylation of Replication Protein A by S-phase checkpoint kinases. *DNA Repair (Amst),* Vol. 5, No. 3 (pp. 369-380), 1568-7864 (Print) 1568-7856 (Linking)

Liu, Y., Zhou, J., Omelchenko, M. V., et al. (2003). Transcriptome dynamics of *Deinococcus radiodurans* recovering from ionizing radiation. *Proc Natl Acad Sci U S A,* Vol. 100, No. 7 (pp. 4191-4196), 0027-8424 (Print) 0027-8424 (Linking)

Lohman, T. M., & Ferrari, M. E. (1994). *Escherichia coli* single-stranded DNA-binding protein: multiple DNA-binding modes and cooperativities. *Annu Rev Biochem*, Vol. 63, (pp. 527-570), 0066-4154 (Print) 0066-4154 (Linking)

Longhese, M. P., Neecke, H., Paciotti, V., et al. (1996). The 70 kDa subunit of Replication Protein A is required for the G1/S and intra-S DNA damage checkpoints in budding yeast. *Nucleic Acids Res*, Vol. 24, No. 18 (pp. 3533-3537), 0305-1048 (Print) 0305-1048 (Linking)

Lu, D., & Keck, J. L. (2008). Structural basis of *Escherichia coli* single-stranded DNA-binding protein stimulation of exonuclease I. *Proc Natl Acad Sci U S A*, Vol. 105, No. 27 (pp. 9169-9174), 1091-6490 (Electronic) 0027-8424 (Linking)

Luo, X., Schwarz-Linek, U., Botting, C. H., et al. (2007). CC1, a novel crenarchaeal DNA binding protein. *J Bacteriol*, Vol. 189, No. 2 (pp. 403-409), 0021-9193 (Print) 0021-9193 (Linking)

Machwe, A., Lozada, E., Wold, M. S., et al. (2011). Molecular cooperation between the Werner syndrome protein and Replication Protein A in relation to replication fork blockage. *J Biol Chem*, Vol. 286, No. 5 (pp. 3497-3508), 1083-351X (Electronic) 021-9258 (Linking)

Machwe, A., Xiao, L., Groden, J., et al. (2006). The Werner and Bloom syndrome proteins catalyze regression of a model replication fork. *Biochemistry*, Vol. 45, No. 47 (pp. 13939-13946), 0006-2960 (Print) 0006-2960 (Linking)

Machwe, A., Xiao, L., Lloyd, R. G., et al. (2007). Replication fork regression *in vitro* by the Werner syndrome protein (WRN): holliday junction formation, the effect of leading arm structure and a potential role for WRN exonuclease activity. *Nucleic Acids Res*, Vol. 35, No. 17 (pp. 5729-5747), 1362-4962 (Electronic) 0305-1048 (Linking)

Majka, J., Binz, S. K., Wold, M. S., et al. (2006). Replication Protein A directs loading of the DNA damage checkpoint clamp to 5'-DNA junctions. *J Biol Chem*, Vol. 281, No. 38 (pp. 27855-27861), 0021-9258 (Print) 0021-9258 (Linking)

Maniar, H. S., Wilson, R., & Brill, S. J. (1997). Roles of Replication Protein-A subunits 2 and 3 in DNA replication fork movement in *Saccharomyces cerevisiae*. *Genetics*, Vol. 145, No. 4 (pp. 891-902), 0016-6731 (Print) 0016-6731 (Linking)

Marwedel, T., Ishibashi, T., Lorbiecke, R., et al. (2003). Plant-specific regulation of Replication Protein A2 (OsRPA2) from rice during the cell cycle and in response to ultraviolet light exposure. *Planta*, Vol. 217, No. 3 (pp. 457-465), 0032-0935 (Print) 0032-0935 (Linking)

Mason, A. C., Haring, S. J., Pryor, J. M., et al. (2009). An alternative form of Replication Protein A prevents viral replication *in vitro*. *J Biol Chem*, Vol. 284, No. 8 (pp. 5324-5331), 0021-9258 (Print) 0021-9258 (Linking)

Mason, A. C., Roy, R., Simmons, D. T., et al. (2010). Functions of alternative Replication Protein A in initiation and elongation. *Biochemistry*, Vol. 49, No. 28 (pp. 5919-5928), 1520-4995 (Electronic) 0006-2960 (Linking)

McCready, S., Muller, J. A., Boubriak, I., et al. (2005). UV irradiation induces homologous recombination genes in the model archaeon, *Halobacterium* sp. NRC-1. *Saline Systems*, Vol. 1, (pp. 3)

McInerney, P., & O'Donnell, M. (2007). Replisome fate upon encountering a leading strand block and clearance from DNA by recombination proteins. *J Biol Chem*, Vol. 282, No. 35 (pp. 25903-25916), 0021-9258 (Print) 0021-9258 (Linking)

Mer, G., Bochkarev, A., Gupta, R., et al. (2000). Structural basis for the recognition of DNA repair proteins UNG2, XPA, and RAD52 by replication factor RPA. *Cell*, Vol. 103, No. 3 (pp. 449-456), 0092-8674 (Print) 0092-8674 (Linking)

Meyer, R. R., & Laine, P. S. (1990). The single-stranded DNA-binding protein of *Escherichia coli*. *Microbiol Rev*, Vol. 54, No. 4 (pp. 342-380), 0146-0749 (Print) 0146-0749 (Linking)

Mijakovic, I., Petranovic, D., Macek, B., et al. (2006). Bacterial single-stranded DNA-binding proteins are phosphorylated on tyrosine. *Nucleic Acids Res*, Vol. 34, No. 5 (pp. 1588-1596), 1362-4962 (Electronic) 0305-1048 (Linking)

Naue, N., Fedorov, R., Pich, A., et al. (2011). Site-directed mutagenesis of the $\chi$ subunit of DNA polymerase III and single-stranded DNA-binding protein of *E. coli* reveals key residues for their interaction. *Nucleic Acids Res*, Vol. 39, No. 4 (pp. 1398-1407), 1362-4962 (Electronic) 0305-1048 (Linking)

Norais, C. A., Chitteni-Pattu, S., Wood, E. A., et al. (2009). DdrB protein, an alternative *Deinococcus radiodurans* SSB induced by ionizing radiation. *J Biol Chem*, Vol. 284, No. 32 (pp. 21402-21411), 0021-9258 (Print) 0021-9258 (Linking)

Nuss, J. E., Patrick, S. M., Oakley, G. G., et al. (2005). DNA damage induced hyperphosphorylation of Replication Protein A. 1. Identification of novel sites of phosphorylation in response to DNA damage. *Biochemistry*, Vol. 44, No. 23 (pp. 8428-8437), 0006-2960 (Print) 0006-2960 (Linking)

Oakley, G. G., Loberg, L. I., Yao, J., et al. (2001). UV-induced hyperphosphorylation of Replication Protein A depends on DNA replication and expression of ATM protein. *Mol Biol Cell*, Vol. 12, No. 5 (pp. 1199-1213), 1059-1524 (Print) 1059-1524 (Linking)

Oakley, G. G., Patrick, S. M., Yao, J., et al. (2003). RPA phosphorylation in mitosis alters DNA binding and protein-protein interactions. *Biochemistry*, Vol. 42, No. 11 (pp. 3255-3264), 0006-2960 (Print) 0006-2960 (Linking)

Oakley, G. G., Tillison, K., Opiyo, S. A., et al. (2009). Physical interaction between Replication Protein A (RPA) and MRN: involvement of RPA2 phosphorylation and the N-terminus of RPA1. *Biochemistry*, Vol. 48, No. 31 (pp. 7473-7481), 1520-4995 (Electronic) 0006-2960 (Linking)

Olszewski, M., Grot, A., Wojciechowski, M., et al. (2010). Characterization of exceptionally thermostable single-stranded DNA-binding proteins from *Thermotoga maritima* and *Thermotoga neapolitana*. *BMC Microbiol*, Vol. 10, (pp. 260), 1471-2180 (Electronic) 1471-2180 (Linking)

Olszewski, M., Mickiewicz, M., & Kur, J. (2008). Two highly thermostable paralogous single-stranded DNA-binding proteins from *Thermoanaerobacter tengcongensis*. *Arch Microbiol*, Vol. 190, No. 1 (pp. 79-87), 0302-8933 (Print) 0302-8933 (Linking)

Ono, Y., Tomita, K., Matsuura, A., et al. (2003). A novel allele of fission yeast *rad11* that causes defects in DNA repair and telomere length regulation. *Nucleic Acids Res*, Vol. 31, No. 24 (pp. 7141-7149), 1362-4962 (Electronic) 0305-1048 (Linking)

Osman, K., Sanchez-Moran, E., Mann, S. C., et al. (2009). Replication protein A (AtRPA1a) is required for class I crossover formation but is dispensable for meiotic DNA break repair. *EMBO J*, Vol. 28, No. 4 (pp. 394-404), 1460-2075 (Electronic) 0261-4189 (Linking)

Overmeer, R. M., Moser, J., Volker, M., et al. (2011). Replication Protein A safeguards genome integrity by controlling NER incision events. *J Cell Biol*, Vol. 192, No. 3 (pp. 401-415), 1540-8140 (Electronic) 0021-9525 (Linking)

Pages, V., & Fuchs, R. P. (2003). Uncoupling of leading- and lagging-strand DNA replication during lesion bypass *in vivo*. *Science*, Vol. 300, No. 5623 (pp. 1300-1303), 1095-9203 (Electronic) 0036-8075 (Linking)

Pan, Z. Q., Park, C. H., Amin, A. A., et al. (1995). Phosphorylated and unphosphorylated forms of human single-stranded DNA-binding protein are equally active in simian virus 40 DNA replication and in nucleotide excision repair. *Proc Natl Acad Sci U S A*, Vol. 92, No. 10 (pp. 4636-4640), 0027-8424 (Print) 0027-8424 (Linking)

Parker, A. E., Clyne, R. K., Carr, A. M., et al. (1997). The *Schizosaccharomyces pombe rad11+* gene encodes the large subunit of Replication Protein A. *Mol Cell Biol*, Vol. 17, No. 5 (pp. 2381-514), 0270-7306 (Print) 0270-7306 (Linking)

Patrick, S. M., Oakley, G. G., Dixon, K., et al. (2005). DNA damage induced hyperphosphorylation of Replication Protein A. 2. Characterization of DNA binding activity, protein interactions, and activity in DNA replication and repair. *Biochemistry*, Vol. 44, No. 23 (pp. 8438-8448), 0006-2960 (Print) 0006-2960 (Linking)

Philipova, D., Mullen, J. R., Maniar, H. S., et al. (1996). A hierarchy of SSB protomers in Replication Protein A. *Genes Dev*, Vol. 10, No. 17 (pp. 2222-2233), 0890-9369 (Print) 0890-9369 (Linking)

Plate, I., Hallwyl, S. C., Shi, I., et al. (2008). Interaction with RPA is necessary for Rad52 repair center formation and for its mediator activity. *J Biol Chem*, Vol. 283, No. 43 (pp. 29077-29085), 0021-9258 (Print) 0021-9258 (Linking)

Pretto, D. I., Tsutakawa, S., Brosey, C. A., et al. (2010). Structural dynamics and single-stranded DNA binding activity of the three N-terminal domains of the large subunit of Replication Protein A from small angle X-ray scattering. *Biochemistry*, Vol. 49, No. 13 (pp. 2880-2889), 1520-4995 (Electronic) 0006-2960 (Linking)

Pugh, R. A., Lin, Y., Eller, C., et al. (2008). *Ferroplasma acidarmanus* RPA2 facilitates efficient unwinding of forked DNA substrates by monomers of FacXPD helicase. *J Mol Biol*, Vol. 383, No. 5 (pp. 982-998), 1089-8638 (Electronic) 0022-2836 (Linking)

Ralf, C., Hickson, I. D., & Wu, L. (2006). The Bloom's syndrome helicase can promote the regression of a model replication fork. *J Biol Chem*, Vol. 281, No. 32 (pp. 22839-22846), 0021-9258 (Print) 0021-9258 (Linking)

Richard, D. J., Bolderson, E., Cubeddu, L., et al. (2008). Single-stranded DNA-binding protein hSSB1 is critical for genomic stability. *Nature*, Vol. 453, No. 7195 (pp. 677-681), 1476-4687 (Electronic) 0028-0836 (Linking)

Richard, D. J., Bolderson, E., & Khanna, K. K. (2009). Multiple human single-stranded DNA binding proteins function in genome maintenance: structural, biochemical and functional analysis. *Crit Rev Biochem Mol Biol*, Vol. 44, No. 2-3 (pp. 98-116), 1549-7798 (Electronic) 1040-9238 (Linking)

Richard, D. J., Cubeddu, L., Urquhart, A. J., et al. (2011). hSSB1 interacts directly with the MRN complex stimulating its recruitment to DNA double-strand breaks and its endo-nuclease activity. *Nucleic Acids Res*, 1362-4962 (Electronic) 0305-1048 (Linking)

Richard, D. J., Savage, K., Bolderson, E., et al. (2011). hSSB1 rapidly binds at the sites of DNA double-strand breaks and is required for the efficient recruitment of the MRN complex. *Nucleic Acids Res*, Vol. 39, No. 5 (pp. 1692-1702), 1362-4962 (Electronic) 0305-1048 (Linking)

Robbins, J. B., McKinney, M. C., Guzman, C. E., et al. (2005). The euryarchaeota, nature's medium for engineering of single-stranded DNA-binding proteins. *J Biol Chem*, Vol. 280, No. 15 (pp. 15325-15339), 0021-9258 (Print) 0021-9258 (Linking)

Robbins, J. B., Murphy, M. C., White, B. A., et al. (2004). Functional analysis of multiple single-stranded DNA-binding proteins from *Methanosarcina acetivorans* and their effects on DNA synthesis by DNA polymerase BI. *J Biol Chem*, Vol. 279, No. 8 (pp. 6315-6326), 0021-9258 (Print) 0021-9258 (Linking)

Rolfsmeier, M. L., & Haseltine, C. A. (2010). The single-stranded DNA binding protein of *Sulfolobus solfataricus* acts in the presynaptic step of homologous recombination. *J Mol Biol*, Vol. 397, No. 1 (pp. 31-45), 1089-8638 (Electronic) 0022-2836 (Linking)

Saijo, M., Takedachi, A., & Tanaka, K. (2011). Nucleotide Excision Repair by Mutant Xeroderma Pigmentosum Group A (XPA) Proteins with Deficiency in Interaction with RPA. *J Biol Chem*, Vol. 286, No. 7 (pp. 5476-5483), 1083-351X (Electronic) 0021-9258 (Linking)

Sakaguchi, K., Ishibashi, T., Uchiyama, Y., et al. (2009). The multi-Replication Protein A (RPA) system--a new perspective. *FEBS J*, Vol. 276, No. 4 (pp. 943-963), 1742-4658 (Electronic) 1742-464X (Linking)

Santocanale, C., Neecke, H., Longhese, M. P., et al. (1995). Mutations in the gene encoding the 34 kDa subunit of yeast Replication Protein A cause defective S phase progression. *J Mol Biol*, Vol. 254, No. 4 (pp. 595-607), 0022-2836 (Print) 0022-2836 (Linking)

Sharma, A., Nitharwal, R. G., Singh, B., et al. (2009). *Helicobacter pylori* single-stranded DNA binding protein--functional characterization and modulation of *H. pylori* DnaB helicase activity. *FEBS J*, Vol. 276, No. 2 (pp. 519-531), 1742-4658 (Electronic) 1742-464X (Linking)

Sheng, D., Zhu, S., Wei, T., et al. (2008). The *in vitro* activity of a Rad55 homologue from *Sulfolobus tokodaii*, a candidate mediator in RadA-catalyzed homologous recombination. *Extremophiles*, Vol. 12, No. 1 (pp. 147-157), 1431-0651 (Print) 1431-0651 (Linking)

Shereda, R. D., Bernstein, D. A., & Keck, J. L. (2007). A central role for SSB in *Escherichia coli* RecQ DNA helicase function. *J Biol Chem*, Vol. 282, No. 26 (pp. 19247-19258), 0021-9258 (Print) 0021-9258 (Linking)

Shereda, R. D., Kozlov, A. G., Lohman, T. M., et al. (2008). SSB as an organizer/mobilizer of genome maintenance complexes. *Crit Rev Biochem Mol Biol*, Vol. 43, No. 5 (pp. 289-318), 1549-7798 (Electronic) 1040-9238 (Linking)

Shultz, R. W., Tatineni, V. M., Hanley-Bowdoin, L., et al. (2007). Genome-wide analysis of the core DNA replication machinery in the higher plants *Arabidopsis* and rice. *Plant Physiol*, Vol. 144, No. 4 (pp. 1697-1714), 0032-0889 (Print) 0032-0889 (Linking)

Soustelle, C., Vedel, M., Kolodner, R., et al. (2002). Replication Protein A is required for meiotic recombination in *Saccharomyces cerevisiae*. *Genetics*, Vol. 161, No. 2 (pp. 535-547), 0016-6731 (Print) 0016-6731 (Linking)

Sowd, G., Wang, H., Pretto, D., et al. (2009). Replication Protein A stimulates the Werner syndrome protein branch migration activity. *J Biol Chem*, Vol. 284, No. 50 (pp. 34682-34691), 1083-351X (Electronic) 0021-9258 (Linking)

Stephan, H., Concannon, C., Kremmer, E., et al. (2009). Ionizing radiation-dependent and independent phosphorylation of the 32-kDa subunit of Replication Protein A during mitosis. *Nucleic Acids Res*, Vol. 37, No. 18 (pp. 6028-6041), 1362-4962 (Electronic) 0305-1048 (Linking)

Sugiman-Marangos, S., & Junop, M. S. (2010). The structure of DdrB from *Deinococcus*: a new fold for single-stranded DNA binding proteins. *Nucleic Acids Res*, Vol. 38, No. 10 (pp. 3432-3440), 1362-4962 (Electronic) 0305-1048 (Linking)

Sugiyama, T., & Kantake, N. (2009). Dynamic regulatory interactions of rad51, rad52, and Replication Protein-A in recombination intermediates. *J Mol Biol*, Vol. 390, No. 1 (pp. 45-55), 1089-8638 (Electronic) 0022-2836 (Linking)

Suhasini, A. N., Sommers, J. A., Mason, A. C., et al. (2009). FANCJ helicase uniquely senses oxidative base damage in either strand of duplex DNA and is stimulated by Replication Protein A to unwind the damaged DNA substrate in a strand-specific manner. *J Biol Chem*, Vol. 284, No. 27 (pp. 18458-18470), 1083-351X (Electronic) 0021-9258 (Linking)

Sun, J., Yu, E. Y., Yang, Y., et al. (2009). Stn1-Ten1 is an Rpa2-Rpa3-like complex at telomeres. *Genes Dev*, Vol. 23, No. 24 (pp. 2900-2914), 1549-5477 (Electronic) 0890-9369 (Linking)

Takashi, Y., Kobayashi, Y., Tanaka, K., et al. (2009). *Arabidopsis* Replication Protein A 70a is required for DNA damage response and telomere length homeostasis. *Plant Cell Physiol*, Vol. 50, No. 11 (pp. 1965-1976), 1471-9053 (Electronic) 0032-0781 (Linking)

Tanaka, M., Earl, A. M., Howell, H. A., et al. (2004). Analysis of *Deinococcus radiodurans*'s transcriptional response to ionizing radiation and desiccation reveals novel proteins that contribute to extreme radioresistance. *Genetics*, Vol. 168, No. 1 (pp. 21-3), 0016-6731 (Print) 0016-6731 (Linking)

Teng, Y., Longhese, M., McDonough, G., et al. (1998). Mutants with changes in different domains of yeast Replication Protein A exhibit differences in repairing the control region, the transcribed strand and the non-transcribed strand of the *Saccharomyces cerevisiae* MFA2 gene. *J Mol Biol*, Vol. 280, No. 3 (pp. 355-363), 0022-2836 (Print) 0022-2836 (Linking)

Theobald, D. L., Mitton-Fry, R. M., & Wuttke, D. S. (2003). Nucleic acid recognition by OB-fold proteins. *Annu Rev Biophys Biomol Struct*, Vol. 32, (pp. 115-133), 1056-8700 (Print) 1056-8700 (Linking)

Theriot, C. A., Hegde, M. L., Hazra, T. K., et al. (2010). RPA physically interacts with the human DNA glycosylase NEIL1 to regulate excision of oxidative DNA base damage in primer-template structures. *DNA Repair (Amst)*, Vol. 9, No. 6 (pp. 643-652), 1568-7856 (Electronic) 1568-7856 (Linking)

Ujaoney, A. K., Potnis, A. A., Kane, P., et al. (2010). Radiation desiccation response motif-like sequences are involved in transcriptional activation of the Deinococcal *ssb* gene by ionizing radiation but not by desiccation. *J Bacteriol*, Vol. 192, No. 21 (pp. 5637-5644), 1098-5530 (Electronic) 0021-9193 (Linking)

Umezu, K., Sugawara, N., Chen, C., et al. (1998). Genetic analysis of yeast RPA1 reveals its multiple functions in DNA metabolism. *Genetics*, Vol. 148, No. 3 (pp. 989-1005), 0016-6731 (Print) 0016-6731 (Linking)

Vassin, V. M., Anantha, R. W., Sokolova, E., et al. (2009). Human RPA phosphorylation by ATR stimulates DNA synthesis and prevents ssDNA accumulation during DNA-replication stress. *J Cell Sci*, Vol. 122, No. Pt 22 (pp. 4070-4080), 1477-9137 (Electronic) 0021-9533 (Linking)

Wadsworth, R. I., & White, M. F. (2001). Identification and properties of the crenarchaeal single-stranded DNA binding protein from *Sulfolobus solfataricus*. *Nucleic Acids Res*, Vol. 29, No. 4 (pp. 914-920), 1362-4962 (Electronic) 0305-1048 (Linking)

Wang, Y., Putnam, C. D., Kane, M. F., et al. (2005). Mutation in Rpa1 results in defective DNA double-strand break repair, chromosomal instability and cancer in mice. *Nat Genet*, Vol. 37, No. 7 (pp. 750-755), 1061-4036 (Print) 1061-4036 (Linking)

Williams, G. J., Lees-Miller, S. P., & Tainer, J. A. (2010). Mre11-Rad50-Nbs1 conformations and the control of sensing, signaling, and effector responses at DNA double-strand breaks. *DNA Repair (Amst)*, Vol. 9, No. 12 (pp. 1299-1306), 1568-7856 (Electronic) 1568-7856 (Linking)

Witte, G., Urbanke, C., & Curth, U. (2003). DNA polymerase III chi subunit ties single-stranded DNA binding protein to the bacterial replication machinery. *Nucleic Acids Res*, Vol. 31, No. 15 (pp. 4434-4440), 1362-4962 (Electronic) 0305-1048 (Linking)

Wold, M. S. (1997). Replication Protein A: a heterotrimeric, single-stranded DNA-binding protein required for eukaryotic DNA metabolism. *Annu Rev Biochem*, Vol. 66, (pp. 61-92), 0066-4154 (Print) 0066-4154 (Linking)

Woodman, I. L., Brammer, K., & Bolt, E. L. (2010). Physical interaction between archaeal DNA repair helicase Hel308 and Replication Protein A (RPA). *DNA Repair (Amst)*, 1568-7856 (Electronic) 1568-7856 (Linking)

Xu, G., Lu, H., Wang, L., et al. (2010). DdrB stimulates single-stranded DNA annealing and facilitates RecA-independent DNA repair in *Deinococcus radiodurans*. *DNA Repair (Amst)*, Vol. 9, No. 7 (pp. 805-812), 1568-7856 (Electronic) 1568-7856 (Linking)

Xu, X., Vaithiyalingam, S., Glick, G. G., et al. (2008). The basic cleft of RPA70N binds multiple checkpoint proteins, including RAD9, to regulate ATR signaling. *Mol Cell Biol*, Vol. 28, No. 24 (pp. 7345-7353), 1098-5549 (Electronic) 0270-7306 (Linking)

Yang, J., Yu, Y., Hamrick, H. E., et al. (2003). ATM, ATR and DNA-PK: initiators of the cellular genotoxic stress responses. *Carcinogenesis*, Vol. 24, No. 10 (pp. 1571-1580), 0143-3334 (Print) 0143-3334 (Linking)

Yuan, J., Ghosal, G., & Chen, J. (2009). The annealing helicase HARP protects stalled replication forks. *Genes Dev*, Vol. 23, No. 20 (pp. 2394-2399), 1549-5477 (Electronic) 0890-9369 (Linking)

Yusufzai, T., Kong, X., Yokomori, K., et al. (2009). The annealing helicase HARP is recruited to DNA repair sites via an interaction with RPA. *Genes Dev*, Vol. 23, No. 20 (pp. 2400-2404), 1549-5477 (Electronic) 0890-9369 (Linking)

Yuzhakov, A., Kelman, Z., Hurwitz, J., et al. (1999). Multiple competition reactions for RPA order the assembly of the DNA polymerase delta holoenzyme. *EMBO J*, Vol. 18, No. 21 (pp. 6189-6199), 0261-4189 (Print) 0261-4189 (Linking)

Yuzhakov, A., Kelman, Z., & O'Donnell, M. (1999). Trading places on DNA--a three-point switch underlies primer handoff from primase to the replicative DNA polymerase. *Cell*, Vol. 96, No. 1 (pp. 153-163), 0092-8674 (Print) 0092-8674 (Linking)

Zernik-Kobak, M., Vasunia, K., Connelly, M., et al. (1997). Sites of UV-induced phosphorylation of the p34 subunit of Replication Protein A from HeLa cells. *J Biol Chem*, Vol. 272, No. 38 (pp. 23896-23904), 0021-9258 (Print) 0021-9258 (Linking)

Zou, L., & Elledge, S. J. (2003). Sensing DNA damage through ATRIP recognition of RPA-ssDNA complexes. *Science*, Vol. 300, No. 5625 (pp. 1542-1548), 1095-9203 (Electronic) 0036-8075 (Linking)

Zou, L., Liu, D., & Elledge, S. J. (2003). Replication Protein A-mediated recruitment and activation of Rad17 complexes. *Proc Natl Acad Sci U S A*, Vol. 100, No. 24 (pp. 13827-13832), 0027-8424 (Print) 0027-8424 (Linking)

# 10

# Recognition and Repair Pathways of Damaged DNA in Higher Plants

Sascha Biedermann[1,2], Sutton Mooney[1] and Hanjo Hellmann[1]
*[1]Washington State University Pullman*
*[2]Angewandte Genetik, Berlin*
*[1]United States of America*
*[2]Germany*

## 1. Introduction

Living organisms are continuously exposed to factors that threaten the integrity of their cells. This includes structural and enzymatic components like lipids or proteins, but also their genomes. Damage to genetic material can be critical as unrecognized and unrepaired DNA damage may cause fatal mutations not only threatening the organism's immediate survival but also that of its descendants. These genotoxic factors can derive from their surrounding environment and may include chemicals or ionizing radiation; but DNA damage can also be caused by reactive oxygen species (ROS) that are byproducts of daily metabolism or result from insufficient protection against abiotic stress conditions.

UV light can cause direct DNA damage by generating 6-4 and CPD photoproducts (example given in Fig. 1 is a thymine dimer). UV like most abiotic stress conditions can also generate ROS production in the cell. ROS have a high potential to damage single bases by oxidation (example give is 8-oxoG (Fig. 1)), but are also capable of introducing single or double strand breaks.

In contrast to most animals, plants are sessile organisms that cannot change their location when exposed to unfavorable conditions such as drought or salinity. Plants also face the difficult situation that they depend on sunlight for photosynthesis, a process that on its own constitutively generates ROS (Asada, 1999; Krieger-Liszkay, 2005; Triantaphylides and Havaux, 2009). Sunlight also contains significant amounts of UV-B light, which can contribute to both ROS production in the nucleus as well as directly affecting the DNA structure. Sunlight and high production rates of ROS are two of the main factors that lead to many mutations in plants. Consequently, the current review will focus on mechanisms that plants have in place to recognize and repair damaged DNA caused by either of these factors. We will provide a brief overview on the different classifications of DNA damage that can be expected, how these damages are repaired, and what is known about regulatory and physiological mechanisms that are in place in plants to recognize and respond to DNA damage. Because plants have taken a different evolutionary path than animals and possess some unique features not found in animals, we will compare selected repair and regulatory pathways in animals and plants. Despite their differences, plants and animals share many aspects in damaged DNA recognition and repair, and for this reason we will conclude this chapter by elaborating on some opinions for using plants as powerful and valuable model organisms for animals to understand the underlying processes of DNA repair.

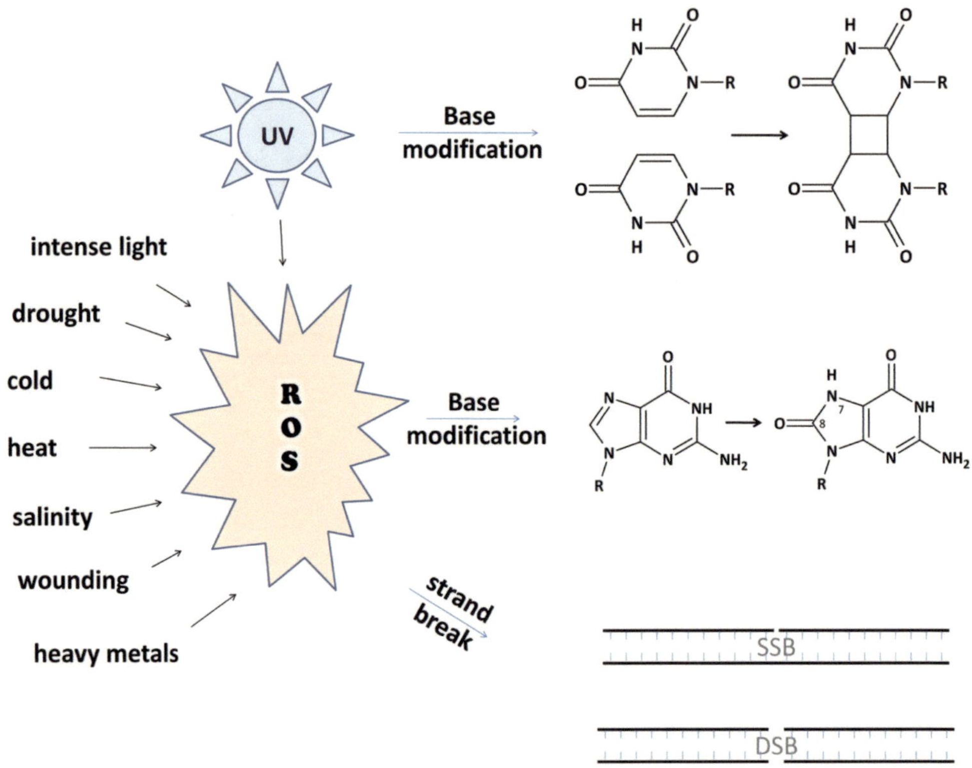


Fig. 1. UV light and ROS as genotoxic stress factors.

## 2. DNA damage caused by exposure to sunlight and abiotic stress

Ironically, although sunlight is obligatory for photosynthesis and survival of plants, it also represents one of the major threats to their genomic integrity. This can be ascribed to at least three reasons:

First, sunlight contains energy rich UV-C (280 to 100 nm), UV-B (290 to 320 nm) and UV-A (320–400 nm) light. Whereas UV-C is filtered out in the atmosphere, UV-B and UV-A can reach earth's surface. Although the amount strongly depends on the latitude and elevation, as well as cloud cover and canopy density, due to their sessile nature plants are exposed throughout the day to this genotoxic stress. UV-light is a strong mutagen that is absorbed by the DNA and may lead to the generation of cyclobutane pyrimidine dimers (CPD) and to a lesser extent pyrimidine (6,4) pyrimidone dimers (Friedberg EC et al., 2006). Both photoproducts are DNA lesions that affect transcriptional processes and result in error-prone replication (Fig. 1) (Friedberg EC et al., 2006). Solar UV light can also indirectly cause DNA damage by ROS production in the nucleus (Iovine et al., 2009). ROS induce a broad range of DNA damage, which includes base and nucleotide modifications, especially in sequences with a high guanosine content, and may even cause strand breaks (Wiseman and Halliwell, 1996; Tuteja et al., 2001; Tuteja and Tuteja, 2001). Although the precise nature of ROS generated by UV-light is not fully resolved, it is well established that oxygenated nucleotides like 8-oxo-guanine that can be caused by the accumulation of hydroxyl radicals (•OH) after prolonged UV exposure in the cell (Yamamoto et al., 1992; Hattori et al., 1996).

Second, ROS are commonly produced as metabolic byproducts in the chloroplasts, peroxisomes, and mitochondria (Foyer and Noctor, 2003). In fact it is estimated for mammals that per day ~180 guanines are oxidized to 8-hydroxyguanine in a single cell (Lindahl, 1993); and it is likely that this rate is even higher in photosynthetically active plants where chloroplasts continuously produce ROS. Furthermore, excessive light exposure as it may occur in mid-day under non-shaded conditions can overexcite the photosynthetic machinery. As a consequence, singlet oxygen ($^1O_2$) can be produced from triplet-state chlorophyll in the light- harvesting complex of photosystem II (PSII). In addition, byproducts of photosynthetic activities are superoxide ($O_2^-$) and hydrogen peroxide ($H_2O_2$) that can derive from water-splitting activities of the oxygen-evolving complex of PSII, and superoxide can be generated on the reducing side of PSI by the Mehler reaction (Noctor et al., 2002) (Fig. 1).

Third, heat from the sunlight can lead to failure of the structural composition and enzymatic machinery within the cell. To prevent cellular collapse, plants have developed a variety of protective mechanisms, the most important being the cooling effect of water transpiration through stomata. However, this dependency on water availability, together with their immobility, make plants highly susceptible to water stress conditions that derive from drought, salinity, or cold. Abiotic stress unbalances metabolic processes including photosynthesis, which ultimately causes a general increase in ROS concentration in the cell (Vinocur and Altman, 2005; Jaspers and Kangasjarvi, 2010). Although ROS detoxifying defense mechanisms are in place in the organelles and the cytosol, under the stress conditions described above, these mechanisms may not provide sufficient protection. To avoid excessive mutations over prolonged exposure to abiotic stress, plant cells depend on efficient repair pathways.

## 3. Major repair mechanisms in plants

### 3.1 Photoreactivation by photolyases

In plants the main repair pathway for direct DNA damage caused by UV-light that leads to the generation of CPDs and (6–4) photoproducts is based on the activity of photolyases (Jiang et al., 1997). Two types of photolyases have evolved that specifically recognize and repair either type of photodamage. Based on sequence homology, CPD photolyases are grouped into two different classes: while class I CPD photolyases are present in microorganisms, class II enzymes can be found in archaea, eubacteria, some animals (excluding placental mammals), and plants (Kanai et al., 1997). In comparison, (6-4) photolyases have been found in metazoans and plants, and they share sequence similarities with class I CPD photolyases (Kanai et al., 1997).

The structure and reaction mechanisms of photolyases have been intensively studied in the last decade, providing us with plentiful data on their function. Photolyases have two types of chromophoric co-factors that are used for photoreactivation (Huang et al., 2006; Ozturk et al., 2008; Hitomi et al., 2009). One chromophore is $FADH^-$, the two electron reduced form of FAD, while the second one can be either methenyltetrahydrofolate (MTHF) or 7,8-didemethyl-8-hydroxy-5-deazariboflavin (8-HDF). MTHF or 8-HDF function as the light harvesting chromophores that absorb blue light (300-600 nm), and transfer the energy to $FADH^-$ (Moldt et al., 2009; Li et al., 2010; Okafuji et al., 2010). Photolyases bind directly to CPD and (6-4) photoproducts, where an electron is transferred from the excited $FADH^-$ to the dimers generating pyrimidine monomers, upon which the enzyme is released (Li et al., 2010; Okafuji et al., 2010) (Fig. 2).

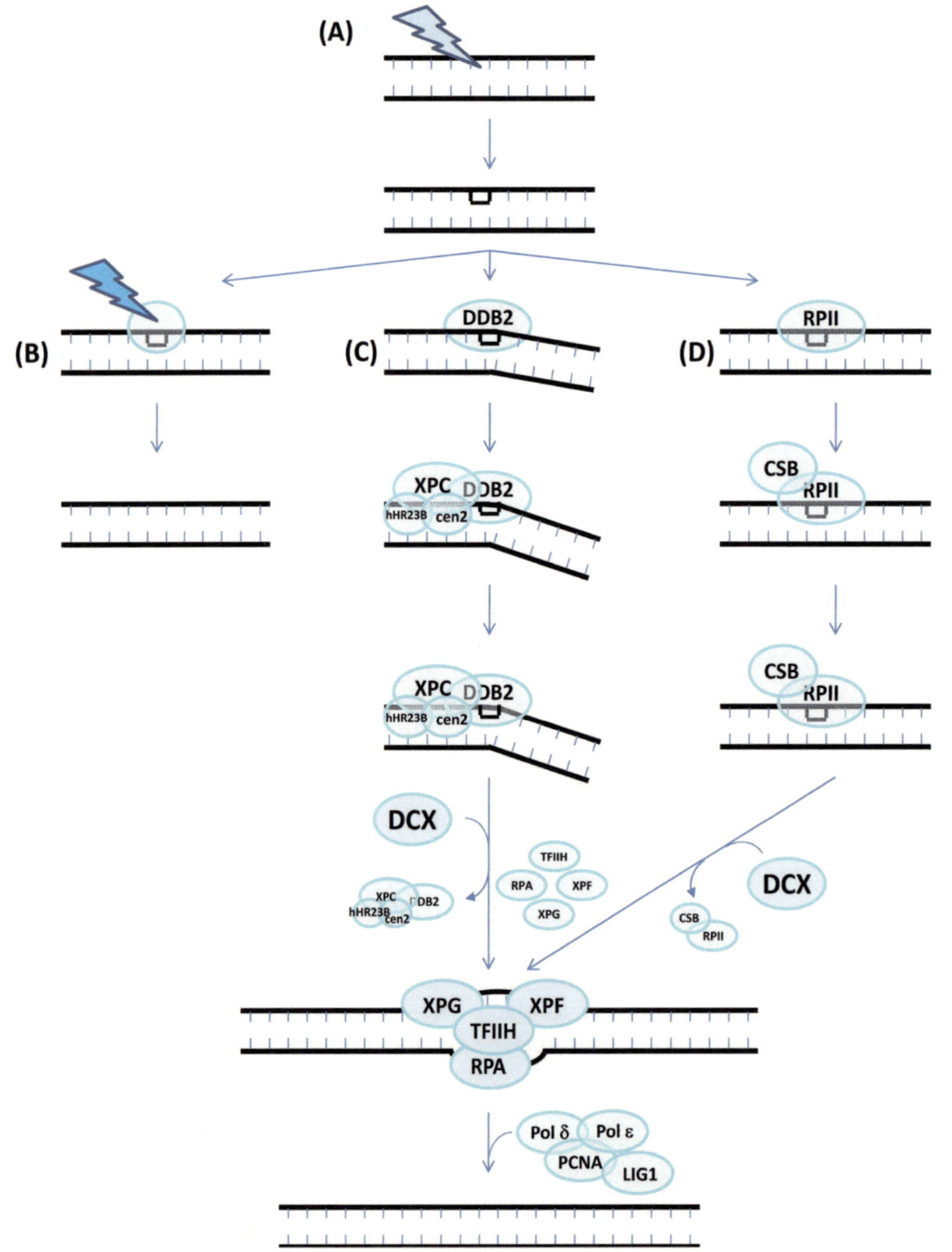


Fig. 2. Photodamage and potential repair pathways in plants.
**(A)** Direct DNA damage caused by UV can be recognized and repaired by **(B)** photolyases in a light-dependent reaction. Alternatively, repair can follow **(C)** the global genome nucleotide excision repair (GGR) or **(D)** the transcription coupled NER (TCR).

Photolyases have been widely described in plants and may often comprise small gene families like, for example, in *Arabidopsis*, which encodes for five members (http://www.arabidopsis.org/). While loss of single members can lead to increased UV-sensitivity (Jiang et al., 1997; Landry et al., 1997; Nakajima et al., 1998; Teranishi et al., 2004), the constitutive expression of CPD photolyases has been demonstrated to markedly improve UV tolerance in higher plants (Hidema et al., 2007; Kaiser et al., 2009). Although not much is known about their regulatory aspects, it has been demonstrated in rice that phosphorylation may play a role in regulating photolyase activities (Teranishi et al., 2008) and a few reports show that light increases photolyase expression (Chen et al., 1994; Waterworth et al., 2002). It was recently indicated that in darkness basal transcription of the photolyase genes *UVR3* and *PHR1* is sustained by the light signaling transcription factors HY5 and HYH and is limited by the actions of COP1 and DET1 dependent E3 ligases (Castells et al., 2010). Upon light exposure and during photomorphogenesis, COP1 leaves the nucleus and expression of *PHR1* is greatly induced by HY5 and HYH while the repression through DET1 remains in place. These observations suggest that photoreactivation is controlled by the photomorphogenisis pathway, and the activation of the PHR1 is dependent on photomorphogenetic regulators.

### 3.2 Nucleotide excision repair

A mechanism that can substitute for photolyase activities in plants, and which is required for photodamage repair in mammals, is the nucleotide excision repair (NER) pathway. NER is light-independent and, hence, sometimes referred to as dark repair. In contrast to photoreactivation, which reduces CPDs and 6-4 photoproducts back to pyrimidine monomers, NER is based on a complex recognition and repair machinery that excises and *de novo* synthesizes single DNA strands between 24-32 bp around the lesions. NER is highly conserved among eukaryotes and has two sub-pathways: transcription coupled NER (TCR) and global genome NER (GGR). NER has been intensively studied in animals, but the findings are a model for what is being found in plants, and will be briefly summarized in the following paragraph.

GGR and TCR recruit the same repair proteins; however, they mainly differ in their initial steps of damaged DNA recognition. GGR is genome-wide active, and its initial steps include the xeroderma pigmentosum group C factor (XPC), which is able to sense thermodynamic destabilizations of the Watson-Crick duplex caused by a flipping-out of the affected bases from the strands (Min and Pavletich, 2007). XPC in itself is capable of detecting most bulky DNA lesions, but for the recognition of CPDs it is supported by WD-40 protein Damaged DNA Binding 2 (DDB2) (Aboussekhra et al., 1995; Mu et al., 1995; Mu et al., 1996; Moser et al., 2005; Min and Pavletich, 2007; Scrima et al., 2008). DDB2 binds with high affinity to photoproducts, induces a bending of the DNA to approximately 40° and facilitates the flipping of the affected bases that are recognized and bound by the XPC/hHR23B complex, which further introduces structural changes into the DNA (Min and Pavletich, 2007; Scrima et al., 2008). DDB2 is part of a DDB1-CUL4-RBX1 (DCX) E3 ligase that mediates the polyubiquitination of histones, XPC and DDB2 itself (Rapic-Otrin et al., 2002; Fitch et al., 2003; Sugasawa et al., 2005; Chen et al., 2006; Kapetanaki et al., 2006; Wang et al., 2006). As a consequence, DDB2 is degraded via the 26S proteasome clearing the way for later repair stages (Rapic-Otrin et al., 2002; Fitch et al., 2003; Chen et al., 2006). Interestingly ubiquitination has the opposite effect on XPC leading to its stabilization and activation (Sugasawa et al., 2005). The DDB2-dependent ubiquitination of histones H2A, H3, and H4 may be necessary for the loosening of the DNA structure to allow the binding of other repair proteins (Kapetanaki et al., 2006; Wang et al., 2006). In a similar way the recently observed ability of DDB2 to recruit histone modifying proteins to specific DNA sequences could contribute to accessibility of the DNA for XPC and other factors (Minig et al., 2009; Roy et al., 2010). XPC is then needed for the recruitment of the core NER repair factors XPA, TFIIH, and RPA (Evans et al., 1997; Araujo et al., 2001; Thoma and Vasquez, 2003). XPA and the basal transcription factor complex TFIIH bind to the damaged site and unwind the DNA around the lesion (Reardon and Sancar, 2003; Maltseva et al., 2006; Yang et al., 2006; Kesseler et al., 2007; Krasikova et al., 2008). Unwinding is specifically performed by two subunits of TFIIH, the helicases XPB (ERCC3) and XPD (ERCC2). RPA is a heterotrimeric DNA binding protein, and while it prevents incision of the non-damaged DNA strand, together with XPA, it stabilizes the opened double helix (Blackwell et al., 1996; Camenisch et al., 2006; Maltseva et al., 2006; Yang et al., 2006). Incisions are performed by the endonucleases XPF (ERCC1) and XPG which nick the damaged DNA strand 5′ and 3′ around the lesion. After the damaged strand is excised, the gap is filled and ligated by the concerted activities of replication factors Proliferating Cell Nuclear Antigen (PCNA), Replication Factor C (RFC), Replication Protein A (RPA), DNA polymerases δ and ε, and DNA ligase 1 (LIG1) (Nichols and Sancar, 1992; Shivji et al., 1992; Green and Almouzni, 2003; Ogi et al., 2010). In contrast to GGR, TCR is specifically connected to DNA lesions in transcriptionally active regions. Here, RNA polymerase 2 (RP2) becomes stalled at CPD or (6-4) photoproduct containing sites (Selby and Sancar, 1997; Tornaletti and Hanawalt, 1999). Recognition of stalled RP2 has not been fully resolved. However, a critical role has been shown for Cockayne Syndrome factor B (CSB), a member of the SWI/SNF family of helicases (Selby and Sancar, 1997; van Gool et al., 1997; Citterio et al., 2000; Kamiuchi et al., 2002; Fousteri et al., 2006; Cazzalini et al., 2008). CSB binds to the stalled RP2, and this binding is a necessary trigger for recruitment of the same core repair proteins as described for GGR. Comparable to DDB2, CSB becomes a target of the DCX E3 ligase, which is mediated by another WD-40 protein, CSA. This interaction ultimately results in degradation of CSA, CSB and possibly also RP2 (Groisman et al., 2006).

Most of the proteins that play a role in GGR or TCR can be found in animals and plants, while only a few members, like XPA and TF2H3, a subunit of TFIIH, appear to be absent in plants (Kimura and Sakaguchi, 2006). It is currently open whether plants encode for functional analogs of XPA and TF23H that would perform tasks similar to these proteins. For most of the other NER proteins that are conserved among animals and plants, a role in DNA repair has been demonstrated, frequently by reverse genetic studies in *Arabidopsis thaliana*. Here, proteins shown to be involved in damaged DNA recognition in animals, such as DCX-E3 ligases, DDB2 and CSA, have also been recently described by several groups in plants (Bernhardt et al., 2006; Molinier et al., 2008; Al Khateeb and Schroeder, 2009; Bernhardt et al., 2010; Biedermann and Hellmann, 2010; Zhang et al., 2010; Zhang and Schroeder, 2010; Castells et al., 2011). While plants affected in ATCSA-1, the Arabidopsis CSA ortholog, do not display an abnormal development (Biedermann and Hellmann, 2010), loss of CUL4 or DDB2 cause a dwarf-like phenotype (Bernhardt et al., 2006; Koga et al., 2006). Interestingly, Arabidopsis *ddb2* or *atcsa-1* mutants are UV-hypersensitive but only when brought into the dark right after UV treatment, demonstrating that plants primarily rely on photoreactivation rather than NER (Biedermann and Hellmann, 2010). However, when kept in the dark both mutants have reduced repair activities when compared to wild type (Biedermann and Hellmann, 2010). CSB-like helicases are also present in plants

(Kimura et al., 2004; Shaked et al., 2006), and although they are not biochemically characterized, studies in Arabidopsis demonstrate their critical role for UV tolerance (Shaked et al., 2006). Other mutants directly affected in NER factors such as Arabidopsis mutants *atcen2* and *uvh3–1/xpg,* also show decreased repair activities *in vitro* and behave hypersensitive towards UV-C exposure, respectively (Liu et al., 2000; Molinier et al., 2004b). Loss of the TFIIH transcription factor complex subunits XPB/UVH6 and XPD is lethal; however, *uvh6-1* plants expressing a mutated but potentially partially functional XPB protein already show decreased repair rates of UV-induced 6–4 photoproducts (Liu et al., 2003). Overall the current findings strongly indicate that the basic mechanisms of UV-induced damaged DNA recognition and NER based repair are comparable and highly conserved among plants and animals.

### 3.3 Base excision repair

Not all nucleotide modifications can be repaired by NER, and many DNA lesions generated by reactive oxygen species (ROS) are not recognized by the NER proteins. Thus as an additional mechanism to ensure genomic integrity, cells utilize other repair mechanisms like base excision repair (BER). Because ROS are continuously produced as metabolic byproducts or by ionizing radiation, they represent a considerable source of the daily DNA damage. ROS-induced DNA lesions include for example 8-hydroxyguanine (8-oxoG), formamidopyrimidines, and 5-hydroxyuracil, which can potentially lead to miscoding during replication and transcription.

As a general rule BER requires the activities of DNA glycosylases, which cleave the N-glycosyl bond between the base and the sugar at the lesion site. This releases the base and leaves an abasic or apurinic/apyrimidinic (AP) site. In bacteria, fungi, plants and animals, several DNA glycosylases have been described that either specifically or broadly recognize certain lesions. For example, the mammalian DNA glycosylase OGG1 has a high affinity to 8-oxoG and some formamidopyrimidines, while another mammalian DNA glycosylase, NEIL1, efficiently repairs formamidopyrimidines but only poorly 8-oxoG (Morland et al., 2002; Parsons et al., 2005). DNA glycosylases are classified as either being mono- or bifunctional. Monofunctionally they only perform the cleavage reaction of the glycosylic bond between the deoxyribose and the target base to generate an AP site. Bifunctional DNA glycosylases/lyases, to which OGG1 and NEIL1 belong, are able to catalyze the release of the oxidized base and the cleavage of the DNA backbone at the AP site (Hazra et al., 2001).

Although there is currently no evidence that plants have NEIL1 orthologs, which are common in bacteria and animals and required in part for excision of oxidized purines and pyrimidines, most other DNA glycosylases have been found. For example, plants encode for orthologs of OGG1 (Roldan-Arjona and Ariza, 2009), and their activity in excising oxidized purines has been demonstrated for the *Arabidopsis* AtOGG1 (Dany and Tissier, 2001; Garcia-Ortiz et al., 2001; Morales-Ruiz et al., 2003). In addition to OGG1, plants also encode for proteins related to the bifunctional Endonuclease III/Nth from *E. coli*, yeast, and animals, which remove a broad range of damaged pyrimidines (Breimer and Lindahl, 1980; Boorstein et al., 1989; Hatahet et al., 1994; Phadnis et al., 2006; Guay et al., 2008). Like their bacterial counterparts, *Arabidopsis* AtNTH1 also shows a broad substrate specificity and DNA glycosylase activity for DNA lesions containing modified pyrimidines (Krokan et al., 1997; Roldan-Arjona et al., 2000). Furthermore, plants encode for proteins related to MutM/Fpg, an original model DNA glycosylase/lyase from *E. coli* that excises 8-oxo-guanine and other oxidized purines from damaged DNA (Tchou et al., 1991; Tchou et al., 1993; Bhagwat and

Gerlt, 1996; Ohtsubo et al., 1998; Murphy and Gao, 2001; Roldan-Arjona and Ariza, 2009). Although enzymatic function for all three types of plant DNA glycosylases is established, there is unfortunately no information available on how loss of these proteins affects development or ROS sensitivity of mutant plants.

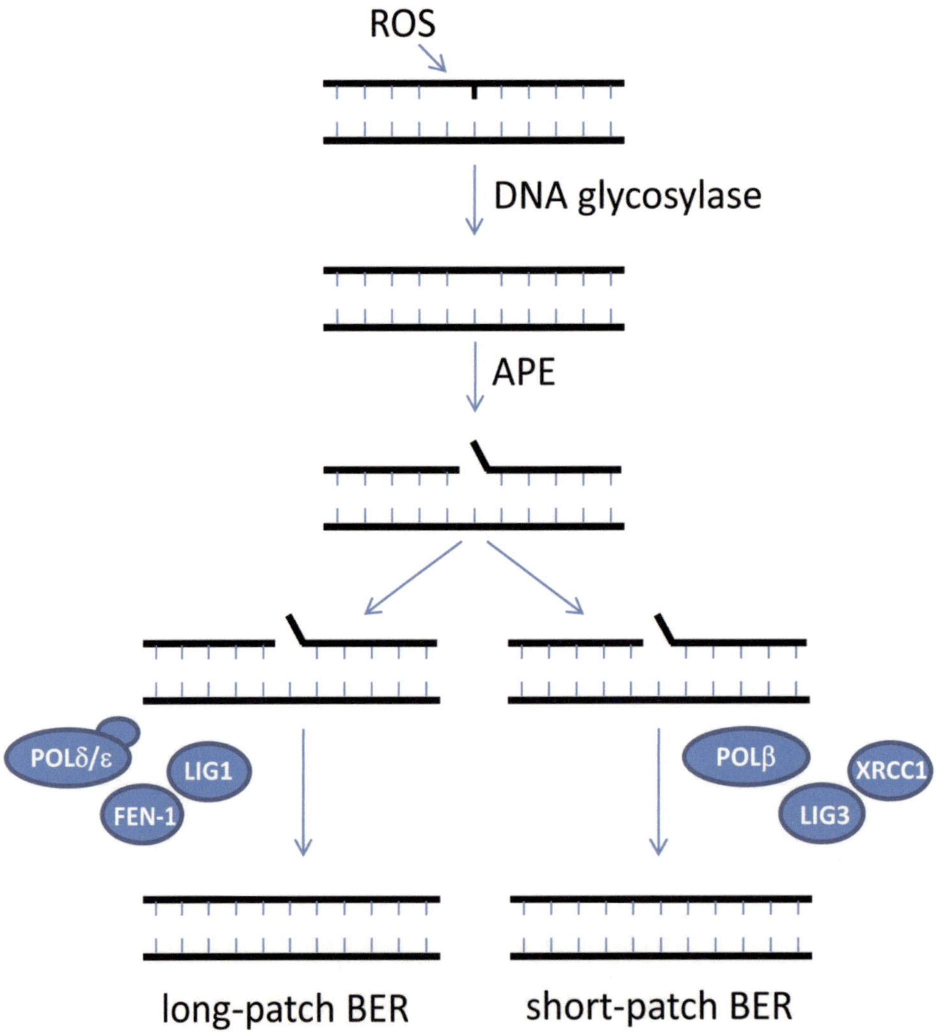


Fig. 3. Schematic model for base excision repair (BER).

DNA lesions caused by ROS are recognized and modified by the concerted activities of a DNA glycosylase and APE, after which cells can either take the route of long-patch repair or alternatively the short-patch repair pathway. Currently evidence indicates for plants that the long-patch repair is employed for BER.

Plant OGG1 and NTH proteins generate 3′ phospho α,β-unsaturated aldehydes (3′ dRP) at the strand breaks, and these need to be removed to generate free 3′ hydroxyl ends to allow gap-filling repair mediated by a DNA polymerase (Demple and Harrison, 1994; Roldan-Arjona et al., 2000; Garcia-Ortiz et al., 2001). Removal of 3′dRP is mediated in plants and animals by AP endonucleases (APE) which also work on AP sites generated by either monofunctional DNA glycosylases or those that occurred through spontaneous degradation of the DNA (Babiychuk et al., 1994; Demple et al., 1997; Pascucci et al., 2002) (Fig. 3).

Subsequently to APE, two separate BER repair pathways can become active in mammalian cells. First, the short-patch repair pathway, which relies on the concerted activities of DNA polymerase β (Polβ), X-ray repair cross-complementing protein 1 (XRCC1), and the DNA ligase 3 (LIG3). Polβ has an intrinsic 3′dRP activity and can remove deoxyribose sugar itself if required (Caldecott, 2001). XRCC1 interacts with LIG3 and other BER proteins and may function as a repair coordinating protein (Vidal et al., 2001) (Fig. 3). Alternatively, the long patch-repair pathway can be employed in mammalian cells, which requires activities of DNA polymerases δ and ε, RFC, PCNA, and flap endonuclease 1 (FEN1) to remove and resynthesize up to 10 nucleotides 3′ to the AP site, while the nick is ligated by LIG1 (Matsumoto, 2001) (Fig. 3).

While most proteins are present in plants that can participate in long-patch repair (Kimura and Sakaguchi, 2006), it is currently open whether a short-patch pathway exists in plants since no obvious homologs of POLβ and LIG3 are identified so far (Kimura and Sakaguchi, 2006; Roldan-Arjona and Ariza, 2009). In addition, plant XRCC1-like proteins lack domains that are necessary for complex assembly with POLβ and LIG3, and it is therefore currently open whether the protein participates in BER (Vidal et al., 2001; Taylor et al., 2002). Although no POLβ proteins are described in plants so far, it is possible that their function is conducted by POLλ. Both polymerases belong to the X superfamily of DNA polymerases and several amino acid residues are conserved between POLβ and λ (Garcia-Diaz et al., 2000; Uchiyama et al., 2004). In addition, POLλ has been demonstrated in rice to possess intrinsic 3′dRP activity and its expression is mainly found in meristematic and proliferating tissues (Uchiyama et al., 2004).

An important role in the recognition and repair of SSB and activation of BER involves poly(ADP-ribose) polymerases (PARP). PARP proteins belong to small protein families with, for example, 18 members in human, and they are highly conserved among eukaryotes (Ame et al., 2004); however, it is PARP1 and PARP2 that have been brought in context with damaged DNA recognition and DNA repair processes. PARP1 is a 113 kDa protein that contains a modular set of domains that enable it to fulfill multiple functions in the cell. At its N-terminal region PARP1 contains a DNA break recognition fold that is composed of a duplicated zinc finger similar to DNA ligase III. A BRCT motif is present in the center that can be found in many proteins connected with maintenance of genomic integrity and cell cycle checkpoints. The motif also functions as the main interface for protein–protein interactions. Finally, at its COOH-terminal region, PARP1 has motifs with different catalytic activities including $NAD^+$ hydrolysis as well as initiation, elongation, branching and termination of ADP-ribose polymers (Citarelli et al., 2010). It has been shown in mammalian cells that, upon binding a DNA lesion PARP1 poly(ADP)ribosylates itself as well as nearby histones (H1 and H2B), which relaxes the chromatin structure allowing better access for XRCC1 and other repair proteins to the damaged site (Poirier et al., 1982; Masson et al., 1998; Pleschke et al., 2000). Plant PARP1 and PARP2 are nuclear localized like their animal counterparts, and they become transcriptionally activated upon genotoxic stress conditions such as ionizing radiation or oxidative stress (Puchta et al., 1995; Babiychuk et al., 1998;

Doucet-Chabeaud et al., 2001; Chen et al., 2003). However, although a similar role of plant PARP1 and PARP2 in damaged DNA recognition and initiation of DNA repair is likely, a detailed *in planta* functional description is still missing for these proteins.

### 3.4 DSB repair: Nonhomologous end joining and homologous recombination

ROS, especially •OH generated by ionizing radiation or via the Fenton reaction (Karanjawala et al., 2003; Clark, 2008), also have a high potential to cause double-strand breaks (DSB) (Karanjawala et al., 2002; Karanjawala et al., 2003). DSB require repair mechanisms distinct from photolyases, NER and BER. Therefore cells primarily depend on either the nonhomologous DNA end joining pathway (NHEJ) or homologous recombination (HR). NHEJ is an error-prone repair pathway, which directly ligates the free DNA ends together. In animals, the pathway is discussed to start with the binding of the heterodimeric Ku70/Ku80 complex to a DNA end. This step is required for employment of DNA-dependent protein kinase (DNA-PK) and Artemis endonuclease that process the DNA ends (Ma et al., 2002), while rejoining and ligation is performed by the XRCC4/LIG4/XLF complex (Grawunder et al., 1997; Barnes et al., 1998) (Fig. 4). The processing of the DNA ends can result in deletions or insertions and is the reason why NHEJ based repair often results in mutations in the repaired DNA. Current research in plants indicates that the NHEJ pathway is conserved among plants and animals. Ku70 and Ku80 related proteins as well as the Artemis-like protein SNM1/PSO1 are expressed in *Arabidopsis* and rice, and *Arabidopsis* mutants affected in these proteins become hypersensitive to γ-irradiation and the chemotherapeutic agent bleomycin, a double-strand break inducing chemical, which is in agreement with their roles in NHEJ (Tamura et al., 2002; Friesner and Britt, 2003; Gallego et al., 2003; Molinier et al., 2004a; Kimura et al., 2005; Kimura and Sakaguchi, 2006; Charbonnel et al., 2010). Likewise, XRCC4 and Lig4 homologues have been described in plants, and functionally connected to NHEJ (West et al., 2000; Friesner and Britt, 2003; Kimura and Sakaguchi, 2006; Waterworth et al., 2010).

In contrast to the error prone NHEJ pathway, HR is a more accurate repair mechanism that uses homologous DNA strands as templates for repair activities (Boyko et al., 2006a; Boyko et al., 2006b; Li and Ma, 2006; Osman et al., 2011). Several alternative pathways may exist that allow HR based repair of DSBs, however, good evidence is provided for at least two alternative pathways in plants. One is the synthesis-dependent strand annealing (SDSA) mechanism which involves the meiotic recombination11/Rad50/X-ray sensitive 2 (MRN) complex (Waterworth et al., 2007; Ronceret et al., 2009; Amiard et al., 2010). The MRN complex is discussed to function as a first sensor of double strand breaks. It generates single strand DNA at the DSB sites that can be used as templates to mediate HR by RecA and Rad51 homologues (Lin et al., 2006; Li et al., 2007; Markmann-Mulisch et al., 2007; Odahara et al., 2007; Vignard et al., 2007; Waterworth et al., 2007; Odahara et al., 2009; Ronceret et al., 2009; Amiard et al., 2010; Chittela and Sainis, 2010; Devisetty et al., 2010; Ko et al., 2010; Schaefer et al., 2010; Wang et al., 2010; Ko et al., 2011) (Fig. 4). However, the precise subsequent steps of Holliday structure formation, cleavage by endonucleases and dissociation into two DNA chains is only poorly understood in plants. Alternatively to SDSA, plants also use the single strand annealing (SSA) mechanism (Tissier et al., 1995; Ayora et al., 2002; Blanck et al., 2009; Mannuss et al., 2010). SSA requires a double strand break between two repeated sequences that are oriented in the same direction. Adjacent to the break, single-stranded DNA is created so that the repeated sequences can be used as complementary strands to anneal the ends of the break, after which non-homologous tails are detached and nicks can be ligated (Tissier et al., 1995; Puchta, 2005; Blanck et al., 2009; Mannuss et al., 2010). Because HR is less likely to cause changes in the genetic information than NHEJ, it is likely that the extent to which either NHEJ or HR repair pathways are employed in DSB repair may impact genome evolution in living organisms.

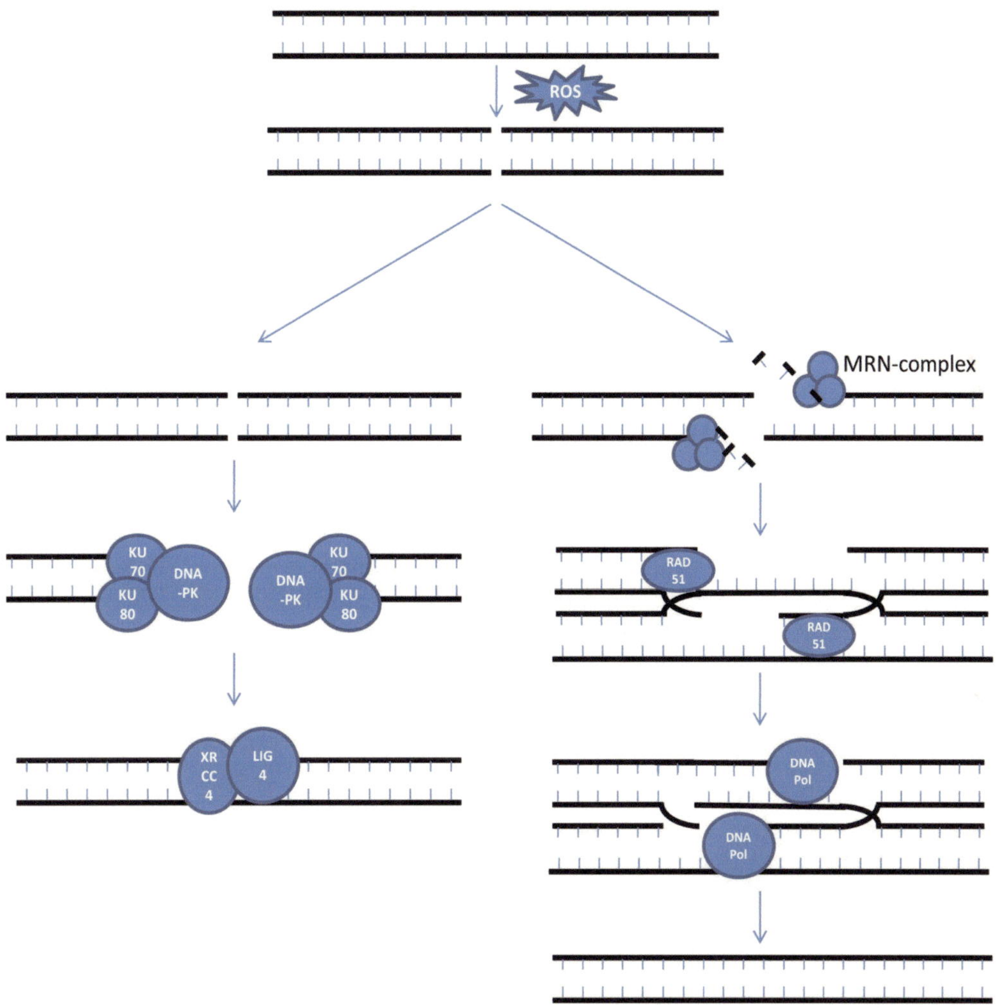


Fig. 4. ROS induced repair of double-strand breaks.

Two alternative pathways for which strong evidence is present to exist in plants are shown. Double-strand breaks can either be repaired by nonhomologous DNA end joining pathway (NHEJ; left hand side), or by homologous recombination (HR; right hand side).

### 3.5 DNA repair in chloroplasts

Based on their high metabolic activities in respiration and photosynthesis, organelles are centers of ROS production. Both mitochondria and chloroplasts possess their own repair pathways, and it appears to be that they have most of the repair pathways that are also found in the nucleus (for an excellent review about mitochondrial repair see (Boesch et al., 2011). We will focus here on chloroplast repair and briefly summarize recent findings.

The chloroplast genome is in general relative small, but gene numbers can vary significantly between species ranging from, for example, 54 in *Helicosporidium sp. ex Simulium jonesii* and up to 301 in *Pinus koraiensis* (http://chloroplast.cbio.psu.edu/); (Cui et al., 2006). These genes and their corresponding proteins are crucial for proper functioning of the organelle and hence survival of the plant and it is not surprising that chloroplasts have several repair pathways.

A recent report described a rice CPD photolyase to mediate repair of direct DNA damage caused by UV light (Takahashi et al., 2011), and also an earlier report describes PHR2, a class II photolyase predicted to be in chloroplasts of *C. reinhardtii* (Petersen et al., 1999). There is also strong evidence in *Arabidopsis* for two bifunctional DNA glycosylase/lyase of the *E. coli* Endonuclease III/Nth type and an APE to be involved in repair of ROS based DNA damage (Gutman and Niyogi, 2009). The authors can show specific localization of the three proteins to the chloroplast and specific activities *in vitro*. However, single or even triple mutants affected in the three proteins do not display any apparent developmental defects or increased sensitivities to photo-oxidative stress (e.g. UV- and high light or methyl viologen), from which the authors concluded that additional, yet unknown BER repair pathways exist in chloroplast (Gutman and Niyogi, 2009).

Currently no clear data are available for NER activities in the chloroplasts and only poor evidence is currently present on whether or how chloroplasts repair DSBs. Work on the green algae *Chlamydomonas reinhardtii* showed presence of a chloroplast-located RecA homolog, which is inducible in expression by DNA-damaging reagents (Nakazato et al., 2003). In addition, *Arabidopsis* T-DNA insertion mutants affected in a chloroplast localized RecA (*cpRecA*) homolog have increased amounts of single-strand DNA, altered structures of chloroplast DNA, and chloroplasts showed signs of reduced function after four generations post T-DNA insertion (Rowan et al., 2010). Yet, further data for additional repair proteins is still missing, as well as strong evidence for HR or NHEJ activities in chloroplasts of higher plants. Recent findings, however, indicate that chloroplasts repair DSBs using microhomology-mediated end joining (MMEJ) (Kwon et al., 2010). This repair mechanism requires only very short (2–14 bp) regions of homology, and is discussed as a potential backup to NHEJ in eukaryotes (Heacock et al., 2004; Bennardo et al., 2008). Although Kwon and co-workers provide strong evidence for MMEJ in chloroplasts, it is currently open which proteins mediate this repair.

### 3.6 Physiological responses after UV and ROS exposure

Besides immediate repair processes, it is also critical for plant cells to generate a physiological environment in which further DNA damage is prevented or at least reduced. A common physiological response to UV exposure in plants appears to be the accumulation of anthocyanin and flavonoids, potentially as a photoprotective or ROS quenching mechanism (Ng et al., 1964 ; Yatsuhashi et al., 1982; Takeda and Abe, 1992; Ye et al., 2010). It is interesting to note that some plants like grape vine (*Vitis vinifera*) or common bean (*Phaseolus vulgaris*) accumulate resveratrol or coumestrol, respectively, in response to UV exposure (Langcake and Pryce, 1977; Beggs et al., 1985). Resveratrol is a protective phytoalexin that is produced primarily under biotic stress conditions, while coumestrol is a phytoestrogen with unknown function. Both compounds are associated with effecting cell proliferation, cell cycle, and apoptosis of mammalian cells (Ndebele et al., 2010; Delmas et al., 2011) and may be signaling molecules in plants to trigger specific responses upon UV exposure.

A critical factor that is discussed as a regulator of DNA repair pathways in response to increased ROS accumulation in the cell appears to be ADP-Ribose/NADH Pyrophosphohydrolase AtNUDX7 (Ishikawa et al., 2009). AtNUDX7 belongs to the family of Nudix hydrolyases, which catalyze the hydrolysis of dinucleoside polyphosphates, nucleoside di- and triphosphates, nucleotide sugars, and coenzymes in plants and animals (McLennan, 2006; Kraszewska, 2008). AtNUDX7 substrates are ADP-Ribose (ADP-Rib) and NADH which are converted to AMP plus ribose 5-phosphate and nicotinamide mononucleotide (NMNH) plus AMP, respectively (Ogawa et al., 2005). The protein may have a central function for the homeostasis of $NAD^+$ pools by supplying ATP via nucleotide recycling from free ADP-Ribose molecules. This may be critical for the cell since substantial PARP activity can significantly lower $NAD^+$ and ATP levels; such a depletion of cellular energy can result in necrotic cell death (Ha and Snyder, 1999; Virag and Szabo, 2002; De Block et al., 2005). As discussed for BER, DNA damaged-induced, PARP-dependent poly(ADP)-ribosylation of proteins is considered a critical step for recognition of damage to be converted into intracellular signals that can trigger DNA repair programs or cell death. Consequently, AtNUDX7 is up-regulated upon abiotic stress (salinity, drought, high light, paraquat), and plants constitutively overexpressing AtNUDX7 become less susceptible to these stress conditions (Ishikawa et al., 2009).

A microarray study has shown that UV-C, bleomycin, or biotic stress factors elicit a hypersensitive response and increased $H_20_2$ levels in the cell (Molinier et al., 2005). Although each stress elicited specific responses, the authors could also find 209 genes that were commonly up-regulated, while 54 were similarly down-regulated by all three stress treatments. Among the commonly regulated genes were components of signaling pathways, transcription factors, and genes connected with an oxidative stress or defense response. Cell-cycle genes were also down-regulated after genotoxic stress exposure, as was earlier noted for animals (Dasika et al., 1999). However, the authors also noted that in Arabidopsis expression of only a comparably few number of repair genes was induced, and concluded that the plant must be mainly relying on existing synthesized proteins. It will be interesting to see whether results are broadly applicable to other plant species or whether the tested conditions and responses are specific for Arabidopsis.

### 3.7 ATM/ATR dependent regulation of DNA repair

A central regulator of the fate of damaged cells between apoptosis or cell cycle arrest and DNA repair in animals is the tumor-suppressing p53, sometimes dubbed the "guardian of the genome". This transcription factor controls not only cell cycle genes like p21 and apoptosis factors like PUMA, NOXA, and BAX but also various components of major DNA repair pathways such as CSB, DDB2 and XPC (NER); FANCC (DNA crosslink repair) and MSH2, MLH1, and PMS2 (mismatch repair) (Gatz and Wiesmuller, 2006; Brady and Attardi, 2010). There is also evidence that it has a more direct role in BER, interacting with APE1 and OGG1 and thereby enhancing the excision of oxidized DNA bases (Gatz and Wiesmuller, 2006; Vigneron and Vousden, 2010). Additionally p53 seems to recognize and bind directly to certain DNA structures e.g. Holliday junctions and mismatches where it represses the

activities of HR and NHEJ (Bakalkin et al., 1994; Subramanian and Griffith, 2005; Gatz and Wiesmuller, 2006).
Activation of p53 after DNA damaging conditions is achieved by phosphorylation by the checkpoint kinases ATAXIA TELANGIECTASIA MUTATED (ATM) and ATAXIA TELANGIECTASIA AND RAD3 RELATED (ATR) (Canman et al., 1998; Tibbetts et al., 1999). While recent studies imply that ATM is a sensor for the redox state of the cell, it is mainly known to be activated by the above-mentioned DSB sensing MRN-complex (Bakkenist and Kastan, 2003; Falck et al., 2005; Kruger and Ralser, 2011; Perry and Tainer, 2011). ATR, on the other hand, is recruited to RPA-coated UV-induced lesions by the ATR INTERACTING PROTEIN (ATRIP) (Wright et al., 1998; Cortez et al., 2001; Ball and Cortez, 2005; Warmerdam et al., 2010). Once activated both kinases phosphorylate p53 and the effector kinases CHK1 and CHK2 regulating cell cycle and DNA repair (Brady and Attardi, 2010).
Curiously no plant homologues of p53 have been identified in any of the model organisms. This is probably linked to the absence of the core apoptotic machinery as we know it from animals. In contrast most of the DNA repair targets of p53, as well as ATM and ATR, are very well conserved in plants. Where loss of one of the checkpoint kinases in animals is lethal, the existence of viable *atr* and *atm* mutant plants in Arabidopsis make it an ideal model for their investigation. Both are involved in the response to ionizing radiation (IR) and necessary for the IR-induced transcription activation of many genes participating in DNA repair, cell cycle control, transcription, and replication (Culligan et al., 2006; Ricaud et al., 2007; Yoshiyama et al., 2009; Furukawa et al., 2010).
This raises the question if there is a factor that is functioning as a p53 analog mediating the DNA damage response between ATM/ATR and the downstream repair factors. An answer to that could be SUPPRESSOR OF GAMMA RESPONSE 1 (SOG1). Though unrelated to p53 and unique to plants, this transcription factor, discovered in a screen for suppressor mutants of the γ-irradiation induced cell cycle arrest of Arabidopsis *uvh1* seeds, is necessary for the activation of genes downstream of both ATM and ATR in response to γ-irradiation (Preuss and Britt, 2003; Yoshiyama et al., 2009; Furukawa et al., 2010). SOG1, ATM, and ATR were also found to trigger plant programmed cell death (PCD) in root meristems after γ- or UV-B irradiation, a mechanism that was recently shown to be distinct from animal apoptosis (Fulcher and Sablowski, 2009; Furukawa et al., 2010). Hence, SOG1 is a good candidate to control repair processes in a p53-like fashion, at least by activating transcription of the plant homologues of factors like DDB2, MSH2 and XPC in response to UV and IR stresses.
Current research indicates that plants and animals share roughly similar repair pathways. But for some repair proteins that have been described in animals no homologues have been found in plants, as yet. However, with ongoing research, it seems plausible that plant counterparts will be identified that can substitute for missing animal orthologs as it appears to be the case with p53 and SOG1.

## 4. Plants as model organisms to study DNA repair

Plants and animals share a surprisingly high degree of conservation among their abilities to repair damaged DNA (please also see Table 1 at the end of this passage for an overview of genes involved in DNA repair in the model plant *Arabidopsis thaliana*). While mammalian researchers have very valid and scientifically relevant reasons to use animal subjects, plants can and should be considered as excellent and viable alternatives to investigate the fundamentals of DNA repair processes. Tolerance towards mutations and abiotic stresses along with the relative ease of upkeep and propagation of the research organisms are two factors that we will briefly discuss in this final section of the review.

Due to their inability to elude many constantly damaging influences, plants need to utilize efficient ways to cope with these stresses. One strategy plants seem to have adopted to manage the higher demands on DNA repair is redundancy. For instance, genes of every pathway discussed here were found to be duplicated in Arabidopsis or rice (Singh et al., 2010). Additionally the existence of both 8-oxo-guanine glycosylases, OGG1, as well as MutM/Fpg in Arabidopsis demonstrate functional redundancy of independent, alternative repair pathways, which may have originated from the incorporation of chloroplast and mitochondrial genes into the nuclear genome (Boesch et al., 2009; Singh et al., 2010; Rowan et al., 2010).

Probably because of these gene duplications, functional redundancies, and more efficient or alternative pathways in comparison to animals, plants often have greater flexibilities in how they can respond to and potentially tolerate damaged DNA and mutations. For example a homozygous mutant in ATR kinase, which would be lethal in mammals, can in plants be investigated for the impact on DNA repair, control of apoptosis or gene expression profiles. In order to see the global effects of genotoxic stressors on a model organism, the subjects need to be exposed to different degrees of damaging agents. Here, plants are ideal models because of their sessile nature. They can be cultivated under very steady and reproducible conditions, while stress exposure is highly controlled. In addition, from an ethical point of view, plants can be taken to the edge of survival with very harsh treatments such as high levels of UV-light or toxin applications that for some may be not comfortable to perform on animals.

In comparison to animals, plants are low cost organisms that only require minimal monitoring along with water and occasionally fertilizer. Small plants like the moss *Physcomitrella patens* or *Arabidopsis thaliana* can be cultivated to great numbers within in a few square feet while by comparison animals require adequate space and regular food, water, and cleaning. While mutant lines are readily available for many animal and plant systems, shipment and propagation of plant resources can be quite straightforward. Seeds can be harvested for immediate propagation of the next generation or stored long-term, even at room temperature, before use months or even years later. Sending seed material to colleagues around the world is technically simple since no special transport accommodations need to be made. Generating transgenic *Arabidopsis* lines using *Agrobacterium* infection is a standard lab procedure, and allows for rapid complementation of mutant lines to verify protein functionality and observation of response and recovery. Also generation time of Arabidopsis plants is very short with just two months from seed to seed.

In addition to using plants as basic models to understand DNA repair processes, there are also practical reasons why this area of research urgently needs to be expanded. With the increase in food shortages for increasing populations, the recognition of environmental toxins and the growing evidence of impending and occurring climate changes across the world, it becomes critical to rapidly develop plants that can better cope with environmental stress. As such, stress tolerant crop plants generated either by genetic engineering or classical breeding will become increasingly important resources to guarantee stable food supplies to the human population in an expected changing environment.

| Repair pathway | Representative Gene Model | Gene in Arabidopsis | Function | Acc. No. | Reference |
|---|---|---|---|---|---|
| **Photore-activation** | | *PHR1/UVR2* | repair of CPDs | AT1G12370 | Ahmad et al., 1997; Landry et al., 1997 |
| | | *PHR2* | repair of CPDs | AT2G47590 | Ahmad et al., 1998; Petersen et al., 1999 |
| | | *UVR3* | repair of 6-4PPs | AT3G15620 | Jiang et al., 1997; Nakajima et al., 1998 |
| **NER** | *XPC* | *AtRAD4* | recognition of CPDs and 6-4PPs, GGR | AT5G16630 | Kunz et al., 2005; Liang et al., 2006 |
| | *HHR23A,B/RAD23* | *RAD23A* | recognition of CPDs and 6-4PPs, GGR | AT1G16190 | Molinier et al., 2005; Kunz et al., 2005; Farmer et al., 2010 |
| | | *RAD23B* | | AT1G79650 | Molinier et al., 2004b Kunz et al., 2005; Farmer et al., 2010 |
| | | *RAD23C* | | AT3G02540 | Molinier et al., 2004b; Kunz et al., 2005; Farmer et al., 2010 |
| | | *RAD23D* | | AT5G38470 | Molinier et al., 2004b; Kunz et al., 2005; Farmer et al., 2010 |
| | *CEN2* | *AtCEN2* | recognition of CPDs and 6-4PPs, GGR | AT4G37010 | Molinier et al., 2004b; Liang et al., 2006 |
| | *ROC1/RBX1* | *RBX1A* | activation of CUL4-dependent ligases | AT5G20570 | Lechner et al., 2002; Gray et al., 2002 |
| | | *RBX1B* | | AT3G42830 | Lechner et al., 2002; Gray et al., 2002 |
| | *CUL4* | *CUL4* | Ubiquitylation of targets | AT5G46210 | Molinier et al., 2008; (Biedermann and Hellmann, 2010 |
| | *DDB1* | *AtDDB1a* | Ubiquitylation of targets | AT4G05420 | Molinier et al., 2008; (Biedermann and Hellmann, 2010 |
| | | *AtDDB1b* | | AT4G21100 | Bernhardt et al., 2006; Bernhardt et al., 2010 |
| | *DDB2* | *DDB2* | recognition of CPDs and 6-4PPs, GGR, substrate recognition for CUL4-dependent ubiquitination | At5g58760 | Koga et al., 2006; Molinier et al., 2008 |
| | *TFIIH1* | *AtTFB1-1* | TFIIH subunit p62 | At1g55750 | Kunz et al., 2005; Singh et al., 2010 |
| | | *AtTFB1-2* | | At1g55680 | Kunz et al., 2005; Singh et al., 2010 |
| | | *AtTFB1-3* | | At3g61420 | Kunz et al., 2005; Singh et al., 2010 |

| Repair pathway | Representative Gene Model | Gene in Arabidopsis | Function | Acc. No. | Reference |
|---|---|---|---|---|---|
| | *TFIIH2* | *AtGTF2H2* | TFIIH subunit p44 | At1g05050 | Kunz et al., 2005; Singh et al., 2010 |
| | *TFIIH3* | *AtTFB4* | TFIIH subunit p34 | AT1G18340 | Kunz et al., 2005; Singh et al., 2010 |
| | *TFIIH4* | *AtTFB2* | TFIIH subunit p52 | At4g17020 | Kunz et al., 2005; Singh et al., 2010 |
| | *TFIIH5* | *AtTFB5* | TFIIH subunit | AT1G12400 | Kunz et al., 2005; Singh et al., 2010 |
| | | | | AT1G62886 | Singh et al., 2010 |
| | *CDK7* | *CAK3AT/CDKD1;1* | cyclin activating kinase-subcomplex of THIIH | AT1G73690 | Singh et al., 2010 |
| | | *CAK4AT/CDKD1;2* | | AT1G66750 | Singh et al., 2010 |
| | | *CAK2AT/CDKD1;3* | | AT1G18040 | Singh et al., 2010 |
| | *XPB/RAD25/ERCC3* | *AtXPB1* | helicase subunit of TFIIH | AT5G41370 | Costa et al., 2001 |
| | | *AtXPB2* | | AT5G41360 | Morgante et al., 2005 |
| | *XPD/RAD3/ERCC2* | *AtXPD/UVH6* | helicase subunit of TFIIH | AT1G03190 | Jenkins et al., 1995; Liu et al., 2003 |
| | *XPF/RAD1/ERCC4* | *AtRAD1/UVH1* | 5'-endonuclease | AT5G41150 | Harlow et al., 1994; Jenkins et al., 1995 |
| | *XPG/RAD2/ERCC5* | *UVH3/UVR1* | 3'-endonuclease | AT3G28030 | Jenkins et al., 1995; Liu et al., 2003 |
| | *CSA/RAD28/ERCC8* | *ATCSA-1/CSAat1A* | substrate recognition for CUL4-dependent ubiquitination, TCR | AT1G27840 | Biedermann and Hellmann, 2010; Zhang et al., 2010 |
| | | *ATCSA-2/CSAat1B* | | AT1G19750 | Kunz et al., 2005; Zhang et al., 2010 |
| | *CSB/RAD26/ERCC6* | *CHR8* | binding of stalled RNA polymerase, recruitment of repair machinery, TCR | AT2G18760 | Shaked et al., 2006 |
| | | *CHR24* | | AT5G63950 | Shaked et al., 2006 |
| **BER** | *OGG1* | *AtOGG1* | 8-oxoguanine DNA glycosylase | AT1G21710 | Garcia-Ortiz et al., 2001; Dany and Tissier, 2001 |
| | *MutM* | *AtFPG/MMH* | formamidopyrimidine DNA glycosylase | AT1G52500 | Ohtsubo et al., 1998 |
| | *NTH* | *AtNTH1* | DNA glycosylase and apyrimidinic (AP) lyase/endonuclease | AT2G31450 | Gutman and Niyogi, 2009 |
| | | *AtNTH2* | | AT1G05900 | Gutman and Niyogi, 2009 |

| Repair pathway | Representative Gene Model | Gene in Arabidopsis | Function | Acc. No. | Reference |
|---|---|---|---|---|---|
| | *APE* | *ARP/APE1* | apurinic/apyrimidinic (AP) endonuclease | AT2G41460 | Babiychuk et al., 1994; Gutman and Niyogi, 2009 |
| | | *APE2* | | AT4G36050 | Singh et al., 2010 |
| | *XRCC1* | *AtXRCC1* | co-factor of DNA ligase 3 | AT1G80420 | Petrucco et al., 2002; Singh et al., 2010 |
| | *FEN* | *FEN1* | flap endonuclease | AT5G26680 | Singh et al., 2010 |
| **NHEJ/HR** | *KU70/XRCC6* | *AtKU70* | binding of DNA double strand break ends | AT1G16970 | Riha et al., 2002 |
| | *KU80/XRCC5* | *AtKU80* | binding of DNA double strand break ends | AT1G48050 | Riha et al., 2002 |
| | *XRCC4* | *XRCC4* | co-factor of DNA ligase 4 | AT3G23100 | West et al., 2000 |
| | *LIG4* | *AtLIG4* | DNA ligation | AT5G57160 | West et al., 2000 |
| | *MRE11* | *AtMRE11* | subunit of the MRN complex, damage recognition, generation of single-stranded DNA | AT5G54260 | Hartung and Puchta, 1999; Daoudal-Cotterell et al., 2002 |
| | *RAD50* | *AtRAD50* | subunit of the MRN complex, damage recognition, generation of single-stranded DNA | AT2G31970 | Gallego and White, 2001 |
| | *NBS1* | *AtNBS1* | subunit of the MRN complex, damage recognition, generation of single-stranded DNA | AT3G02680 | Bleuyard et al., 2006; Waterworth et al., 2007 |
| | *RECA (E. Coli)* | *AtRECA1/cp RecA* | DNA binding, mediation of inter-strand-pairing | AT1G79050 | Cerutti et al., 1992; Cao Cao et al., 1997; Shedge et al., 2007; Rowan et al., 2010 |
| | | *AtRECA2* | | AT2G19490 | Shedge et al., 2007 |
| | | *AtRECA3* | | AT3G10140 | Khazi et al., 2003; Shedge et al., 2007 |
| | | | | AT3G32920 | Shedge et al., 2007 |
| | | *DRT100* | | AT3G12610 | Pang et al., 1992; Pang et al., 1993 |
| | *RAD51* | *AtRAD51/RAD51A* | DNA binding, mediation of inter-strand-pairing | AT5G20850 | Doutriaux et al., 1998 |
| | | *RAD51B* | | AT2G28560 | Bleuyard et al., 2005; Osakabe et al., 2005 |
| | | *RAD51C* | | AT2G45280 | Bleuyard et al., 2005 |
| | | *RAD51D/SSN1* | | AT1G07745 | Bleuyard et al., 2005; Osakabe et al., 2006 |
| | *BRCA1* | *AtBRCA1* | supports homology pairing | AT4G21070 | Lafarge and Montane, 2003 |

| Repair pathway | Representative Gene Model | Gene in Arabidopsis | Function | Acc. No. | Reference |
|---|---|---|---|---|---|
| | *BRCA2* | *AtBRCA2A* | supports homology pairing | AT4G00020 | Siaud et al., 2004; Dray et al., 2006 |
| | | *AtBRCA2B* | | AT5G01630 | Siaud et al., 2004; Dray et al., 2006 |
| **Other** | *ATM* | *AtATM* | checkpoint kinase | AT3G48190 | Garcia et al., 2000) |
| | *ATR/RAD3* | *AtATR/AtRAD3* | checkpoint kinase | AT5G40820 | Culligan et al., 2004 |
| | *PCNA* | *AtPCNA1* | DNA polymerase processivity factor activity | AT1G07370 | Strzalka et al., 2009 |
| | | *AtPCNA2* | | AT2G29570 | Strzalka et al., 2009 |
| | *LIG1* | *AtLIG1* | DNA ligation | AT1G08130 | Taylor et al., 1998 |
| | | | | AT1G49250 | Singh et al., 2010 |
| | *PARP* | *AtPARP1* | damage recognition, poly(ADP)ribosylation | AT4G02390 | Lepiniec et al., 1995 |
| | | *AtPARP2* | | AT2G31320 | Doucet-Chabeaud et al., 2001 |
| | | *AtPARP3* | | AT5G22470 | Singh et al., 2010 |
| | *RPA1* | *AtRPA1A/AtRPA1-3/RPA70A* | stabilization of single-stranded DNA intermediates | AT2G06510 | Ishibashi et al., 2005; Chang et al., 2009 |
| | | *AtRPA1-1* | | AT4G19130 | Kunz et al., 2005; Singh et al., 2010 |
| | | *AtRPA1-5/RPA70B* | | AT5G08020 | Kunz et al., 2005; Singh et al., 2010 |
| | | *AtRPA1-2/RPA70C* | | AT5G45400 | Kunz et al., 2005; Singh et al., 2010 |
| | | *AtRPA1-4/RPA70D* | | AT5G61000 | Kunz et al., 2005; Singh et al., 2010 |
| | *RPA2* | *AtRPA2-1/ATRPA32A* | | AT2G24490 | Kunz et al., 2005 |
| | | *AtRPA2-2/ATRPA32B* | | AT3G02920 | Kunz et al., 2005 |
| | *RPA3* | | | AT3G52630 | Singh et al., 2010 |
| | | | | AT4G18590 | Singh et al., 2010 |

Table 1. Overview of genes involved in DNA repair in the model plant *Arabidopsis thaliana*.

## 5. References

Aboussekhra, A., Biggerstaff, M., Shivji, M.K., Vilpo, J.A., Moncollin, V., Podust, V.N., Protic, M., Hubscher, U., Egly, J.M., and Wood, R.D. (1995). Mammalian DNA nucleotide excision repair reconstituted with purified protein components. Cell 80, 859-868.

Ahmad, M., Jarillo, J.A., and Cashmore, A.R. (1998). PHR2: a novel Arabidopsis gene related to the blue-light photoreceptor/photolyase family. Plant Physiol 117.

Ahmad, M., Jarillo, J.A., Klimczak, L.J., Landry, L.G., Peng, T., Last, R.L., and Cashmore, A.R. (1997). An enzyme similar to animal type II photolyases mediates photoreactivation in Arabidopsis. Plant Cell 9, 199-207.

Al Khateeb, W.M., and Schroeder, D.F. (2009). Overexpression of Arabidopsis damaged DNA binding protein 1A (DDB1A) enhances UV tolerance. Plant Mol Biol 70, 371-383.

Ame, J.C., Spenlehauer, C., and de Murcia, G. (2004). The PARP superfamily. Bioessays 26, 882-893.

Amiard, S., Charbonnel, C., Allain, E., Depeiges, A., White, C.I., and Gallego, M.E. (2010). Distinct roles of the ATR kinase and the Mre11-Rad50-Nbs1 complex in the maintenance of chromosomal stability in Arabidopsis. Plant Cell 22, 3020-3033.

Araujo, S.J., Nigg, E.A., and Wood, R.D. (2001). Strong functional interactions of TFIIH with XPC and XPG in human DNA nucleotide excision repair, without a preassembled repairosome. Mol Cell Biol 21, 2281-2291.

Asada, K. (1999). THE WATER-WATER CYCLE IN CHLOROPLASTS: Scavenging of Active Oxygens and Dissipation of Excess Photons. Annu Rev Plant Physiol Plant Mol Biol 50, 601-639.

Ayora, S., Piruat, J.I., Luna, R., Reiss, B., Russo, V.E., Aguilera, A., and Alonso, J.C. (2002). Characterization of two highly similar Rad51 homologs of Physcomitrella patens. J Mol Biol 316, 35-49.

Babiychuk, E., Kushnir, S., Van Montagu, M., and Inze, D. (1994). The Arabidopsis thaliana apurinic endonuclease Arp reduces human transcription factors Fos and Jun. Proc Natl Acad Sci U S A 91, 3299-3303.

Babiychuk, E., Cottrill, P.B., Storozhenko, S., Fuangthong, M., Chen, Y., O'Farrell, M.K., Van Montagu, M., Inze, D., and Kushnir, S. (1998). Higher plants possess two structurally different poly(ADP-ribose) polymerases. Plant J 15, 635-645.

Bakalkin, G., Yakovleva, T., Selivanova, G., Magnusson, K.P., Szekely, L., Kiseleva, E., Klein, G., Terenius, L., and Wiman, K.G. (1994). p53 binds single-stranded DNA ends and catalyzes DNA renaturation and strand transfer. Proc Natl Acad Sci U S A 91, 413-417.

Bakkenist, C.J., and Kastan, M.B. (2003). DNA damage activates ATM through intermolecular autophosphorylation and dimer dissociation. Nature 421, 499-506.

Ball, H.L., and Cortez, D. (2005). ATRIP oligomerization is required for ATR-dependent checkpoint signaling. J Biol Chem 280, 31390-31396.

Barnes, D.E., Stamp, G., Rosewell, I., Denzel, A., and Lindahl, T. (1998). Targeted disruption of the gene encoding DNA ligase IV leads to lethality in embryonic mice. Curr Biol 8, 1395-1398.

Beggs, C.J., Stolzer-Jehle, A., and Wellmann, E. (1985). Isoflavonoid formation as an indicator of UV stress in bean (Phaseolus vulgaris L.) leaves. Plant Physiol 79, 630-634.

Bennardo, N., Cheng, A., Huang, N., and Stark, J.M. (2008). Alternative-NHEJ is a mechanistically distinct pathway of mammalian chromosome break repair. PLoS Genet 4, e1000110.

Bernhardt, A., Mooney, S., and Hellmann, H. (2010). Arabidopsis DDB1a and DDB1b are critical for embryo development. Planta 232, 555-566.

Bernhardt, A., Lechner, E., Hano, P., Schade, V., Dieterle, M., Anders, M., Dubin, M.J., Benvenuto, G., Bowler, C., Genschik, P., and Hellmann, H. (2006). CUL4 associates with DDB1 and DET1 and its downregulation affects diverse aspects of development in Arabidopsis thaliana. Plant J 47, 591-603.

Bhagwat, M., and Gerlt, J.A. (1996). 3'- and 5'-strand cleavage reactions catalyzed by the Fpg protein from Escherichia coli occur via successive beta- and delta-elimination mechanisms, respectively. Biochemistry 35, 659-665.

Biedermann, S., and Hellmann, H. (2010). The DDB1a interacting proteins ATCSA-1 and DDB2 are critical factors for UV-B tolerance and genomic integrity in Arabidopsis thaliana. Plant J 62, 404-415.

Blackwell, L.J., Borowiec, J.A., and Mastrangelo, I.A. (1996). Single-stranded-DNA binding alters human replication protein A structure and facilitates interaction with DNA-dependent protein kinase. Mol Cell Biol 16, 4798-4807.

Blanck, S., Kobbe, D., Hartung, F., Fengler, K., Focke, M., and Puchta, H. (2009). A SRS2 homolog from Arabidopsis thaliana disrupts recombinogenic DNA intermediates and facilitates single strand annealing. Nucleic Acids Res 37, 7163-7176.

Bleuyard, J.Y., Gallego, M.E., and White, C.I. (2006). Recent advances in understanding of the DNA double-strand break repair machinery of plants. DNA Repair (Amst) 5, 1-12.

Boesch, P., Weber-Lotfi, F., Ibrahim, N., Tarasenko, V., Cosset, A., Paulus, F., Lightowlers, R.N., and Dietrich, A. (2011). DNA repair in organelles: Pathways, organization, regulation, relevance in disease and aging. Biochim Biophys Acta 1813, 186-200.

Boorstein, R.J., Hilbert, T.P., Cadet, J., Cunningham, R.P., and Teebor, G.W. (1989). UV-induced pyrimidine hydrates in DNA are repaired by bacterial and mammalian DNA glycosylase activities. Biochemistry 28, 6164-6170.

Boyko, A., Filkowski, J., Hudson, D., and Kovalchuk, I. (2006a). Homologous recombination in plants is organ specific. Mutat Res 595, 145-155.

Boyko, A., Zemp, F., Filkowski, J., and Kovalchuk, I. (2006b). Double-strand break repair in plants is developmentally regulated. Plant Physiol 141, 488-497.

Brady, C.A., and Attardi, L.D. (2010). p53 at a glance. J Cell Sci 123, 2527-2532.

Breimer, L., and Lindahl, T. (1980). A DNA glycosylase from Escherichia coli that releases free urea from a polydeoxyribonucleotide containing fragments of base residues. Nucleic Acids Res 8, 6199-6211.

Caldecott, K.W. (2001). Mammalian DNA single-strand break repair: an X-ra(y)ted affair. Bioessays 23, 447-455.

Camenisch, U., Dip, R., Schumacher, S.B., Schuler, B., and Naegeli, H. (2006). Recognition of helical kinks by xeroderma pigmentosum group A protein triggers DNA excision repair. Nat Struct Mol Biol 13, 278-284.

Canman, C.E., Lim, D.S., Cimprich, K.A., Taya, Y., Tamai, K., Sakaguchi, K., Appella, E., Kastan, M.B., and Siliciano, J.D. (1998). Activation of the ATM kinase by ionizing radiation and phosphorylation of p53. Science 281, 1677-1679.

Cao, J., Combs, C., and Jagendorf, A.T. (1997). The chloroplast-located homolog of bacterial DNA recombinase. Plant Cell Physiol 38, 1319-1325.

Castells, E., Molinier, J., Drevensek, S., Genschik, P., Barneche, F., and Bowler, C. (2010). det1-1-induced UV-C hyposensitivity through UVR3 and PHR1 photolyase gene over-expression. Plant J.

Castells, E., Molinier, J., Benvenuto, G., Bourbousse, C., Zabulon, G., Zalc, A., Cazzaniga, S., Genschik, P., Barneche, F., and Bowler, C. (2011). The conserved factor DE-ETIOLATED 1 cooperates with CUL4-DDB1(DDB2) to maintain genome integrity upon UV stress. EMBO J 30, 1162-1172.

Cazzalini, O., Perucca, P., Savio, M., Necchi, D., Bianchi, L., Stivala, L.A., Ducommun, B., Scovassi, A.I., and Prosperi, E. (2008). Interaction of p21(CDKN1A) with PCNA regulates the histone acetyltransferase activity of p300 in nucleotide excision repair. Nucleic Acids Res 36, 1713-1722.

Cerutti, H., Osman, M., Grandoni, P., and Jagendorf, A.T. (1992). A homolog of Escherichia coli RecA protein in plastids of higher plants. Proc Natl Acad Sci U S A 89, 8068-8072.

Chang, Y., Gong, L., Yuan, W., Li, X., Chen, G., Zhang, Q., and Wu, C. (2009). Replication protein A (RPA1a) is required for meiotic and somatic DNA repair but is dispensable for DNA replication and homologous recombination in rice. Plant Physiol 151, 2162-2173.

Charbonnel, C., Gallego, M.E., and White, C.I. (2010). Xrcc1-dependent and Ku-dependent DNA double-strand break repair kinetics in Arabidopsis plants. Plant J 64, 280-290.

Chen, H., Shen, Y., Tang, X., Yu, L., Wang, J., Guo, L., Zhang, Y., Zhang, H., Feng, S., Strickland, E., Zheng, N., and Deng, X.W. (2006). Arabidopsis CULLIN4 Forms an E3 Ubiquitin Ligase with RBX1 and the CDD Complex in Mediating Light Control of Development. Plant Cell 18, 1991-2004.

Chen, I.P., Haehnel, U., Altschmied, L., Schubert, I., and Puchta, H. (2003). The transcriptional response of Arabidopsis to genotoxic stress - a high-density colony array study (HDCA). Plant J 35, 771-786.

Chen, J.J., Mitchell, D.L., and Britt, A.B. (1994). A Light-Dependent Pathway for the Elimination of UV-Induced Pyrimidine (6-4) Pyrimidinone Photoproducts in Arabidopsis. Plant Cell 6, 1311-1317.

Chittela, R.K., and Sainis, J.K. (2010). Plant DNA recombinases: a long way to go. J Nucleic Acids 2010.

Citarelli, M., Teotia, S., and Lamb, R.S. (2010). Evolutionary history of the poly(ADP-ribose) polymerase gene family in eukaryotes. BMC Evol Biol 10, 308.

Citterio, E., Van Den Boom, V., Schnitzler, G., Kanaar, R., Bonte, E., Kingston, R.E., Hoeijmakers, J.H., and Vermeulen, W. (2000). ATP-dependent chromatin remodeling by the Cockayne syndrome B DNA repair-transcription-coupling factor. Mol Cell Biol 20, 7643-7653.

Clark, R.A.F. (2008). Oxidative Stress and "Senescent" Fibroblasts in Non-Healing Wounds as Potential Therapeutic Targets. J Invest Dermatol 128, 2361–2364.

Cortez, D., Guntuku, S., Qin, J., and Elledge, S.J. (2001). ATR and ATRIP: partners in checkpoint signaling. Science 294, 1713-1716.

Costa, R.M., Morgante, P.G., Berra, C.M., Nakabashi, M., Bruneau, D., Bouchez, D., Sweder, K.S., Van Sluys, M.A., and Menck, C.F. (2001). The participation of AtXPB1, the XPB/RAD25 homologue gene from Arabidopsis thaliana, in DNA repair and plant development. Plant J 28, 385-395.

Cui, L., Veeraraghavan, N., Richter, A., Wall, K., Jansen, R.K., Leebens-Mack, J., Makalowska, I., and dePamphilis, C.W. (2006). ChloroplastDB: the Chloroplast Genome Database. Nucleic Acids Res 34, D692-696.

Culligan, K., Tissier, A., and Britt, A. (2004). ATR regulates a G2-phase cell-cycle checkpoint in Arabidopsis thaliana. Plant Cell 16, 1091-1104.

Culligan, K.M., Robertson, C.E., Foreman, J., Doerner, P., and Britt, A.B. (2006). ATR and ATM play both distinct and additive roles in response to ionizing radiation. Plant J 48, 947-961.

Dany, A.L., and Tissier, A. (2001). A functional OGG1 homologue from Arabidopsis thaliana. Mol Genet Genomics 265, 293-301.

Daoudal-Cotterell, S., Gallego, M.E., and White, C.I. (2002). The plant Rad50-Mre11 protein complex. FEBS Lett 516, 164-166.

Dasika, G.K., Lin, S.C., Zhao, S., Sung, P., Tomkinson, A., and Lee, E.Y. (1999). DNA damage-induced cell cycle checkpoints and DNA strand break repair in development and tumorigenesis. Oncogene 18, 7883-7899.

De Block, M., Verduyn, C., De Brouwer, D., and Cornelissen, M. (2005). Poly(ADP-ribose) polymerase in plants affects energy homeostasis, cell death and stress tolerance. Plant J 41, 95-106.

Delmas, D., Aires, V., Limagne, E., Dutartre, P., Mazue, F., Ghiringhelli, F., and Latruffe, N. (2011). Transport, stability, and biological activity of resveratrol. Ann N Y Acad Sci 1215, 48-59.

Demple, B., and Harrison, L. (1994). Repair of oxidative damage to DNA: enzymology and biology. Annu Rev Biochem 63, 915-948.

Demple, B., Harrison, L., Wilson, D.M., 3rd, Bennett, R.A., Takagi, T., and Ascione, A.G. (1997). Regulation of eukaryotic abasic endonucleases and their role in genetic stability. Environ Health Perspect 105 Suppl 4, 931-934.

Devisetty, U.K., Mayes, K., and Mayes, S. (2010). The RAD51 and DMC1 homoeologous genes of bread wheat: cloning, molecular characterization and expression analysis. BMC Res Notes 3, 245.

Doucet-Chabeaud, G., Godon, C., Brutesco, C., de Murcia, G., and Kazmaier, M. (2001). Ionising radiation induces the expression of PARP-1 and PARP-2 genes in Arabidopsis. Mol Genet Genomics 265, 954-963.

Dray, E., Siaud, N., Dubois, E., and Doutriaux, M.P. (2006). Interaction between Arabidopsis Brca2 and its partners Rad51, Dmc1, and Dss1. Plant Physiol 140, 1059-1069.

Evans, E., Moggs, J.G., Hwang, J.R., Egly, J.M., and Wood, R.D. (1997). Mechanism of open complex and dual incision formation by human nucleotide excision repair factors. EMBO J 16, 6559-6573.

Falck, J., Coates, J., and Jackson, S.P. (2005). Conserved modes of recruitment of ATM, ATR and DNA-PKcs to sites of DNA damage. Nature 434, 605-611.

Farmer, L.M., Book, A.J., Lee, K.H., Lin, Y.L., Fu, H., and Vierstra, R.D. (2010). The RAD23 family provides an essential connection between the 26S proteasome and ubiquitylated proteins in Arabidopsis. Plant Cell 22, 124-142.

Fitch, M.E., Cross, I.V., Turner, S.J., Adimoolam, S., Lin, C.X., Williams, K.G., and Ford, J.M. (2003). The DDB2 nucleotide excision repair gene product p48 enhances global genomic repair in p53 deficient human fibroblasts. DNA Repair (Amst) 2, 819-826.

Fousteri, M., Vermeulen, W., van Zeeland, A.A., and Mullenders, L.H. (2006). Cockayne syndrome A and B proteins differentially regulate recruitment of chromatin remodeling and repair factors to stalled RNA polymerase II in vivo. Mol Cell 23, 471-482.

Foyer, C.H., and Noctor, G. (2003). Redox sensing and signalling associated with reactive oxygen in chloroplasts, peroxisomes and mitochondria Physiol Plant 119, 355-364.

Friedberg EC, Walker GC, Siede W, Wood RD, Schultz RA, and ., E.E. (2006). DNA repair and mutagenesis. (ASM Press, Washington, DC).

Friesner, J., and Britt, A.B. (2003). Ku80- and DNA ligase IV-deficient plants are sensitive to ionizing radiation and defective in T-DNA integration. Plant J 34, 427-440.

Fulcher, N., and Sablowski, R. (2009). Hypersensitivity to DNA damage in plant stem cell niches. Proc Natl Acad Sci U S A 106, 20984-20988.

Furukawa, T., Curtis, M.J., Tominey, C.M., Duong, Y.H., Wilcox, B.W., Aggoune, D., Hays, J.B., and Britt, A.B. (2010). A shared DNA-damage-response pathway for induction of stem-cell death by UVB and by gamma irradiation. DNA Repair (Amst) 9, 940-948.

Gallego, M.E., and White, C.I. (2001). RAD50 function is essential for telomere maintenance in Arabidopsis. Proc Natl Acad Sci U S A 98, 1711-1716.

Gallego, M.E., Bleuyard, J.Y., Daoudal-Cotterell, S., Jallut, N., and White, C.I. (2003). Ku80 plays a role in non-homologous recombination but is not required for T-DNA integration in Arabidopsis. Plant J 35, 557-565.

Garcia-Diaz, M., Dominguez, O., Lopez-Fernandez, L.A., de Lera, L.T., Saniger, M.L., Ruiz, J.F., Parraga, M., Garcia-Ortiz, M.J., Kirchhoff, T., del Mazo, J., Bernad, A., and Blanco, L. (2000). DNA polymerase lambda (Pol lambda), a novel eukaryotic DNA polymerase with a potential role in meiosis. J Mol Biol 301, 851-867.

Garcia-Ortiz, M.V., Ariza, R.R., and Roldan-Arjona, T. (2001). An OGG1 orthologue encoding a functional 8-oxoguanine DNA glycosylase/lyase in Arabidopsis thaliana. Plant Mol Biol 47, 795-804.

Garcia, V., Salanoubat, M., Choisne, N., and Tissier, A. (2000). An ATM homologue from Arabidopsis thaliana: complete genomic organisation and expression analysis. Nucleic Acids Res 28, 1692-1699.

Gatz, S.A., and Wiesmuller, L. (2006). p53 in recombination and repair. Cell Death Differ 13, 1003-1016.

Grawunder, U., Wilm, M., Wu, X., Kulesza, P., Wilson, T.E., Mann, M., and Lieber, M.R. (1997). Activity of DNA ligase IV stimulated by complex formation with XRCC4 protein in mammalian cells. Nature 388, 492-495.

Gray, W.M., Hellmann, H., Dharmasiri, S., and Estelle, M. (2002). Role of the Arabidopsis RING-H2 protein RBX1 in RUB modification and SCF function. Plant Cell 14, 2137-2144.

Green, C.M., and Almouzni, G. (2003). Local action of the chromatin assembly factor CAF-1 at sites of nucleotide excision repair in vivo. EMBO J 22, 5163-5174.

Groisman, R., Kuraoka, I., Chevallier, O., Gaye, N., Magnaldo, T., Tanaka, K., Kisselev, A.F., Harel-Bellan, A., and Nakatani, Y. (2006). CSA-dependent degradation of CSB by the ubiquitin-proteasome pathway establishes a link between complementation factors of the Cockayne syndrome. Genes Dev 20, 1429-1434.

Guay, D., Garand, C., Reddy, S., Schmutte, C., and Lebel, M. (2008). The human endonuclease III enzyme is a relevant target to potentiate cisplatin cytotoxicity in Y-box-binding protein-1 overexpressing tumor cells. Cancer Sci 99, 762-769.

Gutman, B.L., and Niyogi, K.K. (2009). Evidence for base excision repair of oxidative DNA damage in chloroplasts of Arabidopsis thaliana. J Biol Chem 284, 17006-17012.

Ha, H.C., and Snyder, S.H. (1999). Poly(ADP-ribose) polymerase is a mediator of necrotic cell death by ATP depletion. Proc Natl Acad Sci U S A 96, 13978-13982.

Harlow, G.R., Jenkins, M.E., Pittalwala, T.S., and Mount, D.W. (1994). Isolation of uvh1, an Arabidopsis mutant hypersensitive to ultraviolet light and ionizing radiation. Plant Cell 6, 227-235.

Hartung, F., and Puchta, H. (1999). Isolation of the Complete cDNA of the Mre11 Homologue of Arabidopsis (Accession No. AJ243822) Indicates Conservation of DNA Recombination Mechanisms Between Plants and Other Eucaryotes. Plant Physiol 121, 312.

Hatahet, Z., Kow, Y.W., Purmal, A.A., Cunningham, R.P., and Wallace, S.S. (1994). New substrates for old enzymes. 5-Hydroxy-2'-deoxycytidine and 5-hydroxy-2'-deoxyuridine are substrates for Escherichia coli endonuclease III and formamidopyrimidine DNA N-glycosylase, while 5-hydroxy-2'-deoxyuridine is a substrate for uracil DNA N-glycosylase. J Biol Chem 269, 18814-18820.

Hattori, Y., Nishigori, C., Tanaka, T., Uchida, K., Nikaido, O., Osawa, T., Hiai, H., Imamura, S., and Toyokuni, S. (1996). 8-hydroxy-2'-deoxyguanosine is increased in epidermal cells of hairless mice after chronic ultraviolet B exposure. J Invest Dermatol 107, 733-737.

Hazra, T.K., Hill, J.W., Izumi, T., and Mitra, S. (2001). Multiple DNA glycosylases for repair of 8-oxoguanine and their potential in vivo functions. Prog Nucleic Acid Res Mol Biol 68, 193-205.

Heacock, M., Spangler, E., Riha, K., Puizina, J., and Shippen, D.E. (2004). Molecular analysis of telomere fusions in Arabidopsis: multiple pathways for chromosome end-joining. EMBO J 23, 2304-2313.

Hidema, J., Taguchi, T., Ono, T., Teranishi, M., Yamamoto, K., and Kumagai, T. (2007). Increase in CPD photolyase activity functions effectively to prevent growth inhibition caused by UVB radiation. Plant J 50, 70-79.

Hitomi, K., DiTacchio, L., Arvai, A.S., Yamamoto, J., Kim, S.T., Todo, T., Tainer, J.A., Iwai, S., Panda, S., and Getzoff, E.D. (2009). Functional motifs in the (6-4) photolyase crystal structure make a comparative framework for DNA repair photolyases and clock cryptochromes. Proc Natl Acad Sci U S A 106, 6962-6967.

Huang, Y., Baxter, R., Smith, B.S., Partch, C.L., Colbert, C.L., and Deisenhofer, J. (2006). Crystal structure of cryptochrome 3 from Arabidopsis thaliana and its implications for photolyase activity. Proc Natl Acad Sci U S A 103, 17701-17706.

Iovine, B., Nino, M., Irace, C., Bevilacqua, M.A., and Monfrecola, G. (2009). Ultraviolet B and A irradiation induces fibromodulin expression in human fibroblasts in vitro. Biochimie 91, 364-372.

Ishibashi, T., Koga, A., Yamamoto, T., Uchiyama, Y., Mori, Y., Hashimoto, J., Kimura, S., and Sakaguchi, K. (2005). Two types of replication protein A in seed plants. FEBS J 272, 3270-3281.

Ishikawa, K., Ogawa, T., Hirosue, E., Nakayama, Y., Harada, K., Fukusaki, E., Yoshimura, K., and Shigeoka, S. (2009). Modulation of the poly(ADP-ribosyl)ation reaction via the Arabidopsis ADP-ribose/NADH pyrophosphohydrolase, AtNUDX7, is involved in the response to oxidative stress. Plant Physiol 151, 741-754.

Jaspers, P., and Kangasjarvi, J. (2010). Reactive oxygen species in abiotic stress signaling. Physiol Plant 138, 405-413.

Jenkins, M.E., Harlow, G.R., Liu, Z., Shotwell, M.A., Ma, J., and Mount, D.W. (1995). Radiation-sensitive mutants of Arabidopsis thaliana. Genetics 140, 725-732.

Jiang, C.Z., Yee, J., Mitchell, D.L., and Britt, A.B. (1997). Photorepair mutants of Arabidopsis. Proc Natl Acad Sci U S A 94, 7441-7445.

Kaiser, G., Kleiner, O., Beisswenger, C., and Batschauer, A. (2009). Increased DNA repair in Arabidopsis plants overexpressing CPD photolyase. Planta 230, 505-515.

Kamiuchi, S., Saijo, M., Citterio, E., de Jager, M., Hoeijmakers, J.H., and Tanaka, K. (2002). Translocation of Cockayne syndrome group A protein to the nuclear matrix: possible relevance to transcription-coupled DNA repair. Proc Natl Acad Sci U S A 99, 201-206.

Kanai, S., Kikuno, R., Toh, H., Ryo, H., and Todo, T. (1997). Molecular evolution of the photolyase-blue-light photoreceptor family. J Mol Evol 45, 535-548.

Kapetanaki, M.G., Guerrero-Santoro, J., Bisi, D.C., Hsieh, C.L., Rapic-Otrin, V., and Levine, A.S. (2006). The DDB1-CUL4ADDB2 ubiquitin ligase is deficient in xeroderma pigmentosum group E and targets histone H2A at UV-damaged DNA sites. Proc Natl Acad Sci U S A 103, 2588-2593.

Karanjawala, Z.E., Hsieh, C.L., and Lieber, M.R. (2003). Overexpression of Cu/Zn superoxide dismutase is lethal for mice lacking double-strand break repair. DNA Repair (Amst) 2, 285-294.

Karanjawala, Z.E., Murphy, N., Hinton, D.R., Hsieh, C.L., and Lieber, M.R. (2002). Oxygen metabolism causes chromosome breaks and is associated with the neuronal apoptosis observed in DNA double-strand break repair mutants. Curr Biol 12, 397-402.

Kesseler, K.J., Kaufmann, W.K., Reardon, J.T., Elston, T.C., and Sancar, A. (2007). A mathematical model for human nucleotide excision repair: damage recognition by random order assembly and kinetic proofreading. J Theor Biol 249, 361-375.

Khazi, F.R., Edmondson, A.C., and Nielsen, B.L. (2003). An Arabidopsis homologue of bacterial RecA that complements an E. coli recA deletion is targeted to plant mitochondria. Mol Genet Genomics 269, 454-463.

Kimura, S., and Sakaguchi, K. (2006). DNA repair in plants. Chem Rev 106, 753-766.

Kimura, S., Saotome, A., Uchiyama, Y., Mori, Y., Tahira, Y., and Sakaguchi, K. (2005). The expression of the rice (Oryza sativa L.) homologue of Snm1 is induced by DNA damages. Biochem Biophys Res Commun 329, 668-672.

Kimura, S., Tahira, Y., Ishibashi, T., Mori, Y., Mori, T., Hashimoto, J., and Sakaguchi, K. (2004). DNA repair in higher plants; photoreactivation is the major DNA repair pathway in non-proliferating cells while excision repair (nucleotide excision repair and base excision repair) is active in proliferating cells. Nucleic Acids Res 32, 2760-2767.

Ko, J.C., Su, Y.J., Lin, S.T., Jhan, J.Y., Ciou, S.C., Cheng, C.M., and Lin, Y.W. (2010). Suppression of ERCC1 and Rad51 expression through ERK1/2 inactivation is essential in emodin-mediated cytotoxicity in human non-small cell lung cancer cells. Biochem Pharmacol 79, 655-664.

Ko, J.C., Tsai, M.S., Kuo, Y.H., Chiu, Y.F., Weng, S.H., Su, Y.C., and Lin, Y.W. (2011). Modulation of Rad51, ERCC1, and thymidine phosphorylase by emodin result in synergistic cytotoxic effect in combination with capecitabine. Biochem Pharmacol 81, 680-690.

Koga, A., Ishibashi, T., Kimura, S., Uchiyama, Y., and Sakaguchi, K. (2006). Characterization of T-DNA insertion mutants and RNAi silenced plants of Arabidopsis thaliana UV-damaged DNA binding protein 2 (AtUV-DDB2). Plant Mol Biol 61, 227-240.

Krasikova, Y.S., Rechkunova, N.I., Maltseva, E.A., Petruseva, I.O., Silnikov, V.N., Zatsepin, T.S., Oretskaya, T.S., Scharer, O.D., and Lavrik, O.I. (2008). Interaction of nucleotide excision repair factors XPC-HR23B, XPA, and RPA with damaged DNA. Biochemistry (Mosc) 73, 886-896.

Kraszewska, E. (2008). The plant Nudix hydrolase family. Acta Biochim Pol 55, 663-671.

Krieger-Liszkay, A. (2005). Singlet oxygen production in photosynthesis. J Exp Bot 56, 337 - 346.

Krokan, H.E., Standal, R., and Slupphaug, G. (1997). DNA glycosylases in the base excision repair of DNA. Biochem J 325 ( Pt 1), 1-16.

Kruger, A., and Ralser, M. (2011). ATM Is a Redox Sensor Linking Genome Stability and Carbon Metabolism. Sci Signal 4, pe17.

Kunz, B.A., Anderson, H.J., Osmond, M.J., and Vonarx, E.J. (2005). Components of nucleotide excision repair and DNA damage tolerance in Arabidopsis thaliana. Environ Mol Mutagen 45, 115-127.

Kwon, T., Huq, E., and Herrin, D.L. (2010). Microhomology-mediated and nonhomologous repair of a double-strand break in the chloroplast genome of Arabidopsis. Proc Natl Acad Sci U S A 107, 13954-13959.

Lafarge, S., and Montane, M.H. (2003). Characterization of Arabidopsis thaliana ortholog of the human breast cancer susceptibility gene 1: AtBRCA1, strongly induced by gamma rays. Nucleic Acids Res 31, 1148-1155.

Landry, L.G., Stapleton, A.E., Lim, J., Hoffman, P., Hays, J.B., Walbot, V., and Last, R.L. (1997). An Arabidopsis photolyase mutant is hypersensitive to ultraviolet-B radiation. Proc Natl Acad Sci U S A 94, 328-332.

Langcake, P., and Pryce, R.J. (1977). The production of resveratrol and the viniferins by grapevines in response to UV radiation. Phytochemistry 16, 1193-1196.

Lechner, E., Xie, D., Grava, S., Pigaglio, E., Planchais, S., Murray, J.A., Parmentier, Y., Mutterer, J., Dubreucq, B., Shen, W.H., and Genschik, P. (2002). The AtRbx1 protein is part of plant SCF complexes, and its down-regulation causes severe growth and developmental defects. J Biol Chem 277, 50069-50080.

Lepiniec, L., Babiychuk, E., Kushnir, S., Van Montagu, M., and Inze, D. (1995). Characterization of an Arabidopsis thaliana cDNA homologue to animal poly(ADP-ribose) polymerase. FEBS Lett 364, 103-108.

Li, J., Liu, Z., Tan, C., Guo, X., Wang, L., Sancar, A., and Zhong, D. (2010). Dynamics and mechanism of repair of ultraviolet-induced (6-4) photoproduct by photolyase. Nature 466, 887-890.

Li, J., Harper, L.C., Golubovskaya, I., Wang, C.R., Weber, D., Meeley, R.B., McElver, J., Bowen, B., Cande, W.Z., and Schnable, P.S. (2007). Functional analysis of maize RAD51 in meiosis and double-strand break repair. Genetics 176, 1469-1482.

Li, W., and Ma, H. (2006). Double-stranded DNA breaks and gene functions in recombination and meiosis. Cell Res 16, 402-412.

Liang, L., Flury, S., Kalck, V., Hohn, B., and Molinier, J. (2006). CENTRIN2 interacts with the Arabidopsis homolog of the human XPC protein (AtRAD4) and contributes to efficient synthesis-dependent repair of bulky DNA lesions. Plant Mol Biol 61, 345-356.

Lin, Z., Kong, H., Nei, M., and Ma, H. (2006). Origins and evolution of the recA/RAD51 gene family: evidence for ancient gene duplication and endosymbiotic gene transfer. Proc Natl Acad Sci U S A 103, 10328-10333.

Lindahl, T. (1993). Instability and decay of the primary structure of DNA. Nature 362, 709-715.

Liu, Z., Hossain, G.S., Islas-Osuna, M.A., Mitchell, D.L., and Mount, D.W. (2000). Repair of UV damage in plants by nucleotide excision repair: Arabidopsis UVH1 DNA repair gene is a homolog of Saccharomyces cerevisiae Rad1. Plant J 21, 519-528.

Liu, Z., Hong, S.W., Escobar, M., Vierling, E., Mitchell, D.L., Mount, D.W., and Hall, J.D. (2003). Arabidopsis UVH6, a homolog of human XPD and yeast RAD3 DNA repair genes, functions in DNA repair and is essential for plant growth. Plant Physiol 132, 1405-1414.

Ma, Y., Pannicke, U., Schwarz, K., and Lieber, M.R. (2002). Hairpin opening and overhang processing by an Artemis/DNA-dependent protein kinase complex in nonhomologous end joining and V(D)J recombination. Cell 108, 781-794.

Maltseva, E.A., Rechkunova, N.I., Petruseva, I.O., Silnikov, V.N., Vermeulen, W., and Lavrik, O.I. (2006). Interaction of nucleotide excision repair factors RPA and XPA with DNA containing bulky photoreactive groups imitating damages. Biochemistry (Mosc) 71, 270-278.

Mannuss, A., Dukowic-Schulze, S., Suer, S., Hartung, F., Pacher, M., and Puchta, H. (2010). RAD5A, RECQ4A, and MUS81 have specific functions in homologous recombination and define different pathways of DNA repair in Arabidopsis thaliana. Plant Cell 22, 3318-3330.

Markmann-Mulisch, U., Wendeler, E., Zobell, O., Schween, G., Steinbiss, H.H., and Reiss, B. (2007). Differential requirements for RAD51 in Physcomitrella patens and Arabidopsis thaliana development and DNA damage repair. Plant Cell 19, 3080-3089.

Masson, M., Niedergang, C., Schreiber, V., Muller, S., Menissier-de Murcia, J., and de Murcia, G. (1998). XRCC1 is specifically associated with poly(ADP-ribose) polymerase and negatively regulates its activity following DNA damage. Mol Cell Biol 18, 3563-3571.

Matsumoto, Y. (2001). Molecular mechanism of PCNA-dependent base excision repair. Prog Nucleic Acid Res Mol Biol 68, 129-138.

McLennan, A.G. (2006). The Nudix hydrolase superfamily. Cell Mol Life Sci 63, 123-143.

Min, J.H., and Pavletich, N.P. (2007). Recognition of DNA damage by the Rad4 nucleotide excision repair protein. Nature 449, 570-575.

Minig, V., Kattan, Z., van Beeumen, J., Brunner, E., and Becuwe, P. (2009). Identification of DDB2 protein as a transcriptional regulator of constitutive SOD2 gene expression in human breast cancer cells. J Biol Chem 284, 14165-14176.

Moldt, J., Pokorny, R., Orth, C., Linne, U., Geisselbrecht, Y., Marahiel, M.A., Essen, L.O., and Batschauer, A. (2009). Photoreduction of the folate cofactor in members of the photolyase family. J Biol Chem 284, 21670-21683.

Molinier, J., Stamm, M.E., and Hohn, B. (2004a). SNM-dependent recombinational repair of oxidatively induced DNA damage in Arabidopsis thaliana. EMBO Rep 5, 994-999.

Molinier, J., Ramos, C., Fritsch, O., and Hohn, B. (2004b). CENTRIN2 modulates homologous recombination and nucleotide excision repair in Arabidopsis. Plant Cell 16, 1633-1643.

Molinier, J., Lechner, E., Dumbliauskas, E., and Genschik, P. (2008). Regulation and role of Arabidopsis CUL4-DDB1A-DDB2 in maintaining genome integrity upon UV stress. PLoS Genet 4, e1000093.

Molinier, J., Oakeley, E.J., Niederhauser, O., Kovalchuk, I., and Hohn, B. (2005). Dynamic response of plant genome to ultraviolet radiation and other genotoxic stresses. Mutat Res 571, 235-247.

Morales-Ruiz, T., Birincioglu, M., Jaruga, P., Rodriguez, H., Roldan-Arjona, T., and Dizdaroglu, M. (2003). Arabidopsis thaliana Ogg1 protein excises 8-hydroxyguanine and 2,6-diamino-4-hydroxy-5-formamidopyrimidine from oxidatively damaged DNA containing multiple lesions. Biochemistry 42, 3089-3095.

Morgante, P.G., Berra, C.M., Nakabashi, M., Costa, R.M., Menck, C.F., and Van Sluys, M.A. (2005). Functional XPB/RAD25 redundancy in Arabidopsis genome: characterization of AtXPB2 and expression analysis. Gene 344, 93-103.

Morland, I., Rolseth, V., Luna, L., Rognes, T., Bjoras, M., and Seeberg, E. (2002). Human DNA glycosylases of the bacterial Fpg/MutM superfamily: an alternative pathway for the repair of 8-oxoguanine and other oxidation products in DNA. Nucleic Acids Res 30, 4926-4936.

Moser, J., Volker, M., Kool, H., Alekseev, S., Vrieling, H., Yasui, A., van Zeeland, A.A., and Mullenders, L.H. (2005). The UV-damaged DNA binding protein mediates efficient targeting of the nucleotide excision repair complex to UV-induced photo lesions. DNA Repair (Amst) 4, 571-582.

Mu, D., Hsu, D.S., and Sancar, A. (1996). Reaction mechanism of human DNA repair excision nuclease. J Biol Chem 271, 8285-8294.

Mu, D., Park, C.H., Matsunaga, T., Hsu, D.S., Reardon, J.T., and Sancar, A. (1995). Reconstitution of human DNA repair excision nuclease in a highly defined system. J Biol Chem 270, 2415-2418.

Murphy, T.M., and Gao, M.J. (2001). Multiple forms of formamidopyrimidine-DNA glycosylase produced by alternative splicing in Arabidopsis thaliana. J Photochem Photobiol B 61, 87-93.

Nakajima, S., Sugiyama, M., Iwai, S., Hitomi, K., Otoshi, E., Kim, S.T., Jiang, C.Z., Todo, T., Britt, A.B., and Yamamoto, K. (1998). Cloning and characterization of a gene (UVR3) required for photorepair of 6-4 photoproducts in Arabidopsis thaliana. Nucleic Acids Res 26, 638-644.

Nakazato, E., Fukuzawa, H., Tabata, S., Takahashi, H., and Tanaka, K. (2003). Identification and expression analysis of cDNA encoding a chloroplast recombination protein REC1, the chloroplast RecA homologue in Chlamydomonas reinhardtii. Biosci Biotechnol Biochem 67, 2608-2613.

Ndebele, K., Graham, B., and Tchounwou, P.B. (2010). Estrogenic activity of coumestrol, DDT, and TCDD in human cervical cancer cells. Int J Environ Res Public Health 7, 2045-2056.

Ng, Y.L., Thimann, K.V., and Gordon, S.A. (1964 ). The biogenesis of anthocyanins. X. The action spectrum for anthocyanin formation in *Spirodela oligorrhiza*. Arch Biochem Biophys 107, 550-558.

Nichols, A.F., and Sancar, A. (1992). Purification of PCNA as a nucleotide excision repair protein. Nucleic Acids Res 20, 2441-2446.

Noctor, G., Veljovic-Jovanovic, S., Driscoll, S., Novitskaya, L., and Foyer, C.H. (2002). Drought and oxidative load in the leaves of C3 plants: a predominant role for photorespiration? Ann Bot 89 Spec No, 841-850.

Odahara, M., Kuroiwa, H., Kuroiwa, T., and Sekine, Y. (2009). Suppression of repeat-mediated gross mitochondrial genome rearrangements by RecA in the moss Physcomitrella patens. Plant Cell 21, 1182-1194.

Odahara, M., Inouye, T., Fujita, T., Hasebe, M., and Sekine, Y. (2007). Involvement of mitochondrial-targeted RecA in the repair of mitochondrial DNA in the moss, Physcomitrella patens. Genes Genet Syst 82, 43-51.

Ogawa, T., Ueda, Y., Yoshimura, K., and Shigeoka, S. (2005). Comprehensive analysis of cytosolic Nudix hydrolases in Arabidopsis thaliana. J Biol Chem 280, 25277-25283.

Ogi, T., Limsirichaikul, S., Overmeer, R.M., Volker, M., Takenaka, K., Cloney, R., Nakazawa, Y., Niimi, A., Miki, Y., Jaspers, N.G., Mullenders, L.H., Yamashita, S., Fousteri, M.I., and Lehmann, A.R. (2010). Three DNA polymerases, recruited by different mechanisms, carry out NER repair synthesis in human cells. Mol Cell 37, 714-727.

Ohtsubo, T., Matsuda, O., Iba, K., Terashima, I., Sekiguchi, M., and Nakabeppu, Y. (1998). Molecular cloning of AtMMH, an Arabidopsis thaliana ortholog of the Escherichia coli mutM gene, and analysis of functional domains of its product. Mol Gen Genet 259, 577-590.

Okafuji, A., Biskup, T., Hitomi, K., Getzoff, E.D., Kaiser, G., Batschauer, A., Bacher, A., Hidema, J., Teranishi, M., Yamamoto, K., Schleicher, E., and Weber, S. (2010). Light-induced activation of class II cyclobutane pyrimidine dimer photolyases. DNA Repair (Amst) 9, 495-505.

Osman, K., Higgins, J.D., Sanchez-Moran, E., Armstrong, S.J., and Franklin, F.C. (2011). Pathways to meiotic recombination in Arabidopsis thaliana. New Phytol.

Ozturk, N., Kao, Y.T., Selby, C.P., Kavakli, I.H., Partch, C.L., Zhong, D., and Sancar, A. (2008). Purification and characterization of a type III photolyase from Caulobacter crescentus. Biochemistry 47, 10255-10261.

Pang, Q., Hays, J.B., and Rajagopal, I. (1992). A plant cDNA that partially complements Escherichia coli recA mutations predicts a polypeptide not strongly homologous to RecA proteins. Proc Natl Acad Sci U S A 89, 8073-8077.

Pang, Q., Hays, J.B., Rajagopal, I., and Schaefer, T.S. (1993). Selection of Arabidopsis cDNAs that partially correct phenotypes of Escherichia coli DNA-damage-sensitive mutants and analysis of two plant cDNAs that appear to express UV-specific dark repair activities. Plant Mol Biol 22, 411-426.

Parsons, J.L., Zharkov, D.O., and Dianov, G.L. (2005). NEIL1 excises 3' end proximal oxidative DNA lesions resistant to cleavage by NTH1 and OGG1. Nucleic Acids Res 33, 4849-4856.

Pascucci, B., Maga, G., Hubscher, U., Bjoras, M., Seeberg, E., Hickson, I.D., Villani, G., Giordano, C., Cellai, L., and Dogliotti, E. (2002). Reconstitution of the base excision repair pathway for 7,8-dihydro-8-oxoguanine with purified human proteins. Nucleic Acids Res 30, 2124-2130.

Perry, J.J., and Tainer, J.A. (2011). All Stressed Out Without ATM Kinase. Sci Signal 4, pe18.

Petersen, J.L., Lang, D.W., and Small, G.D. (1999). Cloning and characterization of a class II DNA photolyase from Chlamydomonas. Plant Mol Biol 40, 1063-1071.

Petrucco, S., Volpi, G., Bolchi, A., Rivetti, C., and Ottonello, S. (2002). A nick-sensing DNA 3'-repair enzyme from Arabidopsis. J Biol Chem 277, 23675-23683.

Phadnis, N., Mehta, R., Meednu, N., and Sia, E.A. (2006). Ntg1p, the base excision repair protein, generates mutagenic intermediates in yeast mitochondrial DNA. DNA Repair (Amst) 5, 829-839.

Pleschke, J.M., Kleczkowska, H.E., Strohm, M., and Althaus, F.R. (2000). Poly(ADP-ribose) binds to specific domains in DNA damage checkpoint proteins. J Biol Chem 275, 40974-40980.

Poirier, G.G., de Murcia, G., Jongstra-Bilen, J., Niedergang, C., and Mandel, P. (1982). Poly(ADP-ribosyl)ation of polynucleosomes causes relaxation of chromatin structure. Proc Natl Acad Sci U S A 79, 3423-3427.

Preuss, S.B., and Britt, A.B. (2003). A DNA-damage-induced cell cycle checkpoint in Arabidopsis. Genetics 164, 323-334.

Puchta, H. (2005). The repair of double-strand breaks in plants: mechanisms and consequences for genome evolution. J Exp Bot 56, 1-14.

Puchta, H., Swoboda, P., Gal, S., Blot, M., and Hohn, B. (1995). Somatic intrachromosomal homologous recombination events in populations of plant siblings. Plant Mol Biol 28, 281-292.

Rapic-Otrin, V., McLenigan, M.P., Bisi, D.C., Gonzalez, M., and Levine, A.S. (2002). Sequential binding of UV DNA damage binding factor and degradation of the p48 subunit as early events after UV irradiation. Nucleic Acids Res 30, 2588-2598.

Reardon, J.T., and Sancar, A. (2003). Recognition and repair of the cyclobutane thymine dimer, a major cause of skin cancers, by the human excision nuclease. Genes Dev 17, 2539-2551.

Ricaud, L., Proux, C., Renou, J.P., Pichon, O., Fochesato, S., Ortet, P., and Montane, M.H. (2007). ATM-mediated transcriptional and developmental responses to gamma-rays in Arabidopsis. PLoS One 2, e430.

Riha, K., Watson, J.M., Parkey, J., and Shippen, D.E. (2002). Telomere length deregulation and enhanced sensitivity to genotoxic stress in Arabidopsis mutants deficient in Ku70. EMBO J 21, 2819-2826.

Roldan-Arjona, T., and Ariza, R.R. (2009). Repair and tolerance of oxidative DNA damage in plants. Mutat Res 681, 169-179.

Roldan-Arjona, T., Garcia-Ortiz, M.V., Ruiz-Rubio, M., and Ariza, R.R. (2000). cDNA cloning, expression and functional characterization of an Arabidopsis thaliana homologue of the Escherichia coli DNA repair enzyme endonuclease III. Plant Mol Biol 44, 43-52.

Ronceret, A., Doutriaux, M.P., Golubovskaya, I.N., and Pawlowski, W.P. (2009). PHS1 regulates meiotic recombination and homologous chromosome pairing by controlling the transport of RAD50 to the nucleus. Proc Natl Acad Sci U S A 106, 20121-20126.

Rowan, B.A., Oldenburg, D.J., and Bendich, A.J. (2010). RecA maintains the integrity of chloroplast DNA molecules in Arabidopsis. J Exp Bot 61, 2575-2588.

Roy, N., Stoyanova, T., Dominguez-Brauer, C., Park, H.J., Bagchi, S., and Raychaudhuri, P. (2010). DDB2, an essential mediator of premature senescence. Mol Cell Biol 30, 2681-2692.

Schaefer, D.G., Delacote, F., Charlot, F., Vrielynck, N., Guyon-Debast, A., Le Guin, S., Neuhaus, J.M., Doutriaux, M.P., and Nogue, F. (2010). RAD51 loss of function abolishes gene targeting and de-represses illegitimate integration in the moss Physcomitrella patens. DNA Repair (Amst) 9, 526-533.

Scrima, A., Konickova, R., Czyzewski, B.K., Kawasaki, Y., Jeffrey, P.D., Groisman, R., Nakatani, Y., Iwai, S., Pavletich, N.P., and Thoma, N.H. (2008). Structural basis of UV DNA-damage recognition by the DDB1-DDB2 complex. Cell 135, 1213-1223.

Selby, C.P., and Sancar, A. (1997). Cockayne syndrome group B protein enhances elongation by RNA polymerase II. Proc Natl Acad Sci U S A 94, 11205-11209.

Shaked, H., Avivi-Ragolsky, N., and Levy, A.A. (2006). Involvement of the Arabidopsis SWI2/SNF2 chromatin remodeling gene family in DNA damage response and recombination. Genetics 173, 985-994.

Shedge, V., Arrieta-Montiel, M., Christensen, A.C., and Mackenzie, S.A. (2007). Plant mitochondrial recombination surveillance requires unusual RecA and MutS homologs. Plant Cell 19, 1251-1264.

Shivji, K.K., Kenny, M.K., and Wood, R.D. (1992). Proliferating cell nuclear antigen is required for DNA excision repair. Cell 69, 367-374.

Siaud, N., Dray, E., Gy, I., Gerard, E., Takvorian, N., and Doutriaux, M.P. (2004). Brca2 is involved in meiosis in Arabidopsis thaliana as suggested by its interaction with Dmc1. EMBO J 23, 1392-1401.

Singh, S.K., Roy, S., Choudhury, S.R., and Sengupta, D.N. (2010). DNA repair and recombination in higher plants: insights from comparative genomics of Arabidopsis and rice. BMC Genomics 11, 443.

Strzalka, W., Oyama, T., Tori, K., and Morikawa, K. (2009). Crystal structures of the Arabidopsis thaliana proliferating cell nuclear antigen 1 and 2 proteins complexed with the human p21 C-terminal segment. Protein Sci 18, 1072-1080.

Subramanian, D., and Griffith, J.D. (2005). Modulation of p53 binding to Holliday junctions and 3-cytosine bulges by phosphorylation events. Biochemistry 44, 2536-2544.

Sugasawa, K., Okuda, Y., Saijo, M., Nishi, R., Matsuda, N., Chu, G., Mori, T., Iwai, S., Tanaka, K., and Hanaoka, F. (2005). UV-induced ubiquitylation of XPC protein mediated by UV-DDB-ubiquitin ligase complex. Cell 121, 387-400.

Takahashi, M., Teranishi, M., Ishida, H., Kawasaki, J., Takeuchi, A., Yamaya, T., Watanabe, M., Makino, A., and Hidema, J. (2011). Cyclobutane pyrimidine dimer (CPD) photolyase repairs ultraviolet-B-induced CPDs in rice chloroplast and mitochondrial DNA. Plant J.

Takeda, J., and Abe, S. (1992). Light-induced synthesis of anthocyanin in carrot cells in suspension. IV. The action spectrum. Photochem Photobiol 56, 69-74.

Tamura, K., Adachi, Y., Chiba, K., Oguchi, K., and Takahashi, H. (2002). Identification of Ku70 and Ku80 homologues in Arabidopsis thaliana: evidence for a role in the repair of DNA double-strand breaks. Plant J 29, 771-781.

Taylor, R.M., Thistlethwaite, A., and Caldecott, K.W. (2002). Central role for the XRCC1 BRCT I domain in mammalian DNA single-strand break repair. Mol Cell Biol 22, 2556-2563.

Taylor, R.M., Hamer, M.J., Rosamond, J., and Bray, C.M. (1998). Molecular cloning and functional analysis of the Arabidopsis thaliana DNA ligase I homologue. Plant J 14, 75-81.

Tchou, J., Michaels, M.L., Miller, J.H., and Grollman, A.P. (1993). Function of the zinc finger in Escherichia coli Fpg protein. J Biol Chem 268, 26738-26744.

Tchou, J., Kasai, H., Shibutani, S., Chung, M.H., Laval, J., Grollman, A.P., and Nishimura, S. (1991). 8-oxoguanine (8-hydroxyguanine) DNA glycosylase and its substrate specificity. Proc Natl Acad Sci U S A 88, 4690-4694.

Teranishi, M., Iwamatsu, Y., Hidema, J., and Kumagai, T. (2004). Ultraviolet-B sensitivities in Japanese lowland rice cultivars: cyclobutane pyrimidine dimer photolyase activity and gene mutation. Plant Cell Physiol 45, 1848-1856.

Teranishi, M., Nakamura, K., Morioka, H., Yamamoto, K., and Hidema, J. (2008). The native cyclobutane pyrimidine dimer photolyase of rice is phosphorylated. Plant Physiol 146, 1941-1951.

Thoma, B.S., and Vasquez, K.M. (2003). Critical DNA damage recognition functions of XPC-hHR23B and XPA-RPA in nucleotide excision repair. Mol Carcinog 38, 1-13.

Tibbetts, R.S., Brumbaugh, K.M., Williams, J.M., Sarkaria, J.N., Cliby, W.A., Shieh, S.Y., Taya, Y., Prives, C., and Abraham, R.T. (1999). A role for ATR in the DNA damage-induced phosphorylation of p53. Genes Dev 13, 152-157.

Tissier, A.F., Lopez, M.F., and Signer, E.R. (1995). Purification and characterization of a DNA strand transferase from broccoli. Plant Physiol 108, 379-386.

Tornaletti, S., and Hanawalt, P.C. (1999). Effect of DNA lesions on transcription elongation. Biochimie 81, 139-146.

Triantaphylides, C., and Havaux, M. (2009). Singlet oxygen in plants: production, detoxification and signaling. Trends Plant Sci 14, 219-228.

Tuteja, N., and Tuteja, R. (2001). Unraveling DNA repair in human: molecular mechanisms and consequences of repair defect. Crit Rev Biochem Mol Biol 36, 261-290.

Tuteja, N., Singh, M.B., Misra, M.K., Bhalla, P.L., and Tuteja, R. (2001). Molecular mechanisms of DNA damage and repair: progress in plants. Crit Rev Biochem Mol Biol 36, 337-397.

Uchiyama, Y., Kimura, S., Yamamoto, T., Ishibashi, T., and Sakaguchi, K. (2004). Plant DNA polymerase lambda, a DNA repair enzyme that functions in plant meristematic and meiotic tissues. Eur J Biochem 271, 2799-2807.

van Gool, A.J., Citterio, E., Rademakers, S., van Os, R., Vermeulen, W., Constantinou, A., Egly, J.M., Bootsma, D., and Hoeijmakers, J.H. (1997). The Cockayne syndrome B protein, involved in transcription-coupled DNA repair, resides in an RNA polymerase II-containing complex. EMBO J 16, 5955-5965.

Vidal, A.E., Boiteux, S., Hickson, I.D., and Radicella, J.P. (2001). XRCC1 coordinates the initial and late stages of DNA abasic site repair through protein-protein interactions. EMBO J 20, 6530-6539.

Vignard, J., Siwiec, T., Chelysheva, L., Vrielynck, N., Gonord, F., Armstrong, S.J., Schlogelhofer, P., and Mercier, R. (2007). The interplay of RecA-related proteins and the MND1-HOP2 complex during meiosis in Arabidopsis thaliana. PLoS Genet 3, 1894-1906.

Vigneron, A., and Vousden, K.H. (2010). p53, ROS and senescence in the control of aging. Aging (Albany NY) 2, 471-474.

Vinocur, B., and Altman, A. (2005). Recent advances in engineering plant tolerance to abiotic stress: achievements and limitations. Curr Opin Biotechnol 16, 123-132.

Virag, L., and Szabo, C. (2002). The therapeutic potential of poly(ADP-ribose) polymerase inhibitors. Pharmacol Rev 54, 375-429.

Wang, H., Zhai, L., Xu, J., Joo, H.Y., Jackson, S., Erdjument-Bromage, H., Tempst, P., Xiong, Y., and Zhang, Y. (2006). Histone H3 and H4 ubiquitylation by the CUL4-DDB-

ROC1 ubiquitin ligase facilitates cellular response to DNA damage. Mol Cell 22, 383-394.

Wang, S., Durrant, W.E., Song, J., Spivey, N.W., and Dong, X. (2010). Arabidopsis BRCA2 and RAD51 proteins are specifically involved in defense gene transcription during plant immune responses. Proc Natl Acad Sci U S A 107, 22716-22721.

Warmerdam, D.O., Kanaar, R., and Smits, V.A. (2010). Differential Dynamics of ATR-Mediated Checkpoint Regulators. J Nucleic Acids 2010.

Waterworth, W.M., Jiang, Q., West, C.E., Nikaido, M., and Bray, C.M. (2002). Characterization of Arabidopsis photolyase enzymes and analysis of their role in protection from ultraviolet-B radiation. J Exp Bot 53, 1005-1015.

Waterworth, W.M., Masnavi, G., Bhardwaj, R.M., Jiang, Q., Bray, C.M., and West, C.E. (2010). A plant DNA ligase is an important determinant of seed longevity. Plant J 63, 848-860.

Waterworth, W.M., Altun, C., Armstrong, S.J., Roberts, N., Dean, P.J., Young, K., Weil, C.F., Bray, C.M., and West, C.E. (2007). NBS1 is involved in DNA repair and plays a synergistic role with ATM in mediating meiotic homologous recombination in plants. Plant J 52, 41-52.

West, C.E., Waterworth, W.M., Jiang, Q., and Bray, C.M. (2000). Arabidopsis DNA ligase IV is induced by gamma-irradiation and interacts with an Arabidopsis homologue of the double strand break repair protein XRCC4. Plant J 24, 67-78.

Wiseman, H., and Halliwell, B. (1996). Damage to DNA by reactive oxygen and nitrogen species: role in inflammatory disease and progression to cancer. Biochem J 313 ( Pt 1), 17-29.

Wright, J.A., Keegan, K.S., Herendeen, D.R., Bentley, N.J., Carr, A.M., Hoekstra, M.F., and Concannon, P. (1998). Protein kinase mutants of human ATR increase sensitivity to UV and ionizing radiation and abrogate cell cycle checkpoint control. Proc Natl Acad Sci U S A 95, 7445-7450.

Yamamoto, F., Nishimura, S., and Kasai, H. (1992). Photosensitized formation of 8-hydroxydeoxyguanosine in cellular DNA by riboflavin. Biochem Biophys Res Commun 187, 809-813.

Yang, Z., Roginskaya, M., Colis, L.C., Basu, A.K., Shell, S.M., Liu, Y., Musich, P.R., Harris, C.M., Harris, T.M., and Zou, Y. (2006). Specific and efficient binding of xeroderma pigmentosum complementation group A to double-strand/single-strand DNA junctions with 3'- and/or 5'-ssDNA branches. Biochemistry 45, 15921-15930.

Yatsuhashi, H., Hashimoto, T., and Shimizu, S. (1982). Ultraviolet action spectrum for anthocyanin formation in broom sorghum first internodes. Plant Physiol 70, 735-741.

Ye, J., Meng, X., Yan, C., and Wang, C. (2010). Effect of purple sweet potato anthocyanins on beta-amyloid-mediated PC-12 cells death by inhibition of oxidative stress. Neurochem Res 35, 357-365.

Yoshiyama, K., Conklin, P.A., Huefner, N.D., and Britt, A.B. (2009). Suppressor of gamma response 1 (SOG1) encodes a putative transcription factor governing multiple responses to DNA damage. Proc Natl Acad Sci U S A 106, 12843-12848.

Zhang, C., Guo, H., Zhang, J., Guo, G., Schumaker, K.S., and Guo, Y. (2010). Arabidopsis cockayne syndrome A-like proteins 1A and 1B form a complex with CULLIN4 and damage DNA binding protein 1A and regulate the response to UV irradiation. Plant Cell 22, 2353-2369.

Zhang, Y., and Schroeder, D.F. (2010). Effect of overexpression of Arabidopsis damaged DNA-binding protein 1A on de-etiolated 1. Planta 231, 337-348.

# 11

# DNA Damage Protection and Induction of Repair by Dietary Phytochemicals and Cancer Prevention: What Do We Know?

Alice A. Ramos[1], Cristóvão F. Lima[2] and Cristina Pereira-Wilson[1]
[1]*CBMA – Molecular and Environmental Biology Centre*
[2]*CITAB – Centre for the Research and Technology of Agro-Environmental and Biological Sciences*
*Department of Biology, School of Sciences, University of Minho, Campus de Gualtar, Braga, Portugal*

## 1. Introduction

DNA damage accumulates in cells over time as a result of exposure to a variety of exogenous and endogenous agents. These damages, if not repaired properly, can generate mutations in somatic or germline cells, which are involved in the pathogenesis of many diseases, such as cancer. To maintain genomic integrity generation after generation, organisms possess multiple mechanisms such as inhibition of carcinogen uptake into the cells, induction of detoxification enzymes, increased cellular defenses that prevent DNA damage, enhancement of DNA repair, increased anti-inflammatory activity, inhibition of cell proliferation, and modulation of apoptosis through effects on signal transduction pathways (de Kok *et al.*, 2008); (Pan *et al.*, 2008). In the last decades, several dietary constituents have been shown to modulate all these processes. Epidemiological studies as well as laboratory data suggest that consumption of fruits and vegetables is associated with a reduced risk of developing a wide range of cancers. It has been estimated that 30-40% of all tumours can be prevented with a correct lifestyle and diet, in particular colon cancer (Rajamanickam and Agarwal, 2008). Multiple mechanisms have been proposed to explain the chemopreventive effects of phytochemicals. Protection of DNA from damage and modulation of DNA repair assume an important role on prevention of mutations and consequently of the carcinogenic process. The comet assay or single cell gel electrophoresis (SCGE) assay is a rapid, sensitive and relatively simple method for assessing DNA damage and its repair in individual cells. The standard comet assay measures DNA breaks and alkali-labile sites that are converted to strand breaks. With its widespread use, several modifications on the comet assay have been made that allow the quantification of other types of DNA damage as well as DNA repair rates. With the inclusion of an extra step on the comet assay by using specific DNA repair enzymes, different base lesions can be identified by the introduction of breaks at sites of base damage. In this regard, Endonuclease III, FPG and AlkA have been used to detect oxidized pyrimidines, modified purines and alkylpurines bases, respectively. With these modifications the comet assay can be used to estimate oxidative and alkylating DNA damage. Cells' DNA repair capacity can also be measured by using modified protocols of the comet assay, such as following the repair kinetics by the cellular repair assay, or in vitro by using cellular substrates with specific damages to measure base excision repair (BER) and nucleotide excision repair (NER) (Collins *et al.*, 2001b; Collins, 2004). These different modifications of the comet assay have been successfully used to evaluate the chemopreventive potential of several phytochemicals present in our diet. In this review, we will show evidence that dietary agents can protect DNA from oxidative and alkylating agents as well modulate DNA repair in eukaryotic cells, by using the comet assay. Data from different experimental systems, including primary cell cultures, human cell lines, animal models and human biomonitoring studies, will be discussed in order to provide an overview of effects of dietary phytochemicals on DNA damage and repair with particular emphasis on colon cancer chemoprevention. Recently, we have shown that dietary phytochemicals such as quercetin, rutin, rosmarinic acid, luteolin and others not only protect DNA damage but also stimulate DNA repair in liver and colon cell lines (Lima *et al.*, 2006; Ramos *et al.*, 2008; Ramos *et al.*, 2010b; Ramos *et al.*, 2010a). These effects may contribute to their anti-carcinogenic effects. Effects of phytochemicals through DNA repair modulation and their interaction with alkylating agents used as chemotherapeutic drugs will also be referred.

## 2. DNA damage and genomic stability

Cells of all organisms are under continual attack from reactive oxygen species (ROS) and alkylanting species generated by environmental pollutants, drugs, radiation, cigarette smoke and endogenous metabolism. Theses endogenous and exogenous agents can induce harmful effects if the cell's defense mechanisms are not enough to maintain cellular redox homeostasis. Protection and repair of DNA damage represent two important mechanisms to maintain genomic stability.

### 2.1 Oxidative DNA damage

Endogenous and exogenous agents can induce disruption of the cellular redox homeostasis in favor of oxidant state. This imbalance is described as oxidative stress. As a consequence, different types of molecules such as proteins, lipids and nucleic acids, can be damaged, resulting in severe metabolic dysfunction (including lipid peroxidation, protein oxidation, membrane disruption and DNA damage) (Aherne *et al.*, 2007). Oxidative stress has been involved in the development of several pathologies such as certain cancers, once it may lead to mutations that activate oncogenes or inactivate tumor suppressor genes (Allen and Tresini, 2000; Maynard *et al.*, 2009). In tumor cells, oxidative stress can act as a selective factor in favour of these cells, through induction of DNA damage that may generate more mutations; activation of growth-promoting transcription factors and modulation of genes involved in apoptosis and proliferation (Allen and Tresini, 2000; Karihtala and Soini, 2007). A significant consequence of oxidative stress is DNA damage, which may result in genomic instability. It has been estimated that around $10^4$ lesions are induced in a mammalian cell genome every day (Hegde *et al.*, 2008). There are several types of oxidative DNA damage, such as oxidized bases, abasic sites (also called apurinic/apyrimidinic (AP)) and DNA strand breaks. Hydroxylation of guanine at C-8 position, 8-oxoGua (8-Oxo-7,8-

dihydroguanine) is one of the most abundant forms of DNA oxidation and can cause G to T transversions through mispairing in replication.

Tumor cells are characterized by high levels of ROS. Some studies showed that human tumor cells have an increase of levels of 8-oxoG relative to normal cells. Also, low levels of antioxidant have been found in tumor cells (Maynard et al., 2009).

### 2.2 Alkylating DNA damage

The removal of oxidative lesions by cellular repair processes is essential for maintaining genome integrity and survival limiting mutagenesis. However, there are a number of studies indicating that oxidative DNA damage could not account entirely by itself for tumor development, since elevated levels of 8-oxoGua have been shown not to reflect reflect increased cancer rates. In fact, oxidative damage is the most studied DNA damage, however, alkylating DNA damage is not less important. Human exposure to alkylating agents can arise from diet (e.g. presence of heterocyclic amines on food), environment (e.g. exposure to cigarette smoke and fuel combustion), or produced endogenously (e.g. nitrosation of amides and amines mediated by enteric bacteria) (Wirtz et al., 2010).

Alkylating agents can cause a wide spectrum of DNA adducts, including N-alkylated adducts, such as $N^7$-methylguanine ($N^7$MeG), $N^3$-methyladenine ($N^3$MeA) and $N^3$-methylguanine ($N^3$MeG), and O-alkylated adducts, such as $O^6$-methylguanine ($O^6$MeG) and $O^4$-methylthymine ($O^4$MeT). N-alkylated adducts correspond to more than 80% of alkylated bases and exhibit different stabilities. For example, $N^7$MeG (correspond aprox. 70%) is the most stable N-methylation adduct in vitro with 80hr of half-life. $N^3$MeA and $N^3$MeG are less abundant with 9 and 2%, respectively, of total methylation adducts. $O^6$MeG vary from 0.3% (for methyl methanesulfonate) to 8% (for methylnitrosourea) of the total DNA methyl adducts and it is stable in the absence of the DNA repair protein $O^6$-methylguanine-DNA methyltransferase (MGMT). $O^4$MeT is produced in very low amounts (<0.4% of the total DNA methyl adducts) and its mutagenicity and cytotoxicity are unclear. In general, O-alkylations are highly mutagenic and genotoxic, whereas N-alkylations are cytotoxic, but less mutagenic (Drablos *et al.*, 2004; Kondo *et al.*, 2010). $O^6$MeG is the major pre-mutagenic, pre-carcinogenic and pre-cytotoxic DNA lesion induced by methylating agents (Wirtz et al., 2010).

Prevention of DNA damage and modulation of DNA repair by dietary phytochemicals phytochemicals is the main focus of this review but first a brief overview of DNA repair mechanisms will be presented. Effects on chemoprevention of colon cancer will be addressed.

## 3. Mechanisms of DNA repair

Maintainance of genomic integrity is complex due to great diversity of damage that can occur in DNA. In contrast to other biomolecules, DNA cannot be replaced, only repaired. To avoid the deleterious consequences of damage accumulation, cells have a variety of DNA repair pathways, each recognize and repair specific types of DNA damage. Base excision repair (BER), nucleotide excision repair (NER), mismatch repair (MMR), homologous recombination (HR), non-homologous end-joining repair (NHEJ) and direct damage reversal repair are some of the most important pathways used by cells to repair oxidative and alkylating DNA damage (Table I). These cellular repair pathways are not completely independent from one another. Some studies have show physical interactions between some repair proteins from different repair pathways, suggesting that regulation of DNA repair involves protein cross-talk (Knudsen *et al.*, 2009). Protein expression, pos-translational modifications and nuclear translocation of DNA repair proteins have been referred as essential in the regulation of DNA repair activity and to maintain genomic stability. However, these subjects need to be clarified in the future (Knudsen *et al.*, 2009; Tudek, 2007). When DNA damage is not repaired, the cell by a complex network that collectively forms the DNA damage response (DDR) machinery delays cell-cycle progression, acting on cell cycle checkpoints. This delay gives the DNA repair machinery more time, allowing correct repair of the damage. DDR machinery can induce other mechanisms such as apoptosis or necrosis to avoid that altered cells continue to proliferate and result in disease (Bartek *et al.*, 2007; Maynard *et al.*, 2009).

### 3.1 Base Excision Repair

BER is the major pathway involved in the repair of oxidation and alkylation DNA damage and occurs in both the nucleus and mitochondria (D'Errico *et al.*, 2008). BER recognizes and repairs AP sites, DNA SSBs and different types of base modifications, such as oxidized/reduced bases (e.g. 8-oxoG or formamidopyrimidines), alkylated bases, deaminated bases (e.g. uracil) or base mismatches (Maynard et al., 2009). BER pathway involves steps as recognition, excision, filling and ligation that are carried out by four or five enzymes. Briefly, the repair process is initiated by one of several DNA glycosylases, each recognizing a specific DNA lesion (e.g. OGG1, NTH, NEIL and MYH recognize oxidation damage; deamination damages are recognized by UDG, MED1, UNG, and TDG, and MPG initiate alkylation repair) (Knudsen et al., 2009). These DNA glycosylases excise the damaged base (by cleave of N-glycosidic bond between the sugar and the base), generating an AP site. An AP endonuclease, as APE1, cleaves the AP site, to generate 3′ OH and 5′ deoxyribose phosphate (dRP) terminus. The third step is carried through DNA polymerase that fills the nucleotide gap generated due to lesion base removal. Finally, DNA ligase seals the nick on DNA (Hegde *et al.*, 2008; Evans *et al.*, 2004). Several other protein factors have been identified as interacting with the essential BER proteins and/or the DNA to modulate BER activity. BER pathway is described in detail in the several reviews (Fortini *et al.*, 2003; Hegde *et al.*, 2008; Robertson *et al.*, 2009; Fortini *et al.*, 2003).

Hydroxylation of guanine at C-8 position, 8-oxoGua (8-Oxo-7,8-dihydroguanine) is one of the most abundant forms of DNA oxidation and the most studied because of its mutagenic potential. If not properly repaired, 8-oxoG can pair with cytosine or adenine. Replication of 8-oxoG paired with C by DNA polymerases is a non-mutagenic process. However, replication of 8-oxoG paired with A results in GC to TA or TA to GC transversions that are strong mutagenic DNA lesions (Pastoriza Gallego and Sarasin, 2003). In mammalian cells 8-oxoGua is predominantly recognized and excised by a specific DNA glycosylases. hOGG1 removes 8-oxoG when paired with a cytosine and the glycosylase hMYH removes adenine when mispaired with 8-oxoG, both through the BER pathway. Activity of OGG1 is enhanced by cofactors such as human apurinic/apyrimidinic endonuclease (APE1), Xeroderma Pigmentosum complementation group C (XPC) and human endonuclease VIII-like (NEIL1) (D'Errico et al., 2008).

$N^7$alkylG adducts can be repaired by spontaneous depurination resulting in abasic sites that are often correctly repaired by BER. If not repaired, abasic sites may result in single-stranded gaps that can stall replication forks resulting in double stranded breaks. $N^7$alkylG adducts are also recognized and removed from DNA by N-methylpurine-DNAglycoslase

(MPG). MPG is responsible for enzymatic hydrolysis of the N-glycosylic bond resulting an abasic site in the DNA that is repaired by other enzymes of BER pathway. Over expression of MPG may produce an imbalance between abasic sites formation and repair in favor of abasic sites formation leading an increase of alkylating agents cytotoxicity (Doak et al., 2008).

It has been estimated that a large number of AP sites are generated per cell per day. AP sites are unstable and are highly mutagenic because they result in non-template DNA and RNA synthesis. However, the number of mutations is extremely low, which demonstrate the efficient repair of this damage by the repair mechanisms (Jaiswal and Narayan, 2008). The ability of one glycosylase to recognize more than one type of damage, and the fact that each damage may be recognized by more than one type of glycosylases, give a degree of redundancy in the DNA repair processes which contribute to efficient damage repair (Maynard et al., 2009). Several studies have been showed that post-translational modifications, such as phosphorylation, acetylation and sumoylation may modulate repair activity of BER enzymes, influencing repair efficiencies (Tudek, 2007).

Decrease on BER activity can predispose humans to development of certain cancers, such as colon cancer (Jaiswal and Narayan, 2008; Wilson and Bohr, 2007). Otherwise, an increase of BER activity has been associated with resistance to certain cancer treatments (Liu and Gerson, 2006; Marchesi *et al.*, 2007). Nevertheless, the functional significance of BER in prevention, development and treatment of disease remains unclear.

| DNA Repair pathway | DNA damage | Reviews |
|---|---|---|
| Base Excision Repair (BER) | Base modifications (e.g. oxidized and alkylated bases; AP sites; SSBs | Hegde, M. L., et al., 2008<br>Robertson, A.B., et al., 2009 |
| Nucleotide Excision Repair (NER) | DNA adducts (e.g. thymidine dimers and 6-4 photoproducts) induced by UV radiation or electrophilic chemicals | Hanawalt, P.C., 2002<br>Nouspikel, T., 2009 |
| Mismatch Repair (MMR) | Mispaired nucleotides and insertion/deletion loops (IDLs) | Jiricny J., 2006 |
| Direct damage reversal repair | $O^6$MeG lesions | Kondo N., et al., 2010<br>Kaina, B., et al., 2007 and 2010 |
| Homologous recombination (HR) and non-homologous end-joining repair (NHEJ) | Double strand breaks | Dudas and Chovanec, 2004<br>Helleday et al., 2007 |

Table 1. The main DNA repair pathways and types of DNA damage repaired.

### 3.2 Nucleotide Excision Repair

NER is another important repair pathway involved in DNA adduct repair (e.g. thymidine dimers and 6-4 photoproducts) that are induced by ultraviolet radiation, chemicals or ROS (Benhamou and Sarasin, 2000). These adducts change the normal structure of the DNA helix, breaking transcription and replication processes. Two distinct NER sub-pathways, transcription coupled repair (TCR) and global genomic repair (GGR), have been described. Briefly, TCR repair transcription-blocking lesions present in transcribed DNA strands; and GGR pathway repairs lesions over the bulk genome including non-transcribed strands of active genes (Knudsen et al., 2009). Lesions like thymidine dimmers are usually repaired by

TCR, while other lesions as 6-4 photoproducts are efficiently repaired by GGR (for review see Hanawalt, 2002; Nouspikel, 2009).

### 3.3 Mismatch Repair

MMR is a post-replicative DNA repair mechanism that mainly corrects base-base mismatches which are caused by errors of DNA polymerases and insertion/deletion loops (IDLs). Two complexes are responsible for the repair initiation, MutSα (MSH2/MSH6) and MutSβ (MSH2/MSH3) complexes. MutSα recognize base-base mismatches and small IDLs (with one or two extrahelical nucleotides) while MutSβ recognize the larger IDLs. Repair of the new synthesized strand give the DNA polymerase the chance to generate an error-free copy of the template sequence, protecting cells from point mutations and possibly cancer development (Jiricny, 2006; Knudsen *et al.*, 2009). Loss of MMR function prevents the correction of replicative errors, leading to instability of the genome (Davis and Milner, 2007). As more details about NER and MMR pathways are known, relation between deficiencies on these pathways and cancer become stronger (Hegde et al., 2008).
DNA repair pathways have an important role during all carcinogenic process and in its treatment. Defects in DNA-repair pathways, like MMR, BER and NER, lead to an accumulation of mutations and consequently to carcinogenesis (Jiricny and Marra, 2003). Some of these pathways are inactivated due to mutation or epigenetic modifications in some human cancer, for instance, loss of MMR is observed in 15% of sporadic colorectal cancers (Casorelli *et al.*, 2008).

### 3.4 Direct damage reversal repair

Human cells have several DNA repair mechanisms that are capable of correcting specific types of alkylating damage. $O^6$MeG lesions are repaired by direct damage reversal repair carried out by MGMT also referred to as alkylguanine transferase (AGT). Cells with deficient repair of $O^6$MeG by MGMT are hypersensitive to chromosome aberration induced by alkylating agents (Armstrong and Galloway, 1997). MGMT is a key suicide enzyme that efficiently repairs $O^6$MeG before replication, through direct transfer of the adducted methyl group from the oxygen in the guanine to a cysteine residue in the catalytic site of MGMT. $O^6$MeG is highly mutagenic and carcinogenic because it possess a high potential to mispair with thymine during replication. This lesion is read as adenine by DNA polymerases causing GC-AT transitions (Eker *et al.*, 2009). The toxicity of the $O^6$MeG lesion is attributed to the recognition of $O^6$MeG:T mispairs by the MMR pathway that remove the new thymine. In the next round of replication another thymine mispairs with $O^6$MeG that will be removed by MMR. Recognition by MMR creates a gap in DNA by incision on the new replicated strand. If $O^6$MeG remains in one of the template strands the repair process will be repeated, creating a "futile repair loop". This loop will eventually result in toxic double-strand breaks leading to chromosomal aberrations, cell-cycle arrest or apoptosis (Bugni *et al.*, 2009; Kaina *et al.*, 2007; Kaina *et al.*, 2010; Kondo *et al.*, 2010). When both of these systems fail to repair, $O^6$MeG results in point mutations that can possibly initiate the carcinogenic process. Beyond the ability to remove methyl adducts, MGMT can also remove larger adducts such as, ethyl, propyl and butyl adducts, however at a lower efficiency (Doak et al., 2008).
Some authors mention the important role of MGMT in protection against sporadic human colorectal cancer, once that epigenetic silencing of MGMT gene was observed in 50% of these cancers (Lind et al., 2004). MGMT expression in tumor cells have been related with the

resistance of tumors to alkylating agents toxicity (Eker *et al.*, 2009; Nystrom and Mutanen, 2009). Removal of the methyl group from $O^6$MeG by MGMT is dependent on the rate of MGMT syntheses which is induced in response to DNA damage (Doak et al., 2008). Depletion of MGMT by reducing MGMT activity or decreasing gene expression can occur using a specific inhibitor $O^6$-benzylguanine (BG) or through epigenetic silencing, (Eker et al., 2009). Inhibition of MGMT with BG in rats increases azoxymethane (AOM)-induced colon tumors, and transgenic expression of MGMT in mice protects against AOM-induced aberrant crypt foci (ACF) (Bugni *et al.*, 2009; Wali *et al.*, 1999).

### 3.5 Homologous recombination and Non-homologous end-joining repair

In mammalian cells double strand breaks (DSBs), one of the most deleterious damage, can be repaired by two different types of mechanism: 1) non-homologous end-joining (NHEJ) that rejoins the two broken ends in a template independent way with concomitant loss of sequence information. After overlapping of the two DNA ends, the ligase IV complex start the ligation process of the two broken ends; and 2) homologous recombination repair (HR) that uses a homologue undamaged DNA sequence (sister-chromatid or homologous chromosome) to repair the missing sequence between the two DNA ends. HR is an error-free process (Dudas and Chovanec, 2004; Helleday *et al.*, 2007).

If not properly repaired DSB can cause loss of chromosomes and consequently generate mutations with or without induction of cell death (Dudas and Chovanec, 2004). Single-strand breaks repair (SSBR) is a DNA repair pathway extremely important to avoid the deleterious effects of single-strand breaks (for more detail see the review Caldecott, 2007). Since DNA damage is recognized as the initial step in chemical carcinogenesis, inhibition of DNA damage and/or induction of repair would be the first line of defense against cancer caused by carcinogens. Chemoprevention by diet and dietary constituints against oxidative and alkylating agents will be covered by this review.

## 4. Chemopreventive activities of dietary phytochemicals

Diet and lifestyle play crucial roles in cancer aetiology. Nowadays, the idea that prevention of any disease is preferable over treatment is accepted by all. In this context, in the last decades, several studies suggest that regular consumption of fruits, vegetables and spices have health benefits including risk reduction of developing a cancer, namely, colon cancer (Terry et al., 2001). Much of the protective effects have been attributed to phytochemicals such as polyphenols, terpenes and alkaloids, present in low levels in plants (Barth et al., 2005). For instance, flavonoids (polyphenolic compounds) have been reported to possess potential on prevention of several cancers specially cancers of gastrointestinal tract, like oral cavity and colon cancer (Kuo, 1996). The World Cancer Research Fund (WCRF) in its report about diet and prevention of cancer in 2007, mentioned that fruits and vegetables in general probably protect against cancers of the mouth, pharynx, larynx, oesophagus, lung, and stomach and there are limited evidences that suggest protective effects of fruits against cancers of the nasopharynx, pancreas, liver, and colorectum (WCRF, 2007).

The use of plants for the prevention of diseases is an ancient practice. However, it was in the last decades that scientific community started to show interest in the medicinal properties of plants. The first scientific evidences showing that vegetables and fruits might be protective against some cancers emerged in the 1990s. Nevertheless, twenty year on no consensus exists about the real role of diet on cancer prevention, and many questions remain to be answered. Which component(s) of the diet is (are) responsible for the protective effects? Are the protective effects the result of the interactions between different components? What type of interactions exists between them (e.g. synergistic, antagonistic interaction)? What is the mechanism by which they prevent cancer?

Dietary agents have different structural features that are responsible for a great variety of biological activities such as anti-inflammatory, antioxidant, free radical scavenging, anti-mutagenic and enzyme modulating activities. These activities may be responsible for the possible chemopreventive effects of natural compound. Modulation of diet can be used as a possible cancer chemoprevention strategy (Heo *et al.*, 2001; WCRF, 2007).

Chemoprevention is the process of using natural or synthetic compounds to block, reverse, or prevent the development of cancers through the action on multiple cellular mechanisms. Generally, these cellular mechanisms can be grouped in two: 1) Anti-mutagenesis, that includes the inhibition of the uptake, formation/activation of carcinogens, their detoxification, the blockage of carcinogen–DNA binding, and the enhancement of fidelity of DNA repair; 2) Anti-proliferation/anti-progression, that includes modification of signal transduction pathways, inhibition of oncogene activity, promotion of the cellular differentiation, enhancement of apoptosis, inhibition of inflammation and angiogenesis, and modulation of hormone/growth factor activity (Davis, 2007; Moon Y. Yeo et al., 2001). Phytochemicals may alter multiple molecular targets within a specific biological process related with cancer and when in combination with other natural compounds can have an additive or synergistic effect as well as antagonistic interactions. Nowadays, it is accepted that the combination of foods and/or multiple natural compounds may offer increased chemoprevention against cancer as compared to isolated compounds. However, the interactions between the different compounds within the food or with other foods need to be clarified. Furthermore, active compounds of many plants remain uncharacterized, which restrict the knowledge about the role of diet on cancer prevention (Davis and Milner, 2007; Mehta *et al.*, 2010).

In chemoprevention studies several experimental models can be used. However, experience shows that the results may be different depending on the experimental model used and whether the whole plants evaluated or only isolated compounds. Data from cultured cells and animal models may not reflect the response in humans. Also, plants and their isolated compounds may not have similar biological effects (Davis and Milner, 2007; Mehta *et al.*, 2010). Chemopreventive effect of food and/or its compounds depend on absorption, metabolism, distribution and excretion of phytochemicals. Phytochemicals' absorption is dependent on source and the method of food processing. In the same plant species the phytochemicals contents may change depending on the plant genotype, the season of the year and the place where the plant was grown. Intensity and duration of the exposure to dietary components also influence the cellular response. Thus, dose and duration of exposure become fundamental considerations in interpreting findings from nutritional studies (Davis and Milner, 2007).

During the last decades, some long-term intervention studies have been performed to understand the contribution of diet on prevention of diseases. However, this type of studies has the inconvenience of the high time consumption and cost. Several biomarkers have been validated to predict cancer risk and to evaluate the potential chemopreventive effect of food and/or its compounds (Davis and Milner, 2007). In general, biomarkers can be divided in three major types: biomarkers of exposure, which allow the evaluation of whether the intake of dietary components is sufficient to lead to a certain biological response; biomarkers of effect, which give information about the mechanisms of action of dietary components; and biomarkers of susceptibility, which indicate which individuals are susceptible to specific dietary exposures (Davis and Milner, 2007). In this review, we will be focus in one biomarker of exposure assessed by comet assay.

## 5. The comet assay

The comet assay, also called the single cell gel electrophoresis (SCGE) assay was first introduced by Ostling and Johanson in 1984 as a microelectrophoretic technique for the direct visualization of DNA damage in individual cells. In this assay, cells embedded in agarose are placed on a microscope slide, lysed by detergents in high salt solution and submitted to electrophoresis under neutral conditions. It usually accepted that, in neutral condition, DNA migration is due to presence of double-strand breaks (DSB). However, it was demonstrated that DSB as well as single strand breaks (SSB) were detected in this conditions (Collins *et al.*, 1997a; Gedik *et al.*, 1992; Ostling and Johanson, 1984). Singh *et al.*, (1988) introduced the electrophoresis under alkaline (pH >13) conditions for detecting DNA damage in single cells. At alkaline conditions, DNA migration is associated with the presence of strand breaks (single and/or double strand), SSB associated with incomplete excision repair sites, and alkali-labile sites (ALS). The alkaline version of comet assay had more success because it allows the detection of a wide spectrum of damages, and in fact almost all genotoxic agents induce more SSB and/or ALS than DSB (Fairbairn *et al.*, 1995; Tice et al., 2000).

Among the several methods to measure DNA damage including classical cytogenetic tests such as chromosome aberrations, micronuclei and sister chromatid exchanges, the comet assay has become the most commonly used. This assay shows some advantages relatively to other genotoxicity assays such as: 1) evaluates DNA damage at individual cell; 2) requires a small number of cells per sample; 3) any animal tissue can be used, since single cell/nucleus suspension can be obtained; 4) proliferating or non-proliferating cells can be used; 5) detects low levels of DNA damage (high sensitivity); 6) needs small amounts of a test substance; 7) detects several classes of DNA damage such as DSB, SSB, ALS, incomplete repair of a-basic sites and cross-links; 8) low costs; 9) simple and fast tool (Hartmann et al., 2003; Speit *et al.*, 2003). Despite great advantages, some limitations have been attributed to the comet assay: it does not detect high level of DNA damage and DNA fragments smaller than 50 kb, and therefore apoptotic cells detection is very difficult (Nossoni, 2008). The comet assay done with lymphocytes is an important biomarker for early biological effects of exposure to environmental mutagenic agents (Dusinska and Collins, 2008). Angerer *et al.*, (2007) in a review about human biomonitoring refer, however, some problems that should be kept in mind when lymphocytes are used. The major difficulty is the interpretation of data, because the damage levels and capacity to repair of these cells may be different from cells of others tissues. Usually lymphocytes repair their damage very slowly and not all the damage to cells and organs are detectable using lymphocytes. Furthermore, a great intra-individual and inter-individual variability of the basal level of DNA damage it was found that is influenced by a variety of factors such as lifestyle, diet, medication, air pollution, season, climate or exercise. Lymphocytes also show limited survival in vitro, requiring incubation with a mitogen such as phytohaemagglutinin (Collins et al., 2008).

In the last decade, scientific community demonstrated an increasing interest in the alkaline version of comet assay that has brought a rapid increase in the number of papers and reports published using this assay. Comet assay is now used in different research areas such as human and environmental biomonitoring, mechanistic studies of DNA repair, genetic toxicology, nutrition and clinical studies. Below is a detailed description of the standard comet assay and new modifications to detect different DNA damages and DNA repair capacities (fig.1).

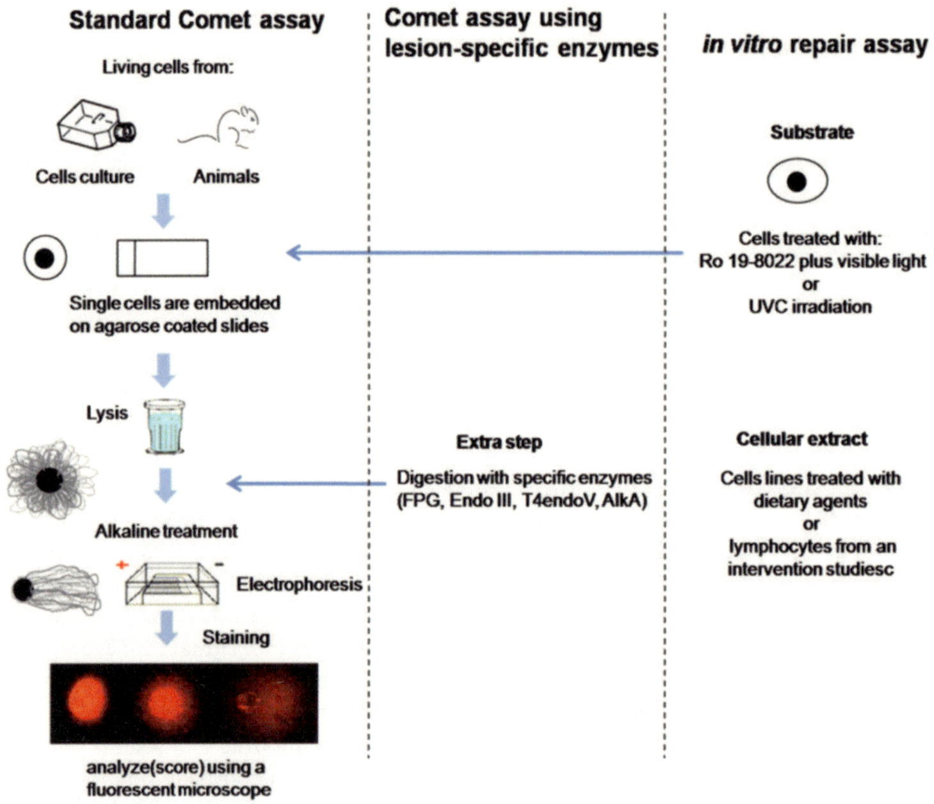


Fig. 1. General steps of the standard comet assay and its modifications.

### 5.1 Standard comet assay

Among the various versions of the comet assay, the alkaline (pH of the unwinding and electrophoresis buffer >13) is the most used.The first step is to cover microscope slides with 1% of normal melting point (NMP) agarose and dry it at room temperature. A second layer composed by cells embedded in 0.5% LMP agarose (at 37°C) is spread above the first layer, covering it with a cover glass and keeping at 4°C during few minutes. After removing cover glass, slides are lysed at least for one hour up to 24h in lysing solution containing detergent and high molarity NaCl (2.5M NaCl, 100mM Na2EDTA, 10mM Tris Base, pH 10 plus 1% Triton X-100). This solution removes membranes and soluble cellular (300mM NaOH, 1mM Na2EDTA, pH >13) constituents, as well as histones, producing nucleoids of supercoiled DNA attached to the nuclear matrix. DNA unwinding occur in alkaline conditions (pH>13) immersing slides in alkaline buffer at 4°C. The time required for unwinding changes based on the cells being examined. In this step, breaks in the DNA relax the supercoiling and allow DNA loops to expand. Electrophoresis occurs under alkaline condition at 0.8V/cm and 300 mA for 20 min.

During electrophoresis, DNA loops containing breaks migrate towards the anode forming in the end DNA structures like a comet, with a head (the nuclear region) and a tail that contain DNA loops that extended during electrophoresis due to breaks. DNA migration is dependent of several parameters, such as, concentration of agarose in the gel, pH, temperature and duration of alkaline unwinding, temperature, voltage, and duration of electrophoresis.
After electrophoresis, slides are neutralized using neutralization buffer, stained with fluorescent agent (e.g. ethidium bromide, SYBRGold), and analyzed (scored) using a fluorescent microscope. The scoring may be done by visual scoring or by computer programs. In visual scoring the researcher scores at least one hundred comets using the following classification: 0 to comet without DNA in tail; 1, 2 and 3 with increasing amount of DNA in tail and 4 to comet were DNA is almost all in the tail. In the end the score of each sample changes between 0 and 400 (arbitrary units). An alternative methodology are the computer programs that allow to measure different parameters of the comets such as tail intensity, tail length, intensity of head, and tail moment. Tail intensity corresponds to the percentage of DNA in the tail of the comet and is the most used parameter. Intensity of tail fluorescence indicates the extent of damage. It is important to use positive and negative controls as well as to blind scoring (Collins et al., 2008; Nossoni, 2008).
Comet assay under standard conditions reflects endogenous DNA damage such as single and double strand breaks and apurinic/apyrimidinic (AP) sites in almost any eukaryotic cell population. There are other modifications that make it even more sensitive and allow to measure oxidised pyrimidines and purines and alkylation DNA damage. These modifications will be explained below.

### 5.2 The use of lesion-specific enzymes

Alkaline version (described above) measures strand DNA breaks and AP sites (that are converted to strand breaks). However, genotoxic agents not only induce breaks and AP sites, but also DNA damage such as base oxidation and others base modifications, that are generated in large scale in cells. Several DNA repair enzymes recognize damaged bases, introducing breaks at sites of the base damage. Thus, inclusion of an extra step of nucleoid DNA digestion with lesion-specific enzymes following lysis, allow detection of modified bases increasing the sensitivity and specificity of the comet assay (Collins, 2009; Hoelzl et al., 2009).
Endonuclease III (EndoIII) was the first enzyme used to recognize oxidized pyrimidines in DNA and to remove them, leaving an AP site that is subsequently converted in breaks at pH13. These breaks that occur at sites of base oxidation increase comet tail intensity (Collins *et al.*, 1993). Formamidopyrimidine DNA glycosylase (FPG) recognizes and breaks modified purines as well as 8-oxoguanine and also ring-opened purines, or formamidopyrimidines (Fapy) (Dusinska and Collins, 1996). T4 endonuclease V recognise UV-induced cyclobutane pyrimidine dimers (Collins *et al.*, 1997b). AlkA is a bacterial repair enzyme whose main substrate is the $N^3$-MeA, an alkylated base and converts it to AP sites (Collins *et al.*, 2001a).
The use of repair enzymes has been particularly useful in estimating oxidative damage of certain pollutants and drugs in several experimental models and in biomonitoring studies, for example to evaluate the role of dietary agents in protection against oxidative DNA damage. However, the specificity of the enzymes is limited, for instance FPG recognizes 8-oxoGua but also detects alkylation damage ($N^7$ MeG) (Speit *et al.*, 2004).
After lysis, in parallel with a slide incubated with a lesion-specific enzyme, a slide incubated without enzyme (only with buffer) is used as a control. Subtraction of control (which contain

SBs and AP sites) to the condition treated with enzyme gives a value that correspond to the damage recognized by the enzyme and is usually referred as 'netenzyme-sensitive sites'.

### 5.3 DNA repair assays

Beside effects on protection against DNA damage, comet assay was also developed to assess DNA repair ability of the cells and effects of diet on DNA damage repair rates. For that, two different methodologies are frequently used:

1. The "cellular repair assay" that measures the ability of cells to rejoin strand breaks induced by a DNA damaging agent. In this assay two different treatment regimens can be used: (A) Pretreatment of cells with dietary agent followed by exposure to DNA damaging agent, and cells allowed to recover in fresh culture medium at 37ºC. At different time points, samples are taken for analysis with the standard comet assay. Thus, we evaluate the effect of preincubation with test extract/compound on the ability of cells to rejoin SBs; and (B) treatment with DNA damaging agent treatment is done before cells are incubated with the test extract/compounds. In this case the aim is to test effects on nonenzymatic repair. Inclusion of lesion-specific enzymes allow to assess repair ability of others damages beyond strand breaks and AP sites.
2. The "in vitro repair assay" was developed by (Collins *et al.*, 2001b) to measure excision repair activity of cell extracts, such as lymphocytes collected in dietary intervention studies or from cells treated with dietary agents. These cell extracts are used as an extra step (similar to the use of lesion-specific enzymes) in DNA substrates containing a specific damage. The first application of this assay was the measurement of repair rates of oxidized bases, called "in vitro BER assay". In this case substrate cells are treated with the photosensitiser Ro 19-8022 (Roche) plus visible light to induce 8-oxoGua, and then cells are embedded in agarose on a slide. After lysis, substrate nucleoids are incubated with a cell extract (e.g. cells incubated with dietary agent) that have enzymes that recognize 8-oxoGua and cut at the place of the lesion. This assay allows to measure the activity of the repair enzyme 8-oxoguanine DNA glycosylase OGG1present in cell extract. A modification of the "in vitro repair assay" was introduced by Langie et al., (2006) to assess nucleotide excision repair (NER), the "in vitro NER assay". In this version cells were treated with benzo(a)pyrene diolepoxide and bulky adducts were formed. In 2009, Gaivao *et al.*, (2009) exposed cells to UVC irradiation inducing cyclobutane pyrimidine dimers and 6-4 photoproducts. Irradiated cells are embedded in agarose on a slide, and lysed to expose the DNA, which is then incubated with the cell extract. Incision at damage sites is detected using the alkaline comet assay and indicates repair ability. In these assays, higher DNA intensity in the tail indicates higher DNA repair activity of the cell extracts. Cell extracts of cells incubated with vehicle are used as control (basal) repair abilities.

### 5.4 Other modifications

The format of comet assay most used is 2 gels per slide. To large numbers of samples new formats have been developed, such as 12 gels per slide, that have several advantages: 1) reduces the number of cells required for each gel (approx. 200 cells/gel); 2) allows different conditions in the same slide (different genotoxic chemicals; enzymes or cell extracts); 3) requires low volume of solutions; 4) increases the number of samples processed at one time. This new format has been used in human biomonitoring studies with a great number of samples, and also when is necessary to use several repair enzymes to detect different kinds of damage (Shaposhnikov et al., 2010).

## 6. Application of the comet assay in chemoprevention studies

Application of the comet assay to the study of the protective effects of diet against oxidative/alkylating DNA damage and repair will be summarized bellow. For more details see the following revisions, (Hoelzl et al., 2009; Moller and Loft, 2002; Wasson *et al.*, 2008 and Wong *et al.*, 2005).

### 6.1 Effect of diet on prevention of oxidative DNA damage

Prevention of DNA damage is one of the cellular mechanisms that may prevent cancer. Diet plays an important role in regulating DNA damage for instance by modulating the antioxidant/oxidant balance. The protective effect observed in many studies could be due, in part, to the presence of phenolic and/or non-phenolic constituents that have ability to act as antioxidant by free radical scavenging and chelating metal ions (Anderson *et al.*, 2000); (Ross and Kasum, 2002). They can also act as indirect antioxidant by increasing levels of antioxidants such as glutathione (GSH) and/or by increasing the activity of antioxidant enzymes such as catalase (CAT), glutathione peroxidase (GPX) and superoxide dismutase (SOD) (Alia *et al.*, 2005; Lima *et al.*, 2005; Lima *et al.*, 2006; Frei and Higdon, 2003). Phytochemicals can also modulate phase I (activating) enzymes and phase II (detoxifying) enzymes involved in xenobiotic metabolism (Chen and Kong, 2004; Ferguson *et al.*, 2004; Moon *et al.*, 2006; Ross and Kasum, 2002).

Phytochemicals are bioactive compounds present in plants where they are produced as secondary metabolites to protect themselves from several pathogenic agents. Their consumption by humans confers protection against some diseases. Most bioactive phytochemicals belong to one of 5 groups: polyphenols, carotenoids, alkaloids, nitrogen-containing compounds, and organosulfur compounds. Polyphenols and carotenoids include several hundreds of compounds and are the most studied groups. Polyphenols may be further classified into 4 groups, according with the number of phenol rings that they contain: Flavonois, phenolic acids, stilbenes, and lignans. The flavonoids may themselves be classified into the follow subgroups: flavonols, flavones, isoflavones, flavanones, flavanols and anthocyanidins (Fig.2).

#### 6.1.1 Polyphenols

Numerous studies have shown the antioxidant and DNA protective properties of polyphenols. Quercetin is a flavonoid found in a variety of foods including apples, onions, wine and tea. Several studies, including our own showed the protective effects of quercetin against oxidative DNA damage in HepG2 cells (Lima et al., 2006; Ramos et al., 2008), Caco-2 cells (Aherne and O'Brien, 1999), HMB-2 cells (Horvathova *et al.*, 2005), human macrophage (U-937 cells) (Kanupriya et al., 2006; Moon et al., 2006); human lymphocytes (healthy volunteers) (Wilms *et al.*, 2007), and murine leukemia L1210 cells (Horvathova *et al.*, 2003). Wilms *et al.*, (2005) reported the protective effects of quercetin against the formation of oxidative DNA damage and bulky DNA adducts in human lymphocytes, induced by $H_2O_2$ and benzo(a)pyrene (B(a)P, respectively. In the same study, results obtained in an in vivo experiments showed that four weeks of quercetin-rich blueberry/apple juice mixture

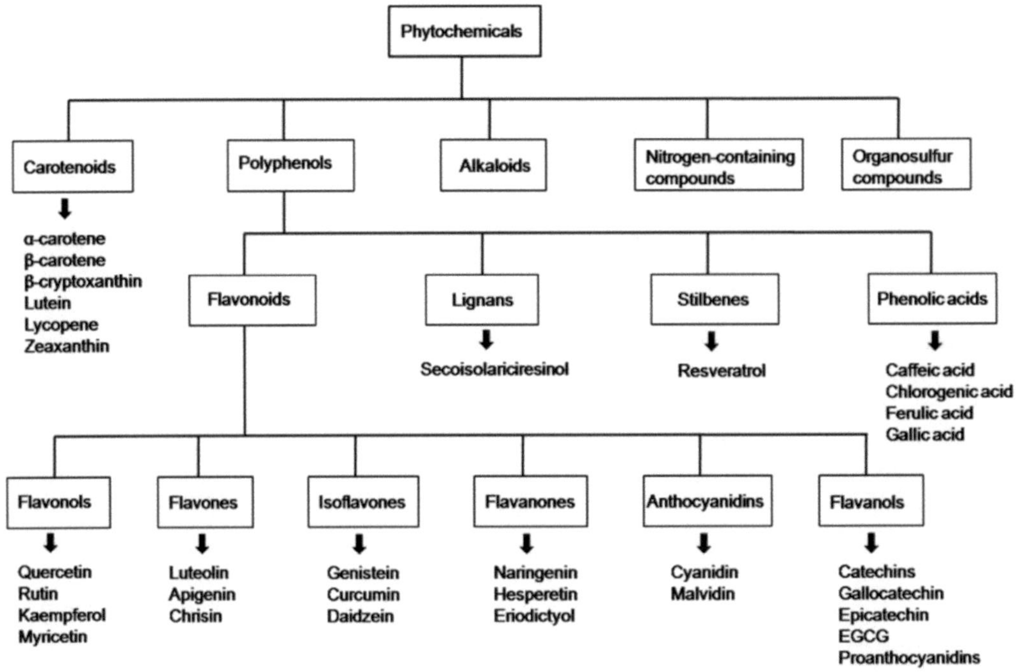


Fig. 2. Classification of phytochemicals and the main natural compounds in each group.

consumption led to a decrease of oxidative DNA damage and BPDE-DNA adduct levels by 41% and 11%, respectively, although the results were not statistically significant. Increases in the total antioxidant capacity of plasma and in plasma quercetin content were observed. Others flavonoids, such as luteolin (Cai *et al.*, 1997; Horvathova et al., 2005; Lima et al., 2006; Min and Ebeler, 2008; Ramos *et al.*, 2010b), rutin (Moon et al., 2006; Ramos et al., 2008), genistein (Cai et al., 1997), catechin and epicatechin (Kanupriya et al., 2006), showed antigenotoxic effects against oxidative DNA damage in several cell models.

In an ex vivo study, lymphocytes from three healthy subjects were pre-incubated with several dietary antioxidants. Quercetin and caffeic acid ( a phenolic acid) protected against $H_2O_2$-induced DNA damage, however in this study no effect was observed when cells were treated with catechin, epicatechin, catechin gallate and epicatechin gallate (Szeto and Benzie, 2002).

Besides quercetin and rutin, we reported that ursolic acid (a triterpenoid) protect against DNA damage induced by tert-butyl hydroperoxide (t-BHP) in HepG2 cells (Ramos et al., 2008). Other reports showed that ursolic acid and/or luteolin protect DNA from damage induced by $H_2O_2$, t-BHP or AZT (3_-azido-3_-dideoxythymidine) in several cell lines, such as leukemic cells, HEI-OC1 auditory cells and PC12 cells (Horvathova et al., 2003; Horvathova *et al.*, 2004; Ovesna *et al.*, 2006; Yu et al., 2009; Noroozi *et al.*, 1998; Silva *et al.*, 2008). Rosmarinic acid (RA), reduced the frequency of micronuclei and the extent of DNA damage induced by doxorubicin in V79 cells (Furtado *et al.*, 2009). Caffeic acid (3,4-dihydroxy cinnamic acid), also a dietary phenolic compound, showed a photoprotective effect (Devipriya *et al.*, 2008; Benkovic et al., 2009). Human blood lymphocytes irradiated with UVB (280-320) after pretreatment with caffeic acid exhibited lower levels of lipid peroxidation markers such as thiobarbituric acid reactive substance (TBARS) and lipid hydroperoxide (LPH) and also a decrease of UVB-induced DNA damage (Prasad *et al.*, 2009).

Naringin, a citrus grapefruit flavonone, showed antigenotoxic properties in V79 cells (Jagetia *et al.*, 2007). 4-Coumaric acid, a phenolic acid present in many foods and drinks, such as wine, tea, berries, apples, spinach and cereals reduced basal oxidative DNA damage in rat colonic mucosa when evaluated by comet assay (Guglielmi *et al.*, 2003). Resveratrol, found in substantial amounts in several types of beverages including red wine and fruits, showed genoprotective effects under conditions of oxidative stress induced by $H_2O_2$ in C6 glioma cells (Quincozes-Santos et al., 2007). Apigenin, a flavonoid widely distributed in many herbs, fruits, and vegetables, has shown chemopreventive activities in several biological systems. Jeyabal *et al.*, (2005) reported the protective role of apigenin against the oxidative stress caused by N-nitrosodiethylamine and phenobarbital in Wistar albino rats. Rusak et al., (2010), showed genoprotective effects of apigenin and other flavonoids (luteolin and kaempferol) in human peripheral lymphocytes against oxidative damage induced by hydrogen peroxide.

### 6.1.2 Carotenoids

Tomato is one of the main sources of lycopene, a carotenoid with antioxidant properties. Pretreatment of rat hepatocytes with lycopene (1.86, 9.31 and 18.62 μM) in culture, showed a significant decrease in the levels of TBARS and DNA damage induced by gamma-radiation. Antioxidant enzymes such as superoxide dismutase (SOD), catalase (CAT) and glutathione peroxidase (GPx), as well as, the levels of GSH, vitamins A, E, C, increased significantly when hepatocytes were pretreated with the carotenoid (Srinivasan et al., 2007). At physiological concentrations (0.3-10 μM) lycopene and beta-carotene also protect Chinese hamster lung fibroblasts against DNA damage induced by 3-morpholinosydnonimine (SIN-1) (Muzandu et al., 2006). In a human intervention study, healthy volunteers were submitted to a supplementation with lycopene during 8 weeks. Consumption of lycopene decreased oxidative DNA damage in lymphocytes and urinary 8-hydroxy deoxoguanosine levels when compared with the basal levels (Devaraj et al., 2008). Also, Zhao *et al.*, (2006) evaluated the protective effect of lycopene and others carotenoids against DNA damage in humans. Here, thirty-seven healthy, nonsmoking postmenopausal women consumed for 56 days a daily dose of mixed carotenoids (lycopene, lutein and beta-carotene; 4 mg each), 12 mg of a single carotenoid (lycopene, lutein or beta-carotene), or placebo. At the end the lymphocytes were isolated and DNA damage measured by comet assay. The results showed that all groups that consumed carotenoids had significantly lower endogenous DNA damage than that found on baseline measurements. No differences were found in placebo group. Lutein also decreased DNA damage induced by cisplatin in mice when evaluated by comet assay and increased GSH levels when compared with a negative control group (Serpeloni *et al.*, 2010). Lorenzo *et al.*, (2009) reported that β-cryptoxanthin at low concentrations, close to those found in plasma, protects Caco-2 and HeLa cells from oxidative DNA damage induced by $H_2O_2$ or by visible light in the presence of a photosensitizer. Consumption of β-carotene decreased the number of strand breaks induced by $H_2O_2$ in lymphocytes (Panayiotidis and Collins, 1997).

Pre-treatment with astaxanthin, a red carotenoid used as a dietary additive, at 12.5, 25 and 50 mg/kg/day for 5 days before cyclophosphamide treatment resulted in the amelioration of antioxidant defenses (glutathione and superoxide dismutase) in the liver and decreased DNA damage evaluated by standard comet assay and using specific-enzymes (FPG and EndoIII) in bone marrow cells and peripheral blood lymphocytes isolated from mice. This carotenoid also reduced the frequency of chromosomal breakage and micronucleus formation in the mouse bone marrow cells and peripheral blood. Astaxanthin, also showed antigenotoxic effects against cyclophosphamide in germ cell from male mice (Tripathi and Jena, 2008).

### 6.1.3 Whole foods

Several studies, including our own with colon cancer cells, have found that polyphenol rich plant extracts inhibit formation of SBs and 8-oxoGua induced by oxidantive agents (Ramos *et al.,* 2010a). Some plants, such as *Salvia officinalis L.* (sage), *Rosmarinus officinalis L.* (rosemary) and *Origanum vulgare L.* (oregano) have antioxidant properties that confer protection against oxidative DNA damage in colon cells as demonstrated by Aherne et al., (2007).

Green tea is rich in polyphenolic antioxidants and their effects on health are the subject of several studies. Green tea decreased DNA oxidation in lymphocytes, colonocytes and hepatocytes when rats ingested 6.5 mg/kg bw per day, 5 days of tea extract (Kager et al., 2010). Evidences of genoprotective effects of green tea appear not only from in vitro and in vivo studies, but also from human supplementation trials. Human lymphocytes isolated from healthy volunteers that took 2 x 150 ml/d of 1% (w/v) green tea showed a decrease of basal oxidation-induced DNA damage with and without FPG enzyme (Han *et al.,* 2011). One of the main constituents of green tea is (-)-epigallocatechin-3-gallate (EGCG) that could be responsible for their beneficial effects. In human peripheral leucocytes treatement with low EGCG concentrations (2-100μM) decreased both bleomycin-induced breaks and endonuclease III sensitive sites (Glei and Pool-Zobel, 2006).

Apple is one of the most consumed fruit, therefore is an important source of polyphenols in humans. Their chemoprotective effects have been shown in vitro and in vivo studies (Koch et al., 2009; Veeriah et al., 2008). Apple juice has been found to possess antioxidant and antiproliferative activities as well as the ability to increase the expression of phase II gene glutathione S-transferase T2 (GSTT2) in human colon cells (Petermann et al., 2009). Apple extract can also protect against oxidative-induced DNA damage in human colon cells, such as LT97 (Miene (Miene *et al.,* 2009), HT29, HCT115 and CaCo-2 cells (McCann et al., 2007; Schaefer et al., 2006). Also, grape juices exhibit antigenotoxic activity (Dani et al., 2009).

The anticarcinogenic properties of olive oil have been attributed to the presence of phenolic compounds. Fabiani et al., (2008) reported that some of its isolated compounds (e.g. hydroxytyrosol, [3,4-dyhydroxyphenyl-ethanol (3,4-DHPEA)] and a complex mixture of phenols extracted from virgin olive oil) protected against H2O2 in human peripheral blood mononuclear cells and promyelocytic leukemia cells (HL60). These results have a great impact not only because of the high level of protection observed (between 80 and 90%) but also because, according to the authors, the concentrations tested could easily be reached with normal intake of olive oil.

Annatto is a native shrub from Tropical America, whose seeds are a rich source of carotenoids, such as bixin, norbixin and phytoene and have antigenotoxic effects against oxidative DNA damage (Kovary et al., 2001).

Results from human intervention trials have demonstrated the protective effect of isolated compounds as well as fruits and vegetables in peripheral lymphocytes. Pool-Zobel *et al.,* (1997) showed a decrease in pyrimidine oxidation during supplementation with carrot juice. Porrini and Riso, (2000) reported that supplementation with tomato that is rich in lycopene, increase protection against $H_2O_2$-induced DNA damage in lymphocytes. Also a diet rich in fruit and vegetables for 14 days showed a DNA protection from oxidative damage in lymphocytes (Thompson et al., 1999). Broccoli intake also decreases oxidative DNA damage in smokers and nonsmokers (Riso *et al.*, 2009). In a recent study, Sprague-Dawley rats fed with a wild-blueberry diet or a control diet for four or eight weeks were used to assess the effect of the consumption of this fruit on the resistance to $H_2O_2$-induced DNA damage. After treatment period, lymphocytes were exposed, ex vivo, to $H_2O_2$ and it was observed that wild-blueberry diet did not change antioxidant capacity in lymphocytes after eight weeks of treatment, but increased DNA protection against oxidative damage (Del Bo et al., 2010). Dulebohn et al., (2008) using the same animal model, reported that blueberries consumption for 3 weeks increase GST activity and decrease oxidative DNA damage in the liver. However, contrarily to in vitro studies, blueberries consumption did not significantly increase phase II enzyme activities in short-term supplementation times.

As described above, many isolated compounds and some plants showed genoprotective effects in several experimental models, however it is important to keep in mind that these dietary agents can also induce DNA damage in certain conditions. The balance between the genoprotective and genotoxic effects of dietary agents is dependent on their concentration, incubation period and types of cells (Rusak et al., 2010).

### 6.2 Effect of diet on prevention of alkylating DNA damage

Alkylation of DNA can be an important initial step in cancer formation. High levels of alkylating damage have been found in human colorectal DNA where high incidence of tumours have been observed (Hall *et al.*, 1991; Povey *et al.*, 2000). To assess antigenotoxic effects of diet against alkylating damage, several experimental models have been developed. Among them, colon tumours induction in rodent models, with carcinogenic chemicals such as 1,2-dimethylhydrazine (DMH) or azoxymethane (AOM) are the most used, and they are believed to be representative of colon carcinogenesis in humans (Barth et al., 2005).

#### 6.2.1 Phytochemicals

Dolara et al., (2005) reported that red wine polyphenols (50 mg/kg) administered to F344 rats for 16 weeks inhibited colon carcinogenesis induced by AOM or DMH. Wine polyphenols also decreased basal level of DNA oxidative damage of the colon mucosa. Supplementation of Wistar male rats with resveratrol showed to significantly decrease DMH-induced leukocyte DNA damage. In this study, an increase of levels of enzymic and non-enzymic antioxidant defense and a decrease in the extent of lipid peroxidation markers were also observed (Sengottuvelan *et al.*, 2009). Other chemopreventive agents, such as quercetin, rutin, curcumin, silymarin, lycopene and farnesol, with antioxidant properties, have been found to inhibit DMH- and AOM-induced colon carcinogenesis and DNA damage in animal models (Kim et al., 1998; Volate *et al.*, 2005). Lupeol, a pentacyclic triterpene present in mango, also protected against DMBA induced DNA alkylation damage in Swiss albino mice (Nigam *et al.*, 2007).

#### 6.2.2 Whole foods

Many whole foods and plant crude extracts have also been found to protect against alkylating damage. The water extract of *Salvia officinalis* prevent formation of aberrant crypt foci (ACFs, a pre-carcinogenic lesion) induced by AOM in rat colon and also protected DNA of colonocytes (unpublished observations). Using the same experimental model, Sengupta *et al.*, (2004 and 2003) reported that tomato and garlic prevent ACFs, induced by AOM in rat colon. Tomato also decreased incidence and progression of 9,10-dimethyl benzanthracene (DMBA)-induced mouse skin tumours (De and Das, 2001). Intake of beer reduced ACF formation and protected against DNA damage induced by AOM in the rat colon mucosa (Nozawa et al., 2004). de Lima *et al.*, (2005) evaluated the effect of aqueous extract of propolis on the formation of DMH-induced ACF and DNA damage in rat colon. Propolis had no effect on ACF formation, however, modulation of DMH-induced DNA damage in colon cells was observed. At lower concentrations (12, 34 and 108 mg/Kg bw/day) aqueous extract of propolis decrease the level of DNA damage. However, the highest concentration (336mg/Kg bw/day) induced DNA damage in rat colon. Dietary agents such as, ginseng, lemon grass and propolis, have been found to inhibit DMH- and AOM-induced colon carcinogenesis and DNA damage in animal model (Bazo et al., 2002; Suaeyun *et al.*, 1997; Volate et al., 2005). Consumption of onion, blueberries (Boateng et al., 2007), and garbanzo beans (Murillo *et al.*, 2004) also decreased the number of AOM-induced ACFs in rats and mice, respectively.

Some studies reported antigenotoxic effects of diet against alkylating DNA damage using cytogenetic assays (micronucleus assay) (Azevedo Bentes Monteiro Neto et al., 2011; Gurbuz *et al.*, 2009). Edenharder *et al.*, (1998) reported that sweet cherries, strawberries, cucumber, tomatoes, bananas, oranges, asparagus, yellow red peppers and specially spinach had a protective effect against clastogenicity of cyclosphosphamide (an alkylating drug) in mice.

Using comet assay some in vivo studies have shown the antigenotoxic effects of dietary agents, namely, artepillin C (a polyphenolic acid found in Brazilian green propolis and Baccharis dracunculifolia) (Azevedo Bentes Monteiro Neto et al., 2011), safranal, (a constituent of Crocus sativus L. stigmas) (Hosseinzadeh and Sadeghnia, 2007), orange juice (Franke *et al.*, 2005b) and vitamin C (Franke *et al.*, 2005a) against DNA damage induced by methyl methanesulfonate (MMS). Also lemongrass protected leukocytes from DNA damage induced by N-methyl-N-nitrosurea (MNU) (Bidinotto *et al.*, 2010). Data from application of comet assay in the assessment of genoprotective effects of diet against alkylating DNA damage is limited. First, AlkA is, as far as we know, the only repair enzyme used for detection of alkylating DNA damage by the comet assay (Collins *et al.*, 2001a). Alk A recognises 3-MeA in DNA, but its specificity is low, detecting other modified bases, some of which are also other alkylated bases. Furthermore, 3-MeA is not the most abundant alkylating damage and it does not represent the alkylating damage with more mutagenic/carcinogenic potential. Other alkylating lesions, like $N^7$MeG, the most abundant lesion, and $O^6$MeG, the most mutagenic, are until now undectectable by comet assay.

### 6.3 Effect of diet on induction of DNA repair

DNA damage can arrest cell cycle progression to allow DNA repair, preventing, therefore, replication of errors, or to induce apoptosis to eliminate cells severely damaged. Defective DNA repair is usually linked to human cancer development. Therefore, enhancement of DNA repair can be understood as a prevention strategy against cancer and an important molecular target for dietary phytochemicals (Davis and Milner, 2007). However, few studies have investigated whether DNA repair activity can be modified by diet in humans.

New modifications of the comet assay have been developed to assess effects of dietary agents on DNA repair ability (as described above). Briefly, the "cellular repair assay" measures the ability of cells to rejoin strand breaks induced by a DNA damaging agent; while the "in vitro repair assay" measures the excision repair activity of a protein extract prepared from cells treated with dietary agents, incubating with a DNA substrate containing a specific type of damage.

### 6.3.1 Polyphenols

Recently, we reported that luteolin and luteolin-7-glucoside increased rejoining of strand breaks after treatment with $H_2O_2$ in Caco-2 cells. Luteolin-7-glucoside also had a BER inductive effect increasing incision activity in Caco-2 cells (Ramos *et al.*, 2010a; Ramos *et al.*, 2010b). Quercetin also increased rejoining of strand breaks induced by *t*-BHP in HepG2 (Ramos et al., 2008). Moreover, dietary agents such as flavonoids, vitamins E and C had been reported as inducers of oxidative DNA damage repair activity (Davis and Milner, 2007).

### 6.3.2 Carotenoids

An in vitro study using HeLa and Caco-2 cells reported that β-cryptoxanthin increased rejoining of strand breaks induced by $H_2O_2$ and increase the repair of oxidised bases. However, increase of repair activity was not related with increase of hOGG1 or APE1expression (Lorenzo et al., 2009). The lack of correlation between activity and mRNA expression of OGG1 and APE1 has also been demonstrated in other studies (Collins *et al.*, 2003; Silva *et al.*, 2009). β-carotene, lutein and lycopene also enhanced strand breaks rejoining in lymphocytes (Fillion *et al.*, 1998; Torbergsen and Collins, 2000). Paz-Elizur *et al.*, (2007) measured OGG1 activity and mRNA expression in 120 healthy individuals and a poor correlation between activity and mRNA was found.

### 6.3.3 Whole foods

Water extracts of Salvia species increased rejoining of strand breaks after treatment with $H_2O_2$ in Caco-2 cells. These water extracts also increased incision activity of a Caco-2 cell extract on a DNA substrate containing specific oxidative damage (8-oxoGua) (Ramos *et al.*, 2010a). Nakamura et al., (2000) reported that aqueous fractions of Fushimi sweet pepper increase repair against ultraviolet-induced cyclobutane pyrimidine dimers in human fibroblasts.

Collins et al., (2003), in a human intervention study, showed that 3 weeks of a dietary supplementation with kiwifruit increased DNA repair capacity measured by "in vitro repair assay". Also Freese, (2006) showed that kiwifruit consumption increased DNA repair capacity in human lymphocytes. Brevik *et al.*, (2011) in a human biomonitoring study, reported that consumption of kiwifruits and antioxidant-rich plant products reduced DNA strand breaks in lymphocytes. Increase of BER activity was observed in the group that consumed antioxidant-rich plant products. However, a reduction of NER activity was observed in both groups. No explanations have been found for this decrease in NER pathway. Diet supplementation with cooked carrots, during 3 weeks, increased in vitro repair activity and strand break rejoining in lymphocytes (Astley *et al.*, 2004).

High dietary folate intake has been associated with a decreased risk of cancer development, such as colorectal cancer. In vitro, rodent and human studies demonstrated that low folate intake increases uracil misincorporation leading to increase of DNA damage, chromosomal breakage and malignant transformation; modulates DNA repair by inhibiting thymidine and purine biosynthesis and induces epigenetic changes leading to global DNA hypomethylation and/or changes in gene-specific methylation and protooncogene activation (Duthie and McMillan, 1997; Duthie, 2010; Duthie *et al.*, 2000; Melnyk et al., 1999). In vivo, folate deficiency induced DNA repair, such as increase of OGG1 and MGMT (Duthie *et al.*, 2010). However, remains unclear if increasing folate intake improve DNA repair. Generaly, the protective role of folate against carcinogenesis is not completely understood.

## 7. Effects of phytochemicals through DNA repair modulation and their interaction with alkylating agents used as chemotherapeutic

Some DNA-damaging agents (specially alkylating agents) are used in cancer therapy due to their ability to induce DNA damage and subsequently apoptosis of tumor cells (Maynard et al., 2009). The efficacy of DNA damage-based cancer therapy is modulated by DNA repair pathways. Therefore these pathways may, attenuate the therapeutic effects of alkylating agents. These drugs are usually classified in two classes: monofunctional (e.g., N-methyl-N_-nitro-N-nitrosoguanidine [MNNG], temozolomide [TMZ] and dacarbazine) and bifunctional alkylating agents (e.g., carmustine [BCNU], cyclophosphamide, lomustine [CCNU] and fotemustine).

BCNU, induces several kinds of DNA damage such as cross-linking, strand breaks and modified bases (Kondo et al., 2010). Between alkylation damage, $N^7$ alkyl-guanine is the most abundant (around 90% of the total alkylation events) and $O^6$ alkyl-guanine is the less frequent. $O^6$ alkyl-guanine, if not repaired before cell division, can form base pairs with T, generating GC→AT transitions mutations by action of MMR pathway. $O^6$ alkyl-guanine is the lesion mainly responsible for the cytotoxic and mutagenic effects of these alkylating drugs. However $O^6$ alkyl-guanine can be repaired by MGMT. In human colorectal adenoma, reduced MGMT activity has been found. Therefore, more mutations occur when cells are treated with alkylating agent (Lees *et al.*, 2004; Lees *et al.*, 2002). However, high levels of MGMT where found in some other tumors (Baer et al., 1993). In the context of therapy with alkylating agents, inhibition of MGMT activity in tumor cells is desirable. The coadjuvant drug $O^6$-benzylguanine ($O^6$-BG) inactivates MGMT, acting as a pseudosubstrate. Effect of $O^6$-BG has been investigated when in combination with an alkylating drug to increase its efficacy (Liu *et al.*, 2002).

$N^7$-alkylG is the most frequent alkylation damage however is not considered to be as mutagenic as $O^6$-alkylG because it is efficiently repaired by BER pathway. N-methylpurine-DNAglycoslase (MPG), the only glycosylase that recognizes alkylation lesions in animal cells, removes $N^7$-alkylG by hydrolysis of the N-glycosylic bond creating an AP site that is repaired by the other enzymes of BER pathway (Drablos et al., 2004). An overexpression of MPG increases the production of AP sites. If the levels of the other enzymes of BER pathway remain unaltered, repair of AP sites is low and accumulation of these lesions becomes cytotoxic and mutagenic. Therefore, an overexpression of MPG or a decrease in other enzymes involved in the subsequent steps in BER pathway, increases cytotoxicity of alkylating drugs. This cytoxicity becomes more relevant when cells are resistant to cytotoxicity from $O^6$-alkylation.

MGMT and MMR have contrasting effects on DNA O6-alkylG. While MGMT is an efficient mechanism of repair, MMR in contrast, does not remove the alkylated base but introduce more lesions like strand break in an attempt to repair the mismatch. Accumulation of strand breaks may activate apoptotic pathways, leading to cell death. In some cells, resistance to alkylating agents can be mediated by MGMT and MMR. Active MGMT and loss of MMR pathway protect cells against the cell death induced by methylating chemotherapeutic drugs (Allan and Travis, 2005). Depletion of MGMT activity (for example, by $O^6$-BG or by epigenetic silencing of the MGMT gene) and intact MMR system results in reversion of resistance with high sensitivity to the cytotoxic effects of alkylating drugs (Casorelli et al., 2008; Esteller et al., 2000; Hegi et al., 2005). Tumors with low MGMT level are more sensitive to alkylating chemotherapy (Bandres et al., 2005). Therefore,DNA repair mechanisms may be understood as a promising target to develop new cancer treatments (Helleday *et al.*, 2008; Jiricny, 2006). Different strategies have been developed to enhance the efficacy of chemotherapy using alkylating agents. In tumor cells, inhibition of MGMT activity and/or BER pathway decreases resistance to alkylating drugs (Drablos et al., 2004; Jaiswal et al., 2011; Middleton and Margison, 2003). Downregulation of DNA repair pathways (except MMR) may increase efficacy of alkylating agents, decreasing the amount of drug needed for chemotherapy and consequently reduction of the side effects (Kondo et al., 2010).

Dietary agents that modulate MGMT expression and/or BER pathway may play an important role in chemotherapy when in combination with alkylating agents. However this subject, in contrast to chemoprevention, has received little attention. Some studies have been that dietary agents may increase MGMT activity. Niture *et al.*, (2006), investigated the potential ability of some Indian medicinal plants extracts to modulate MGMT activity and expression in human peripheral blood lymphocytes and cancer cell lines. The results showed that both the ethanolic and aqueous extracts from neem (*Azadirachta indica*), holy basil (*Ocimum sanctum*), winter cherry (*Withania somnifera*), and oregano (*Origanum majorana*) increased MGMT expression and its activity. Extracts from gooseberry (*Emblica officinalis*), common basil (*Ocimum basilicum*), and spearmint (*Mentha viridis*) also increased MGMT levels, however to a smaller extent. Later, the same author reported that some phytochemicals such as curcumin, silymarin and resveratrol increase protein expression as well as activity of MGMT in lymphocytes and cancer cell lines (Niture *et al.*, 2007). In tumor cells a number of genes are abnormally methylated. Some dietary agents, such as genistein and epigallocatechin-3-gallate showed the ability to reactivate some methylation-silenced genes in cancer cells like MGMT due to a direct inhibition of DNA methyltransferase (Fang et al., 2005; Fang et al., 2003). Recently, Billson et al., (2009), demonstrated that a high vegetable intake in humans decreases MGMT activity in normal colorectal mucosa. To understand the real role of dietary agents on chemotherapy when in combination with alkylating drugs more studies are need.

## 8. Conclusion

Prevention of DNA damage and/or enhanced DNA repair activity by dietary agents constitute an important strategy to prevent mutations and consequently inhibit the carcinogenic process. Diet supplementation with phytochemicals, with beneficial effects, increases their concentrations in the organism. However, effects of supra-physiological concentrations need to be evaluated in each case since a safe phytochemical at physiological concentrations can be toxic at higher concentrations.

The comet assay is a powerful tool to assess the effects of diet on DNA. The immense literature (more than 5500 papers in Pubmed since 1995) that use comet assay (standard and modified versions) demonstrates the real potential of this assay. Some dietary agents have shown ability to prevent DNA damage (oxidative and/or alkylanting) in several experimental models from in vitro to human intervention studies. Less is known about the effect of diet on DNA repair modulation. However, the modifications of comet assay (e.g. use specific-enzymes) gives an opportunity to enhance the knowledge in this field. In spite of the large number of publications much remains to be done. An emergent field is the effect of combinations between diet and drugs used in chemotherapy. In our view, comet assay can be a useful approach also to understand the role of dietary constituents on chemotherapy.

## 9. Acknowledgment

Ramos A.A. is supported by the Foundation for Science and Technology, Portugal, grant SFRH/BD/35672/2007.

## 10. References

Aherne, S. A., Kerry, J. P. & O'Brien, N. M. (2007). Effects of plant extracts on antioxidant status and oxidant-induced stress in Caco-2 cells. Br J Nutr, 97, 321-328.

Aherne, S. A. & O'Brien, N. M. (1999). Protection by the flavonoids myricetin, quercetin, and rutin against hydrogen peroxide-induced DNA damage in Caco-2 and Hep G2 cells. Nutr Cancer, 34, 160-166.

Alia, M., Ramos, S., Mateos, R., Bravo, L. & Goya, L. (2005). Response of the antioxidant defense system to tert-butyl hydroperoxide and hydrogen peroxide in a human hepatoma cell line (HepG2). J Biochem Mol Toxicol, 19, 119-128.

Allan, J. M. & Travis, L. B. (2005). Mechanisms of therapy-related carcinogenesis. Nat Rev Cancer, 5, 943-955.

Allen, R. G. & Tresini, M. (2000). Oxidative stress and gene regulation. Free Radic Biol Med, 28, 463-499.

Anderson, R. F., Amarasinghe, C., Fisher, L. J., Mak, W. B. & Packer, J. E. (2000). Reduction in free-radical-induced DNA strand breaks and base damage through fast chemical repair by flavonoids. Free Radic Res, 33, 91-103.

Angerer, J., Ewers, U. & Wilhelm, M. (2007). Human biomonitoring: state of the art. Int J Hyg Environ Health, 210, 201-228.

Armstrong, M. J. & Galloway, S. M. (1997). Mismatch repair provokes chromosome aberrations in hamster cells treated with methylating agents or 6-thioguanine, but not with ethylating agents. Mutat Res, 373, 167-178.

Astley, S. B., Elliott, R. M., Archer, D. B. & Southon, S. (2004). Evidence that dietary supplementation with carotenoids and carotenoid-rich foods modulates the DNA damage: repair balance in human lymphocytes. Br J Nutr, 91, 63-72.

Azevedo Bentes Monteiro Neto, M., Souza Lima, I. M., Furtado, R. A., Bastos, J. K., Silva Filho, A. A. & Tavares, D. C. (2011). Antigenotoxicity of artepillin C in vivo evaluated by the micronucleus and comet assays. J Appl Toxicol.

Baer, J. C., Freeman, A. A., Newlands, E. S., Watson, A. J., Rafferty, J. A. & Margison, G. P. (1993). Depletion of O6-alkylguanine-DNA alkyltransferase correlates with potentiation of temozolomide and CCNU toxicity in human tumour cells. Br J Cancer, 67, 1299-1302.

Bandres, E., Andion, E., Escalada, A., Honorato, B., Catalan, V., Cubedo, E., Cordeu, L., Garcia, F., Zarate, R., Zabalegui, N. & Garcia-Foncillas, J. (2005). Gene expression profile induced by BCNU in human glioma cell lines with differential MGMT expression. J Neurooncol, 73, 189-198.

Bartek, J., Bartkova, J. & Lukas, J. (2007). DNA damage signalling guards against activated oncogenes and tumour progression. Oncogene, 26, 7773-7779.

Barth, S. W., Fahndrich, C., Bub, A., Dietrich, H., Watzl, B., Will, F., Briviba, K. & Rechkemmer, G. (2005). Cloudy apple juice decreases DNA damage, hyperproliferation and aberrant crypt foci development in the distal colon of DMH-initiated rats. Carcinogenesis, 26, 1414-1421.

Bazo, A. P., Rodrigues, M. A., Sforcin, J. M., de Camargo, J. L., Ribeiro, L. R. & Salvadori, D. M. (2002). Protective action of propolis on the rat colon carcinogenesis. Teratog Carcinog Mutagen, 22, 183-194.

Benhamou, S. & Sarasin, A. (2000). Variability in nucleotide excision repair and cancer risk: a review. Mutat Res, 462, 149-158.

Benkovic, V., Knezevic, A. H., Orsolic, N., Basic, I., Ramic, S., Viculin, T., Knezevic, F. & Kopjar, N. (2009). Evaluation of radioprotective effects of propolis and its flavonoid constituents: in vitro study on human white blood cells. Phytother Res, 23, 1159-1168.

Bidinotto, L. T., Costa, C. A., Salvadori, D. M., Costa, M., Rodrigues, M. A. & Barbisan, L. F. (2010). Protective effects of lemongrass (Cymbopogon citratus STAPF) essential oil on DNA damage and carcinogenesis in female Balb/C mice. J Appl Toxicol.

Billson, H. A., Harrison, K. L., Lees, N. P., Hall, C. N., Margison, G. P. & Povey, A. C. (2009). Dietary variables associated with DNA N7-methylguanine levels and O6-alkylguanine DNA-alkyltransferase activity in human colorectal mucosa. Carcinogenesis, 30, 615-620.

Boateng, J., Verghese, M., Shackelford, L., Walker, L. T., Khatiwada, J., Ogutu, S., Williams, D. S., Jones, J., Guyton, M., Asiamah, D., Henderson, F., Grant, L., DeBruce, M., Johnson, A., Washington, S. & Chawan, C. B. (2007). Selected fruits reduce azoxymethane (AOM)-induced aberrant crypt foci (ACF) in Fisher 344 male rats. Food Chem Toxicol, 45, 725-732.

Brevik, A., Karlsen, A., Azqueta, A., Tirado, A. E., Blomhoff, R. & Collins, A. (2011). Both base excision repair and nucleotide excision repair in humans are influenced by nutritional factors. Cell Biochem Funct, 29, 36-42.

Bugni, J. M., Meira, L. B. and Samson, L. D. (2009) Alkylation-induced colon tumorigenesis in mice deficient in the Mgmt and Msh6 proteins. Oncogene, 28, 734-741.

Cai, Q., Rahn, R. O. & Zhang, R. (1997). Dietary flavonoids, quercetin, luteolin and genistein, reduce oxidative DNA damage and lipid peroxidation and quench free radicals. Cancer Lett, 119, 99-107.

Caldecott, K. W. (2007). Mammalian single-strand break repair: mechanisms and links with chromatin. DNA Repair (Amst), 6, 443-453.

Casorelli, I., Russo, M. T. & Bignami, M. (2008). Role of mismatch repair and MGMT in response to anticancer therapies. Anticancer Agents Med Chem, 8, 368-380.

Chen, C. and Kong, A. N. (2004). Dietary chemopreventive compounds and ARE/EpRE signaling. Free Radic Biol Med, 36, 1505-1516.

Collins, A. R. (2004). The comet assay for DNA damage and repair: principles, applications, and limitations. Mol Biotechnol, 26, 249-261.

Collins, A. R. (2009). Investigating oxidative DNA damage and its repair using the comet assay. Mutat Res, 681, 24-32.

Collins, A. R., Dobson, V. L., Dusinska, M., Kennedy, G. & Stetina, R. (1997a). The comet assay: what can it really tell us? Mutat Res, 375, 183-193.

Collins, A. R., Dusinska, M. & Horska, A. (2001a). Detection of alkylation damage in human lymphocyte DNA with the comet assay. Acta Biochim Pol, 48, 611-614.

Collins, A. R., Dusinska, M., Horvathova, E., Munro, E., Savio, M. & Stetina, R. (2001b). Inter-individual differences in repair of DNA base oxidation, measured in vitro with the comet assay. Mutagenesis, 16, 297-301.

Collins, A. R., Duthie, S. J. & Dobson, V. L. (1993). Direct enzymic detection of endogenous oxidative base damage in human lymphocyte DNA. Carcinogenesis, 14, 1733-1735.

Collins, A. R., Harrington, V., Drew, J. & Melvin, R. (2003). Nutritional modulation of DNA repair in a human intervention study. Carcinogenesis, 24, 511-515.

Collins, A. R., Mitchell, D. L., Zunino, A., de Wit, J. & Busch, D. (1997b). UV-sensitive rodent mutant cell lines of complementation groups 6 and 8 differ phenotypically from their human counterparts. Environ Mol Mutagen, 29, 152-160.

Collins, A. R., Oscoz, A. A., Brunborg, G., Gaivao, I., Giovannelli, L., Kruszewski, M., Smith, C. C. & Stetina, R. (2008). The comet assay: topical issues. Mutagenesis, 23, 143-151.

D'Errico, M., Parlanti, E. & Dogliotti, E. (2008). Mechanism of oxidative DNA damage repair and relevance to human pathology. Mutat Res, 659, 4-14.

Dani, C., Oliboni, L. S., Umezu, F. M., Pasquali, M. A., Salvador, M., Moreira, J. C. & Henriques, J. A. (2009). Antioxidant and antigenotoxic activities of purple grape juice--organic and conventional--in adult rats. J Med Food, 12, 1111-1118.

Davis, C. D. (2007). Nutritional interactions: credentialing of molecular targets for cancer prevention. Exp Biol Med (Maywood), 232, 176-183.

Davis, C. D. & Milner, J. A. (2007). Biomarkers for diet and cancer prevention research: potentials and challenges. Acta Pharmacol Sin, 28, 1262-1273.

de Kok, T. M., van Breda, S. G. & Manson, M. M. (2008). Mechanisms of combined action of different chemopreventive dietary compounds: a review. Eur J Nutr, 47 Suppl 2, 51-59.

de Lima, R. O., Bazo, A. P., Said, R. A., Sforcin, J. M., Bankova, V., Darros, B. R. & Salvadori, D. M. (2005). Modifying effect of propolis on dimethylhydrazine-induced DNA damage but not colonic aberrant crypt foci in rats. Environ Mol Mutagen, 45, 8-16.

De, S. & Das, S. (2001). Protective Effects of Tomato Juice on Mouse Skin Carcinogenesis. Asian Pac J Cancer Prev, 2, 43-47.

Del Bo, C., Martini, D., Vendrame, S., Riso, P., Ciappellano, S., Klimis-Zacas, D. & Porrini, M. (2010). Improvement of lymphocyte resistance against H(2)O(2)-induced DNA damage in Sprague-Dawley rats after eight weeks of a wild blueberry (Vaccinium angustifolium)-enriched diet. Mutat Res, 703, 158-162.

Devaraj, S., Mathur, S., Basu, A., Aung, H. H., Vasu, V. T., Meyers, S. & Jialal, I. (2008). A dose-response study on the effects of purified lycopene supplementation on biomarkers of oxidative stress. J Am Coll Nutr, 27, 267-273.

Devipriya, N., Sudheer, A. R. & Menon, V. P. (2008). Caffeic acid protects human peripheral blood lymphocytes against gamma radiation-induced cellular damage. J Biochem Mol Toxicol, 22, 175-186.

Doak, S. H., Brusehafer, K., Dudley, E., Quick, E., Johnson, G., Newton, R. P. & Jenkins, G. J. (2008). No-observed effect levels are associated with up-regulation of MGMT following MMS exposure. Mutat Res, 648, 9-14.

Dolara, P., Luceri, C., De Filippo, C., Femia, A. P., Giovannelli, L., Caderni, G., Cecchini, C., Silvi, S., Orpianesi, C. & Cresci, A. (2005). Red wine polyphenols influence carcinogenesis, intestinal microflora, oxidative damage and gene expression profiles of colonic mucosa in F344 rats. Mutat Res, 591, 237-246.

Drablos, F., Feyzi, E., Aas, P. A., Vaagbo, C. B., Kavli, B., Bratlie, M. S., Pena-Diaz, J., Otterlei, M., Slupphaug, G. & Krokan, H. E. (2004). Alkylation damage in DNA and RNA--repair mechanisms and medical significance. DNA Repair (Amst), 3, 1389-1407.

Dudas, A. & Chovanec, M. (2004). DNA double-strand break repair by homologous recombination. Mutat Res, 566, 131-167.

Dulebohn, R. V., Yi, W., Srivastava, A., Akoh, C. C., Krewer, G. & Fischer, J. G. (2008). Effects of blueberry (Vaccinium ashei) on DNA damage, lipid peroxidation, and phase II enzyme activities in rats. J Agric Food Chem, 56, 11700-11706.

Dusinska, M. & Collins, A. R. (1996). Detection of oxi-dised purines and UV-induced photoproducts in DNA of single cells, by inclusion of lesion-specific enzymes in the comet assay. Alternative Laboratory Animal, 24, 405-411.

Dusinska, M. & Collins, A. R. (2008). The comet assay in human biomonitoring: gene-environment interactions. Mutagenesis, 23, 191-205.

Duthie, S. J. (2010) Folate and cancer: how DNA damage, repair and methylation impact on colon carcinogenesis. J Inherit Metab Dis, 34, 101-109.

Duthie, S. J., Grant, G., Pirie, L. P., Watson, A. J. and Margison, G. P. (2010) Folate deficiency alters hepatic and colon MGMT and OGG-1 DNA repair protein expression in rats but has no effect on genome-wide DNA methylation. Cancer Prev Res (Phila), 3, 92-100.

Duthie, S. J. and McMillan, P. (1997) Uracil misincorporation in human DNA detected using single cell gel electrophoresis. Carcinogenesis, 18, 1709-1714.

Duthie, S. J., Narayanan, S., Blum, S., Pirie, L. and Brand, G. M. (2000) Folate deficiency in vitro induces uracil misincorporation and DNA hypomethylation and inhibits DNA excision repair in immortalized normal human colon epithelial cells. Nutr Cancer, 37, 245-251.

Edenharder, R., Frangart, J., Hager, M., Hofmann, P. and Rauscher, R. (1998) Protective effects of fruits and vegetables against in vivo clastogenicity of cyclosphosphamide or benzo[a]pyrene in mice. Food Chem Toxicol, 36, 637-645.

Eker, A. P., Quayle, C., Chaves, I. and van der Horst, G. T. (2009) DNA repair in mammalian cells: Direct DNA damage reversal: elegant solutions for nasty problems. Cell Mol Life Sci, 66, 968-980.

Esteller, M., Garcia-Foncillas, J., Andion, E., Goodman, S. N., Hidalgo, O. F., Vanaclocha, V., Baylin, S. B. and Herman, J. G. (2000) Inactivation of the DNA-repair gene MGMT and the clinical response of gliomas to alkylating agents. N Engl J Med, 343, 1350-1354.

Evans, M. D., Dizdaroglu, M. and Cooke, M. S. (2004) Oxidative DNA damage and disease: induction, repair and significance. Mutat Res, 567, 1-61.

Fabiani, R., Rosignoli, P., De Bartolomeo, A., Fuccelli, R., Servili, M., Montedoro, G. F. and Morozzi, G. (2008) Oxidative DNA damage is prevented by extracts of olive oil, hydroxytyrosol, and other olive phenolic compounds in human blood mononuclear cells and HL60 cells. J Nutr, 138, 1411-1416.

Fairbairn, D. W., Olive, P. L. and O'Neill, K. L. (1995) The comet assay: a comprehensive review. Mutat Res, 339, 37-59.

Fang, M. Z., Chen, D., Sun, Y., Jin, Z., Christman, J. K. and Yang, C. S. (2005) Reversal of hypermethylation and reactivation of p16INK4a, RARbeta, and MGMT genes by genistein and other isoflavones from soy. Clin Cancer Res, 11, 7033-7041.

Fang, M. Z., Wang, Y., Ai, N., Hou, Z., Sun, Y., Lu, H., Welsh, W. and Yang, C. S. (2003) Tea polyphenol (-)-epigallocatechin-3-gallate inhibits DNA methyltransferase and reactivates methylation-silenced genes in cancer cell lines. Cancer Res, 63, 7563-7570.

Ferguson, L. R., Philpott, M. and Karunasinghe, N. (2004) Dietary cancer and prevention using antimutagens. Toxicology, 198, 147-159.

Fillion, L., Collins, A. and Southon, S. (1998) Beta-carotene enhances the recovery of lymphocytes from oxidative DNA damage. Acta Biochim Pol, 45, 183-190.

Fortini, P., Pascucci, B., Parlanti, E., D'Errico, M., Simonelli, V. and Dogliotti, E. (2003) The base excision repair: mechanisms and its relevance for cancer susceptibility. Biochimie, 85, 1053-1071.

Franke, S. I., Pra, D., da Silva, J., Erdtmann, B. and Henriques, J. A. (2005a) Possible repair action of Vitamin C on DNA damage induced by methyl methanesulfonate, cyclophosphamide, FeSO4 and CuSO4 in mouse blood cells in vivo. Mutat Res, 583, 75-84.

Franke, S. I., Pra, D., Erdtmann, B., Henriques, J. A. and da Silva, J. (2005b) Influence of orange juice over the genotoxicity induced by alkylating agents: an in vivo analysis. Mutagenesis, 20, 279-283.

Freese, R. (2006) Markers of oxidative DNA damage in human interventions with fruit and berries. Nutr Cancer, 54, 143-147.

Frei, B. and Higdon, J. V. (2003) Antioxidant activity of tea polyphenols in vivo: evidence from animal studies. J Nutr, 133, 3275S-3284S.

Furtado, R. A., de Araujo, F. R., Resende, F. A., Cunha, W. R. and Tavares, D. C. (2009) Protective effect of rosmarinic acid on V79 cells evaluated by the micronucleus and comet assays. J Appl Toxicol, 30, 254-259.

Gaivao, I., Piasek, A., Brevik, A., Shaposhnikov, S. and Collins, A. R. (2009) Comet assay-based methods for measuring DNA repair in vitro; estimates of inter- and intra-individual variation. Cell Biol Toxicol, 25, 45-52.

Gedik, C. M., Ewen, S. W. and Collins, A. R. (1992) Single-cell gel electrophoresis applied to the analysis of UV-C damage and its repair in human cells. Int J Radiat Biol, 62, 313-320.

Glei, M. and Pool-Zobel, B. L. (2006) The main catechin of green tea, (-)-epigallocatechin-3-gallate (EGCG), reduces bleomycin-induced DNA damage in human leucocytes. Toxicol In Vitro, 20, 295-300.

Guglielmi, F., Luceri, C., Giovannelli, L., Dolara, P. and Lodovici, M. (2003) Effect of 4-coumaric and 3,4-dihydroxybenzoic acid on oxidative DNA damage in rat colonic mucosa. Br J Nutr, 89, 581-587.

Gurbuz, N., Ozkul, A. and Burgaz, S. (2009) Effects of vitamin C and N-acetylcysteine against cyclophosphamide-induced genotoxicity in exfoliated bladder cells of mice in vivo. J BUON, 14, 647-652.

Hall, C. N., Badawi, A. F., O'Connor, P. J. and Saffhill, R. (1991) The detection of alkylation damage in the DNA of human gastrointestinal tissues. Br J Cancer, 64, 59-63.

Han, K. C., Wong, W. C. and Benzie, I. F. (2011) Genoprotective effects of green tea (Camellia sinensis) in human subjects: results of a controlled supplementation trial. Br J Nutr, 105, 171-179.

Hanawalt, P. C. (2002) Subpathways of nucleotide excision repair and their regulation. Oncogene, 21, 8949-8956.

Hartmann, A., Agurell, E., Beevers, C., Brendler-Schwaab, S., Burlinson, B., Clay, P., Collins, A., Smith, A., Speit, G., Thybaud, V. and Tice, R. R. (2003) Recommendations for conducting the in vivo alkaline Comet assay. 4th International Comet Assay Workshop. Mutagenesis, 18, 45-51.

Hegde, M. L., Hazra, T. K. and Mitra, S. (2008) Early steps in the DNA base excision/single-strand interruption repair pathway in mammalian cells. Cell Res, 18, 27-47.

Hegi, M. E., Diserens, A. C., Gorlia, T., Hamou, M. F., de Tribolet, N., Weller, M., Kros, J. M., Hainfellner, J. A., Mason, W., Mariani, L., Bromberg, J. E., Hau, P., Mirimanoff, R. O., Cairncross, J. G., Janzer, R. C. and Stupp, R. (2005) MGMT gene silencing and benefit from temozolomide in glioblastoma. N Engl J Med, 352, 997-1003.

Helleday, T., Lo, J., van Gent, D. C. and Engelward, B. P. (2007) DNA double-strand break repair: from mechanistic understanding to cancer treatment. DNA Repair (Amst), 6, 923-935.

Helleday, T., Petermann, E., Lundin, C., Hodgson, B. and Sharma, R. A. (2008) DNA repair pathways as targets for cancer therapy. Nat Rev Cancer, 8, 193-204.

Heo, M. Y., Sohn, S. J. and Au, W. W. (2001) Anti-genotoxicity of galangin as a cancer chemopreventive agent candidate. Mutat Res, 488, 135-150.

Hoelzl, C., Knasmuller, S., Misik, M., Collins, A., Dusinska, M. and Nersesyan, A. (2009) Use of single cell gel electrophoresis assays for the detection of DNA-protective effects of dietary factors in humans: recent results and trends. Mutat Res, 681, 68-79.

Horvathova, K., Chalupa, I., Sebova, L., Tothova, D. and Vachalkova, A. (2005) Protective effect of quercetin and luteolin in human melanoma HMB-2 cells. Mutat Res, 565, 105-112.

Horvathova, K., Novotny, L., Tothova, D. and Vachalkova, A. (2004) Determination of free radical scavenging activity of quercetin, rutin, luteolin and apigenin in H2O2-treated human ML cells K562. Neoplasma, 51, 395-399.

Horvathova, K., Novotny, L. and Vachalkova, A. (2003) The free radical scavenging activity of four flavonoids determined by the comet assay. Neoplasma, 50, 291-295.

Hosseinzadeh, H. and Sadeghnia, H. R. (2007) Effect of safranal, a constituent of Crocus sativus (saffron), on methyl methanesulfonate (MMS)-induced DNA damage in mouse organs: an alkaline single-cell gel electrophoresis (comet) assay. DNA Cell Biol, 26, 841-846.

Jagetia, A., Jagetia, G. C. and Jha, S. (2007) Naringin, a grapefruit flavanone, protects V79 cells against the bleomycin-induced genotoxicity and decline in survival. J Appl Toxicol, 27, 122-132.

Jaiswal, A. S., Banerjee, S., Aneja, R., Sarkar, F. H., Ostrov, D. A. and Narayan, S. (2011) DNA polymerase beta as a novel target for chemotherapeutic intervention of colorectal cancer. PLoS One, 6, e16691.

Jaiswal, A. S. and Narayan, S. (2008) A novel function of adenomatous polyposis coli (APC) in regulating DNA repair. Cancer Lett, 271, 272-280.

Jeyabal, P. V., Syed, M. B., Venkataraman, M., Sambandham, J. K. and Sakthisekaran, D. (2005) Apigenin inhibits oxidative stress-induced macromolecular damage in N-nitrosodiethylamine (NDEA)-induced hepatocellular carcinogenesis in Wistar albino rats. Mol Carcinog, 44, 11-20.

Jiricny, J. (2006) The multifaceted mismatch-repair system. Nat Rev Mol Cell Biol, 7, 335-346.

Jiricny, J. and Marra, G. (2003) DNA repair defects in colon cancer. Curr Opin Genet Dev, 13, 61-69.

Kager, N., Ferk, F., Kundi, M., Wagner, K. H., Misik, M. and Knasmuller, S. (2010) Prevention of oxidative DNA damage in inner organs and lymphocytes of rats by green tea extract. Eur J Nutr, 49, 227-234.

Kaina, B., Christmann, M., Naumann, S. and Roos, W. P. (2007) MGMT: key node in the battle against genotoxicity, carcinogenicity and apoptosis induced by alkylating agents. DNA Repair (Amst), 6, 1079-1099.

Kaina, B., Margison, G. P. and Christmann, M. (2010) Targeting O-methylguanine-DNA methyltransferase with specific inhibitors as a strategy in cancer therapy. Cell Mol Life Sci, 67, 3663-3681.

Kanupriya, Dipti, P., Sharma, S. K., Sairam, M., Ilavazhagan, G., Sawhney, R. C. and Banerjee, P. K. (2006) Flavonoids protect U-937 macrophages against tert-butylhydroperoxide induced oxidative injury. Food Chem Toxicol, 44, 1024-1030.

Karihtala, P. and Soini, Y. (2007) Reactive oxygen species and antioxidant mechanisms in human tissues and their relation to malignancies. APMIS, 115, 81-103.

Kim, J. M., Araki, S., Kim, D. J., Park, C. B., Takasuka, N., Baba-Toriyama, H., Ota, T., Nir, Z., Khachik, F., Shimidzu, N., Tanaka, Y., Osawa, T., Uraji, T., Murakoshi, M., Nishino, H. and Tsuda, H. (1998) Chemopreventive effects of carotenoids and curcumins on mouse colon carcinogenesis after 1,2-dimethylhydrazine initiation. Carcinogenesis, 19, 81-85.

Knudsen, N. O., Andersen, S. D., Lutzen, A., Nielsen, F. C. and Rasmussen, L. J. (2009) Nuclear translocation contributes to regulation of DNA excision repair activities. DNA Repair (Amst), 8, 682-689.

Koch, T. C., Briviba, K., Watzl, B., Fahndrich, C., Bub, A., Rechkemmer, G. and Barth, S. W. (2009) Prevention of colon carcinogenesis by apple juice in vivo: impact of juice constituents and obesity. Mol Nutr Food Res, 53, 1289-1302.

Kondo, N., Takahashi, A., Ono, K. and Ohnishi, T. (2010) DNA damage induced by alkylating agents and repair pathways. J Nucleic Acids, 2010, 543531.

Kovary, K., Louvain, T. S., Costa e Silva, M. C., Albano, F., Pires, B. B., Laranja, G. A., Lage, C. L. and Felzenszwalb, I. (2001) Biochemical behaviour of norbixin during in vitro DNA damage induced by reactive oxygen species. Br J Nutr, 85, 431-440.

Kuo, S. M. (1996) Antiproliferative potency of structurally distinct dietary flavonoids on human colon cancer cells. Cancer Lett, 110, 41-48.

Langie, S. A., Knaapen, A. M., Brauers, K. J., van Berlo, D., van Schooten, F. J. and Godschalk, R. W. (2006) Development and validation of a modified comet assay to phenotypically assess nucleotide excision repair. Mutagenesis, 21, 153-158.

Lees, N. P., Harrison, K. L., Hall, C. N., Margison, G. P. and Povey, A. C. (2004) Reduced MGMT activity in human colorectal adenomas is associated with K-ras GC->AT transition mutations in a population exposed to methylating agents. Carcinogenesis, 25, 1243-1247.

Lees, N. P., Harrison, K. L., Hill, E., Hall, C. N., Margison, G. P. and Povey, A. C. (2002) Longitudinal variation in O(6)-alkylguanine DNA-alkyltransferase activity in the human colon and rectum. Br J Cancer, 87, 168-170.

Lima, C. F., Andrade, P. B., Seabra, R. M., Fernandes-Ferreira, M. and Pereira-Wilson, C. (2005) The drinking of a Salvia officinalis infusion improves liver antioxidant status in mice and rats. J Ethnopharmacol, 97, 383-389.

Lima, C. F., Fernandes-Ferreira, M. and Pereira-Wilson, C. (2006) Phenolic compounds protect HepG2 cells from oxidative damage: relevance of glutathione levels. Life Sci, 79, 2056-2068.

Lind, G. E., Thorstensen, L., Lovig, T., Meling, G. I., Hamelin, R., Rognum, T. O., Esteller, M. and Lothe, R. A. (2004) A CpG island hypermethylation profile of primary colorectal carcinomas and colon cancer cell lines. Mol Cancer, 3, 28.

Liu, L. and Gerson, S. L. (2006) Targeted modulation of MGMT: clinical implications. Clin Cancer Res, 12, 328-331.

Liu, L., Schwartz, S., Davis, B. M. and Gerson, S. L. (2002) Chemotherapy-induced O(6)-benzylguanine-resistant alkyltransferase mutations in mismatch-deficient colon cancer. Cancer Res, 62, 3070-3076.

Lorenzo, Y., Azqueta, A., Luna, L., Bonilla, F., Dominguez, G. and Collins, A. R. (2009) The carotenoid beta-cryptoxanthin stimulates the repair of DNA oxidation damage in addition to acting as an antioxidant in human cells. Carcinogenesis, 30, 308-314.

Marchesi, F., Turriziani, M., Tortorelli, G., Avvisati, G., Torino, F. and De Vecchis, L. (2007) Triazene compounds: mechanism of action and related DNA repair systems. Pharmacol Res, 56, 275-287.

Maynard, S., Schurman, S. H., Harboe, C., de Souza-Pinto, N. C. and Bohr, V. A. (2009) Base excision repair of oxidative DNA damage and association with cancer and aging. Carcinogenesis, 30, 2-10.

McCann, M. J., Gill, C. I., G, O. B., Rao, J. R., McRoberts, W. C., Hughes, P., McEntee, R. and Rowland, I. R. (2007) Anti-cancer properties of phenolics from apple waste on colon carcinogenesis in vitro. Food Chem Toxicol, 45, 1224-1230.

Mehta, R. G., Murillo, G., Naithani, R. and Peng, X. (2010) Cancer chemoprevention by natural products: how far have we come? Pharm Res, 27, 950-961.

Melnyk, S., Pogribna, M., Miller, B. J., Basnakian, A. G., Pogribny, I. P. and James, S. J. (1999) Uracil misincorporation, DNA strand breaks, and gene amplification are associated with tumorigenic cell transformation in folate deficient/repleted Chinese hamster ovary cells. Cancer Lett, 146, 35-44.

Middleton, M. R. and Margison, G. P. (2003) Improvement of chemotherapy efficacy by inactivation of a DNA-repair pathway. Lancet Oncol, 4, 37-44.

Miene, C., Klenow, S., Veeriah, S., Richling, E. and Glei, M. (2009) Impact of apple polyphenols on GSTT2 gene expression, subsequent protection of DNA and modulation of proliferation using LT97 human colon adenoma cells. Mol Nutr Food Res, 53, 1254-1262.

Min, K. and Ebeler, S. E. (2008) Flavonoid effects on DNA oxidation at low concentrations relevant to physiological levels. Food Chem Toxicol, 46, 96-104.

Moller, P. and Loft, S. (2002) Oxidative DNA damage in human white blood cells in dietary antioxidant intervention studies. Am J Clin Nutr, 76, 303-310.

Moon, H. K., Yang, E. S. and Park, J. W. (2006) Protection of peroxynitrite-induced DNA damage by dietary antioxidants. Arch Pharm Res, 29, 213-217.

Murillo, G., Choi, J. K., Pan, O., Constantinou, A. I. and Mehta, R. G. (2004) Efficacy of garbanzo and soybean flour in suppression of aberrant crypt foci in the colons of CF-1 mice. Anticancer Res, 24, 3049-3055.

Muzandu, K., Ishizuka, M., Sakamoto, K. Q., Shaban, Z., El Bohi, K., Kazusaka, A. and Fujita, S. (2006) Effect of lycopene and beta-carotene on peroxynitrite-mediated cellular modifications. Toxicol Appl Pharmacol, 215, 330-340.

Nakamura, Y., Tomokane, I., Mori, T., Tanaka, A., Koutani, J., Matsuo, T., Okamoto, S., Sato, K. and Ohtsuki, K. (2000) DNA repair effect of traditional sweet pepper Fushimi-togarashi: seen in suppression of UV-induced cyclobutane pyrimidine dimer in human fibroblast. Biosci Biotechnol Biochem, 64, 2575-2580.

Nigam, N., Prasad, S. and Shukla, Y. (2007) Preventive effects of lupeol on DMBA induced DNA alkylation damage in mouse skin. Food Chem Toxicol, 45, 2331-2335.

Niture, S. K., Rao, U. S. and Srivenugopal, K. S. (2006) Chemopreventative strategies targeting the MGMT repair protein: augmented expression in human lymphocytes and tumor cells by ethanolic and aqueous extracts of several Indian medicinal plants. Int J Oncol, 29, 1269-1278.

Niture, S. K., Velu, C. S., Smith, Q. R., Bhat, G. J. and Srivenugopal, K. S. (2007) Increased expression of the MGMT repair protein mediated by cysteine prodrugs and chemopreventative natural products in human lymphocytes and tumor cell lines. Carcinogenesis, 28, 378-389.

Noroozi, M., Angerson, W. J. and Lean, M. E. (1998) Effects of flavonoids and vitamin C on oxidative DNA damage to human lymphocytes. Am J Clin Nutr, 67, 1210-1218.

Nossoni, F. (2008) Single-Cell Gel Electrophoresis (Comet Assay): Methodology, Potential Applications, and Limitations in Cancer Research. MMG 445 Basic Biotechnology eJournal, 4, 30-35.

Nouspikel, T. (2009) DNA repair in mammalian cells : Nucleotide excision repair: variations on versatility. Cell Mol Life Sci, 66, 994-1009.

Nozawa, H., Yoshida, A., Tajima, O., Katayama, M., Sonobe, H., Wakabayashi, K. and Kondo, K. (2004) Intake of beer inhibits azoxymethane-induced colonic carcinogenesis in male Fischer 344 rats. Int J Cancer, 108, 404-411.

Nystrom, M. and Mutanen, M. (2009) Diet and epigenetics in colon cancer. World J Gastroenterol, 15, 257-263.

Ostling, O. and Johanson, K. J. (1984) Microelectrophoretic study of radiation-induced DNA damages in individual mammalian cells. Biochem Biophys Res Commun, 123, 291-298.

Ovesna, Z., Kozics, K. and Slamenova, D. (2006) Protective effects of ursolic acid and oleanolic acid in leukemic cells. Mutat Res, 600, 131-137.

Pan, M. H., Ghai, G. and Ho, C. T. (2008) Food bioactives, apoptosis, and cancer. Mol Nutr Food Res, 52, 43-52.

Panayiotidis, M. and Collins, A. R. (1997) Ex vivo assessment of lymphocyte antioxidant status using the comet assay. Free Radic Res, 27, 533-537.

Pastoriza Gallego, M. and Sarasin, A. (2003) Transcription-coupled repair of 8-oxoguanine in human cells and its deficiency in some DNA repair diseases. Biochimie, 85, 1073-1082.

Paz-Elizur, T., Elinger, D., Leitner-Dagan, Y., Blumenstein, S., Krupsky, M., Berrebi, A., Schechtman, E. and Livneh, Z. (2007) Development of an enzymatic DNA repair assay for molecular epidemiology studies: distribution of OGG activity in healthy individuals. DNA Repair (Amst), 6, 45-60.

Petermann, A., Miene, C., Schulz-Raffelt, G., Palige, K., Holzer, J., Glei, M. and Bohmer, F. D. (2009) GSTT2, a phase II gene induced by apple polyphenols, protects colon epithelial cells against genotoxic damage. Mol Nutr Food Res, 53, 1245-1253.

Pool-Zobel, B. L., Bub, A., Muller, H., Wollowski, I. and Rechkemmer, G. (1997) Consumption of vegetables reduces genetic damage in humans: first results of a human intervention trial with carotenoid-rich foods. Carcinogenesis, 18, 1847-1850.

Porrini, M. and Riso, P. (2000) Lymphocyte lycopene concentration and DNA protection from oxidative damage is increased in women after a short period of tomato consumption. J Nutr, 130, 189-192.

Povey, A. C., Hall, C. N., Badawi, A. F., Cooper, D. P. and O'Connor, P. J. (2000) Elevated levels of the pro-carcinogenic adduct, O(6)-methylguanine, in normal DNA from the cancer prone regions of the large bowel. Gut, 47, 362-365.

Prasad, N. R., Jeyanthimala, K. and Ramachandran, S. (2009) Caffeic acid modulates ultraviolet radiation-B induced oxidative damage in human blood lymphocytes. J Photochem Photobiol B, 95, 196-203.

Quincozes-Santos, A., Andreazza, A. C., Nardin, P., Funchal, C., Goncalves, C. A. and Gottfried, C. (2007) Resveratrol attenuates oxidative-induced DNA damage in C6 Glioma cells. Neurotoxicology, 28, 886-891.

Rajamanickam, S. and Agarwal, R. (2008) Natural products and colon cancer: current status and future prospects. Drug Dev Res, 69, 460-471.

Ramos, A. A., Azqueta, A., Pereira-Wilson, C. and Collins, A. R. (2010a) Polyphenolic compounds from Salvia species protect cellular DNA from oxidation and stimulate DNA repair in cultured human cells. J Agric Food Chem, 58, 7465-7471.

Ramos, A. A., Lima, C. F., Pereira, M. L., Fernandes-Ferreira, M. and Pereira-Wilson, C. (2008) Antigenotoxic effects of quercetin, rutin and ursolic acid on HepG2 cells: evaluation by the comet assay. Toxicol Lett, 177, 66-73.

Ramos, A. A., Pereira-Wilson, C. and Collins, A. R. (2010b) Protective effects of ursolic acid and luteolin against oxidative DNA damage include enhancement of DNA repair in Caco-2 cells. Mutat Res, 692, 6-11.

Riso, P., Martini, D., Visioli, F., Martinetti, A. and Porrini, M. (2009) Effect of broccoli intake on markers related to oxidative stress and cancer risk in healthy smokers and nonsmokers. Nutr Cancer, 61, 232-237.

Robertson, A. B., Klungland, A., Rognes, T. and Leiros, I. (2009) DNA repair in mammalian cells: Base excision repair: the long and short of it. Cell Mol Life Sci, 66, 981-993.

Ross, J. A. and Kasum, C. M. (2002) Dietary flavonoids: bioavailability, metabolic effects, and safety. Annu Rev Nutr, 22, 19-34.

Rusak, G., Piantanida, I., Masic, L., Kapuralin, K., Durgo, K. and Kopjar, N. (2010) Spectrophotometric analysis of flavonoid-DNA interactions and DNA damaging/protecting and cytotoxic potential of flavonoids in human peripheral blood lymphocytes. Chem Biol Interact, 188, 181-189.

Schaefer, S., Baum, M., Eisenbrand, G., Dietrich, H., Will, F. and Janzowski, C. (2006) Polyphenolic apple juice extracts and their major constituents reduce oxidative damage in human colon cell lines. Mol Nutr Food Res, 50, 24-33.

Sengottuvelan, M., Deeptha, K. and Nalini, N. (2009) Resveratrol ameliorates DNA damage, prooxidant and antioxidant imbalance in 1,2-dimethylhydrazine induced rat colon carcinogenesis. Chem Biol Interact, 181, 193-201.

Sengupta, A., Ghosh, S. and Das, S. (2003) Tomato and garlic can modulate azoxymethane-induced colon carcinogenesis in rats. Eur J Cancer Prev, 12, 195-200.

Sengupta, A., Ghosh, S. and Das, S. (2004) Modulatory influence of garlic and tomato on cyclooxygenase-2 activity, cell proliferation and apoptosis during azoxymethane induced colon carcinogenesis in rat. Cancer Lett, 208, 127-136.

Serpeloni, J. M., Grotto, D., Mercadante, A. Z., de Lourdes Pires Bianchi, M. and Antunes, L. M. (2010) Lutein improves antioxidant defense in vivo and protects against DNA damage and chromosome instability induced by cisplatin. Arch Toxicol, 84, 811-822.

Shaposhnikov, S., Azqueta, A., Henriksson, S., Meier, S., Gaivao, I., Huskisson, N. H., Smart, A., Brunborg, G., Nilsson, M. and Collins, A. R. (2010) Twelve-gel slide format optimised for comet assay and fluorescent in situ hybridisation. Toxicol Lett, 195, 31-34.

Silva, J. P., Gomes, A. C. and Coutinho, O. P. (2008) Oxidative DNA damage protection and repair by polyphenolic compounds in PC12 cells. Eur J Pharmacol, 601, 50-60.

Silva, J. P., Gomes, A. C., Proenca, F. and Coutinho, O. P. (2009) Novel nitrogen compounds enhance protection and repair of oxidative DNA damage in a neuronal cell model: comparison with quercetin. Chem Biol Interact, 181, 328-337.

Singh, N. P., McCoy, M. T., Tice, R. R. and Schneider, E. L. (1988) A simple technique for quantitation of low levels of DNA damage in individual cells. Exp Cell Res, 175, 184-191.

Speit, G., Schutz, P., Bonzheim, I., Trenz, K. and Hoffmann, H. (2004) Sensitivity of the FPG protein towards alkylation damage in the comet assay. Toxicol Lett, 146, 151-158.

Speit, G., Witton-Davies, T., Heepchantree, W., Trenz, K. and Hoffmann, H. (2003) Investigations on the effect of cigarette smoking in the comet assay. Mutat Res, 542, 33-42.

Srinivasan, M., Sudheer, A. R., Pillai, K. R., Kumar, P. R., Sudhakaran, P. R. and Menon, V. P. (2007) Lycopene as a natural protector against gamma-radiation induced DNA damage, lipid peroxidation and antioxidant status in primary culture of isolated rat hepatocytes in vitro. Biochim Biophys Acta, 1770, 659-665.

Suaeyun, R., Kinouchi, T., Arimochi, H., Vinitketkumnuen, U. and Ohnishi, Y. (1997) Inhibitory effects of lemon grass (Cymbopogon citratus Stapf) on formation of azoxymethane-induced DNA adducts and aberrant crypt foci in the rat colon. Carcinogenesis, 18, 949-955.

Szeto, Y. T. and Benzie, I. F. (2002) Effects of dietary antioxidants on human DNA ex vivo. Free Radic Res, 36, 113-118.

Terry, P., Giovannucci, E., Michels, K. B., Bergkvist, L., Hansen, H., Holmberg, L. and Wolk, A. (2001) Fruit, vegetables, dietary fiber, and risk of colorectal cancer. J Natl Cancer Inst, 93, 525-533.

Thompson, H. J., Heimendinger, J., Haegele, A., Sedlacek, S. M., Gillette, C., O'Neill, C., Wolfe, P. and Conry, C. (1999) Effect of increased vegetable and fruit consumption on markers of oxidative cellular damage. Carcinogenesis, 20, 2261-2266.

Tice, R. R., Agurell, E., Anderson, D., Burlinson, B., Hartmann, A., Kobayashi, H., Miyamae, Y., Rojas, E., Ryu, J. C. and Sasaki, Y. F. (2000) Single cell gel/comet assay: guidelines for in vitro and in vivo genetic toxicology testing. Environ Mol Mutagen, 35, 206-221.

Torbergsen, A. C. and Collins, A. R. (2000) Recovery of human lymphocytes from oxidative DNA damage; the apparent enhancement of DNA repair by carotenoids is probably simply an antioxidant effect. Eur J Nutr, 39, 80-85.

Tripathi, D. N. and Jena, G. B. (2008) Astaxanthin inhibits cytotoxic and genotoxic effects of cyclophosphamide in mice germ cells. Toxicology, 248, 96-103.

Tudek, B. (2007) Base excision repair modulation as a risk factor for human cancers. Mol Aspects Med, 28, 258-275.

Veeriah, S., Balavenkatraman, K. K., Bohmer, F., Kahle, K., Glei, M., Richling, E., Scheppach, W. and Pool-Zobel, B. L. (2008) Intervention with cloudy apple juice results in altered biological activities of ileostomy samples collected from individual volunteers. Eur J Nutr, 47, 226-234.

Volate, S. R., Davenport, D. M., Muga, S. J. and Wargovich, M. J. (2005) Modulation of aberrant crypt foci and apoptosis by dietary herbal supplements (quercetin, curcumin, silymarin, ginseng and rutin). Carcinogenesis, 26, 1450-1456.

Wali, R. K., Skarosi, S., Hart, J., Zhang, Y., Dolan, M. E., Moschel, R. C., Nguyen, L., Mustafi, R., Brasitus, T. A. and Bissonnette, M. (1999) Inhibition of O(6)-methylguanine-DNA methyltransferase increases azoxymethane-induced colonic tumors in rats. Carcinogenesis, 20, 2355-2360.

Wasson, G. R., McKelvey-Martin, V. J. and Downes, C. S. (2008) The use of the comet assay in the study of human nutrition and cancer. Mutagenesis, 23, 153-162.

WCRF (2007) Food, Nutrition, Physical Activity and the Prevention of Cancer: A Global Perspective. American Institute for Cancer Research, London.

Wilms, L. C., Claughton, T. A., de Kok, T. M. and Kleinjans, J. C. (2007) GSTM1 and GSTT1 polymorphism influences protection against induced oxidative DNA damage by quercetin and ascorbic acid in human lymphocytes in vitro. Food Chem Toxicol, 45, 2592-2596.

Wilms, L. C., Hollman, P. C., Boots, A. W. and Kleinjans, J. C. (2005) Protection by quercetin and quercetin-rich fruit juice against induction of oxidative DNA damage and formation of BPDE-DNA adducts in human lymphocytes. Mutat Res, 582, 155-162.

Wilson, D. M., 3rd and Bohr, V. A. (2007) The mechanics of base excision repair, and its relationship to aging and disease. DNA Repair (Amst), 6, 544-559.

Wirtz, S., Nagel, G., Eshkind, L., Neurath, M. F., Samson, L. D. and Kaina, B. (2010) Both base excision repair and O6-methylguanine-DNA methyltransferase protect against methylation-induced colon carcinogenesis. Carcinogenesis, 31, 2111-2117.

Wong, V. W. C., Szeto, Y. T., Collins, A. R. and Benzie, I. F. F. (2005) THE COMET ASSAY: a biomonitoring tool for nutraceutical research. Current Topics in Nutraceutical Research, 3, 1-14.

Yu, H. H., Hur, J. M., Seo, S. J., Moon, H. D., Kim, H. J., Park, R. K. and You, Y. O. (2009) Protective effect of ursolic acid from Cornus officinalis on the hydrogen peroxide-induced damage of HEI-OC1 auditory cells. Am J Chin Med, 37, 735-746.

Zhao, X., Aldini, G., Johnson, E. J., Rasmussen, H., Kraemer, K., Woolf, H., Musaeus, N., Krinsky, N. I., Russell, R. M. and Yeum, K. J. (2006) Modification of lymphocyte DNA damage by carotenoid supplementation in postmenopausal women. Am J Clin Nutr, 83, 163-169.

# 12

# The Nuclear Compartmentation of Glutathione: Effect on Cell Cycle Progression

Jelena Markovic, Nancy Mora, Amparo Gimeno, Consuelo Burguete, José Luis García-Gimenez and Federico V. Pallardó
*University of Valencia School of Medicine, Spain*

## 1. Introduction

The oxidizing environment, shared by all aerobic organisms and crucial for their survival, poses a continuous threat to cellular structures all the living beings are made of. Structural proteins and lipids, and cellular membranes they compose, nucleic acids and enzymes that govern vital cellular processes are all susceptible to oxidative damage. Dealing with this inevitable and constant danger is one of the greatest challenges the living being with aerobic metabolism has to meet.

## 2. The implication of cellular redox balance in cell proliferation

### 2.1 Reactive oxidative species in cell proliferation

Classical work of Kelvin Davies (Davies, 1999), more than ten years ago, showed that the cells show a whole range of responses to oxidative stress that depends on the intensity of the stress. Low level of hydrogen peroxide induced mitogenic responses and stimulation of proliferation; this observation was firstly reported by Oberly (Oberly et al., 1981) who have described that oxidative stimuli, such as superoxide and hydrogen peroxide, could activate signalling pathways that lead to proliferation. Davies et al. further assert that considerable increase in the oxidant concentrations caused temporary growth arrest which became permanent with a progressive increase. When high $H_2O_2$ concentrations were used, apoptosis took place and at very high oxidant levels the cells were killed by necrosis. A year later, (Pani et al., 2000) demonstrate a causal link between redox changes and growth control by cell density: they show that low level of oxygen species in the environment of proliferating cells was not only stimulating but necessary for the correct mitogenic signaling. This study was immediately followed by the work of Menon et al., 2003 who suggested that an oxidation event early in G1 phase may be a critical regulatory step in the progression of the cells into S phase. This lead to the development of the model of the "redox cycle within a cell cycle" proposed by the same group several years later (Menon & Goswami 2007).

According to this model, the transient change in ROS could modify the redox state of cell cycle regulatory proteins, at their critical cysteine residues, and thus determine progression or arrest in the proliferation. Antioxidant mechanism could scavenge ROS and reverse the process. In accordance to these reports, Barry Halliwell (Halliwell, 2007) draw a complete view of the present knowledge of the role of oxidative stress in promoting cancer, its damaging effects to DNA, and its action on cell proliferation and apoptosis. Malignant cells produce more radical species and, although antioxidant defence could also be induced in these cells, they display a pro-oxidant state. However, apparently the oxidative stress generated in these high proliferative cells does not exceed the level where oxidative damage becomes so severe that cell function is impaired. This finding is in line with previously cited reports and many others that support the role of reactive oxidative species mediated signalling in the promotion of cell growth.

### 2.2 The bridge between the oxidative stress and cell proliferation - Glutathione

Glutathione (GSH) is the most abundant non-protein thiol in mammalian cells (Meister & Anderson, 1983). It is considered essential for survival in mammalian cells (Viña, 1990) and yeast Meister & Anderson, 1983; Viña et al., 1978), but not in prokaryotic cells. The exact nature of this important difference has not been elucidated. Glutathione was discovered in 1888 by Rey Pailhade as "organic hydrogenate of sulphur" (Rey Paihade, 1988) and "rediscovered" and fully described by Sir Frederic Gowland Hopkins in the 1920s (Hopkins, 1929) and quoted by Sies several years later (Sies, 1999).

Glutathione has attracted the scientific interest with variable intensity along the century since its discovery and many important cellular functions of this tripeptide were revealed along the years. Glutathione shows a widespread localization within cells and considerably high concentration in cells and tissues (up to 10 mM) (Tateishi et al., 1974). Examples of normal physiological functions of glutathione known for a long time include regulation of the transport of certain amino acids (Viña & Viña, 1983) control of cytoskeleton assembly (Burchil et al. 1978) and regulation of enzymatic activity (Ernst et al., 1978; Ziegler, 1985). During 1960s, GSH was demonstrated to be a co-substrate for a number of important enzymatic reactions: GSH-S-transferase was described (Booth, 1961) and its role in a first-line defence against electrophilic insult, obviously dependent on glutathione, was suggested (Boyland, 1969). These pioneer works became the bases for many studies that lead to the development of concepts such as drug and foreign compound detoxification, and multidrug resistance (Smith, 1977) of crucial importance in the modern cancer therapy. Glutathione, as it lacks toxicity linked to cysteine (Viña et al., 1983), is considered perfect as a cellular thiol "redox buffer" with a purpose to maintain a given thiol/disulfide redox potential (Sies, 1999). Therefore, the redox properties and abundance that characterize this molecule grant it a major role in protecting the cell against oxidants and electrophiles, and during 1980s this particular role of glutathione is central in many research efforts.

Association of redox regulation with toxicity events lead to the introduction of the concept of "oxidative stress" at biochemical and cellular level (Sies & Cadenas, 1985). Oxidative stress is generally defined as an imbalance between prooxidants and antioxidants with a considerable effect on other cellular components, including redox sensitive functional groups of proteins. Nowadays, with the increasing awareness of the importance of ROS and glutathione in cellular signalling, and the cellular redox environment in fundamental physiological processes, a new definition of oxidative stress is proposed. According to Jones, 2006, oxidative stress may be better defined as a disruption of redox signaling and control. Interestingly, more than 10 years ago, searching for a molecular link between oxidative stress and cell proliferation, Cotgrave IA and Gerdes RG recommended similar term: "oxidant mediated regulation" (Cortgreave and Gerdes, 1998).

### 2.3 Glutathione in cell proliferation

Several studies from more than 20 years ago have suggested that changes in low molecular weight thiols (LMWT) are associated with regulation of cell growth. Harris and Patt published (Harris & Pat, 1969) that nonproliferating mouse tumour cells contained LMWT than proliferating cells and in early eighties various authors report similar results: human lung and ovarian tumour cells during the exponential growth demonstrate higher GSH levels than during nondividing state (Harris & Pat, 1969; Post, 1983). In accordance to these findings, Kosower and Kosower (Kosower & Kosower, 1978) have demonstrated that decrease of GSH biosynthesis in vivo inhibits tumour growth rate. Moreover, it was suggested that cellular GSH may have to reach certain critical levels before proliferation can be initiated and that variations in the protein sulphydryl redox status may directly relate to regulation of cell growth (Atzori et al. 1990).

Defining the intrinsic cellular redox environment by estimation of glutathione (GSH)/glutathione disulfide (GSSG) redox state, the group of Dean P. Jones (Nkabyo et al. 2002) concluded that each phase in the life of the cell is characterized by the certain redox state. Proliferating cells are in the most reduced state, with the values of Eh between -260mV and -230mV (Schafer & Buettner, 2001). Upon a growth arrest caused by differentiation (Nkabyo et al. 2002) or contact inhibition (Schafer & Buettner, 2001) cells are 40 mV more oxidised (-220mV to -190mV) while the apoptotic process is accompanied by further oxidation up to -165mV (Sun & Oberley, 1996).

Therefore, while the cell progresses from proliferation, through contact inhibition, differentiation, and finally apoptosis, there is an intrinsic and natural progression from more reduced to more oxidised cellular redox environment. The universality of this model which applies to various cells from different organisms (reviewed in Schafer & Buettner, 2001) inspired a daring hypothesis of Schafer and Buettner on the implication and function of thiols and disulfides as nano-switches. The GSSG/2GSH couple is imagined as a switchboard that move the cell from proliferation through differentiation towards programmed cell death, if the redox environment could not be maintained, or necrosis when the oxidative insult is to severe.

### 2.4 Glutathiolation of regulatory proteins as a link between a stimulating oxidative event and reduced cell environment in cell proliferation

During the last two decades the increasing body of evidence reveals that several transcription factors undergo oxidant modification necessary for their activation. For instance, the property of binding DNA and thus regulate gene expression of AP1, NfkB, p53, and SP1 depends on the redox status of cysteinyl thiols in their structures (Sun & Oberley, 1996). Thus, the idea of protein glutathiolation as a regulatory mechanism of importance in cell proliferation came into sight.

Glutathiolation is a protein modification which consists in the covalent union of the tripeptide glutathione to the SH group of the cysteine residue. For a long time this reaction was considered to be a consequence of the equilibrium between protein thiols and GSSG inevitably related to oxidative stress. From this point of view, glutathiolation fulfills two important functions. Firstly, its reversibility enables the preservation of glutathione in the cell and serves as a buffer for the reduction potential; otherwise, GSSG efflux would cause the loss of GSH from the cell, decreasing the reducing capacity which could be recovered only by the synthesis of new GSH (Schafer & Buettner, 2001). Secondly, it provides protection for protein-SH against irreversible modifications and protein damage in response to higher levels of oxidative stress (Dalle-Donne et al., 2007). Interestingly, it was demonstrated that glutathiolation as a posttranslational modification occurs not only during oxidative stress, but also under basal conditions and is involved in regulating distinct transcription factors, such as NF-kB (Pineda-Molina et al., 2001), its inhibitor factor IKK (Reynaert et al., 2006) and c-Jun (Canela et al. 2007). Apparently, the binding capacity of these proteins to DNA or other proteins is modulated by glutathiolation. This relatively recent focus on the implication of glutathiolation modulatory effects on protein function yielded important breakthrough in elucidation of the implication of this modification in various physiological and pathological situations (Giustarini et al. 2004) and raises interesting questions about its possible implications in cell proliferation.

### 2.4.1 The role of glutathione in DNA synthesis

Among the important roles that GSH plays in cellular physiology, and among the first to be described, was its role in DNA synthesis. The pentose phosphate pathway is a cellular source of NADPH that is involved in reductive biosynthesis. In this process, ribose-5-phosphate is formed and subsequently used for the synthesis of RNA, DNA and nucleotide coenzymes. Apart from the synthesis of nucleotides, NADPH is also required for the formation of amino acids, fatty acids, cholesterol, neurotransmitters and nitric oxide (NO). Furthermore, NADPH is the source of electrons in the process of reduction of ribonucleotides to deoxyribonucleotides catalyzed by the ribonucleotide reductase (Thelander & Reichard, 1979).

The route is initialized by two distinct but complemented systems, the thioredoxin system and the glutaredoxin system. Thioredoxin operates by transferring the electrons to ribonucleotide reductase, and they are supplied by the thioredoxin reductase and NADPH. The glutaredoxin system is initialized by the glutathione reductase, which reduces the GSSG to GSH using the NADPH as source of electrons. GSH is used by the glutaredoxin to provide the reducing power to the ribonucleotide reductase (Zahedi et al., 2009).

The crucial role of glutathione in DNA synthesis has been extensively documented (Thelander & Reichard, 1979; Holmgren, 1976). For instance, Dethlefsen and co-workers (Dethlefsen et al. 1988) showed that glutathione depletion inhibits DNA synthesis in mammary carcinoma cells. In addition, the vital importance of GSH in this process has also been demonstrated in human T lymphocytes (Suthanthiran et al., 1990). As mentioned above GSH is an indispensable requirement in eukaryotes. In contrast, it does not demonstrate the same importance in prokariotes. It has been shown that E. Coli lacking gshA, the rate limiting enzyme in the synthesis of GSH, can grow without GSH supplementation (Greenberg & Demple, 1986; Miranda-Vizuete et al., 1996). On the contrary, in yeast, the depletion of GSH does affect cell proliferation on the level different from DNA synthesis: mutants deficient in GCS after GSH withdrawal arrest cells in G1, whereas a strain with a defect in ribonucleotide reduction arrest cells in S phase (Wang et al., 1997). Since other possible explanations, such as protection against oxidative stress or protection against non-native protein disulfides, have been discarded (Spector el al., 2001), it appears that the essential function of GSH in yeast is related to the redox properties of its thiol group. Consequently, glutathione can be replaced by dithiothreitol, but not with a GSH analog where a thiol group has been substituted by a methyl group (Grant et al., 1996). Since GSH is the reductant for glutaredoxin as explained previously, and glutaredoxin is also essential (Rodriguez-Manzaneque et al., 1999) presumably their vital importance may be interdependent. Then GSH seems to be important in S phase. During the process of DNA replication, errors, such as double-strand breaks (DSBs) that arise from stalled replication forks, require attention by the DNA damage response proteins. Thus, the correct control of DNA synthesis and probably essential molecules, such as GSH, are necessary for the correct DNA processing.

One of the most important proteins involved in DNA damage signaling pathway is the ataxia-telangiectasa mutated protein (ATM). This central signaling protein, mainly for DSBs, is involved in the repairing DNA process necessary after replication stress. Thus cells lacking ATM fail to execute many of the cellular responses to DNA damage (Zhou & Elledge, 2000). In addition, control of ATM responses after DNA replication may be necessary for the correct cell cycle control. In that way, ATM is a central component in the cell cycle regulation. Therefore, patients with ataxia telangiectasia have reduction in DNA synthesis (Painter & Young, 1980). Furthermore, a recent work published by Guo Z. and coworkers describes using a series of elegant experiments how ATM sense the redox changes to modulate their activity (Guo et al, 2010). Interestingly, these authors propose that ATM may regulate global cellular responses to oxidative stress, remarking the essential link between redox control and DNA interacting, remodeling or repairing proteins. In Fanconi anemia for instance, Castillo and coworkers have shown that ATM dependent phosphorylation of FANCD2, one of the main proteins in the Fanconi anemia pathway of DNA repair, is necessary for normal S-phase checkpoint activation after oxidative stress (Castillo et al, 2011).

#### 2.4.2 Regulation of telomerase activity by glutathione

The eukaryotic chromosomes are capped by telomeres, which consist of TTAGGG DNA sequences repeated in tandem, associated with several proteins, which protect the final regions of chromosomes. These structures play an important role in the stability and the complete replication of the chromosomes. Conventional DNA polymerases cannot fully replicate the 3′-end of the lagging strand of linear molecules, and therefore in every cell division telomeric sequences are lost (Komberg, 1969). Telomerase is an important enzyme that ensures the maintenance of normal telomere length. This activity is high in human cancers (Kim et al., 1994), but virtually absent in normal human tissues, except germinal cells (Harley et al., 1990). Telomerase regulation is not completely understood, but its changes are related to both cancer and aging (Sharpless & Depinho, 2004). Studies carried out by Jady et al. show that human telomeres are more accessible during the S-phase (Jady et al., 2006) and that the telomerase assembly with telomeres takes place at this specific moment of the cell cycle (Jady et al., 2006; Tomlison et al., 2006). Telomerase plays a key role in cellular homeostasis, because it maintains the length of the telomeres. This especially important in germinal cells in which it is necessary to keep a normal telomeric length after many cellular divisions. Important contributions about the epigenetic control of telomeres have been reported recently (Koziel et al., 2011). In that way, Maria Blasco has suggested that telomeres are under epigenetic control (García-Cao et al., 2004). Mammalian telomeres and subtelomeric regions are enriched in epigenetic marks that are characteristic of heterochromatin. In addition, histone deacetylase enzymes, such as Sirt6, regulate the telomeric chromatin conformation in order to allow the interaction of WRN protein with these chromosomal regions (Michishita et al., 2008).

There are evidence that point to a role of redox environment in a short term regulation of the activity of this important enzyme. Minamino et al., 2001, using vascular smooth muscle cells, reported that hypoxia up-regulates telomerase activity. Hypoxia is known to lower oxidative stress and thus to increase levels of glutathione. A specific inhibitor of telomerase, 2-[3-(trifluoromethyl) phenyl]isothiazolin-3-one, reacts with a key cysteine residue, which is essential for telomerase activity and must be kept reduced. Consequently, it has been reported that dithiothreitol reverses this inhibition (Hayakawa et al., 1999). Furthermore, antioxidants have been shown to inhibit nuclear export of telomerase reverse transcriptase and thus delay replicative senescence of endothelial cells (Haendeler et al., 2004). In conclusion, a critical cysteine residue must be kept reduced in order to maintain full telomerase activity. It is likely that the glutathione redox potential may be important in this process.
Previous findings of our group showed that telomerase is regulated by the shift in glutathione redox potential within values similar to those found *in* vivo and alterations in telomerase activity are coordinated with changes in critical cell cycle proteins, particularly Id2 and E2F4 (Borras et al., 2004).

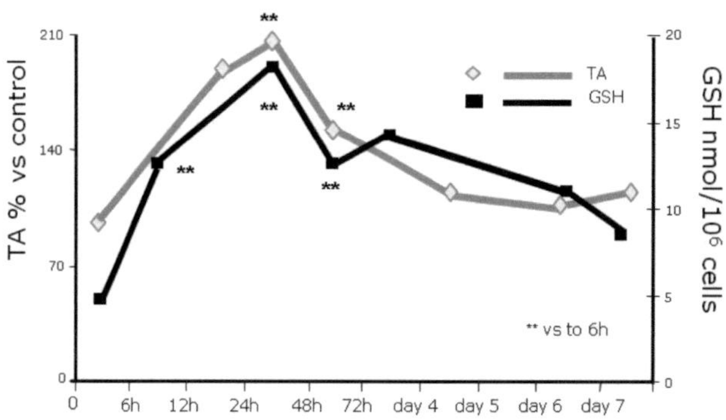


Fig. 1. Reduced glutathione regulates telomerase activity in 3T3 fibroblasts.

Thus, physiological variations in glutathione level induce changes in telomerase activities that are in concordance with changes in cell cycle regulatory proteins. A number of reports have shown similar results. Brown et al., 2007 demonstrated for the first time *in vivo* that high hepatic glutathione levels correlate with increased telomerase activity. Also, the importance of glutathione regulation in telomerase activity has been proved in endothelial progenitor cells (EPC): impairment of antioxidant defences in EPC promoted oxidant mediated apoptosis and telomerase inactivation which subsequently lead to development and/or progression of atherothrombosis (Fujii et al., 2006).
Recent data suggest that telomerase activity is regulated and ordered by telomere structure and telomerase assembly. Experimental evidence suggests that the telomere structure may change in a cell cycle-dependent manner to restrict telomerase activity to S phase (Hug & Ligner, 2006). In addition, telomere structure and specially the telomeric G-overhangs generation are strictly regulated during S phase and prolonged to other cell cycle phases depending on whether are telomeres from the lagging or the leading telomere (Dai et al., 2010). For this to happen, the precise control of the changes not only in telomerase conformation, but in chromatin structure (i.e. in its compactation level) as well, is of vital

importance. This finding that telomere length, and, therefore, telomere structure, is tightly regulated in telomerase proficient cells invokes a connection between cell cycle, telomerase and telomere structure (Blasco, 2002). In other words, the mechanism that lies beneath telomerase regulation might be related with the mechanism that control cell proliferation. This opens a highly significant area for exploratory study and the diversity of processes and control mechanisms that could be involved in this phenomenon remain to be elucidated.

## 3. Compartmentalization of glutathione

### 3.1 The physiological importance of compartmentalization of glutathione

Pioneer work from Meister, (Meister & Anderson, 1983) correlated GSH synthesis and its degradation throughout the so-called $\gamma$-glutamyl cycle, and defined it as a cytosolic processes. The importance of cellular compartmentalization of GSH is two fold, first because it plays an important role in fighting against radical oxygen species (ROS). It is well known that these molecules have a very short half life and exert their action close to the place they were produced. Thus, the presence or absence of GSH could determine the development of localized oxidative damage for the cell structure or metabolic function developed in the vicinity. Secondly, GSH compartmentalization is of vital importance because of its role as a cellular detoxifying agent; it is known that tumours that have high glutathione levels are more resistant to chemotherapy, and the importance of nuclear (Voheringer et al., 1998) and mitochondrial (Benlloch et al. 2005) compartmentalization of GSH has been pointed out.

The overview of compartmentalization of glutathione in mammal cells is a complicated matter. This is due to the presence in the literature of a number of contradictory reports. The reason for the controversy is mainly methodological. Until very recently most reports were mainly based on cell-fractionation techniques. Those techniques appear to be reliable for mitochondrial studies; however their usefulness in nuclear or even endoplasmic reticulum measurements is at least controversial.

#### 3.1.1 Nucleus

Although the role of nuclear GSH in the synthesis of DNA (Thelander & Reichard, 1979) and in protection against oxidative damage or ionizing radiation (Biaglow et al., 1983) is well established, little is known about the concentration of GSH in the nucleus and its regulation. This is due to two main factors. The first is methodological: it is impossible to determine the nuclear concentration of GSH using standard cell fractionation and analytical approaches (for a review see Söderdahl et al., 2003). The second factor is that most, if not all, of the reports share the common view of nuclear GSH distribution in a static situation. Cells are usually studied under steady state conditions *i.e.* when they are confluent ($G_0/G_1$ phase of the cell cycle). The nuclear membrane dissolves during mitosis and is formed again around newly replicated DNA packed in chromosomes; this spectacular change involves a variety of regulatory mechanisms. Therefore, if the nuclear GSH distribution is studied, the cell cycle physiology should be carefully considered.

The role of GSH in cell cycle regulation has been addressed mainly from the point of view of its overall cellular content. This is surprising since it is in the nucleus where most cell cycle progression events take place. The nucleus changes dramatically during the different phases of cell cycle, and failing to consider the corresponding changes in its redox environment could confer an important disadvantage in elucidating the actual importance of glutathione in the control of cell proliferation.

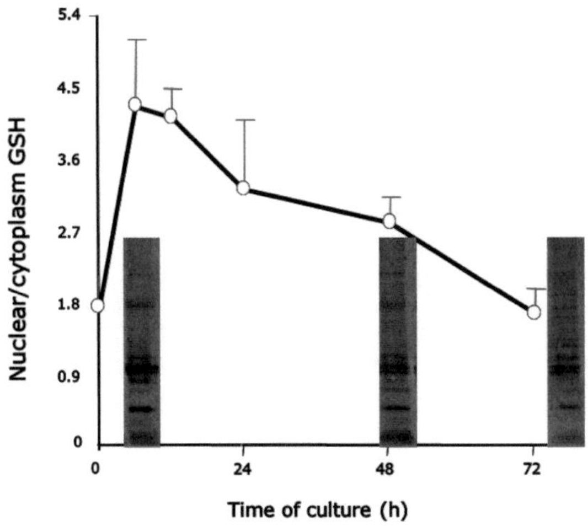


Fig. 2. Modifications of nuclear proteins along the cell cycle.

Our results, in general, are in accordance with the work of Hutter at al, (Hutter et al., 1997), who have studied the redox potential (E) in the normal and malignant cells along the cell cycle. The E of normal cells fluctuates during the cell cycle; for the proliferation to start it has to decrease at least 30mV comparing to its level in the $G_0$ phase (where the cells are 100% confluent). On the contrary, in cancer cells, the E remains low throughout the complete cell cycle, even at a high cell density (Hutter et al., 1997). Our evaluation of the GSH levels along the cell cycle in different models indirectly confirms these findings.

The work of Hutter et al. was further developed and completed by Hoffman et al. (Hoffman et al., 2008), who proposed recently a novel redox model of cell proliferation. They postulate the existence of a redox switch that helps regulate the proliferation within normal cells; its absence in cancer cells enables the bypass of the restriction point and leads to the loss of the control of cell cycle. The authors offer this model as a base to understand the aberrant cellular proliferation that leads to malignant transformation.

According to "redox model of cell proliferation", in normal cells exist a threshold value (θ) of $E \leq 207 \pm 11$mV which initiates the phosphorylation of different regulatory proteins associated with different phases of the cell cycle and, consequently, cell proliferation. When $E > \theta$ cell enters G1/G0 phase. However, when cancer cells are concerned, Hoffman does not take into account the fluctuations in the E level. In our hands, the increase in GSH level along the cell cycle (before the onset of the proliferation comparing to the GSH level at the final time point) is, indeed, less striking than in 3T3 fibroblasts; two-fold comparing to four-fold, respectively. The author hypothesizes, though, the existence of a reductive limit of -260mV which normal cell could not survive, but would not jeopardise cancer cell.

It was proposed previously that the proliferation occurs within the range of ROS levels, concentrations above or below this range could lead to growth arrest or cell death; hence ROS could act like a dual-edged sword (Davies, 1999).

### 3.2 Glutathione controls the cell cycle regulatory proteins

#### 3.2.1 Id2 as a redox sensitive protein

The study of the expression of the Id2 along the cell cycle gave further support to this premise. The family of helix-loop-helix proteins denominated Id (inhibitor of DNA binding or inhibitor of differentiation) was demonstrated to be of considerable importance in the regulation of cell growth, differentiation and cancer in many mammalian tissues (Norton, 2000; Yokota & Mori, 2002). Id2, in particular, was shown to disrupt antiproliferative effects of tumour suppressor proteins of the Rb family, thus allowing cell cycle progression (Lasorella et al., 1996). Indeed, the pattern of the Id2 expression detected by Western blotting, confirmed the distribution of the phases of the cell proliferation detected by flow cytometry. This observation was previously published by our group suggesting a redox regulation of this protein (Borras et al., 2004). In addition, the studies of liver regeneration, process that involves DNA synthesis and cell proliferation, gave further support to our findings.

It was demonstrated that when the increase of GSH after partial hepatectomy was prevented, the liver regeneration was delayed and the total liver amount of the DNA was lower than in the control group (Huang et al., 2001). Furthermore, an early increase in Id2 gene has been demonstrated as well as the contribution of Id2 in the control of hepatocyte priming through modulation of c-myc expression (Rodriguez et al., 2006). All these support our notion that Id2 could be an excellent candidate as a protein marker of the redox regulation of cell proliferation in our models.

### 3.2.2 PCNA as a possible redox sensor in the onset of DNA synthesis

PCNA, a proliferating cell nuclear antigen, is a central protein in both DNA replication and repair. It's a "sliding clamp" that localizes proteins, such as DNA polymerase, to DNA and thus enables the correct DNA replication.

Replication of mammalian genome starts at thousands of origins, called replication foci, which contain PCNA and are activated at different times during S phase. The dynamics of replication foci is still a matter of debate; there are contradictory reports on the organization of the DNA replication sites in diverse cell types attributable to the differences in the technical approach (Dimitrova & Gilbert, 2000; Kennedy et al., 2000). According to Dimitrova, SD and Berezney, R (Dimitrova & Berezney, 2002) there is no fundamental difference in the spatiotemporal organization of the DNA replication in primary, immortalized and malignant mammalian cells. On the contrary, Kennedy's group (Kennedy et al, 2000), observed different patterns of replication foci in primary versus immortalized cell lines, as well as their perinuclear localization in the contact-inhibited cells prior to cell cycle exit (Barbie et al., 2004). Another fundamental question was weather the replication foci are moving along the DNA in the process of the replication, or the DNA is spooling through fixed replication factories. It seems that the important body of evidence is accumulating supporting the fixed-replication-site model (Dimitrova & Gilbert, 2000; Leonhard et al., 2000). The replication machinary bind to DNA, but they are also tethered to an underlying framework called nuclear matrix or skeleton (Leonhardt et al., 2000). Regardless of the discrepancies in their findings, all the authors call attention to the importance of the preserving nuclear architecture in order to guarantee the correct development of the process of DNA replication (Dimitrova & Gilbert, 2000; Barbie et al., 2004; Leonhardt et al., 2000). In addition, it has been shown that chromosome territory organization depends on association with the nuclear skeleton (Leonhardt et al., 2000). More than 20 years ago, Dijkwell et al. (Dijkwell & Wenink, 1986) postulated that the maintenance of the nuclear matrix, especially nuclear lamina, by preserving disulphide bonds depended on the level of nuclear thiols. In accordance to this work, Oleinick et al. (Oleinik et al., 1987) reported that DNA-protein cross links, present at basal level as normal associations of chromosomal loops with the nuclear matrix proteins, can be increased by ionising radiation and removal of intracellular glutathione, and decreased by hydroxyl radical scavengers. The importance of the GSH in cell proliferation could be extrapolated to the safeguarding of the nuclear architecture, providing in that way a proper milieu for the DNA replication. Our results could provide support to the hypothesis of Bellomo et al (Bellomo et al., 1997) that reduced nuclear glutathione may modulate the structural organization of chromatin. It is tempting to speculate that the high nuclear GSH level we observed before (late G1 phase) and at the onset of cell proliferation (S phase) could provide the redox environment that stimulates chromatin decompaction by reducing disulfide bonds.

### 3.3 Nuclear compartmentalization of glutathione as an important feature of proliferating cell: reduce to replicate

The functional compartmentalization is an obvious characteristic of eukaryotic cell. The organelles, visible by light microscopy, are surrounded by membranes, which, although permitting communication, provide unique and defined environment in each one, which guarantee its accurate function. Probably the most remarkable examples of compartmentalization are oxidative phosphorylation in mitochondria, protein folding in endoplasmic reticulum and, for the purpose of this study the most interesting of all, DNA synthesis. It is interesting to note that, when the first two organelles are concerned, the dependence of their function on the correct GSH level has been thoroughly studied. The high intramitochondrial concentration of GSH is maintained by an active multicomponent transport system "pumping" glutathione from the cytosol into the matrix (Matensson et al., 1990). On the contrary, for the correct folding of proteins into a native structure by disulfide bond formation, the GSH level and the ratio GSH/GSSG in the endoplasmic reticulum is maintained at extremely low level by the limited permeability of the vesicle membrane to GSH (Hwang et al., 1992). However, in the case of nuclear compartmentalization of glutathione the reports were scarce and contradictory over the years. This could be attributed to two main factors: methodological difficulties in measuring nuclear glutathione content and the focus of the research generally limited to confluent cells.

### 3.4 Modifications of nuclear proteins along the cell cycle

Various studies have demonstrated that the nucleus is more reduced than the cytosol (15mM GSH vs. 11 mM, respectively) (Bellomo et al., 1997; Schafer & Buettner, 2001; Soboll et al., 1995). An important number of nuclear proteins, including transcription factors, require a reduced environment to bind to DNA. More than 62 proteins are involved directly in transcription, nucleotide metabolism, (de)phosphorylation, or (de)ubiquitinylation, which are all essential processes for cell cycle progression (Connour et al., 2004). For instance, it appears that, at the onset of cell proliferation in the early G1 phase, an increase of ROS in the cytoplasm is necessary for the initiation of the phosphorylation cascade mediated by epidermal growth factor (EGF) that, subsequently, activates DNA replication and the cell division (Carpentes & Cohen, 1990). According to Jang and Surh (Jang & Surh, 2003) nuclear GSH may act as a transcriptional regulator of NF-κB, AP-1, and p53 by altering their nuclear redox state. The transcription factor NF-κB is an example of distinct redox-sensitive activation and DNA binding (Hansen et al., 2006); it is activated by various physiological stimuli known to produce ROS; on the contrary, to permit DNA binding, similar to Fos, Jun, and Nrf2, cysteine residue within DNA binding domain must be reduced. Both processes are guaranteed by the adequate redox state of the cytosolic and nuclear environment, respectively.

Interestingly, the nuclear proteins underwent stronger glutathionylation before and at the onset of cell proliferation than at quiescence. It is not surprising if we bear in mind that high level of GSH in the nucleus could provide protection to the proteins against the oxidative threat coming from the cytoplasm at the early phase of cell proliferation, and that glutathiolation, as it is a reversible modification, could be just the way. On the other hand, based on the simplicity of the redox transition from thiol to disulfide and on the fact that the reversibility was energetically favourable, Cotgrave IA and Gerdes RG (Cortgreave & Gerdes, 1998) more than 10 years ago have proposed glutathionylation as a posttranscriptional modification with the regulative finality. They state that it offers "a strong possibility for transducing "oxidative information" from intracellular oxidants via the GSH redox buffer to individual proteins containing "regulatory thiols". Also, recently, this posttranslational modification was proposed as a likely molecular mechanism for redox dependent signalling mediated by GSH (Fratelli et al., 2005). Thus, high level of GSH in the nucleus, observed before and at the onset of cell proliferation, could provide the "GSH redox buffer" necessary for the progressing of oxidant stimulated mitogenesis. It is encouraging to see that the findings of the present study have provided some support to the assumption that a dynamic intracellular redox environment directs the cell proliferation through redox sensitive cell cycle proteins.

## 4. The depletion of nuclear glutathione hampers the cell cycle progression

With the intention of providing further evidence of the importance of nuclear GSH in the initiation of cell proliferation, we have found ourselves in front of a challenge of depleting nuclear glutathione. A number of reports have focused on the consequences of the depletion of cellular glutathione levels on changes in cellular proliferation (Thomas et al., 1995; Hansen et al., 2006). However, all those reports were performed measuring cellular or total glutathione levels, but there is no information relating cellular proliferation with nuclear glutathione levels. A number of studies have indicated the existence of a nuclear GSH pool that resists depletion after exposure of cells to BSO (Thomas et al., 1995). BSO treatment resulted in the concentration dependent depletion of cytoplasmic GSH, while the depletion of mitochondrial and nuclear pool of GSH required concentrations higher than 100 μM, which induced DNA damage (Green et al., 2006). Spyrou and Holmgren (Spyrou & Holmgren, 1996) showed that inhibition of glutathione synthesis by 0.1 mM BSO was able to decrease GSH synthesis after treatment for 12 hours, but GSH-depleted cells grew as well as control 3T6 cells with no decrease in DNA synthesis. Thus, incubation of cells with low concentration of BSO, although decreases glutathione levels, does not change cell proliferation. On the other hand, Thomas *et al.* (Thomas et al., 1995) showed that non toxic concentrations of N-ethyl maleimide or DEM decreased the GSH level in the nucleus and cytoplasm to a similar extent, whereas the nuclear pool of GSH was much more resistant to BSO depletion.

Based on this findings, we have designed a model to study the effects on the cell proliferation parameters caused by GSH depletion both in the nucleus and the cytoplasm, using 100μM DEM, comparing to the administration of 10 μM BSO when nuclear GSH level is preserved.

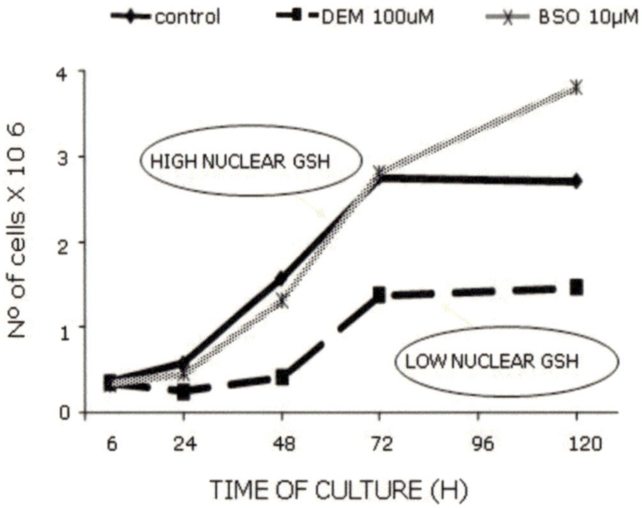


Fig. 3. Changes in cell proliferation caused by GSH depletion.

As reported previously by various authors (Britten et al., 1991; Green et al., 2006; Thomas et al., 1995) nuclear GSH pool was preserved. By contrast, depletion of glutathione levels by DEM induces a marked decrease in nuclear glutathione levels.

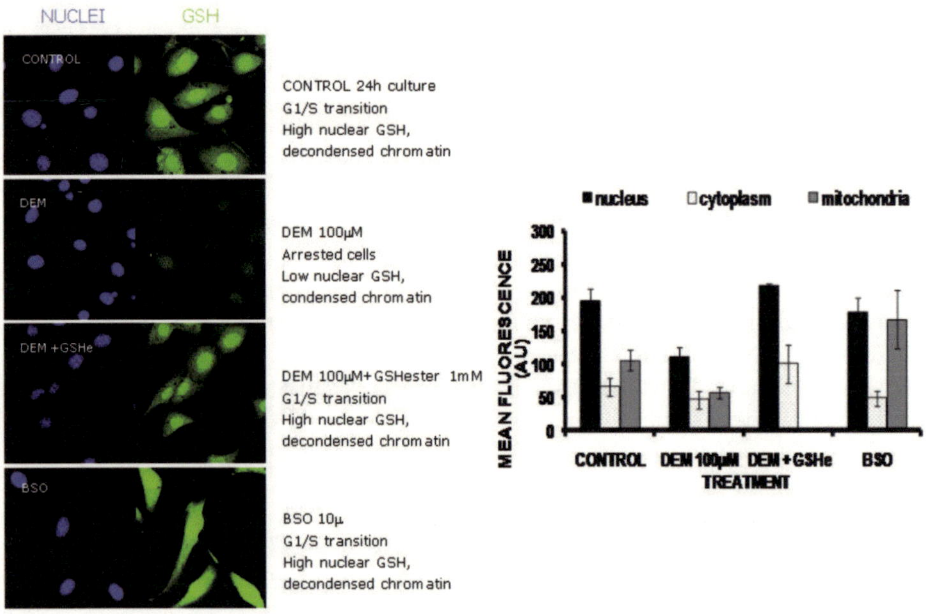


Fig. 4. The depletion of GSH in the nucleus.

The compartmentalization of glutathione depletion could explain the observed differences in the inhibition of cell proliferation. Indeed, our results show that inhibition of glutathione levels by DEM strongly impairs cell proliferation. This difference could be due to the fact that DEM decreases both nuclear and cytosolic glutathione levels in opposition to BSO, which only decreases cytosolic glutathione. It is worth mentioning that the impairment of cell proliferation could not be attributed to the alkylating properties of DEM, since the simultaneous administration of GSHe completely prevented it, nor to the toxicity of the treatment because the cell death was not significantly augmented.

In addition, we have observed the delay in the cell cycle progression caused by DEM, when both nuclear and cytoplasmic GSH was depleted, which is absent in the treatment with BSO when nuclear GSH pool was preserved. Interestingly, Esposito *et al.* (Esposito et al., 2002) showed that direct administration of DEM on the nuclear extracts of COS7 cells induces cell cycle arrest. So, it is daring to speculate that, despite the depletion of cytoplasmic GSH with DEM could not be overlooked, the effect on the cell cycle progression could be attributed to the depletion of the nuclear GSH. Moreover, as Esposito shows, the depletion of nuclear GSH strongly induces a p53-independent accumulation of p21, which causes a cell cycle arrest. In our study, the expression of cell cycle regulatory protein, suggested previously to be under redox control, Id2, was decreased when the level of nuclear GSH was depleted.

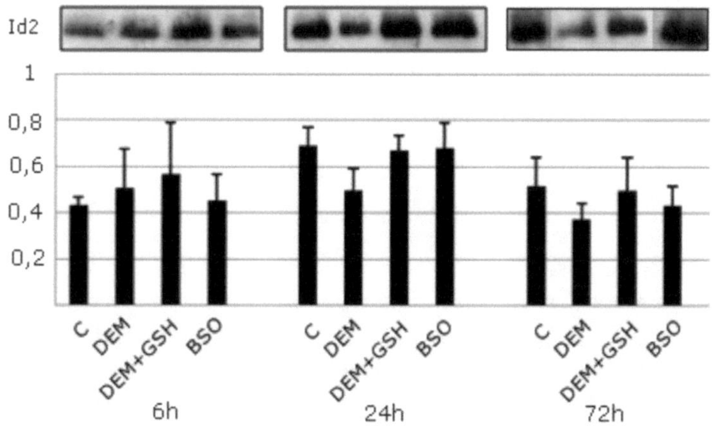


Fig. 5. Nuclear GSH depletion affects Id2 expression.

It has been known that cell proliferation is regulated by a variety of mechanisms working to allow the activation and repression of growth stimulatory genes, one of them being the transcription factors. Previous *in vitro* reports show that the activity of transcription factors is related to its redox environment. In addition, change in the redox potential could induce variations in the activity of those transcription factors. Alterations as small as ± 15 mV in the redox potential can result in transcription factor translocation and activation or deactivation, depending on the direction of the redox shift (Hutter et al., 1997; Sen & Packer, 1996; Sun & Oberley, 1996). Recently Reddy *et al.* (Reddy et al., 2008) have shown that Nrf2 deficiency leads to oxidative stress and DNA lesions, accompanied by impairment of cell-cycle progression, mainly G(2)/M-phase arrest. Both N-acetylcysteine and glutathione (GSH) supplementation ablated the DNA lesions and DNA damage-response pathways in Nrf2 (-/-) cells; however only GSH could rescue the impaired co-localization of mitosis-promoting factors and the growth arrest. Our results demonstrate for the first time that it is nuclear GSH levels, and not total cellular glutathione levels, that specifically correlate with cellular proliferation. Glutathione is considered essential for survival in mammary cells and other eukaryotic cells, but not prokaryotic cells. However, although a number of important functions have been attributed to GSH, its outstanding role in nucleated, but not in prokaryotic cells, remains unknown. Our results underscore the important role of nuclear glutathione in cell physiology and suggest that manipulation of nuclear GSH levels could be of paramount importance during development and cancer.

## 5. The occurrence of the glutathione in the nucleus; active transport, de novo synthesis, diffusion or something else

How GSH enters the nucleus and how it is regulated during the different phases of the cell cycle is still a matter of debate. The regulation of such interactions is also unclear. According to Smith and colleagues (Smith et al., 1996), the possible biochemical mechanisms responsible for the turnover of nuclear GSH are the following: 1.GSH may be taken up from the cytoplasm into the nuclei either passively or through energy-dependent processes 2.GSH may be synthesized *de novo* in the nucleus by the enzymes glutamate cysteine ligase and GSH synthetase 3.GSH may function to transport γ-glu-cys-cys.

### 5.1 ATP dependent sequestration of the GSH to the nucleus

The role of ATP-dependent mechanisms in maintaining the nuclear/cytoplasmic GSH concentration in hepatocytes was demonstrated by Bellomo and co-workers (Bellomo et al., 1997). After 20 min of incubation with the uncoupler protonophore carbonyl cyanide m-chlorophenylhydrazone (CCCP) the nuclear/cytoplasmic GSH gradient disappeared, but the total GSH content remain unchanged. This study was questioned by Briviba et al (Briviba et al., 1993) because of the use of monochlorobimane (BmCl). Despite its high specificity for glutathione this fluorochrome was found to be of no value in the study of cellular GSH distribution; once GSH-BmCl conjugate is formed it demonstrates an increased tendency of nuclear compartmentalization. Indeed, in our study using CMFDA, we have not found an ATP-dependent mechanism of nuclear GSH compartmentalization in 3T3 fibroblasts. Ho and Guenthner, 1997 using nuclear fractions concluded that GSH is taken up by the nucleus by passive diffusion and no evidence for an ATP-dependent mechanism for GSH concentration was observed.

### 5.2 Nuclear synthesis of glutathione

Glutamate cysteine ligase (GCL) and GSH synthetase activities have been reported in nuclei, and a portion of 4-8% of cell GSH synthetic activity is considered capable of maintaining nuclear GSH levels (Ho and Guenthner, 1997). However, we could not find GCL expression in nuclei of 3T3 fibroblasts. In addition as previously reported BSO, a specific inhibitor of GCL was unable of decreasing nuclear glutathione levels. Thus, at least under our experimental conditions, the possible "de novo" synthesis of nuclear glutathione seems improbable in 3T3 fibroblasts.

### 5.3 GSH enters nucleus via nuclear pores

The nuclear pore complex is the biochemical machinery that controls the molecular traffic across the nuclear envelope (Feldherr & Akin, 1990; Nigg, 1997). Ions and small hydrophilic molecules, like glutathione, are considered to move by free and fast diffusion across the nuclear pore (Ribbeck & Gorlich, 2001); nevertheless ion gradients and transnuclear ATP-dependent membrane potential have also been reported (Nigg, 1997). In a series of creative experiments published in early 1990ies, Feldherr CM and Akin D (Feldherr & Akin, 1990; Feldherr & Akin, 1993), shown that permeability of nuclear envelope and nuclear transport were higher in proliferating than in quiescent cells. Reported seven fold reduce in the nuclear transport capacity was induced by the alterations in the characteristics of the pores and not by the changes within the cytoplasm, specifically, the decrease in ATP concentration. One pore forming protein that has been brought into the connection to nuclear glutathione content is Bcl-2. Voehringer and colleagues (Voehringer et al., 1998) showed that over-expression of Bcl-2 recruits GSH to the nucleus. The presence of this protein at the nuclear envelope was demonstrated (Krajewski et al., 1993) and the association with the nuclear pore complexes was suggested. Moreover, Zimmermann et al. (Zimmermann et al., 2007) demonstrated that GSH binds to Bcl-2 in mitochondria, providing a molecular basis for its antioxidant function.

A clear picture emerges showing that the presence of a reduced nuclear environment, probably provided by glutathione, glutaredoxin and thioredoxin mainly, is of paramount importance in the physiology of cell cycle, underscoring the role of oxidative stress in cell proliferation.

## 6. References

Atzori, L.; Dypbukt, J.M.; Sundqvist, K.; Cotgreave, I.; Edman, C.C.; Moldéus, P. & Grafström, R.C. (1990). Growth-associated modifications of low-molecular-weight thiols and protein sulfhydryls in human bronchial fibroblasts. *Journal of Cellular Physiology*, 143, 1, (April 1990), pp. 165-171, ISSN 0021-9541.

Barbie, D.A.; Kudlow, B.A.; Frock, R.; Zhao, J.; Johnson, B.R.; Dyson, N.; Harlow, E. & Kennedy, B.K. (2004). Nuclear reorganization of mammalian DNA synthesis prior to cell cycle exit. *Molecular and cellular biology*. 24, 2, (January, 2004), pp. 595-607, ISSN 0270-7306.

Benlloch, M.; Ortega, A.; Ferrer, P.; Segarra, R.; Obrador, E.; Asensi, M.; Carretero, J. & Estrela, J.M. (2005). Acceleration of glutathione efflux and inhibition of gamma-glutamyltranspeptidase sensitize metastatic B16 melanoma cells to endothelium-induced cytotoxicity. *Journal of Biological Chemistry*, 280, 8, (February 2005), pp. 6950-6959, ISSN 0021-9258.

Bellomo, G.; Palladini, G. & Vairetti, M. (1997). Intranuclear distribution, function and fate of glutathione and glutathione-S-conjugate in living rat hepatocytes studied by fluorescence microscopy. *Microscopy Research and Technique*. 36, 4, (February 1997), pp. 243-52, ISSN 1059-910X.

Biaglow, J.E.; Varnes, M.E.; Clark, E.P. & Epp, E.R. (1983). The role of thiols in cellular response to radiation and drugs. *Radiation Research*, 95, 3, (September 1983), pp. 437-455, ISSN 0449-3060.

Blasco, M.A. (2002). Telomerase beyond telomeres. *Nature Reviews Cancer*, 2, 8, (August 2002), pp. 627-33, ISSN 1474-175X.

Borrás, C.; Esteve, J.M.; Viña, J.R.; Sastre, J.; Viña, J. & Pallardó, F.V. (2004). Glutathione regulates telomerase activity in 3T3 fibroblasts. *Journal of Biological Chemistry*, 279, 33, (August 2004), pp. 34332-34335, ISSN 0021-9258.

Boyland, E. & Chasseaud L.F. (1969). Glutathione S-aralkyltransferase. *The Biochemical Journal*. 115, 5, (Decembre 1969), pp. 985-991, ISSN 0264-6021.

Britten, R.A.; Green, J.A.; Broughton, C.; Browning, P.G.; White, R. & Warenius H. M. (1991). The relationship between nuclear glutathione levels and resistance to melphalan in human ovarian tumour cells. *Biochemical Pharmacology*, 41, 4, (February 1991) pp. 647-649, ISSN 0006-2952.

Briviba, K.; Fraser, G.; Sies, H. & Ketterer, B. (1993). Distribution of the monochlorobimane-glutathione conjugate between nucleus and cytosol in isolated hepatocytes. *The Biochemical Journal*, 294, Pt 3, (September 1993), pp. 631-633, ISSN 0264-6021.

Brown, K.E.; Meleah Mathahs, M.; Broadhurst, K.A.; Coleman, M.C.; Ridnour, L.A.; Schmidt, W.N. & Spitz, D.R. (2007). Increased hepatic telomerase activity in a rat model of iron overload: a role for altered thiol redox state? *Free Radical Biology Medicine*, 42, 2, (January 2007), pp. 228-235, ISSN 0891- 5849.

Burchill, B.R.; Oliver, J.M.; Pearson, C.B.; Leinbach, E.D. & Berlin, R.D. (1978). Microtubule dynamics and glutathione metabolism in phagocytizing human polymorphonuclear leukocytes. *Journal of Cellular Physiology*, 76, 2, (February 1978), pp. 439-447, ISSN 0021-9541.

Canela, A.; Vera, E.; Klatt, P. & Blasco, M.A. (2007). High-throughput telomere length quantification by FISH and its application to human population studies. *Proceedings of the National Academy of Sciences of the United States of America*, 104, 13 (March 2007), pp.5300-5305, ISSN 0027-8424.

Carpenter, G.& Cohen, S. (1990). Epidermal growth factor. *The Journal of Biological Chemistry*, 265, 14 (May 1990), pp. 7709-7712, ISSN 0021-9258.

Castillo, P.; Bogliolo, M. & Surralles J. (2011). Coordinated action of the Fanconi anemia and ataxia telangiectasia pathways in response to oxidative damage. *DNA Repair(Amst)*. 10, 5 (May 2011), pp. 518-525, ISSN 1568-7864.

Conour, J.E.; Graham, W.V. & Gaskins, H.R. (2004). A combined in vitro/bioinformatic investigation of redox regulatory mechanisms governing cell cycle progression. *Physiological Genomics*, 18, 2 (July 2004), pp. 196-205, ISSN 1094-8341.

Cotgreave, I.A. & Gerdes, R.G. (1998). Recent trends in glutathione biochemistry--glutathione-protein interactions: a molecular link between oxidative stress and cell proliferation? *Biochemical and biophysical research communications*, 242, 1, (January 1998), pp. 1-9, ISSN 0006-291X.

Dai, X.; Huang, C.; Bhusari, A., Sampathi, S.; Schubert, K. & Chai, W. (2010). Molecular steps of G-overhang generation at human telomeres and its function in chromosome end protection. *The EMBO Journal*, 29, 16 (August 2010), pp. 2788-2801, ISSN 0261-4189.

Dalle-Donne, I.; Rossi, R.; Giustarini, D.; Colombo, R. & Milzani, A. (2007). S-glutathionylation in protein redox regulation. *Free Radical Biology Medicine*, 43, 6, (September 2007), pp. 883-898, ISSN 0891-5849.

Davies, K.J. (1999). The broad spectrum of responses to oxidants in proliferating cells: a new paradigm for oxidative stress. *IUBMB Life*, 48, 1, (July 1999), pp. 41-47, ISSN 1521-6543.

De Rey Pailhade, M. (1988). Sur un corps d'origine organique hydrogénant le soufre á froid. *C.R. Acad. Sci.* , 106, pp. 1683-1684, ISSN 1287-4620.

Dethlefsen, L.A.; Lehman, C.M.; Biaglow, J.E. & Peck, V.M. (1988). Toxic effects of acute glutathione depletion by buthionine sulfoximine and dimethylfumarate on murine mammary carcinoma cells. *Radiation Research*, 114, 2, (November 1988), pp. 215-224, ISSN 0449-3060.

Dijkwel, P.A. & Wenink, P.W. (1986). Structural integrity of the nuclear matrix: differential effects of thiol agents and metal chelators. *Journal of cell science*, 84, (August 1986) pp. 53-67, ISSN 0021-9533.

Dimitrova, D.S. & Gilbert, D.M. (2000). Temporally coordinated assembly and disassembly of replication factories in the absence of DNA synthesis. *Nature cell biology*, 2, 10, (October 2000), pp. 686-694, ISSN 1465-7392.

Dimitrova, D.S. & Berezney, R. (2002). The spatio-temporal organization of DNA replication sites is identical in primary, immortalized and transformed mammalian cells. *Journal of cell science*, 115, Pt 21, (November 2002) pp. 4037-4051, ISSN 0021-9533.

Ernst, V.; Levin, D.H. & London, I.M. (1978.) Inhibition of protein synthesis initiation by oxidized glutathione: activation of a protein kinase that phosphorylates the alpha subunit of eukaryotic initiation factor 2. *Proceedings of the National Academy of Sciences of the United States of America*, 75, 9, (September 1978), pp. 4110-4114, ISSN 0027-8424.

Esposito, F., Russo, T. & Cimino, F. (2002). Generation of prooxidant conditions in intact cells to induce modifications of cell cycle regulatory proteins. *Methods in Enzymology*, 352, pp. 258-268, ISSN 0076-6879.

Fratelli, M,; Goodwin, L.O.; Ørom, U.A., Lombardi, S., Tonelli, R., Mengozzi, M. & Ghezzi, P. (2005). Gene expression profiling reveals a signaling role of glutathione in redox regulation. *Proccedings of the National Academy of Science of the United States of America*, 102, 39, (September 2005) pp. 13998-14003, ISSN 0027-8424.

Feldherr, C.M. & Akin, D. (1990). The permeability of the nuclear envelope in dividing and nondividing cell cultures. *The Journal of cell biology*, 111, 1 (July 1990) pp. 1-8 ISSN 0021-9525.

Feldherr, C.M. & Akin, D. (1993). Regulation of nuclear transport in proliferating and quiescent cells. *Experimental cell research*, 205, 1, (March 1993), pp. 179-186, ISSN 0014-4827.

Fujii, H.; Li, S.H.; Szmitko, P.E.; Fedak, P.W. & Verma, S. (2006). C-reactive protein alters antioxidant defenses and promotes apoptosis in endothelial progenitor cells. *Arteriosclerosis, thrombosis, and vascular biology*, 26, 11, (November 2006), pp. 2476-2482 ISSN 1079-5642.

García-Cao, M.; O'Sullivan, R.; Peters, A.H.; Jenuwein, T. & Blasco, M.A. (2004). Epigenetic regulation of telomere length in mammalian cells by the Suv39h1 and Suv39h2 histone methyltransferases. *Nature Genetics*, 36, 1, (January 2004), pp. 94-99, ISSN 1061-4036.

Giustarini, D.; Rossi, R.; Milzani, A.; Colombo, R. & Dalle-Donne, I. (2004). S-glutathionylation: from redox regulation of protein functions to human diseases. *Journal of cellular and molecular medicine*, 8, 2, (April 2004), pp. 201-212, ISSN 1582-1838.

Grant, C.M.; MacIver, F.H. & Dawes, I. W. (1996). Glutathione is an essential metabolite required for resistance to oxidative stress in the yeast Saccharomyces cerevisiae. *Current Genetics*, 29, 6, (May 1996), pp. 511-515, ISSN 0172-8083.

Green, R.M.; Graham, M.; O'Donovan, M.R., Chipman, J.K. & Hodges, N.J. (2006). Subcellular compartmentalization of glutathione: correlations with parameters of oxidative stress related to genotoxicity. *Mutagenesis*, 21, 6, (Novembre 2006), pp. 383-390, ISSN 0267-8357.

Greenberg, J.T. & Demple, B. (1986). Glutathione in Escherichia coli is dispensable for resistance to H2O2 and gamma radiation. *Journal of Bacteriology*, 168, 2, (November 1986), pp. 1026-1029, ISSN 0021-9193.

Guo, Z.; Kozlov, S.; Lavin, M.F.; Person, M.D. & Paull T. (2010)ATM Activation by Oxidative Stress. *Science*. 22, 330, (October, 2010), pp. 517-521 ISSN 0193-4511.

Haendeler, J.; Hoffmann, J.; Diehl, J.F.; Vasa, M.; Spyridopo ulos, I.; Zeiher, A.M. & Dimmeler, S. (2004). Antioxidants inhibit nuclear export of telomerase reverse transcriptase and delay replicative senescence of endothelial cells. *Circulation Research*, 94, 6, (April 2004), pp. 768-775, ISSN 0009-7330.

Halliwell, B. (2007). Oxidative stress and cancer: have we moved forward?. *Biochemical Journal*, 401, 1, (January 2007), pp. 1-11, ISSN 0264-6021.

Hansen, J.M.; Go, Y.M. & Jones, D.P. (2006). Nuclear and mitochondrial compartmentalization of oxidative stress and redox signaling. *Annual Review of Pharmacology and Toxicol*ogy 46, (XXX 2006), pp. 215-234. ISSN 0362-1642.

Harley, C.B.; Futcher, A.B. & Greider, C.W. (1990). Telomeres shorten during ageing of human fibroblasts. *Nature*, 345, 6274, (May 1990), pp. 458-460, ISSN 0028-0836.

Harris, J.W. and Patt, H.M. (1969). Non-protein sulfhydryl content and cell-cycle dynamics of Ehrlich ascites tumor. *Experimental Cell Research*, 56, 1, (July 1969), pp. 134-141, ISSN 0014-4827.

Hayakawa, N.; Nozawa, K.; Ogawa, A.; Kato, N.; Yoshida, K.; Akamatsu, K.; Tsuchiya, M.; Nagasaka, A. & Yoshida, S. (1999). Isothiazolone derivatives selectively inhibit telomerase from human and rat cancer cells in vitro. *Biochemistry*, 38, 35, (August 1999), pp. 11501-11507, ISSN 0006-2960.

Ho, Y.F. & Guenthner, T.M. (1997). Isolation of liver nuclei that retain functional trans-membrane transport. *Journal of Pharmacological and Toxicological Methods*, 38, 3, (Novembre 1997), pp. 163-168, ISSN 1056-8719.

Hoffman, A.; Spetner, L.M. & Burke, M. (2008). Ramifications of a redox switch within a normal cell: its absence in a cancer cell. *Free Radical Biology and Meicine*, 45, 3, (August 2008), pp. 265-268, ISSN 0891-5849.

Holmgren, A. (1976). Hydrogen donor system for Escherichia coli ribonucleoside-diphosphate reductase dependent upon glutathione. *Proceedings of the National Academy of Sciences of the United States of America*, 73, 7, (July 1976), pp. 2275-2279, ISSN 0027-8424.

Hopkins, F. (1929). On glutathione: a reinvestigation. *Journal of Biological Chemistry*, 84, (1929), pp. 269-320, ISSN 0021-9258.

Huang, Z.Z.; Chen, C.; Zeng, Z.; Yang, H., Oh, J.; Chen, L, & Lu, S.C. (2001). Mechanism and significance of increased glutathione level in human hepatocellular carcinoma and liver regeneration. *The Faseb Journal*, 15, 1, (January 2001), pp. 19-21, ISSN 0892-6638.

Hug, N. & Lingner, J. (2006). Telomere length homeostasis. *Chromosoma*, 115, 6, (December 2006), pp. 413-25, ISSN 0009-5915.

Hutter, D.E.; Till, B.G. & Greene, J.J. (1997). Redox state changes in density-dependent regulation of proliferation. *Experimental Cell Research*, 232, 2, (May 1997), pp. 435-438, ISSN 0014-4827.

Hwang, C., A.J. Sinskey, and H.F. Lodish, (1992). Oxidized redox state of glutathione in the endoplasmic reticulum. *Science*, 257, 5076, (September 1992), pp. 1496-1502, ISSN 0193-4511.

Jády, B.E.; Richard, P.; Bertrand, E. & Kiss, T. (2006). Cell cycle-dependent recruitment of telomerase RNA and Cajal bodies to human telomeres. *Molecular Biology of the Cell*, 17, 2, (February 2006), pp. 944-954, ISSN 1059-1524.

Jang, J.H. &. Surh, Y.J. (2003). Potentiation of cellular antioxidant capacity by Bcl-2: implications for its antiapoptotic function. *Biochemical Pharmacology*, 66, 8, (October 2003), pp. 1371-1379, ISSN 0006-2952.

Jones, D.P. (2006). Redefining oxidative stress. *Antioxidants & Redox Signaling*, 8, 9-10, (September-October 2006), pp. 1865-1879, ISSN 1523-0864.

Kennedy BK, Barbie DA, Classon M, Dyson N, Harlow E. (2000). Nuclear organization of DNA replication in primary mammalian cells. *Genes and Development*, 14, 22, (Novembre 2000), pp. 2855-2568, ISSN 0890-9369.

Kim, N.W.; Piatyszek, M.A.; Prowse, K.R.; Harley, C.B.; West, M.D.; Ho, P.L.; Coviello, G.M.; Wright, W.E.; Weinrich, S.L. & Shay, J.W. (1994). Specific association of human telomerase activity with immortal cells and cancer. *Science*, 266, 5193, (December 1994), pp. 2011-2015, ISSN 0036-8075.

Krajewski, S.; Tanaka, S.; Takayama, S.M.; Schibler, M.J.; Fenton, W. & Reed J.C. (1993). Investigation of the subcellular distribution of the Bcl-2 oncoprotein: residence in the nuclear envelope, endoplasmic reticulum, and outer mitochondrial membranes. *Cancer Research*, 53, 19, (October 1993), pp. 4701-4714, ISSN 0008-5472.

Kornberg, A. (1969). Active center of DNA polymerase. *Science*, 163, 874, (March 1969), pp. 1410-1418, ISSN 0036-8075.

Kosower, N.S. & Kosower, E.M. (1978). The glutathione status of cells. *International Review Cytology*, 54, (1978), pp. 109-160, ISNN 0074-7696.

Koziel. J.E.; Fox, M.J.; Steding, C.E.; Sprouse, A.A. & Herbert, B.S. (2011). . Medical genetics and epigenetics of telomerase. *Journal of cellular and molecular medicine*, 15, 3, (March, 2011), pp. 457-467 ISNN 1582-1838.

Lasorella, A.; Iavarone, A. & Israel, M.A. (1996). Id2 specifically alters regulation of the cell cycle by tumor suppressor proteins. *Molecular and cellular biology*, 16, 6, (June 1996), pp. 2570-2578, ISSN 0270-7306.

Leonhardt, H.; Rahn, H.P.; Weinzierl, P.; Sporbert, A.; Cremer, T.; Zink, D. & Cardoso M.C. (2000). Dynamics of DNA replication factories in living cells. *The Journal of Cellular Biology*, 149, 2, (April 2000), pp. 271-280, ISSN 0021-9525.

Martensson, J.; Lai, J.C. & Meister, A. (1990). High-affinity transport of glutathione is part of a multicomponent system essential for mitochondrial function. *Proccedings of the National Academy of Sciences of the United States of America*, 87, 18, (September 1990), pp. 7185-7189, ISSN 0027-8424.

Meister, A. & Anderson, M. E. (1983). Glutathione. *Annual Review of Biochemistry*, 52, (1983), pp. 711-760, ISSN 0066-4154.

Menon, S.G.; Sarsour, E.H.; Spitz, D.R.; Higashikubo, R.; Sturm, M.; Zhang, H. & Goswami, P.C. (2003). Redox regulation of the G1 to S phase transition in the mouse embryo fibroblast cell cycle. *Cancer Research*, 63, 9, (May 2003), pp. 2109-2117 ISSN 1078-0432.

Menon, S.G. & Goswami, P.C. (2007). A redox cycle within the cell cycle: ring in the old with the new. *Oncogene*, 26, 8, (February 2007), pp. 1101-1109, ISSN 0950-9232.

Michishita, E.; McCord, R.A.; Berbe,r E., Kioi, M., Padilla-Nash, H., Damian, M., Cheung, P.; Kusumoto, R., Kawashara, T.L.; Barrett, JC.; Chang, H.Y.; Bohr, V.A.; Ried, T.; Gozani, O. & Chua, K.E. (2008). SIRT6 is a histone H3 lysine 9 deacetylase that modulates telomeric chromatin. *Nature*. 452, 7186, (March 2008), pp. 492-496, ISSN 0028- 0836.

Minamino, T.; Mitsialis, S.A. & Kourembanas, S. (2001). Hypoxia extends the life span of vascular smooth muscle cells through telomerase activation. *Molecular and Cellular Biology*, 21, 10, (May 2001), pp. 3336-3342, ISSN 0270-7306.

Miranda-Vizuete, A.; Rodríguez-Ariza, A.; Toribio, F.; Holmgren, A.; López-Barea, J. & Pueyo, C. (1996). The levels of ribonucleotide reductase, thioredoxin, glutaredoxin 1, and GSH are balanced in Escherichia coli K12. *Journal of Biology Chemistry*, 271, 32, (August 1996), pp. 19099-19103, ISSN 0042-6989.

Nigg, E.A. (1997). Nucleocytoplasmic transport: signals, mechanisms and regulation. *Nature*, 386, 6627, (April 1997), pp. 779-787, ISSN 0028- 0836.

Nkabyo, Y.S.; Ziegler, T.R.; Gu, L.H.; Watson, W.H. & Jones, D.P. (2002). Glutathione and thioredoxin redox during differentiation in human colon epithelial (Caco-2) cells. *American journal of physiology: Gastrointestinal and liver physiology*, 283, 6, (December 2002), pp. G1352-1359, ISSN 0193-1857.

Norton, J.D. (2000). ID helix-loop-helix proteins in cell growth, differentiation and tumorigenesis. *Journal of Cell Science*, 113, Pt 22, (November 2000), pp. 3897-905, ISSN 0021-9533.

Oberley, L.W.; Oberley, T.D. & Buettner, G.R. (1981). Cell division in normal and transformed cells: the possible role of superoxide and hydrogen peroxide. *Medical Hypotheses*, 7, 1, (January 1981), pp. 21-42, ISSN 0306-9877.

Oleinick, N.L.; Chiu, S.M.; Ramakrishnan, N. & Xue, L.Y. (1987). The formation, identification, and significance of DNA-protein cross-links in mammalian cells. *The British Journal of Cancer Supplement*, 8, (June 1987), pp. 135-140, ISSN 0306-9443.

Painter, R. B. & Young, B. R. (1980). Radiosensitivity in ataxia-telangiectasia: A new explanation. *Proceedings of the National Academy of Sciences of the United States of America*, 77, 12 (December 1980), pp. 127315-7317 ISSN 0027-8424.

Pani, G.; Colavitti, R.; Bedogni, B.; Anzevino, R.; Borrello, S. & Galeotti, T. (2000). A redox signaling mechanism for density-dependent inhibition of cell growth. *Journal of Biology Chemistry*, 275, 49, (December 2000), pp. 38891-38899, ISSN 0042-6989.

Pineda-Molina, E.; Klatt, P.; Vázquez, J.; Marina, A.; García de Lacoba, M.; Pérez-Sala, D. & Lamas, S. (2001). Glutathionylation of the p50 subunit of NF-kappaB: a mechanism for redox-induced inhibition of DNA binding. *Biochemistry*, 40, 47, (November 2001), pp. 14134-14142, ISSN 0006-2960.

Post, G.B., Keller, DA.; Connor, K.A. & Menzel, D.B. (1983) Effects of culture conditions on glutathione content in A549 cells. *Biochemical and Biophysical Research Communication*, 114, 2, (July 1983), pp. 737-742, ISSN 0006-291X.

Reddy, N.M.; Kleeberger, S.R.; Bream, .JH.; Fallon, P.G.; Kensler, T.W.; Yamamoto, M. & Reddy, S.P. (2008). Genetic disruption of the Nrf2 compromises cell-cycle progression by impairing GSH-induced redox signaling. *Oncogene*, 27, 44, (October 2008), pp. 5821-5832, ISSN 0950-9232.

Reynaert, N.L.; van der Vliet, A.; Guala, A.S.; McGovern, T.; Hristova, M.; Pantano, C.; Heintz, N.H.; Heim, J.; Ho, Y.S.; Matthews, D.E.; Wouters, E.F. & Janssen-Heininger, Y.M. (2006). Dynamic redox control of NF-kappaB through glutaredoxin-regulated S-glutathionylation of inhibitory kappaB kinase beta. *Proceedings of the National Academy of Sciences of the United States of America*, 103, 35, (August 2006), pp. 13086-13091, ISNN 0027-8424.

Ribbeck, K. & Gorlich, D. (2001). Kinetic analysis of translocation through nuclear pore complexes. *The EMBO Journal*, 20, 6, (March 2001): pp. 1320-1330, ISSN 0261-4189.

Rodriguez, J.L.; Sandoval, J.; Serviddio, G.; Sastre, J.; Morante, M.; Perrelli, M.G.; Martínez-Chantar, M.L.; Viña, J.; Viña, J.R.; Mato, J.M.; Avila, M.A.; Franco, L.; López-Rodas, G.& Torres, L. (2006). Id2 leaves the chromatin of the E2F4-p130-controlled c-myc promoter during hepatocyte priming for liver regeneration. *The Biochemical Journal*, 398, 3, (September 2006) pp. 431-437, ISSN 0264-6021.

Rodríguez-Manzaneque, M.T.; Ros, J.; Cabiscol, E.; Sorribas, A. & Herrero, E. (1999). Grx5 gluta redoxin plays a central role in protection against protein oxidative damage in Saccharomyces cerevisiae. *Molecular and Cellular Biology*, 19, 12, (December 1999), pp. 8180-8190, ISNN 0270- 7306.

Schafer, F.Q. & Buettner, G.R. (2001). Redox environment of the cell as viewed through the redox state of the glutathione disulfide/glutathione couple. *Free Radical Biology Medicine*, 30, 11, (June 2001), pp. 1191-212, ISSN 0891- 5849.

Sen, C.K. & Packer, L. (1996). Antioxidant and redox regulation of gene transcription. *The FASEB Journal*, 10, 7, (May 1996) pp. 709-720, ISSN 0892-6638.

Sharpless, N.E. & DePinho, R. A. (2004). Telomeres, stem cells, senescence, and cancer. *Journal of Clinical Investigation*, 113, 2, (January 2004), pp. 160-168, ISSN 0021-9738.

Sies, H. & Cadenas, E. (1985). Oxidative stress: damage to intact cells and organs. *Philosophical transactions of the Royal Society of London. Series B, Biological sciences*, 311, 1152, (December 1985), pp. 617-631, ISSN 0962-8436.

Sies, H. (1999). Glutathione and its role in cellular functions. *Free Radical Biology Medicine*, 27, 9-10, (November 1999), pp. 916-921, ISSN 0891- 5849.

Smith, J.E. (1977). Elevated erythrocyte glutathione associatd with elevated substrate in high-and low-glutathione sheep. *Biochemica et Biophysica Acta*, 496, 2, (February 1977), pp. 516-520, ISSN 006-3002.

Smith, C.V.; Jones, D.P.; Guenthner, T.M.; Lash, L.H. & Lauterburg, B.H. (1996). Compartmentalization of glutathione: implications for the study of toxicity and disease. *Toxicology and Applied Pharmacology*, 140, 1, (September 1996), pp. 1-12, ISSN 0041-008X.

Soboll, S.; Gründel, S.; Harris, J.; Kolb-Bachofen. V.; Ketterer, B. & Sies, H. (1995). The content of glutathione and glutathione S-transferases and the glutathione peroxidase activity in rat liver nuclei determined by a non-aqueous technique of cell fractionation. *The Biochemical Journal*, 311, Pt 3, (November 1995), pp. 889-894, ISSN 0264-6021.

Söderdahl ,T.; Enoksson, M.; Lundberg, M.; Holmgren, A.; Ottersen, O.P.; Orrenius, S.; Bolcsfoldi, G. & Cotgreave, I.A. (2003). Visualization of the compartmentalization of glutathione and protein-glutathione mixed disulfides in cultured cells. *Faseb Journal*, 17, 1, (January 2003), pp. 124-126, ISSN 0892-6638.

Spector, D.; Labarre, J. & Toledano, M.B. (2001). A genetic investigation of the essential role of glutathione: mutations in the proline biosynthesis pathway are the only suppressors of glutathione auxotrophy in yeast. *Journal of Biology Chemistry*, 276, 10, (March 2001), pp. 7011-7016, ISSN 0042-6989.

Spyrou, G. & Holmgren, A. (1996). Deoxyribonucleoside triphosphate pools and growth of glutathione-depleted 3T6 mouse fibroblasts. *Biochemical and Biophysical Research Communications*, 220, 1, (March 1996), pp. 42-46, ISSN 0006-291X.

Sun, Y. & Oberley, L.W. (1996). Redox regulation of transcriptional activators. *Free Radical Biology Medicine*, 21, 3, (1996), pp. 335-348, ISSN 0891- 5849.

Suthanthiran, M.; Anderson, M.E.; Sharma, V.K. & Meister, A. (1990). Glutathione regulates activation-dependent DNA synthesis in highly purified normal human T lymphocytes stimulated via the CD2 and CD3 antigens. *Proceedings of the National Academy of Sciences of the United States of America*, 87, 9, (May 1990), pp. 3343-3347, ISSN 0027-8424.

Tateishi, N.; Higashi, T.; Shinya, S.; Naruse, A. & Sakamoto, Y. (1974). Studies on the regulation of glutathione level in rat liver. *Journal of Biochemistry*, 75, 1, (January 1974), pp. 93-103, ISSN 0021-9258.

Thelander, L. & Reichard, P. (1979). Reduction of ribonucleotides. *Annual Review Biochemistry*, 48, (1979), pp. 133-158, ISSN 0066-4154.

Thomas, M.; Nicklee, T. & Hedley, D.W. (1995). Differential effects of depleting agents on cytoplasmic and nuclear non-protein sulphydryls: a fluorescence image cytometry study. *British Journal of Cancer*, 72, 1, (July 1995), pp. 45-50, ISSN 0007-0929.

Tomlinson, R.L.; Ziegler, T.D.; Supakorndej, T.; Terns, R.M. & Terns, M.P. (2006). Cell cycle-regulated trafficking of human telomerase to telomeres. *Molecular and Cellular Biology*, 17, 2, (February 2006), pp. 955-965, ISSN 0270- 7306.

Vina, J.; Hems, R. & Krebs, H.A. (1978). Maintenance of glutathione content is isolated hepatocyctes. *Biochemical Journal*, 170, 3, (March 1978), pp. 627-630, ISSN 0264-6021.

Viña, J.; Saez, G.T.; Wiggins, D.; Roberts, A.F.; Hems, R. and Krebs, H.A. (1983). The effect of cysteine oxidation on isolated hepatocytes. *Biochemical Journal*, 212, 1, (April 1983), pp. 39-44, ISSN 0264-6021.

Vina, J. &.Vina, J.R. (1983). Role of gamma glutamil traspeptidase in the regulation of amino acid uptake by mammary gland of the lactating rat., in Functions of glutathione. Biochemical, physiological, Toxicological and clinical aspects, A.L.e. al, Editor. 1983, Raven press New York. p. 23-30, ISBN 10:0890049084.

Viña, J. (1990). Glutathione: Metabolism and Physiological Function. *CRC Press Boston,* ISBN 10:0849332745.

Voehringer, D.W.; McConkey, D.J.; McDonnell, T.J.; Brisbay, S. & Meyn, R.E. (1998). Bcl-2 expression causes redistribution of glutathione to the nucleus *Proceedings of the National Academy of Sciences of the United States of America*, 95, 6, (March 1998), pp. 2956-2960, ISSN 0027-8424.

Wang, P.J.; Chabes, A.; Casagrande, R.; Tian, X.C.; Thelander, L. & Huffaker, T.C. (1997). Rnr4p, a novel ribonucleotide reductase small-subunit protein. *Molecular and Cellular Biology*, 17, 10, (October 1997), pp. 6114-6121, ISSN 0270- 7306.

Yokota, Y. & Mori, S. (2002). Role of Id family proteins in growth control. *Journal of Cellular Physiology*, 190, 1, (January 2002) pp. 21-28, ISSN 0021-9541.

Zahedi, A.V. & Homgren A. (2009). Molecular mechanisms of thioreoxin and glutaredoxin as hydrogen donors for Mammalian S Phase ribonucleotide reductase. *The Journal of Biological Chemistry*, 284, 13, (March 2009), pp. 8233-8240, ISSN 0021-9258.

Ziegler, D.M. (1985). Role of reversible oxidation-reduction of enzyme thiols-disulfides in metabolic regulation. *Annual Review Biochemistry*, 54, (1985), pp. 305-329, ISSN 0066-4154.

Zimmermann, A.K.; Loucks, F.A.; Schroeder, E.K.; Bouchard, R.J.; Tyler, K.L. & Linseman D.A. (2007). Glutathione binding to the Bcl-2 homology-3 domain groove: a molecular basis for Bcl-2 antioxidant function at mitochondria. *The Journal of Biological Chemistry*, 282, 40, (October 2007), pp. 29296-29304, ISSN 0021-9258.

Zhou, B-B.S. & Elledge, S. (2000). The DNA damage response: putting checkpoints in perspective. *Nature*, 408, 6811 (November 2000) pp. 433-439, ISSN 0028-0836.

13

# Role for PKCδ on Apoptosis in the DNA Damage Response

Kiyotsugu Yoshida
*Medical Research Institute, Tokyo Medical and Dental University, Tokyo, Japan*

## 1. Introduction

Genotoxic stress induces cell cycle arrest, DNA repair, and apoptotic cell death. The decision by cells either to repair DNA lesions and continue through the cell cycle or to undergo apoptosis is relevant to the incidence of mutagenesis and, subsequently, carcinogenesis. In this regard, incomplete repair of DNA damage prior to replication or mitosis can result in the accumulation of heritable genetic changes. Therapeutic anti-cancer treatments that use genotoxic agents must strike a balance between induction of repair and apoptosis in order to maximize the therapeutic effect. However, the nature of the cellular signaling response that determines cell fate such as survival or death is far from being understood. Certain insights have been derived from the finding that diverse isozymes of the protein kinase C (PKC) family are activated in response to DNA damage. PKC-mediated signaling pathway modulates destiny of cells following genotoxic insults (Yoshida 2007a, Yoshida 2008a). In particular, recent studies have shown that certain isozyme of PKC controls function of the p53 tumor suppressor in induction of cell cycle arrest, DNA repair, and apoptosis. In the past 10 years, understanding the molecular mechanisms of apoptosis mediated by PKC has advanced considerably, and the primary focus of this review is to provide an overview of PKC and p53, its mode of action and its physiological role in DNA damage-induced apoptosis.

## 2. Protein kinase C

The protein kinase C (PKC) family of serine-threonine kinases was first described as a calcium-activated, phospholipid-dependent serine/threonine protein kinase (Takai et al. 1977). PKC is activated diacylglycerol (DAG) hydrolyzed from phosphatidylinositol (PI) by phospholipase C (PLC) under a different cell-signaling system (Nishizuka 1984, Nishizuka 1988, Nishizuka 1992, Nishizuka 1995). It has attracted attention as an intracellular receptor for tumor-promotor phorbol esters, such as 12-O-tetradecanoyl-13-phorbol acetate (TPA) (Niedel et al. 1983). Although PKC had been recognized as a protein kinase, subsequent studies have revealed that it belongs to a family of serine/threonine-specific protein kinases and is activated by diverse stimuli and participates in various cellular processes, such as growth, differentiation, apoptosis, and cellular senescence (Casabona 1997, Clemens et al. 1992, Goodnight et al. 1994, Hofmann 1997, Hug and Sarre 1993, Nishizuka 1984, Nishizuka 1988, Nishizuka 1992, Nishizuka 1995). PKC consists of at least 11 isozymes (α, βI, βII, γ, δ, ε, ζ, η, θ, ι/λ and μ) with selective tissue distribution, activators, and substrates. PKC isozymes have been categorized into three groups: i) the classical/conventional PKCs (cPKCs: α, βI, βII γ), which are calcium dependent and activated by DAG; ii) the novel PKCs (nPKCs: δ, ε, θ, μ), which are calcium-independent and activated by DAG; and iii) the atypical PKCs (aPKCs: ζ, λ), which are calcium-independent and not activated by DAG (Casabona 1997, Goodnight et al. 1994, Hug and Sarre 1993, Nishizuka 1988, Nishizuka 1992, Nishizuka 1995). The cell-specific expression and subcellular localization of individual PKC isozymes indicate important isozyme-specific functions. To elucidate these functions, it should be necessary to study the individual features of each isozyme, such as expression, post-translational modification, substrate specificity, subcellular localization and signaling cross-talk with other proteins. Moreover, the involvement of a PKC isozyme in a signaling pathway resulting in a specific cellular response can be investigated by diverse distinct methods such as overexpression or inhibition of enzyme.

## 3. PKC and apoptotic cell death upon genotoxic insults

Novel PKCδ, θ, and μ are substrates for the effector caspase-3, and proteolytic activation of these novel PKCs has been associated with cell death (Datta et al. 1997, Emoto et al. 1995, Endo et al. 2000). However, recent studies have shown that PKC acts upstream of caspases to regulate cell death. For example, PKC activators enhanced caspase activation, whereas an inhibitor of PKC prevented caspase activation in response to DNA damage (Basu et al. 2001). In particular, studies with PKCδ-/- mice suggest that PKCδ plays pivotal roles in the regulation of cell proliferation and apoptosis (Humphries et al. 2006, Leitges et al. 2001). PKCδ is activated by a variety of stimuli including ionizing radiation, anti-cancer agents, reactive oxygen species (ROS), ultraviolet radiation, growth factors and cytokines (Carpenter et al. 2002, Chen et al. 1999, Denning et al. 1996, Konishi et al. 2001, Reyland et al. 1999, Yoshida and Kufe 2001, Yoshida et al. 2002). Molecular mechanisms such as tyrosine phosphorylation and proteolytic cleavage by caspase-3 are of importance to understand the pro-apoptotic role for PKCδ activation. PKC isozymes have been implicated in the growth factor signal transduction pathway (Nishizuka 1992). By contrast, activation of PKCδ inhibits cell cycle progression and down-regulation of PKCδ is linked to tumor promotion, suggesting that PKCδ may have a negative effect on cell survival (Lu et al. 1997, Watanabe et al. 1992). In many cases, the growth-inhibitory effects of PKCδ have been linked to changes in the expression of factors that influence cell cycle progression. Furthermore, PKCδ plays a pivotal role in the genotoxic stress response leading to apoptosis in various cell types (Brodie and Blumberg 2003, Reyland 2007, Yoshida 2007a). In addition, cells derived from PKCδ-/- mice were shown to be defective in mitochondria-dependent apoptosis (Humphries et al. 2006, Leitges et al. 2001). These findings thus support our proposition of a pro-genotoxic role for PKCδ. PKCδ is activated in response to diverse cellular stimuli by various processes, including membrane translocation (Joseloff et al. 2002, Wang et al. 1999), protein-protein interaction (Benes et al. 2005), tyrosine phosphorylation (Denning et al. 1996, Kaul et al. 2005), and proteolytic cleavage (Emoto et al. 1995, Ghayur et al. 1996, Yoshida 2007a, Yoshida et al. 2003). The translocation of PKCδ to discrete subcellular compartments and/or proteolytic cleavage can be induced by numerous stimuli, such as ceramide, TNFα, UV irradiation, ionizing radiation, oxidative stress, and etoposide (DeVries et al. 2002, Majumder et al. 2000, Matassa et al. 2001, Reyland et al. 1999, Yamaguchi et al. 2007b, Yoshida 2007a, Yoshida et al. 2006a, Yoshida et al. 2002, Yoshida et al. 2003, Yoshida et al. 2006b). Importantly, recent studies have shown that genotoxin-induced PKCδ activation is in part dependent upon Ataxia telangiectasia mutated (ATM) (Yoshida et al. 2003). Whereas ATM activates c-Abl, and c-Abl activates PKCδ, a potential explanation is that DNA damage induces an ATM→c-Abl→PKCδ pathway (Yoshida 2007b, Yoshida and Miki 2005, Yoshida et al. 2005). Alternatively, ATM may directly activate PKCδ in the DNA damage response. In either case, nuclear targeting of PKCδ is pre-requisite for ATM-mediated full activation of PKCδ.

## 4. Nuclear translocation of PKCδ in the apoptotic responses

Translocation of PKCδ into the nucleus has been demonstrated in various cells (Blass et al. 2002, DeVries et al. 2002, DeVries-Seimon et al. 2007, Eitel et al. 2003, Scheel-Toellner et al. 1999, Yoshida et al. 2003, Yuan et al. 1998). Recent study showed that PKCδ translocates to nucleus after exposure of cells with 1-β-D-arabinofuranosylcytosine (ara-C) (Yoshida et al. 2003). Moreover, pretreatment with PKCδ inhibitor, rottlerin, attenuates nuclear targeting of PKCδ (Yoshida et al. 2003), suggesting that its kinase activity is required for nuclear translocation. A putative nuclear localization signal has been identified at the C-terminus of the catalytic domain of PKCδ (DeVries et al. 2002). Numerous PKCδ targets and substrates, including the p53 tumor suppressor, are nuclear proteins that function in induction of apoptosis.

## 5. Role for p53 in response to DNA damage

The tumor suppressor protein p53 plays a central role in mediating stress and DNA damage-induced cell cycle arrest and apoptosis (Vogelstein et al. 2000). The p53 protein controls normal responses to DNA damage and other forms of genotoxic stress and is an indispensable element in maintaining genomic stability (Vogelstein et al. 2000). In fact, *p53* is the most frequently mutated gene in human cancers (Nigro et al. 1989). The level of p53 protein is mostly undetectable in normal cells but rapidly increases in response to a variety of stress stimuli. The mechanism by which the p53 protein is stabilized is not completely understood, but post-translational modification plays a crucial role (Shieh et al. 1997). Mutations in the *p53* gene are frequently correlated with generation of human cancers; however, the p53 pathway can be also derailed by diverse oncogenic molecules (Oren et al. 2002). The *p53* gene knocked-out mice develop tumors with an increased rate (Donehower et al. 1992). It is reasonable that many agents may inhibit the p53 pathway as part of the road toward tumor promotion. However, mechanisms for action of many chemical agents that promote tumor development have not been elucidated. With the central role of p53 in mind, agents that promote tumor formation might block the p53 pathway. Importantly, p53 is regulated primarily via post-translational modifications, especially phosphorylation, and the accumulation of p53 is the first step following cellular stress (Oren 1999). The *mdm2* gene is a transcriptional target of p53, and once synthesized, the MDM2 protein can bind to p53 at its NH2 terminus leading to its rapid degradation through the ubiquitin proteasome-mediated pathway (Kubbutat and Vousden 1998, Oren 1999, Ryan et al. 2001). Upon DNA damage, p53 is phosphorylated at multiple sites at the NH2 terminus, thereby inhibiting MDM2 binding (Burns and El-Deiry 1999, Canman et al. 1998, Kubbutat and Vousden 1998, Oren 1999, Ryan et al. 2001, Siliciano et al. 1997). As a result, p53 degradation stops and p53 accumulates. p53 can also be phosphorylated at its COOH-terminal regulatory domain, which influences its DNA binding

(Meek 1998). In this context, constitutive phosphorylation of p53 by PKC at its COOH-terminal domain can lead to its degradation through ubiquitin proteasome-mediated pathway (Chernov et al. 2001). Moreover, treatment with PKC inhibitors, such as H7 or bisindolylmaleimide I, prohibited COOH-terminal phosphorylation of p53 and increased accumulation of p53 without any effect on the formation of the p53-MDM2 complex (Chernov et al. 2001). However, PKC inhibitors were incapable of p53 accumulation in human papilloma virus-positive HeLa cells (Chernov et al. 2001, Chernov et al. 1998).

## 6. PKCδ regulation of p53

The p53 tumor suppressor is activated following genotoxic stress. Transactivation of p53 target genes dictates cell cycle arrest and DNA repair or apoptosis. Accumulating studies have demonstrated that PKCδ regulates p53 expression at the transcriptional and post-translational levels.

### 6.1 Control at the transcription

Recent reports document that PKCδ transactivates expression of *p53* at the transcriptional level (Abbas et al. 2004, Liu et al. 2007, Yoshida 2008a). The tumor-promoting phorbol ester 12-O-tetradecanoylphorbol-13-acetate (TPA) hinders DNA damage-induced up-regulation of p53 by down-regulating PKCδ. TPA initiates tumor formation in a variety of mice and tissue culture models, and this has been correlated with the down-regulation of PKC (Hansen et al. 1990). TPA initially induces and then diminishes the activity of the diacylglycerol-dependent PKC isoforms (Fournier and Murray 1987, Hansen et al. 1990). Previous studies showed that the tumor-promoting activities of TPA are mediated at least in part by down-regulating PKCδ (Lu et al. 1997). Moreover, transgenic mice over-expressing PKCδ were resistant to tumor promotion by TPA (Reddig et al. 1999). In this regard, previous studies implied that TPA can inhibit the DNA damage-mediated induction of p53 (Magnelli et al. 1995). Moreover, other studies with protein kinase inhibitors suggested that PKCδ regulates the p53 signalsome pathway (Ghosh et al. 1999). Regulation of p53 upon stress most commonly occurs by inhibiting ubiquitination and degradation of the p53 protein. In contrast, repression of p53 by inhibiting PKCδ is caused by the prevention of p53 synthesis, not augmented degradation of p53 protein. Inhibiting PKCδ blocks both basal transcription of the human *p53* gene and initiation of transcription from the human *p53* promoter. The DNA damage-elicited increase in *p53* accumulation is drastically inhibited by pre-treatment with TPA. In addition, the PKCδ inhibitor, rottlerin, is also able to block the DNA damage-mediated induction of *p53*. More importantly, pre-treatment of cells with TPA or treatment with rottlerin results in the inhibition of basal *p53* transcription. In this regard, accumulation of *p53* could not be achieved by any means, including proteasome inhibition, after TPA or rottlerin treatment, since *p53* transcription is hindered. Thus, the tumor-suppressing effects for PKCδ are mediated at least in part through activating *p53* transcription. Suppression of the *p53* promoter has been implied as a mechanism for tumor promotion (Raman et al. 2000, Stuart et al. 1995). Damaged genes in tumor cells are generally the mechanistic drivers toward oncogenesis. However, abrogation of endogenous genes, specifically tumor suppressors, may be also a crucial regulatory mechanism for tumor promotion. In this context, agents that interfere with the activity of PKCδ may inhibit p53 responses.

Recent study also demonstrated that PKCδ induces the promoter activity of p53 via the p53 core promoter element (CPE-p53) and that such induction is enhanced after DNA damage. Upon genotoxic insults, PKCδ is activated and interacts with the death-promoting transcription factor Btf (Bcl-2-associated transcription factor) to co-occupy CPE-p53. Inhibition of PKCδ decreases the affinity of Btf to CPE-p53, thereby reducing *p53* expression. Concomitant with these results, abrogation of Btf-mediated *p53* transcription by RNA interference leads to repression of p53-mediated apoptosis in response to genotoxic stress. These findings demonstrate that activation of *p53* transcription by PKCδ induces p53-dependent apoptosis following DNA damage (Liu et al. 2007).

### 6.2 Control at the post-translation

Recent study demonstrated that both PKCδ and IKKα, but not IKKβ, are targeted to the nucleus after oxidative stress (Yamaguchi et al. 2007a, Yamaguchi et al. 2007b). PKCδ interacts with and activates IKKα. Significantly, upon exposure to oxidative stress, PKCδ-mediated IKKα activation does not contribute to NF-κB activation; rather, nuclear IKK controls transcription activity of p53 by phosphorylation on Ser20. These findings indicate a novel mechanism in which the PKCδ→IKKα signaling pathway contributes to ROS-induced p53 activation. Recent studies have also demonstrated that phosphorylation of p53 at Ser46 induces p53AIP1 expression, resulting in the commitment to the apoptotic cell death (Matsuda et al. 2002, Oda et al. 2000, Taira et al. 2007, Yoshida 2008b). Furthermore, upon genotoxic stress, p53DINP1 is induced and then recruits a kinase(s) to p53, which specifically phosphorylate Ser46 (Okamura et al. 2001). We initially found that PKCδ is associated with Ser46 phosphorylation (Yoshida et al. 2006a). This phosphorylation was required for the interaction of PKCδ to p53. Importantly, p53DINP1 associated with PKCδ in response to anti-cancer agents. In concert with these findings, PKCδ potentiates p53-dependent apoptotic cell death by Ser46 phosphorylation. Taken together, PKCδ controls p53 to induce apoptosis in the cellular response to DNA damage (Yoshida et al. 2006a). Of note, our subsequent studies have demonstrated that another kinase DYRK2 plays a major and direct role on apoptosis induction by phosphorylating p53 at Ser46 in response to DNA damage (Taira et al. 2007, Taira et al. 2010). We also recently found that PKCδ regulates MDM2 expression independently of p53. Given that *Mdm2* mRNA change was detected in p53-proficient, but not deficient cells, PKCδ affected Mdm2 at the post-translational level. In this context, treatment of proteasome inhibitor MG132 restored Mdm2 expression to the steady-state level. Moreover, PKCδ inhibited Mdm2 ubiquitination in p53-deficient cells and loss of PKCδ resulted in an increase in Mdm2 proteasomal degradation. P300/CBP-associated factor (PCAF), an ubiquitin ligase 3 for Mdm2, was observed to participate in Mdm2 ubiquitination by PKCδ inhibition and PCAF silencing rescued Mdm2 diminution. We thus conclude that PKCδ regulates Mdm2 expression distinctively of p53 pathway by affecting Mdm2 ubiquitination and maintenance of Mdm2 expression by PKCδ is important to ensure normal genotoxic cell death response in human cancer cells (Hew et al. 2011).

## 7. Future perspective

PKCδ plays a pivotal role in the control of apoptotic cell death in response to a diverse array of stress stimuli. Thus PKCδ is a pro-apoptotic kinase activated by multiple mechanisms, including subcellular translocation and proteolysis. The proteolytic activation of PKCδ is also important not only in activating the downstream apoptotic cascade including p53, but also in amplifying upstream caspase signaling. Most of the studies mentioned above suggest that the role of PKCδ in the induction of apoptosis is tightly associated with its caspase-dependent cleavage and the regulation of p53. However, functional regulation of p53 by PKCδ remains largely unclear. In this regard, thorough investigation coupled with PKCδ and p53 should be enhanced from multiple views. In the encounter with genotoxic insults, ATM controls various cellular responses, such as cell cycle arrest, transcription, DNA repair, and apoptosis. In this context, DNA damage-induced PKCδ is modulated under ATM, suggesting the notion that establishment of the ATM→PKCδ→p53 signaling cascade provides new mechanistic light on how PKCδ functions as the pro-apoptotic kinase in the nucleus (Figure 1) (Yoshida 2007a, Yoshida 2008a). While dysregulation of the PKCδ signalsome confers resistance to anticancer drugs (Meinhardt et al. 1999), there is little

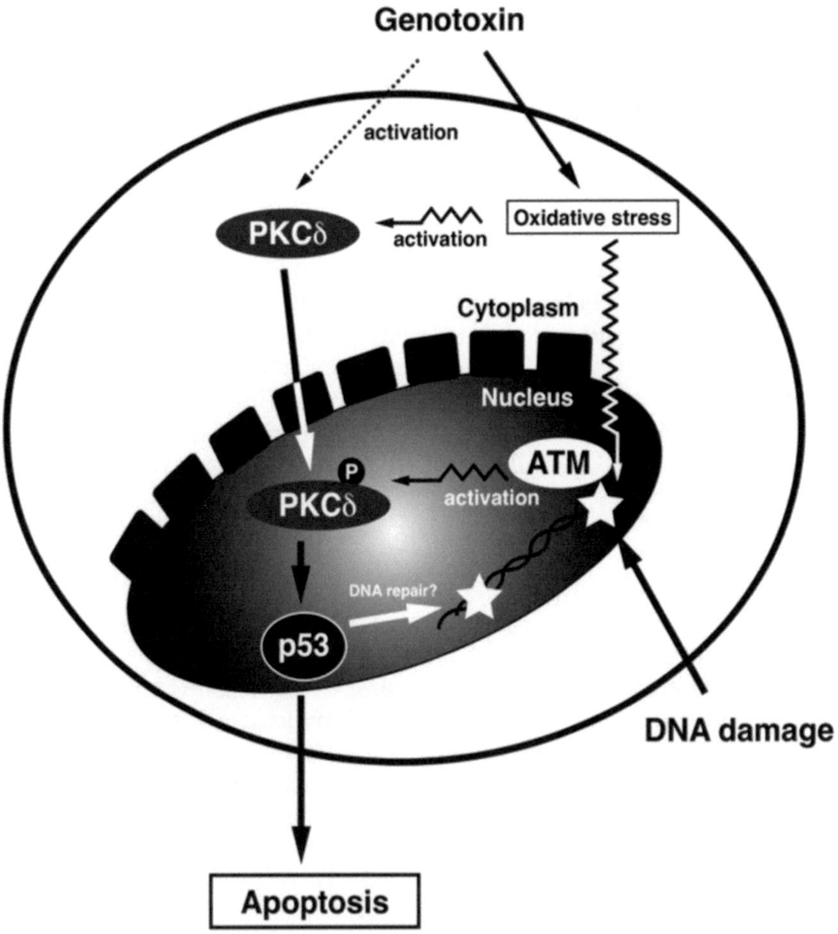


Fig. 1. A hypothetical schema for nuclear targeting of PKCδ in response to DNA damage. Following DNA damage, PKCδ translocates from the cytoplasm into the nucleus. In addition, some genotoxic stress also exerts cytoplasmic oxidative stress to activate PKCδ. In the nucleus, PKCδ is activated by ATM, then induces apoptosis (or DNA repair) in a p53-dependent manner.

understanding of how the PKCδ signaling pathway is influenced when cancer cells acquire resistance to chemotherapeutic drugs. Considering the importance of PKCδ in genotoxic stress-induced apoptosis, a thorough understanding of how it controls apoptosis should benefit cancer therapeutic potentials. Finally, novel PKCδ-based therapy may be used in combination with other agents to confer synergism and prevent the development for drug resistance.

## 8. References


Abbas, T., White, D., Hui, L., Yoshida, K., Foster, D. A., Bargonetti, J. (2004). Inhibition of human p53 basal transcription by down-regulation of protein kinase Cdelta. J Biol Chem 279:9970-7.

Basu, A., Woolard, M. D., Johnson, C. L. (2001). Involvement of protein kinase C-delta in DNA damage-induced apoptosis. Cell Death Differ 8:899-908.

Benes, C. H., Wu, N., Elia, A. E., Dharia, T., Cantley, L. C., Soltoff, S. P. (2005). The C2 domain of PKCdelta is a phosphotyrosine binding domain. Cell 121:271-80.

Blass, M., Kronfeld, I., Kazimirsky, G., Blumberg, P. M., Brodie, C. (2002). Tyrosine phosphorylation of protein kinase Cdelta is essential for its apoptotic effect in response to etoposide. Mol Cell Biol 22:182-95.

Brodie, C., Blumberg, P. M. (2003). Regulation of cell apoptosis by protein kinase c delta. Apoptosis 8:19-27.

Burns, T. F., El-Deiry, W. S. (1999). The p53 pathway and apoptosis. J Cell Physiol 181:231-9.

Canman, C. E., Lim, D. S., Cimprich, K. A. et al. (1998). Activation of the ATM kinase by ionizing radiation and phosphorylation of p53. Science 281:1677-9.

Carpenter, L., Cordery, D., Biden, T. J. (2002). Inhibition of protein kinase C delta protects rat INS-1 cells against interleukin-1beta and streptozotocin-induced apoptosis. Diabetes 51:317-24.

Casabona, G. (1997). Intracellular signal modulation: a pivotal role for protein kinase C. Prog Neuropsychopharmacol Biol Psychiatry 21:407-25.

Chen, N., Ma, W., Huang, C., Dong, Z. (1999). Translocation of protein kinase Cepsilon and protein kinase Cdelta to membrane is required for ultraviolet B-induced activation of mitogen-activated protein kinases and apoptosis. J Biol Chem 274:15389-94.

Chernov, M. V., Bean, L. J., Lerner, N., Stark, G. R. (2001). Regulation of ubiquitination and degradation of p53 in unstressed cells through C-terminal phosphorylation. J Biol Chem 276:31819-24.

Chernov, M. V., Ramana, C. V., Adler, V. V., Stark, G. R. (1998). Stabilization and activation of p53 are regulated independently by different phosphorylation events. Proc Natl Acad Sci U S A 95:2284-9.

Clemens, M. J., Trayner, I., Menaya, J. (1992). The role of protein kinase C isoenzymes in the regulation of cell proliferation and differentiation. J Cell Sci 103 ( Pt 4):881-7.

Datta, R., Kojima, H., Yoshida, K., Kufe, D. (1997). Caspase-3-mediated cleavage of protein kinase C theta in induction of apoptosis. J Biol Chem 272:20317-20.

Denning, M. F., Dlugosz, A. A., Threadgill, D. W., Magnuson, T., Yuspa, S. H. (1996). Activation of the epidermal growth factor receptor signal transduction pathway stimulates tyrosine phosphorylation of protein kinase C delta. J Biol Chem 271:5325-31.

DeVries, T. A., Neville, M. C., Reyland, M. E. (2002). Nuclear import of PKCdelta is required for apoptosis: identification of a novel nuclear import sequence. EMBO J 21:6050-60.

DeVries-Seimon, T. A., Ohm, A. M., Humphries, M. J., Reyland, M. E. (2007). Induction of apoptosis is driven by nuclear retention of protein kinase C delta. J Biol Chem 282:22307-14.

Donehower, L. A., Harvey, M., Slagle, B. L. et al. (1992). Mice deficient for p53 are developmentally normal but susceptible to spontaneous tumours. Nature 356:215-21.

Eitel, K., Staiger, H., Rieger, J. et al. (2003). Protein kinase C delta activation and translocation to the nucleus are required for fatty acid-induced apoptosis of insulin-secreting cells. Diabetes 52:991-7.

Emoto, Y., Manome, Y., Meinhardt, G. et al. (1995). Proteolytic activation of protein kinase C delta by an ICE-like protease in apoptotic cells. EMBO J 14:6148-56.

Endo, K., Oki, E., Biedermann, V. et al. (2000). Proteolytic cleavage and activation of protein kinase C [micro] by caspase-3 in the apoptotic response of cells to 1-beta -D-arabinofuranosylcytosine and other genotoxic agents. J Biol Chem 275:18476-81.

Fournier, A., Murray, A. W. (1987). Application of phorbol ester to mouse skin causes a rapid and sustained loss of protein kinase C. Nature 330:767-9.

Ghayur, T., Hugunin, M., Talanian, R. V. et al. (1996). Proteolytic activation of protein kinase C delta by an ICE/CED 3-like protease induces characteristics of apoptosis. J Exp Med 184:2399-404.

Ghosh, J. C., Suzuki, K., Kodama, S., Watanabe, M. (1999). Effects of protein kinase inhibitors on the accumulation kinetics of p53 protein in normal human embryo cells following X-irradiation. J Radiat Res (Tokyo) 40:23-37.

Goodnight, J., Mischak, H., Mushinski, J. F. (1994). Selective involvement of protein kinase C isozymes in differentiation and neoplastic transformation. Adv Cancer Res 64:159-209.

Hansen, L. A., Monteiro-Riviere, N. A., Smart, R. C. (1990). Differential down-regulation of epidermal protein kinase C by 12-O-tetradecanoylphorbol-13-acetate and diacylglycerol: association with epidermal hyperplasia and tumor promotion. Cancer Res 50:5740-5.

Hew, H. C., Liu, H., Miki, Y., Yoshida, K. (2011). PKCdelta regulates Mdm2 independently of p53 in the apoptotic response to DNA damage. Mol Carcinog.

Hofmann, J. (1997). The potential for isoenzyme-selective modulation of protein kinase C. FASEB J 11:649-69.

Hug, H., Sarre, T. F. (1993). Protein kinase C isoenzymes: divergence in signal transduction? Biochem J 291 ( Pt 2):329-43.

Humphries, M. J., Limesand, K. H., Schneider, J. C., Nakayama, K. I., Anderson, S. M., Reyland, M. E. (2006). Suppression of apoptosis in the protein kinase Cdelta null mouse in vivo. J Biol Chem 281:9728-37.

Joseloff, E., Cataisson, C., Aamodt, H. et al. (2002). Src family kinases phosphorylate protein kinase C delta on tyrosine residues and modify the neoplastic phenotype of skin keratinocytes. J Biol Chem 277:12318-23.

Kaul, S., Anantharam, V., Yang, Y., Choi, C. J., Kanthasamy, A., Kanthasamy, A. G. (2005). Tyrosine phosphorylation regulates the proteolytic activation of protein kinase Cdelta in dopaminergic neuronal cells. J Biol Chem 280:28721-30.

Konishi, H., Yamauchi, E., Taniguchi, H. et al. (2001). Phosphorylation sites of protein kinase C delta in H2O2-treated cells and its activation by tyrosine kinase in vitro. Proc Natl Acad Sci U S A 98:6587-92.

Kubbutat, M. H., Vousden, K. H. (1998). Keeping an old friend under control: regulation of p53 stability. Mol Med Today 4:250-6.

Leitges, M., Mayr, M., Braun, U. et al. (2001). Exacerbated vein graft arteriosclerosis in protein kinase Cdelta-null mice. J Clin Invest 108:1505-12.

Liu, H., Lu, Z. G., Miki, Y., Yoshida, K. (2007). Protein kinase C delta induces transcription of the TP53 tumor suppressor gene by controlling death-promoting factor Btf in the apoptotic response to DNA damage. Mol Cell Biol 27:8480-91.

Lu, Z., Hornia, A., Jiang, Y. W., Zang, Q., Ohno, S., Foster, D. A. (1997). Tumor promotion by depleting cells of protein kinase C delta. Mol Cell Biol 17:3418-28.

Magnelli, L., Cinelli, M., Chiarugi, V. (1995). Phorbol esters attenuate the expression of p53 in cells treated with doxorubicin and protect TS-P53/K562 from apoptosis. Biochem Biophys Res Commun 215:641-5.

Majumder, P. K., Pandey, P., Sun, X. et al. (2000). Mitochondrial translocation of protein kinase C delta in phorbol ester-induced cytochrome c release and apoptosis. J Biol Chem 275:21793-6.

Matassa, A. A., Carpenter, L., Biden, T. J., Humphries, M. J., Reyland, M. E. (2001). PKCdelta is required for mitochondrial-dependent apoptosis in salivary epithelial cells. J Biol Chem 276:29719-28.

Matsuda, K., Yoshida, K., Taya, Y., Nakamura, K., Nakamura, Y., Arakawa, H. (2002). p53AIP1 regulates the mitochondrial apoptotic pathway. Cancer Res 62:2883-9.

Meek, D. W. (1998). Multisite phosphorylation and the integration of stress signals at p53. Cell Signal 10:159-66.

Meinhardt, G., Roth, J., Totok, G., Auner, H., Emmerich, B., Hass, R. (1999). Signaling defect in the activation of caspase-3 and PKCdelta in human TUR leukemia cells is associated with resistance to apoptosis. Exp Cell Res 247:534-42.

Niedel, J. E., Kuhn, L. J., Vandenbark, G. R. (1983). Phorbol diester receptor copurifies with protein kinase C. Proc Natl Acad Sci U S A 80:36-40.

Nigro, J. M., Baker, S. J., Preisinger, A. C. et al. (1989). Mutations in the p53 gene occur in diverse human tumour types. Nature 342:705-8.

Nishizuka, Y. (1984). The role of protein kinase C in cell surface signal transduction and tumour promotion. Nature 308:693-8.

Nishizuka, Y. (1988). The molecular heterogeneity of protein kinase C and its implications for cellular regulation. Nature 334:661-5.

Nishizuka, Y. (1992). Intracellular signaling by hydrolysis of phospholipids and activation of protein kinase C. Science 258:607-14.

Nishizuka, Y. (1995). Protein kinase C and lipid signaling for sustained cellular responses. FASEB J 9:484-96.

Oda, K., Arakawa, H., Tanaka, T. et al. (2000). p53AIP1, a potential mediator of p53-dependent apoptosis, and its regulation by Ser-46-phosphorylated p53. Cell 102:849-62.

Okamura, S., Arakawa, H., Tanaka, T. et al. (2001). p53DINP1, a p53-inducible gene, regulates p53-dependent apoptosis. Mol Cell 8:85-94.

Oren, M. (1999). Regulation of the p53 tumor suppressor protein. J Biol Chem 274:36031-4.

Oren, M., Damalas, A., Gottlieb, T. et al. (2002). Regulation of p53: intricate loops and delicate balances. Biochem Pharmacol 64:865-71.

Raman, V., Martensen, S. A., Reisman, D. et al. (2000). Compromised HOXA5 function can limit p53 expression in human breast tumours. Nature 405:974-8.

Reddig, P. J., Dreckschmidt, N. E., Ahrens, H. et al. (1999). Transgenic mice overexpressing protein kinase Cdelta in the epidermis are resistant to skin tumor promotion by 12-O-tetradecanoylphorbol-13-acetate. Cancer Res 59:5710-8.

Reyland, M. E. (2007). Protein kinase Cdelta and apoptosis. Biochem Soc Trans 35:1001-4.

Reyland, M. E., Anderson, S. M., Matassa, A. A., Barzen, K. A., Quissell, D. O. (1999). Protein kinase C delta is essential for etoposide-induced apoptosis in salivary gland acinar cells. J Biol Chem 274:19115-23.

Ryan, K. M., Phillips, A. C., Vousden, K. H. (2001). Regulation and function of the p53 tumor suppressor protein. Curr Opin Cell Biol 13:332-7.

Scheel-Toellner, D., Pilling, D., Akbar, A. N. et al. (1999). Inhibition of T cell apoptosis by IFN-beta rapidly reverses nuclear translocation of protein kinase C-delta. Eur J Immunol 29:2603-12.

Shieh, S. Y., Ikeda, M., Taya, Y., Prives, C. (1997). DNA damage-induced phosphorylation of p53 alleviates inhibition by MDM2. Cell 91:325-34.

Siliciano, J. D., Canman, C. E., Taya, Y., Sakaguchi, K., Appella, E., Kastan, M. B. (1997). DNA damage induces phosphorylation of the amino terminus of p53. Genes Dev 11:3471-81.

Stuart, E. T., Haffner, R., Oren, M., Gruss, P. (1995). Loss of p53 function through PAX-mediated transcriptional repression. EMBO J 14:5638-45.

Taira, N., Nihira, K., Yamaguchi, T., Miki, Y., Yoshida, K. (2007). DYRK2 is targeted to the nucleus and controls p53 via Ser46 phosphorylation in the apoptotic response to DNA damage. Mol Cell 25:725-38.

Taira, N., Yamamoto, H., Yamaguchi, T., Miki, Y., Yoshida, K. (2010). ATM augments nuclear stabilization of DYRK2 by inhibiting MDM2 in the apoptotic response to DNA damage. J Biol Chem 285:4909-19.

Takai, Y., Kishimoto, A., Inoue, M., Nishizuka, Y. (1977). Studies on a cyclic nucleotide-independent protein kinase and its proenzyme in mammalian tissues. I.

Purification and characterization of an active enzyme from bovine cerebellum. J Biol Chem 252:7603-9.
Vogelstein, B., Lane, D., Levine, A. J. (2000). Surfing the p53 network. Nature 408:307-10.
Wang, Q. J., Bhattacharyya, D., Garfield, S., Nacro, K., Marquez, V. E., Blumberg, P. M. (1999). Differential localization of protein kinase C delta by phorbol esters and related compounds using a fusion protein with green fluorescent protein. J Biol Chem 274:37233-9.
Watanabe, T., Ono, Y., Taniyama, Y. et al. (1992). Cell division arrest induced by phorbol ester in CHO cells overexpressing protein kinase C-delta subspecies. Proc Natl Acad Sci U S A 89:10159-63.
Yamaguchi, T., Kimura, J., Miki, Y., Yoshida, K. (2007a). The deubiquitinating enzyme USP11 controls an IKKalpha -p53 signaling pathway in response to TNFalpha. J Biol Chem 282:33943-8.
Yamaguchi, T., Miki, Y., Yoshida, K. (2007b). Protein kinase C delta activates IkappaB-kinase alpha to induce the p53 tumor suppressor in response to oxidative stress. Cell Signal 19:2088-97.
Yoshida, K. (2007a). PKCdelta signaling: Mechanisms of DNA damage response and apoptosis. Cell Signal 19:892-901.
Yoshida, K. (2007b). Regulation for nuclear targeting of the Abl tyrosine kinase in response to DNA damage. Adv Exp Med Biol 604:155-65.
Yoshida, K. (2008a). Nuclear trafficking of pro-apoptotic kinases in response to DNA damage. Trends Mol Med 14:305-13.
Yoshida, K. (2008b). Role for DYRK family kinases on regulation of apoptosis. Biochem Pharmacol 76:1389-1394.
Yoshida, K., Kufe, D. (2001). Negative regulation of the SHPTP1 protein tyrosine phosphatase by protein kinase C delta in response to DNA damage. Mol Pharmacol 60:1431-8.
Yoshida, K., Liu, H., Miki, Y. (2006a). Protein Kinase C delta regulates Ser46 phosphorylation of p53 tumor suppressor in the apoptotic response to DNA damage. J Biol Chem 281:5734-40.
Yoshida, K., Miki, Y. (2005). Enabling death by the Abl tyrosine kinase: mechanisms for nuclear shuttling of c-Abl in response to DNA damage. Cell Cycle 4:777-9.
Yoshida, K., Miki, Y., Kufe, D. (2002). Activation of SAPK/JNK signaling by protein kinase Cdelta in response to DNA damage. J Biol Chem 277:48372-8.
Yoshida, K., Wang, H. G., Miki, Y., Kufe, D. (2003). Protein kinase Cdelta is responsible for constitutive and DNA damage-induced phosphorylation of Rad9. EMBO J 22:1431-41.
Yoshida, K., Yamaguchi, T., Natsume, T., Kufe, D., Miki, Y. (2005). JNK phosphorylation of 14-3-3 proteins regulates nuclear targeting of c-Abl in the apoptotic response to DNA damage. Nat Cell Biol 7:278-85.
Yoshida, K., Yamaguchi, T., Shinagawa, H., Taira, N., Nakayama, K. I., Miki, Y. (2006b). Protein kinase C delta activates topoisomerase IIalpha to induce apoptotic cell death in response to DNA damage. Mol Cell Biol 26:3414-31.

Yuan, Z. M., Utsugisawa, T., Ishiko, T. et al. (1998). Activation of protein kinase C delta by the c-Abl tyrosine kinase in response to ionizing radiation. Oncogene 16:1643-8.

# 14

# New Players in Recognition of Intact and Cleaved AP Sites: Implication in DNA Repair in Mammalian Cells

Svetlana Khodyreva and Olga Lavrik
*Institute of Chemical Biology and Fundamental Medicine, Siberian Branch of the Russian Academy of Sciences, Russia*

## 1. Introduction

The apurinic/apyrimidinic (AP) sites (called also abasic sites) are common lesion in genomic DNA, arising at a frequency of 10,000 to 50,000 lesions per mammalian cell per day (Lindahl, 1993). Unrepaired AP sites present mutagenic and cytotoxic consequences to the cell (Wilson; & Thompson, 1997). Most of the abasic sites are believed to result directly from spontaneous depurination, or indirectly from deamination of cytosine to uracil, which is then eliminated by uracil glycosylases. AP sites also result from hydrolysis of oxidized or alkylated bases by lesion-specific glycosylases during the early stage of base excision repair (BER) (McCullough et al., 1999). AP sites in isolated DNA are rather stable, but can be converted to single-strand breaks by alkali treatment, heating or nucleophilic attack at the aldehydic C1′ group (Burrows & Muller, 1998). Intact abasic sites are noncoding lesions and *in vivo* can be stable enough to be mutagenic during DNA replication (Loeb & Preston, 1986). To protect genome integrity, eukaryotic organisms have robust enzyme activities, mainly APE1 in mammalian cells (Wilson & Barsky, 2001), that recognize abasic sites and cut the DNA backbone initiating the repair process. The continuous generation and repair of AP sites results in a steady-state levels of AP sites in mammalian cells in the range of approximately 1 site per $10^6$ nucleotides (Atamna et al., 2000, Mohsin Ali et al., 2004). The number of AP sites can increase dramatically under stressful conditions such as X-ray or UV light irradiation or oxidative and alkylating agent exposure (Atamna et al., 2000). Considering the ubiquity of these lesions, it is reasonable to assume that wide range of cellular proteins can interact with abasic sites depending on the physiological state and stages of cell cycle.

The chapter is devoted to search of previously unrecognized proteins capable to interact with intact or cleaved AP sites. We mainly focused on proteins that form Schiff base upon this interaction. In most cases, these proteins are able to process AP sites although less efficiently than previously known counterparts. The biological role of these interactions in providing of backup pathways of DNA repair processes is also discussed.

## 2. Proteins that recognize AP sites

In genomic DNA of higher eukaryotes AP sites irrespectively of their origin are thought to be repaired by base excision repair (Almeida & Sobol, 2007; Hegde et al., 2008).

### 2.1 Base excision repair (overview)

Base excision repair (BER) is one of the major systems of DNA repair, mostly responsible for removing from DNA of non-bulky base lesions that appear in the genome with high frequency (Almeida & Sobol, 2007; Hegde et al., 2008; Schärer, 2003). The base excision repair pathway essentially removes and replaces nucleotides containing aberrant bases in DNA. Metabolically produced reactive nitrogen and oxygen species can modify the DNA bases due to oxidation, deamination and even alkylation at several positions in the base. BER is usually defined as DNA repair initiated by a lesion-specific DNA glycosylase and completed by either of two sub-pathways: short-patch BER; a mechanism whereby only 1 nucleotide is replaced or long-patch BER; a mechanism whereby 2–13 nucleotides are replaced (Frosina et al., 1996; Klungland & Lindahl, 1997).

The majority of BER is currently thought to occur via the short-patch pathway initiated by either a mono-functional or bi-functional DNA glycosylases. The short-patch BER pathway mediated by a mono-functional glycosylase involves removal of aberrant base by the lesion-specific DNA glycosylases, enzymes that hydrolyze cleavage of *N*-glycosylic bond between base and deoxyribose. This results in apurinic/apyrimidinic (also termed abasic) sites (AP sites), which repair is generally initiated through strand incision at its 5'-side by an AP endonuclease, leaving a nick flanked by a 3'-hydroxyl of an undamaged and a deoxyriboso-5'-phosphate (dRP), to which the damaged base was formerly linked. DNA polymerase then inserts a normal deoxyribonucleotide; however, the ligation step to restore intact DNA is blocked because of the dangling dRP moiety. The situation is resolved by a special enzymatic activity, excising dRP moiety (short-patch), or by continuing DNA synthesis with strand displacement, followed by removal of the displaced strand by flap endonuclease 1 (long-patch BER) (Frosina et al., 1996; Klungland & Lindahl, 1997).

In mammalian cells, the major dRP-removing enzyme is DNA polymerase β (Pol β), a multifunctional enzyme consisting of the 8-kDa amino-terminal domain with deoxyribose phosphate (dRP) lyase activity and the 31-kDa carboxy-terminal domain with nucleotidyl transferase activity (Allinson et al., 2001, Matsumoto & Kim, 1995, Piersen et al., 1996, Podlutsky et al., 2001). Thus, Pol β can mediate both steps in single nucleotide BER: insertion of deoxyribonucleotide and removal of dRP moiety preparing the strand for ligation.

Oxidized bases in DNA are manly produced by reactive oxygen species (ROS). ROS are generated as by-products of metabolic processes, primarily oxidative metabolism in the mitochondria (Dawson et al., 1993), and pathological conditions such as inflammation. ROS are also generated by ionizing radiation and some chemotherapeutic drugs (Almeida & Sobol, 2007; Hegde et al., 2008; Schärer, 2003). Oxidized bases are primarily removed by bi-functional DNA glycosylases that have an additional AP site cleavage activity. In addition to oxidation of DNA bases, ROS attack deoxyribose in DNA to generate strand breaks with nonligatable ends. The 3′ blocking groups include 3′ phosphate, 3′ phosphoglycolaldehyde, or 3′ phosphoglycolate (Breen et al., 1995). The 5′ terminus normally contains phosphate but after ROS reaction the nonligatable ends include 5′ OH and 5′ phosphodeoxyribose derivatives such as 2-deoxyribonolactone (Demple et al., 2002). Repair of single-strand breaks (SSBR) with blocked termini utilizes many of the same proteins as the BER process. The principal difference between SSBR and BER is the initiation step. Further both processes may occur at the single nucleotide level (i.e., short-patch repair) or as a long-patch of repair. BER is initiated via DNA glycosylase activity that results in the removal of a damaged base. SSBR is defined specifically for the repair of single-strand breaks in DNA generated by irradiation or ROS (Fan & Wilson, 2005). AP sites appeared via spontaneous base loss and arising from irradiation are also further processed by the BER machinery.

### 2.2 Processing of AP sites

AP sites can be incised by three mechanistically different ways represented in Fig.1.

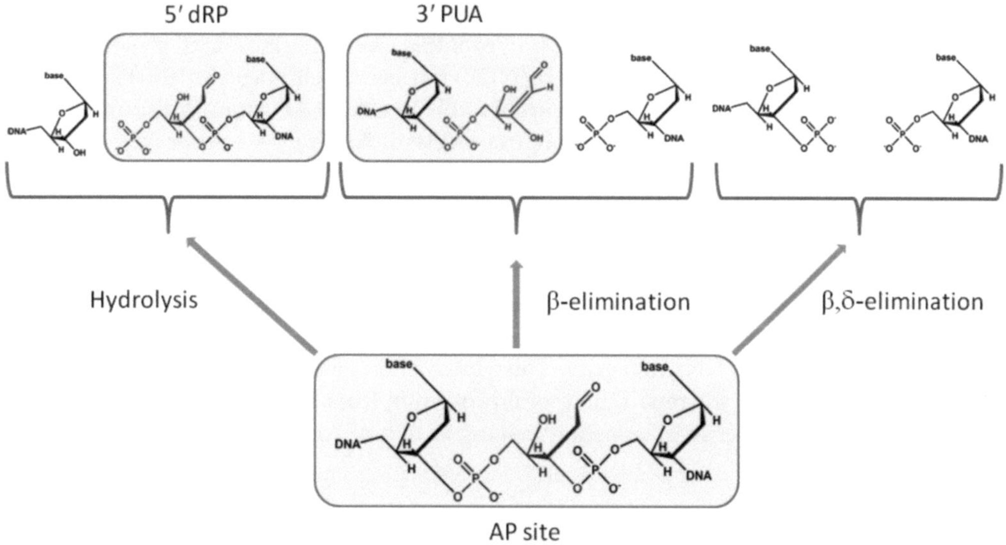


Fig. 1. Structures of intact and cleaved AP sites. DNA structures containing reactive sugar moieties capable of Schiff base formation are marked by grey rectangular boxes.

In mammalian cells, the repair of AP sites is generally initiated through strand incision by APE1, the second enzyme of the canonical BER pathway (Demple et al., 1991). APE1 is thought to process of over 95% of AP sites in mammalian cells (Demple & Harrison, 1994; Wilson & Barsky, 2001). APE1 catalyzes hydrolysis of AP sites by a $Mg^{2+}$-dependent mechanism, resulting in cleavage of the phosphodiester bond 5′ to the AP site and generation of a single-strand break. This reaction produces a 3′-hydroxyl group and a 5′-dRP group flanking the break. This way of AP site processing fits short-patch pathway of the BER process.

Another way of AP site cleavage by the BER machinery involving the action of bi-functional DNA glycosylases is more complicated and requires the 'end cleaning' of termini prior to the further repair reactions may occur. An intermediate reaction step for these enzymes is the formation of a transient Schiff base between the amino group and the C1′ of deoxyribose for both base excision and subsequent DNA strand cleavage. In solution, AP sites exist predominantly as a mixture of ring-closed α- and β-hemiacetals with a minor amount of ring-opened aldehyde and aldehyde hydrate (<1%) (de los Santos et al., 2004). AP sites can be incised through β-elimination using ε-NH2 of a lysine as the active site nucleophile (David & Williams, 1998; McCullough et al., 1999). Strand incision by β-elimination forms a nick with phospho-α,β-unsaturated aldehyde (PUA) at the 3′ margin and phosphate at the 5′ margin (David & Williams, 1998; McCullough et al., 1999) (Fig. 1). While recently discovered mammalian DNA glycosylases, termed NEIL (Nei-like)-1, -2, catalyze the β,δ-elimination reaction with the N-terminal proline being used as the nucleophile (Hazra et al., 2002; Takao et al., 2002, Das et al., 2006). The β,δ-elimination reaction results in a one nucleotide gap flanked with phosphate groups at the 3'- and 5' margins. The products of bi-functional DNA glycosylase activity require the trimming of the 3'-ends to produce 3'-end hydroxyl groups that are indispensable for DNA polymerase activity.

Most of mammalian proteins known to form the Schiff base intermediate with the AP site appear to belong to the BER system. On the other hand, an interaction of AP DNA with proteins not formally involved in BER (for example, human ribosomal protein S3 and nucleoside diphosphate kinase - NM23-H2/NDP) has been well documented (Hegde et al., 2004; Postel et al., 2000). These two proteins are able to cleave AP sites. MutY, unlike other monofuctional DNA glycosylases, is able to interact with AP site via a Schiff base formation (Zharkov & Grollman, 1998) without the concomitant cleavage of AP sites. In this particular case formation of the Schiff base intermediate is considered as a mechanism for temporal protection of AP sites (Zharkov & Grollman, 1998).

Since AP sites in DNA appear to be promiscuous in their binding to many cellular factors and they are constantly generated in high frequency in genomic DNA, it may be important to sequester the AP sites immediately upon formation and further process them by the way that is most favorable for DNA integrity. Thus, interaction of cellular proteins with AP sites might be important for their repair/temporal protection from further degradation or might be involved in damage sensing/signaling making search of AP site reactive proteins a very important task.

### 2.3 Search of new participants of recognition/processing of AP sites

The very promising approach in search for unknown players in AP site recognition is based on a well-known propensity of deoxyribose in AP site, existing in equilibrium between cyclic furanose and acyclic aldehyde forms, to react with amine moieties in its vicinity. The Schiff base intermediate can be reduced by sodium borohydride ($NaBH_4$) or related compounds, forming an irreversible complex between the enzyme and DNA (David & Williams, 1998; Piersen et al., 2000). This reaction is widely used to prove the β-elimination reaction mechanism for the enzymes capable of AP site cleavage (David & Williams, 1998; Piersen et al., 2000), although some proteins (e.g. MutY DNA glycosylase) can form a Schiff base with no further β-elimination (Zharkov & Grollman, 1998). Therefore, upon searching of new players in AP site recognition mediated by the Schiff base formation their ability to cleave AP has to be proved. Along with intact AP site, the product of its cleavage - 3' PUA and 5' dRP moieties (Fig. 1, grey rectangular boxes) are also able to form the Schiff base intermediate with primary amino groups of proteins that allows to use these DNA in search and identification of proteins.

#### 2.3.1 Identification of proteins reactive to AP sites

For identification of protein cross-linked to AP DNA in cell extracts immunochemical and/or mass-spectrometry methods can be used. Identification of proteins reactive to AP sites by combination of cross-linking technique and mass-spectrometry is schematically represented in Fig. 2.

In general, search and identification of proteins reactive to AP sites include the following steps: (1) finding of cellular extract proteins forming covalent adducts with AP sites in DNA; (2) the design of AP-DNA probe containing a functional group providing the selective

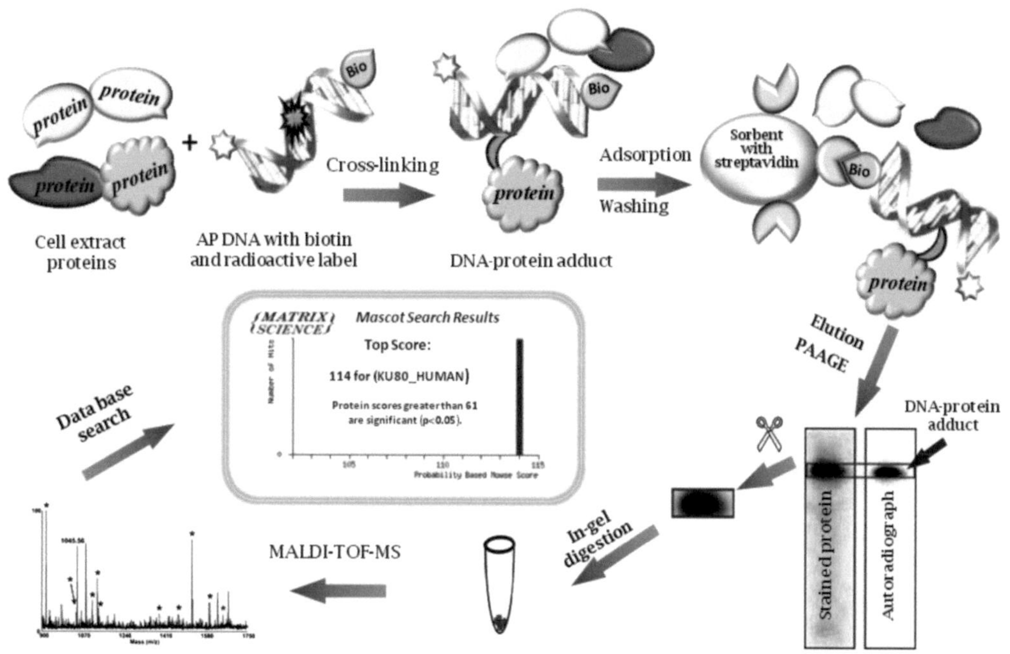


Fig. 2. Workflow of identification of protein cross-linked to DNA containing intact or cleaved AP site.

isolation of cross-linked DNA-protein products; (3) the preparative cross-linking of extract proteins with such DNA; (4) the affinity purification of the resulted products; (5) the identification of the protein in the covalent adduct with DNA using mass-spectrometry methods; (6) the confirmation of the results using purified proteins and/or specific antibodies and the known functions/interactions of the identified protein; and (7) the study of the functional role of the revealed interactions between proteins and AP DNA. A proof-of-principle identification of protein reactive towards AP sites in species from *E. coli* and *S. cerevisiae* was reported in (Rieger et al., 2006).

It should be noted that used protocol includes two steps that increases the selectivity of the method. Affinity purification of cross-linked protein was carried out on commercially available affinity sorbents containing streptavidin, which binds the biotin residue. After adsorption, non-specifically bound proteins were removed by a series of washings. Additional separation of proteins was achieved by electrophoresis under denaturing conditions by the Laemmli method (Laemmli, 1970) followed by staining proteins. The target product was identified by the colocalization in the gel positions of the label in DNA and the stained protein. This approach indicates that only the protein cross-linked to DNA will be subjected to the further analysis. However, one cannot fully exclude the presence of impurity proteins with the same electrophoretic mobility as the target product.

The identification was carried out for a number of proteins forming cross-links with AP sites in extracts of *E. coli* cells at logarithmic and stationary phases of cell growth (Rieger et al., 2006). It should be noted that authors used the previously developed non-enzymatic approach of the creation of AP sites in DNA based on the periodate oxidation of 2,3,5,6-tetrahydroxyhexyl phosphate precursor, which was introduced into an oligonucleotide during the standard phosphoroamidite oligonucleotide synthesis. The periodate oxidation allows one to obtain AP sites in an almost quantitative yield. This method, in the authors' opinion, has several advantages over the more commonly used method that is based on the removal of uracil residues using uracil DNA glycosylase.

The procaryotic proteins AroF, DnaK, MutM, PolA, TnaA, TufA, and UvrA from *E. coli* and eucaryotic ARC1 and Ygl245wp from yeast were identified (Rieger et al., 2006). Protein Ygl245wp with an unknown but essential for cell viability function was prepared in the individual state after its coding sequence was cloned, and the recombinant plasmid was used for the production of the protein in *E. coli* cells followed by its isolation. The obtained protein was shown to bind to AP DNA forming Schiff bases; however, the biological significance of this interaction has not been established. DNA polymerase I, like other DNA polymerases of the A-family, has a weak AP lyase activity and dRP lyase activity (Pinz & Bogenhagen, 2000). However the biological significance of these activities *in vivo* has not been established. The ability of UvrA, the key component of the nucleotide excision repair (NER) in bacteria, to interact with AP sites in the UvrABC complex indicates the possible role of NER as a back-up pathway of AP site repair in bacteria (Showden et al., 1990).

### 2.3.2 Identification of Ku80 subunit of human Ku antigen as a protein reactive to AP sites

Using the same technique we screened mammalian cell extracts for proteins capable of binding AP site-containing DNA. In HeLa cell extract, a 32-bp DNA duplex with an AP site in the middle of the DNA chain was shown to cross-link predominantly to a protein forming a product with an apparent molecular mass of 95 kDa (Fig. 3) (Ilina et al., 2008).

The subsequent analysis of whole cell extracts of human lung fibroblasts, K-562, and MCF-7 cells revealed the products with the same electrophoretic mobility. The preferential cross-linking of this protein reflected extraordinary specificity in light of the multitude of proteins in the cell. If the AP site in DNA is replaced by its analog (the THF residue) or the treatment with NaBH4 is omitted, DNA–protein cross-linked products are not registered (Fig. 3).

In spite of efficient cross-linking of the above mentioned AP DNA to Ku80 polypeptide (as a part of DNA-PK) no cleavage of AP sites was observed (Ilina et al., 2008). Instead Ku80 formed with AP site a long-living Schiff base intermediate without the concomitant AP site cleavage just as was observed for monofunctional DNA glycosylase MutY and considered as a mechanism for temporal protection of AP sites (Zharkov & Grollman, 1998). AP lyase and 5′-dRP activities are distinctive features of the BER process (Almeida & Sobol, 2007; Hegde et al., 2008). The BER 5′-dRP/AP lyases usually function beyond the DS-breaks. But abasic sites associated with double-strand breaks can be generated by ionizing radiation, by treatment with radiomimetic drugs or as a result of attempted BER of complex damages (Yang et al., 2004). These specifically positioned lesions must be removed prior to or in the course of DS break repair. Ku antigen – DS-end binding protein of NHEJ – has been recently shown to act as a 5′-dRP/AP lyase near double-strand breaks (Roberts et al., 2010).

At DSB ends Ku is approximately tenfold more active than Pol β (Roberts et al., 2010), the most known mammalian 5′-dRP lyase (Matsumoto & Kim, 1995). At the same time, Ku was inefficient as AP lyase at AP sites situated at a distance longer than one helix turn from DS breaks just as was reported in (Ilina et al., 2008). $NaBH_4$-dependent cross-linking of

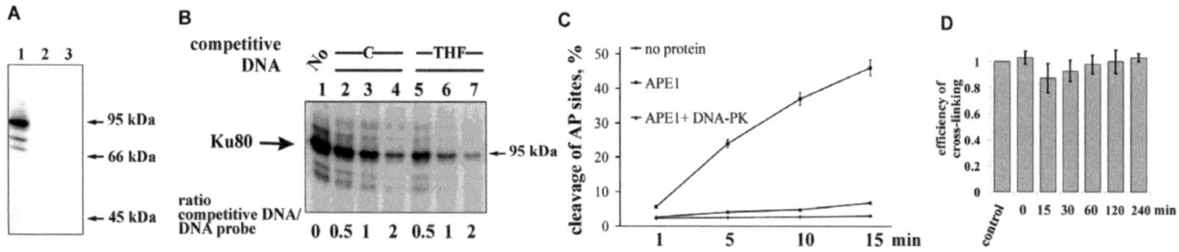


Fig. 3. Interaction of Ku antigen with AP sites (From Ilina et al., 2008). (A) Cross-linking of proteins in HeLa cell extract (lane 1); without borohydride treatment (lane 2); AP DNA probe was replaced by the DNA duplex containing a THF residue (lane 3). (B) Specificity of the Ku80 antigen interaction with AP DNA. Cross-linking of the HeLa cell extract proteins to AP DNA was performed in the absence (lane 1) or presence of competitive DNA at different concentrations (lanes 2-7). The structures of competitive DNAs are shown at the top. Ratio of competitive DNA to DNA probe is shown at the bottom. (C) Influence of DNA-PK on the activity of APE1. (D) Estimation of the stability of Ku complex with AP DNA in HeLa cell extract. AP DNA was preincubated with HeLa cell extract for 15 min at 37°. Then excess of competitive DNA containing a THF residue was added, and the reaction mixture was further incubated at 37° for additional 4 hours. Aliquots at different times were reduced with $NaBH_4$ and analyzed.

appropriate AP lyase substrate and AP lyase activity test in the cell extracts deficient and proficient in Ku antigen unambiguously testify to the role of Ku antigen in processing of AP sites positioned near 5′ termini of DS breaks. Moreover, transfection of Ku deficient or proficient cells with variants of specifically designed substrate DNAs (with natural AP site or its AP lyase-resistant analog or without AP site) followed by PCR amplification of joining products and subsequent restriction analysis of amplicons fully confirmed the necessity of Ku antigen AP lyase activity for removal of near-end AP sites. Altogether the results obtained *in vitro* and *in vivo* testify to use of the 5′-dRP/AP lyase activity of Ku antigen for the excision of near-end abasic sites and explain higher radiosensitivity of mammalian cells deficient in Ku antigen, which is indispensable for classical NHEJ (Schulte-Uentrop et al., 2008). It is worthy of notice, that the same mechanism of AP site cleavage is used by two unrelated DNA repair systems and the suitable positioning of AP sites relative to active site nucleophiles is indispensable for efficient catalysis.

### 2.3.3 AP site recognition by the 5’-dRP/AP lyase in PARP-1

In further screening for proteins that are reactive to AP sites in addition to a linear DNA duplex with an AP site in the middle of the $^{32}$P-5′end-labeled strand, we used circular AP site-containing DNA to exclude interference by Ku80. Circular double-stranded DNA was synthesized, using single-stranded M13 DNA as template, in the presence of dUTP; then, AP sites were generated by uracil DNA glycosylase treatment (Khodyreva et al., 2010a; Khodyreva et al., 2010b). Unlike short duplex DNA with an AP site, that predominantly cross-linked Ku80 in HeLa cell extract (Ilina et al., 2008 and Fig. 4A, lane 5), the use of circular AP site-containing DNA allowed us to detect a novel protein with molecular mass of ~120-kDa that is reactive to AP site (Fig. 4A, lanes 1–4).

To identify the cross-linked protein large-scale cross-linking with the bovine testis nuclear extract (BTNE) and a biotin-containing linear AP DNA was performed. Identification was realized according to the scheme shown in Fig. 2.

Results from the MS analyses were searched against a database, and PARP-1 was identified as the first-rank candidate (Mascot probability score of 248, 38% of coverage).
We tested for and found AP site cross-linking by purified PARP-1 (data not shown). Yet, it was not clear whether the cross-linked complex in the extract resulted from PARP-1's reactivity at the intact AP site or a pre-incised AP site.
We next examined purified PARP-1 cross-linking with a linear DNA containing either an intact AP site or pre-incised AP site; in addition to cross-linking probes, these DNAs are substrates for 5′-dRP and AP lyase enzymatic activity (Fig. 4B).

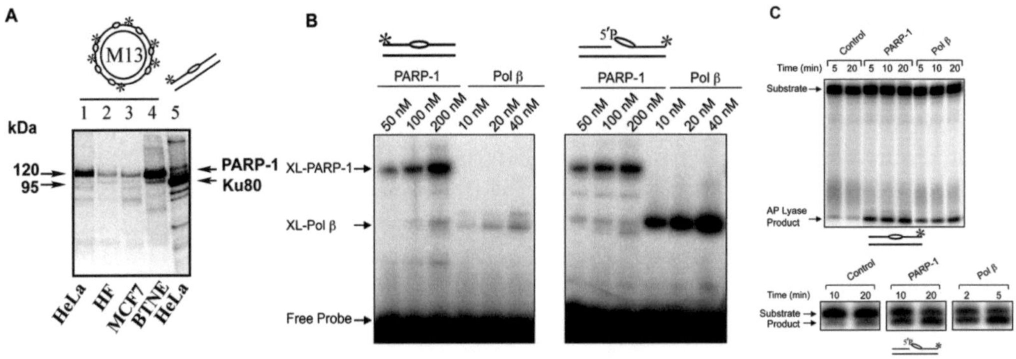


Fig. 4. Interaction of PARP-1 with intact and cleaved AP sites (From Khodyreva et al., 2010b). (A) Cross-linking of mammalian cell extract proteins to circular and linear AP DNA Extracts: whole cell extracts of HeLa, human fibroblasts (HF), MCF-7 and bovine testis nuclear extract (BTNE). (B) Comparison of cross-linking of purified PARP-1 and Pol β with 5′-dRP lyase substrate DNA and AP site-containing DNA. Schematic representations of DNA probes are shown at the top. The * symbol denotes the position of the $^{32}$P-label in the DNA. The bubble-like symbol denotes the presence of the AP site in the DNA. (C) 5′-dRP/AP lyase activities of purified PARP-1. The positions of the substrates and products are indicated, and the DNA is illustrated at the bottom.

Cross-linking of PARP-1 was compared with that of Pol β. PARP-1 and Pol β cross-linked to both of these DNA substrates in a concentration-dependent manner. Pol β has a preference for the pre-incised AP site containing-DNA, as compared to the intact AP site. Conversely, PARP-1 does not show a similar preference, yielding similar cross-linking with both probes. The interaction of PARP-1 with the AP site raised the question of the biological relevance of this finding, including whether PARP-1 binds first to the AP site and protects it until repair proteins are recruited. PARP-1 is well known to become activated by binding to DNA strand breaks (Lindahl et al., 1995). Once the AP site became incised by AP endonuclease, PARP-1 became activated and modified by auto-poly(ADP-ribosyl)ation. First, we examined the specificity of PARP-1 interaction with AP site containing-DNA by competition experiments using two types of competitor DNA. A labeled DNA duplex with a 'natural' AP site was used for PARP-1 cross-linking, and the cross-linking was competed either with a control DNA duplex (without an AP site) or a synthetic AP site-containing DNA, tetrahydrofuran (THF), mimicking the AP site. Cross-linking of PARP-1 was reduced with both control and THF-containing DNA. However, the reduction was stronger in the case of

THF-containing DNA than with control DNA. This suggests that PARP-1 has greater affinity for the THF-containing DNA than for the control DNA (data not shown).

The next question regarding PARP-1's interaction with AP sites was whether the enzyme is activated for poly(ADP-ribose) synthesis upon binding to the intact AP site. PARP-1 is well known to become activated by binding to DNA strand breaks (Lindahl et al., 1995), and to avoid the presence of confounding DNA ends, we prepared a double-hairpin DNA for use as probe. First, using this hairpin DNA with internal $^{32}P$-label, we confirmed the ability of purified PARP-1 to cross-link to the natural AP site. The results showed that double-hairpin DNA bearing the natural AP site was able to cross-link upon $NaBH_4$ reduction, whereas DNA without the AP site (uracil-DNA) failed to yield cross-linked product (data not shown). As expected, THF-containing DNA failed to cross-link. Next, using similar but unlabeled double-hairpin DNA and $^{32}P$-NAD+ as substrate for poly(ADP-ribose) synthesis, we examined the activity of PARP-1. Strong PARP-1 auto-modification was observed only in reaction mixtures containing APE1 (data not shown). PARP-1 auto-modification in reaction mixtures with the natural AP site, but without APE1, was weak; this level, however, was more than the background level (data not shown). Under similar conditions, the THF-containing DNA failed to support poly(ADP-ribose) synthesis, but strong synthesis was observed when APE1 was added. These results indicated that PARP-1 interaction with the intact AP site could result in activation, but this activation involved much less auto-poly(ADP-ribosyl)ation than that observed with APE1-induced strand incision.

Next, to examine PARP-1 auto-modification, purified PARP-1 was first pre-incubated with labeled intact linear AP site-containing DNA. The reaction mixture was then supplemented with $NAD^+$ to allow poly(ADP-ribose) synthesis. Then, the reaction mixture was treated with $NaHB_4$ and analyzed. The results indicated that poly(ADP-ribose) modified enzyme was cross-linked (data not shown). The mechanism of PARP-1 activation was unclear, but presumably involved single strand break formation within the PARP-1 and DNA complex. In light of this result, we were curious to test PARP-1's capacity to conduct strand incision at the AP site via AP lyase activity. As shown in Fig. 4C, PARP-1 was capable of incising AP site-containing DNA, and the activity was similar to that of Pol β. In light of PARP-1's AP lyase activity, we also tested for 5'dRP lyase activity. PARP-1 conducted 5'-dRP lyase activity against a pre-incised AP site (Fig. 4C), but the activity was much lower than that of Pol β. These results suggested that the endogenous PARP-1 AP lyase activity was sufficient to provide poly(ADP-ribose) synthesis activation at the natural AP site.

Interaction of PARP-1 with AP sites appears to be related with regulation of AP site processing. Such a regulation is particularly important for repair of AP sites included in clustered damage, in which chain breaks, oxidized bases and AP sites are grouped within 1-2 turns of DNA helix and can be situated in both DNA chains. During repair of AP sites within clustered damages additional double strand breaks, which are more cytotoxic, may appear (Yang et al., 2004). PARP-1 influence on hydrolysis of AP sites by APE1 on DNA containing AP site either opposite dAMP or synthetic AP site analogues, was tested (Kutuzov et al., 2011). Along with THF residue, which is most widely used to mimic AP sites, the new AP site analogs were tested (Kutuzov et al., 2011). These analogs were residues of diethylene glycol and decane-1,10-diol. The AP site analogs differ in their sensitivity to the APE1 endonuclease activity. PARP-1 interacts more efficiently with AP sites within clusters that leads to stronger cross-linking with AP sites and more considerable inhibition of APE1 activity as compared with AP DNA containing single AP site.

Thus, by virtue of PARP-1's ability to interact with the intact AP sites (single or within cluster) via Schiff base formation, we demonstrated a new role for PARP-1 in regulation of the BER process. PARP-1's interaction at the AP site could recruit this key enzyme and protect the site until APE1 becomes available to initiate strand incision and BER. Alternatively, PARP-1's 5′-dRP/AP lyase activity could perform strand incision and trigger poly(ADP-ribosyl)ation leading to recruitment of other BER factors.

### 2.3.4 New function of Neil1 and Neil2 as 5′dRP lyase

According to current view, in mammalian BER the sub-pathway choice is influenced by the rate-limiting step in SN BER, i.e., removal of the 5′-dRP by the dRP lyase activity of Pol β (Horton et al., 2000; Srivastava et al., 1998). For example, if the 5′-dRP cannot be removed efficiently, continued DNA synthesis will emphasize the LP BER sub-pathway (Horton et al., 2000). Yet, both subpathways appear to operate simultaneously to repair most types of DNA lesions *in vitro* (Horton et al., 2000; Prasad et al., 2000). It has been shown previously that the 5′-dRP BER intermediate is the cytotoxic lesion following exposure to methylating agents, and its removal is a pivotal step in BER *in vivo* (Sobol et al., 2000).

Pol β-deficient mouse cells show little dRPase activity (Sobol et al., 2000), but some residual dRP removal by extracts prepared from these cells is still present (Podlutsky et al., 2001). It is possible that while Pol β carries out the bulk of dRP removal from DNA, other activities could be more specifically employed for certain lesions, cell or tissue types, or at certain points of the cell cycle. In *E. coli*, Fpg (formamidopyrimidine-DNA glycosylase) and to a lesser extent endonuclease VIII (Nei) catalyze β-elimination of dRP moiety (Fig. 1). Three mammalian homologues of bacterial Fpg and Nei termed NEIL (Nei-like)-1, -2, and -3 have been identified (Hazra et al., 2002; Hegde et al., 2008). Based on the similarity of their active sites to those of Fpg and Nei, one could expect that they could also display dRPase activity. We have shown that two of these proteins, NEIL1 and NEIL2, are capable of removing dRP lesions from DNA with the efficiency comparable to that of Pol β, and that they can substitute for Pol β dRPase activity in a reconstituted BER assay (Grin et al., 2006).

dRPase activity can be revealed with 3′-labeled nicked abasic oligonucleotide substrates. Such substrates were prepared by end-filling of a 5′-overhanging oligonucleotide duplexes with $^{32}$P-labeled dATP and the consecutive treatment of the duplex with uracil DNA glycosylase (Ung) and APE1. The resulting dRP site is unstable in nucleophilic buffers and is degraded during migration through Tris-containing polyacrylamide gels, therefore the products were stabilized by sodium borohydride reduction immediately after the dRPase-catalyzed reaction.

Fig. 5A illustrates that both NEIL1 and NEIL2 possess a dRP-removing activity. The dRPase activities of NEIL1 and NEIL2 demonstrated the enzyme concentration and time dependence expected of an enzyme-catalyzed reaction (Fig. 5B and data not shown). Notably, the activity of NEIL1 in these experiments appeared higher than that of NEIL1 (Fig. 5B). Both NEIL1 and NEIL2 excised with similar efficiency when A, C, or T were placed opposite the lesion, and the excision of dRP opposite G was 1.5–2-fold lower; Pol β removed dRP equally well from all opposite-base contexts. To confirm that dRP removal by NEIL1 and NEIL2 proceeds by β-elimination, as in Pol β and Fpg, we have performed the reaction in the presence of sodium borohydride, which reduces the Schiff base covalent complexes formed between the catalytic amine nucleophile of dRP lyases and C1′ of the dRP site during the reaction (Fig. 5C). Such trapped enzyme–DNA complexes are stable enough to be resolved by regular SDS-PAGE. NEIL1 and NEIL2, as well as Fpg and Pol β, formed low-mobility radioactively labeled complexes.

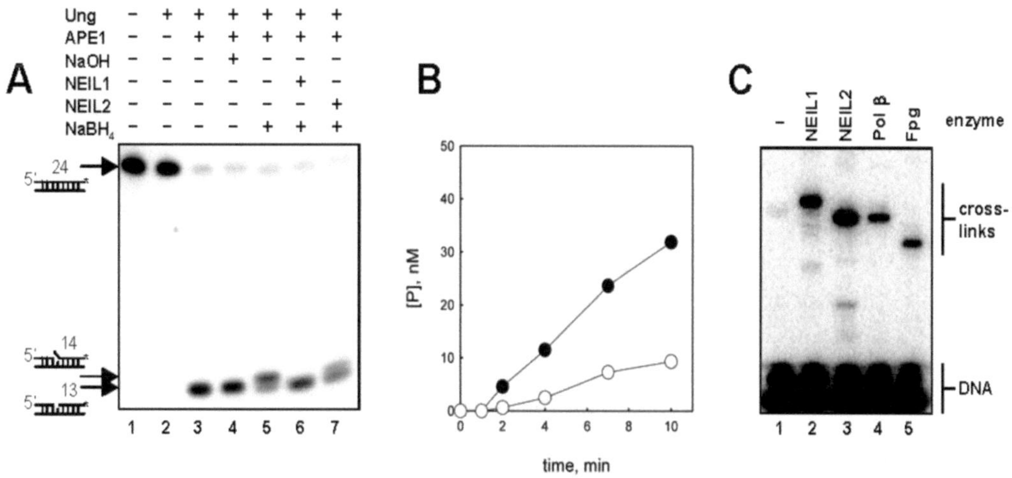


Fig. 5. **dRPase activity of NEIL1 and NEIL2** (From Grin et al., 2006). (A) Cleavage of a dRP moiety by NEIL1 and NEIL2. Lane 1, U-containing oligonucleotide; lane 2, AP-containing oligonucleotide; lanes 3–7, dRP-containing oligonucleotide treated with alkali (lane 4), NEIL1 (lane 6) or NEIL2 (lane 7). In lanes 5–7, the dRP-containing oligonucleotide was stabilized with sodium borohydride to prevent its degradation during electrophoresis. Arrows left to the panels indicate positions of the respective oligonucleotide species after PAGE. (B) Time course of dRP excision by NEIL1 (filled circles) and NEIL2 (open circles). (C) Cross-linking of dRP lyases to a dRP-containing substrate by sodium borohydride: lane 1, no enzyme; lane 2, NEIL1; lane 3, NEIL2; lane 4, Pol β; lane 5, Fpg.

To compare the efficiency of NEIL1 and NEIL2 as dRPases with the same activity of DNA polymerase β, the best-known mammalian dRPase, we have determined steady-state enzyme kinetic constants for all three enzymes. The results of these experiments are summarized in Table 1.

| | $K_M$, μM | $k_{cat}$, min$^{-1}$ | $k_{cat}/K_M$, μM$^{-1}$ min$^{-1}$ |
|---|---|---|---|
| NEIL1 | 0.21±0.03 | 0.65±0.04 | 3.1 |
| NEIL2 | 2.2±0.7 | 1.6±0.1 | 0.74 |
| Pol β | 1.0±0.1 | 3.0±0.1 | 3.0 |

Table 1. Kinetic parameters of the dRPase reaction catalyzed by NEIL1, NEIL2, and DNA polymerase β.

The kinetic data suggest that NEIL1 is as good a dRPase as Pol β, and they both surpassed NEIL2 in their ability to remove dRP from DNA. $K_M$ of NEIL1 was ~5-fold lower than $K_M$ of Pol β, indicating that NEIL1 might bind dRP-containing substrate more tightly; on the other hand, Pol β processed the substrate ~5-fold faster than did NEIL1, resulting in nearly equal specificity constants for both enzymes. NEIL2 had an intermediate catalytic constant and the poorest binding of all three dRP lyases compared in this experiment.

The experiments with individual enzymes suggest that NEIL1 and NEIL2 possess dRP lyase activities and could substitute for Pol β in removing dRP moiety in the BER process. To analyze the proficiency of NEIL1 and NEIL2 dRPase in a multienzyme BER process, we have reconstituted the base-excision, AP site-incision, gap-filling and dRP-excision stages of BER using mammalian enzymes (UNG, OGG1, APE1, Pol β (wild type and K35A/K68A/K72A mutant deficient in dRP lyase activity) and NEIL1 or NEIL2. Both NEIL1 and NEIL2 could rescue BER of uracil lesions driven by a dRP-deficient Pol β. The proficiency of NEIL1 in the full BER was higher compared with NEIL2, in agreement with the kinetic parameters showing that NEIL2 is the worst of the three dRPases. We have also reconstituted the repair of AP sites pre-formed in DNA by action of *E. coli* UDG. No major difference from the repair of U was observed.

Having established that NEIL1 and NEIL2 could substitute for dRPlyase activity of Pol β in the reconstituted BER system, we then studied whether NEIL proteins could manifest their dRPase activity in some particular systems, e.g. in cell extracts lacking Pol β.

#### 2.3.5 Identification of HMGB1 as cofactor of the BER process

To identify proteins that have dRP lyase activity or influence removal of the dRP from BER intermediates in the absence of Pol β, we used Pol β null mouse embryonic fibroblast (MEF) cell extract for sodium borohydride driven cross-linking of the Schiff base dRP lyase intermediate protein-DNA complex (Prasad et al., 2007). The strong labeling of a single species in the Pol β null cell extracts corresponding to an unknown protein-DNA complex of 37 kDa was observed (Fig. 6A).

The preferential cross-linking of this protein reflected extraordinary specificity in light of the multitude of proteins in the cell. Taking into account the molecular masses of NEIL1 and NEIL2 (43.5 kDa and 38.2 kDa, respectively) the product could not be related to glycosylases. It should be noted that an apparent molecular mass of a covalent adduct protein-nucleic acid estimated by electrophoretic mobility is approximately equal to the sum of molecular masses of protein and attached nucleic acid.

For identification of protein we applied the approach schematically depicted in Fig. 2. The DNA probe contained a $^{32}$P-labeled dRP moiety in a single-stranded break and a 3'-biotin tag to facilitate isolation of cross-linked protein-DNA complexes. Eleven of ions observed in MALDI MS spectrum corresponded to peptides of HMGB1. The $(M + H)^+$ ion of m/z 1520.84 was selected automatically during the data dependent acquisition for MS/MS analysis. The values from both the peptide masses and the MS/MS fragment ion masses were used in a database search. The protein was identified as HMGB1 with a Mowse-based score of 102, 32% sequence coverage and a protein score confidence interval of 99.995%. Among the observed ions the ion of m/z 1520.84 corresponds to amino acid residues 113–127 of the mouse HMGB1 and is a 'signature' that distinguishes HMGB1 from the closely related protein, HMGB2 (Bustin & Reeves, 1996). HMGB1 and HMGB2 are nuclear nonhistone DNA-binding proteins that belong to the high-mobility group box family of proteins (Bustin & Reeves, 1996). HMGB1 has an architectural role in the assembly of nucleoprotein complexes and is highly conserved across species (Bustin & Reeves, 1996; Tang et al., 2010 ;Liu et al., 2010; Stros, 2010). HMGB1 binds to DNA in the minor groove without sequence specificity and has the ability to transiently introduce bends or kinks into linear DNA (Liu et al., 2010; Stros, 2010). The intrinsic ability of HMGB1 to alter DNA structures allows it to participate in many biological processes including regulation of chromatin structure, transcription, DNA damage repair and recombination. The importance of HMGB1 in DNA repair was identified in studies that revealed the ability of HMGB1 to bind to a variety of bulky DNA lesions (Liu et al., 2010; Stros, 2010).

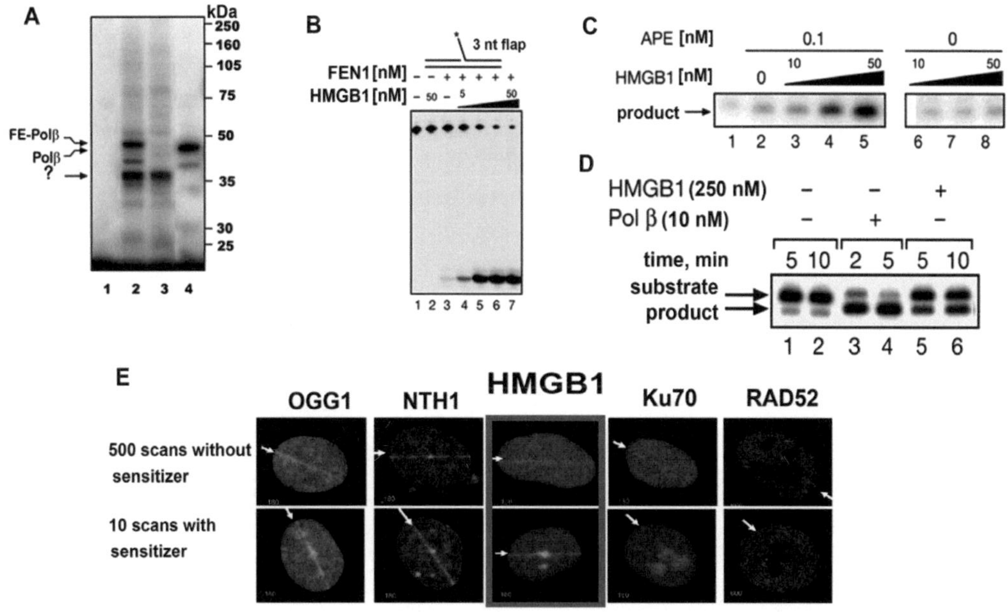


Fig. 6. Identification of HMGB1 as a BER cofactor (from Prasad et al., 2007). (A) Search of extract proteins interacting with the 5'dRP residue in the DNA duplex: lane 2, products of cross-linking between 5' dRP DNA and MEF extract proteins expressing Pol β with flag-epitope (FE), lane 1 control without borohydride treatment. (B) The influence of HMGB1 on FEN1 activity. (C) Influence of HMGB1 on APE1 activity. (D) Comparison of the 5' deoxyribose phosphate lyase activity of HMGB1 and Pol β. (E) Interaction of GFP-HMGB1 in HeLa cells with DNA damage sites induced by scanning laser microirradiation (λ 405 nm) without a sensitizer and in the presence of 8-methoxypsoralen (100 μM). Protein designation: 8-Oxoguanine DNA glycosylase (OGG1); NTH1, DNA glycosylase removing oxidized pyrimidines from DNA; RAD52, protein involved in double-strand break repair, homologous recombination; Ku70, Ku antigen subunit involved in of double-strand break repair, nonhomologous end joining. Arrows show the direction of the scan.

The observed ability of HMGB1 to interact with the BER DNA intermediate poses a question about its role in the process. It was found in the in vitro experiments that HMGB1 isolated from HeLa cells directly interacted with several BER proteins: APE1, Pol β, and FEN1( data not shown) and stimulate the activity of BER enzymes FEN1 and APE1 (Figs. 6B and 6C, respectively). HMGB1 was also revealed to have weak 5' dRP lyase activity (Fig. 6D).
Using HeLa cells expressing HMGB1 in the form of a chimeric protein with green fluorescent protein (GFP-HMGB1), it was found that HMGB1 can be localized in the regions of DNA damage induced by laser microirradiation (Fig. 6E). Irradiation under used conditions generates both single-strand breaks and oxidized bases with high frequency (Lan et al., 2004). Indeed, DNA glycosylases (GFP-OGG1 and GFP-NTH1) efficiently accumulate

in sites of irradiation unlike the proteins recognizing double-strand breaks in DNA (GFP-Ku70 and GFP-RAD52) (Fig. 6E).

Mouse embryonic fibroblasts of the HMGB1+/+ type are more sensitive than HMGB1-/- cells to the combined action of methyl methanesulfonate and methoxyamine, and HMGB1+/+ cells contain a much larger amount of single-strand breaks. The treatment of AP DNA with methoxyamine increases its resistance to APE1 action (Horton et al., 2000).

Another group of researches using two cultivated cell lines of breast cancer found that the increase in the expression level of HMGB1 alters the cells' phenotype by slowing cell growth and increasing the cell sensitivity to ionizing radiation (Jiao et al., 2007).

Interestingly, that in spite of ability of purified NEIL 1/2 to interact with dRP lyase substrate (Grin et al., 2006) we did not reveal abundant products of their cross-linking in the Pol β null MEF extract (Fig. 6 A, lane 2). This interaction appears to be counteracted by effective binding of HMGB1, which is highly abundant in cells.

### 2.3.6 HMGA as cofactor of the BER process

It is interesting to note that dRP- and AP lyase activities were revealed for another group of chromatin proteins (Summer at al., 2009). Mammalian high mobility group proteins are non-histone chromatin architectural factors encoded by two genes, *HMGA1* and *HMGA2*. Alternative mRNA splicing results in at least four protein isoforms involved in chromatin remodeling and gene transcription (Bustin & Reeves, 1996, Reeves, 2001, Cleynen & van de Ven, 2008). HMGA proteins are characterized by the presence of an acidic C-terminal tail and three DNA binding domains containing short basic repeats, the so called AT-hooks, capable to bind in the minor groove of AT-rich sequences in DNA. In humans, HMGA expression is undetectable or very low in differentiated adult tissues, but high HMGA protein levels are associated with human malignant neoplasias (Berner et al., 1997, Abe et al., 2003, Miyazawa et al., 2004, Meyer et al., 2007). In addition, expression of HMGA1 is functionally linked to chemoresistance of some human carcinomas (Liau & Whang, 2008).

Recombinant human HMGA (HMGA1a, HMGA1b and HMGA2) proteins have been shown to efficiently cleave plasmid DNA containing AP sites (Summer et al., 2009). Further analysis revealed that the proteins could be trapped on AP DNA by $NaCNBH_3$ treatment, the mechanism characteristic of AP lyase activity (David & Williams, 1998; McCullough et al.; 1999, Piersen et al., 2000). To determine the chemical nature of DNA ends generated by the HMGA proteins and the efficiency of AP site cleavage, $^{32}P$-labeled double-stranded short DNA duplex containing a single AP site was used as substrate. The analysis revealed that HMGA proteins generated cleavage products, which exhibit the same electrophoretic mobility as those produced by endonuclease III of *E. coli*, an AP lyase catalyzing the β elimination reaction (McCullough et al., 1999; David & Williams, 1998).

To test the possibility that HMGA proteins also possess the related 5'-dRP lyase activity the same DNA duplex bearing label at the 3' end was employed. A 5'-dRP moiety on the labeled strand was produced by endonuclease IV from *E. coli*. To stabilize chemically labile 5'-dRP group and to improve electrophoretic separation of the products, 5'-deoxyribosyl phosphate moiety was adducted with O-benzyl hydroxylamine. The analysis revealed that the HMGA proteins efficiently removed 5'-dRP moiety. Thus, HMGA proteins display the AP/5'-dRP lyase activity characteristic of the BER process.

Having established that the HMGA proteins are lyases, the authors examined the role of this activity in cell context. To this end, cell lines constitutively expressing HMGA2 have been generated. Then using transgenic and parental cell lines and employing a variety of cell-based assays and biochemical approaches, the authors provided evidence that the AP site/dRP lyase activities indeed had important biological functions. First, it has been demonstrated that HMGA2 could be efficiently trapped on genomic DNA. Parental cells A549, which express HMGA2 below detectable level, were exposed to low pH or physiological pH as control. DNA isolated from treated cells was incubated with recombinant HMGA2 under trapping (+$NaCNBH_3$) or non-trapping (+NaCl) conditions. The subsequent dot-blot analysis revealed that HMGA2 could be only trapped by DNA derived from cells exposed to low pH, conditions leading to generation of AP sites. Moreover, HMGA2 expressed in transgenic cell line A549 (1.6) was efficiently trapped in a covalent complex *in vivo* with genomic AP sites generated when the cells were subjected to low pH. Analysis of cytotoxic effects that might result from depurination in parental and transgenic cells caused by exposure to low pH revealed that all transgenic cell lines were substantially more resistant than parental cells.

In order to unravel the role of HMGA2 in response of cells to genotoxic impact, parental and transgenic cells were exposed to hydroxyurea (Hu) or methyl methanesulphonate (MMS). Hu is able to induce base oxidation and depurination (Sakano et al., 2001). MMS produces genomic AP sites through the action of DNA glycosylases, which remove the alkylated bases (Sedgwik et al., 2006). In the case of both reagents expression of HMGA2 resulted in significant protection against cell death leading to increase in cell survival.

Both AP and dRP lyase activities play central roles in the early steps of BER (Hegde et al., 2008). In order to demonstrate that protection from MMS induced DNA damage observed with transgenic cells involves HMGA2 lyase activities the cells were sequentially exposed to MMS and O-benzyl hydroxylamine (BA). BA alone had no effect on the survival of parental or transgenic cells. However, combined action of MMS and BA sensitized HMGA2-containg cells to MMS treatment. BA (analogously to methoxy amine) reacts with the baseless deoxyribose moieties (in intact or cleaved AP sites) rendering them refractory to mammalian AP endonuclease 1 and AP/dRP lyase activities (Horton et al., 2000).

Direct interaction of HMGA2 with APE1 *in vitro* and *in vivo* (Sgarra et al., 2008, Summer et al., 2009, Sgarra et al., 2010) has been reported. However, the influence of HMGA2 on the AP endonuclease 1 activity is still unknown. HMGA2 protects cells against three different genotoxicants, i.e. Hu, MMS and low pH (Summer et al., 2009), which introduce the DNA damages repaired by the BER machinery. It is noteworthy here, that repair of these lesions involves the common intermediates, AP sites and 5′ dRP moieties, which can be processed by HMGA2. This strongly support the idea developed in (Summer et al., 2009) that intrinsic AP/dRP lyase activities of HMGA2 are responsible for the protective action of this protein. However, one could not exclude that in addition to direct action, HMGA2 influences the BER capacity indirectly by enhancing the activity of APE1 as was observed in the case of HMGB1 (Prasad et al., 2007). Activation of APE1 by protein-protein interaction may be involved both in the stage of AP site hydrolysis and removing the 3′ end PUA group. APE1 is known as the main mammalian protein capable to excise this blocking group producing the 3′ end hydroxyl moiety (Wilson & Barsky, 2001; Pascucci et al., 2002).

### 2.3.7 Human ALK B homologue (ABH1) is an AP lyase

Methylated bases in DNA generated by endogenous and environmental alkylating agents can be removed by three distinct strategies. While 3-methyladenine (3-alkyladenine) is

excised by a specific DNA glycosylase that initiates a base excision repair process, 1-methyladenine, 3-methylcytosine and O6-methylguanine are corrected by direct reversal exploring a different mechanism (for more information see a review Sedgwick et al., 2006). One of the strategies of direct reversal involves the activity of DNA dioxygenases, which release the methyl moiety as formaldehyde (Duncan et al., 2002). Although three human DNA dioxygenases - ABH1–ABH3 - catalyze the same oxidative demethylation reaction they display specificity toward methylated base and nucleic acids (DNA or RNA and single- or double-stranded) (Duncan et al., 2002, Westbye et al., 2008, Ougland et al., 2004; Kurowski et al., 2003). Unexpectedly, ABH1 - the closest AlkB *E. coli* homologue - has been shown to display an AP site cleavage activity (Müller et al., 2010).
Intensive study of discovered activity revealed that the DNA cleavage activity of ABH1 did not require added Fe2+ or 2-oxoglutarate, is not inhibited by EDTA, and is unaffected by mutation of the putative metal-binding residues, indicating that this activity arises from an active site distinct from that used for demethylation.
Enzymes that cleave sugar-phosphate backbone at abasic sites can utilize hydrolysis, β- or β,δ-elimination mechanisms (Fig. 1). First, to assess the cleavage mechanism, the activity of ABH1 was examined with DNA containing THF residue, the AP-site analogue, which could not be cleaved by the β-elimination reaction. No AP site cleavage was observed with ABH1 and EndoIII unlike APE1. Second, the electrophoretic mobility of the products resulting from the activities of ABH1, APE1, EndoIII and EndoVIII were examined. Prior to analysis 5′-[$^{32}$P]-labeled ds-oligonucleotides containing the AP site were incubated with the corresponding enzymes. In some samples, the products of AP site cleavage were additionally treated with T4 polynucleotide kinase (PNK) to remove possible 3′-terminal phosphate by this phosphatase. It should be noted that authors used proteinase treatment of the reaction mixtures to stop the reaction and degrade the enzymes prior to separation of oligonucleotides by denaturing PAAG electrophoresis (Fig. 7). The products produced by ABH1 migrate slowly (Fig. 7, lane 1) than the product of the β-elimination reaction (Fig. 7, lane 3) and do not contain the 3′ end phosphate group since the mobility of the products was not changed by PNK treatment (Fig. 7, compare lanes 1 and 2). While the products derived from the EndoVIII activity, which explores the β,δ-elimination mechanism resulting in the 3′ phosphate group, migrate slowly after PNK treatment (Fig. 7, compare lanes 5 and 6). The authors proposed that ABH1 cleaves AP sites by β-elimination with ABH1 being bound with the product in tight complex. They attribute the slight decrease in mobility of the products for the ABH1 samples to tight binding of ABH1 fragments with oligonucleotides. The authors demonstrated that both ABH1 and EndoIII in the presence of $NaBH_4$ are able to generate stable products with single-stranded AP-DNA, double-stranded DNA containing one AP site and double-stranded DNA containing two AP sites, but the important control without reducing agent is missed. Taking into account that ABH1 forms stable adducts with AP DNA without reduction, as observed in the activity test (Fig. 7, lanes 1 and 2), it is questionable whether the trapping of ABH1 is the Schiff base dependent.
ABH1 was shown to display specificity in substrate usage with DNA containing two AP sites being the preferable substrate. Further analysis of AP site cleavage activity at different substrate-to-enzyme ratio demonstrated that concentration of product was always sub-stoichiometric to the enzyme concentration that is in agreement with tight binding of ABH1 with the product.

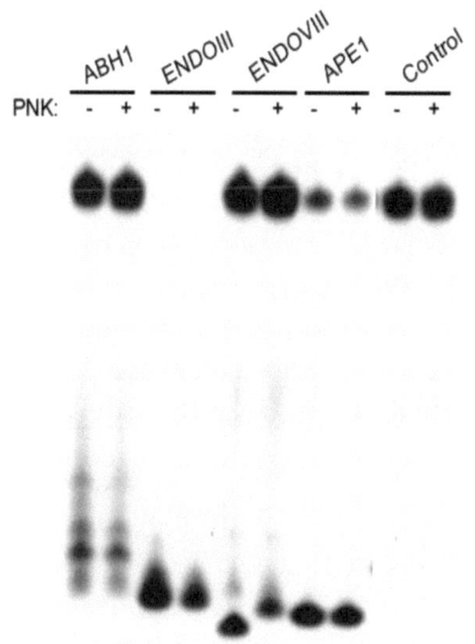


Fig. 7. Comparison of product sizes for ABH1, APE1, ENDOIII, and ENDOVIII, and examination of the effect of phosphatase treatment (from Müller et al., 2010). The uracil containing DNA duplex was cleaved by incubation with ABH1 or the control endonucleases in the presence of UDG for 1 h at 37 °C. Portions of the samples were treated with the phosphatase T4 polynucleotide kinase to remove possible phosphates at the 3′ end of the labeled products. The presence of a 3′-phosphate causes the oligonucleotide to migrate more rapidly than the non-phosphorylated species due to the extra negative charge; removal of the phosphate results in a shift to an apparently larger product, as seen with EndoVIII.

Taking into account ubiquitous expression of APE1 and inefficiency of the ABH1 AP lyase activity, ABH1 hardly play significant role *in vivo* in processing of AP sites. Moreover, the ability of ABH1 to more efficiently cleave opposite AP sites in ds DNA that may result in formation of DS breaks, more toxic for the cells than AP sites, therefore action of ABH1 on clustered AP sites in genomic DNA appears to be dangerous for cells. The authors considered tight binding of ABH1 with the product as a mechanism that protects ends from degradation. On the other hand, tight binding may create hindrances for the repair processes and require special efforts to remove blocking group from the 3′ end. Potentially interesting finding of intrinsic AP lyase activity of ABH1 requires additional studies to draw a conclusion concerning significance of discovered activity *in vivo.*

### 2.3.8 Tyrosyl-DNA-phosphodiesterase mediates the new APE-independent BER pathway in mammals

As mentioned above AP sites can be cleaved by activity of bifunctional DNA glycosylases with associated AP lyase activities via β- or β,δ-elimination mechanism producing DNA intermediates with 3′ end containing 3′-phosphate or 3′-PUA groups (Fig. 1) that have to be removed prior to DNA synthesis may occur. DNA intermediates with blocked 3′end may also appear from action of ROS and as a result of spontaneous decomposition of AP sites.
The 3' PUA is known to be removed by the only AP-endonuclease, APE1, which possesses 3′ phosphodiesterase activity with α-unsaturated aldehydes, producing a single nucleotide gap flanked by a 3′-hydroxyl group and a 5′ phosphate group (Wilson & Barsky, 2001;

Pascucci et al., 2002). However, APE1 is barely active in removing 3' phosphate generated by mammalian DNA glycosylases NEIL1 and NEIL2. The 3' phosphate is efficiently removed by polynucleotide kinase (PNK) and not APE1 (Wiederhold et al., 2004).

Tyrosyl-DNA phosphodiesterase (Tdp1) was discovered as an enzymatic activity from *Saccharomyces cerevisiae* that specifically hydrolyzes the phosphodiester linkage between the O-4 atom of a tyrosine and a DNA 3′ phosphate (Yang et al., 1996). This type of linkage is typical for the covalent reaction intermediate produced upon Topoisomerase 1 cleavage of one DNA strand. Human Tdp1 can also hydrolyze other 3′-end DNA alterations that are covalently linked to the DNA, indicating that it may function as a general 3′-DNA phosphodiesterase and repair enzyme (Dexheimer et al., 2008). Tdp1 can also remove the tetrahydrofuran moiety from the 3'-end of DNA (Interthal et al., 2005). It is conceivable that Tdp1 acts on the 3′ PUA moiety.

To study an ability of Tdp1 to process the 3′ PUA moiety AP DNA was first incubated with Endo III (Fig. 8A, lane 2) (Lebedeva et al., 2011). Following incubation of this product with Tdp1 results in 15-mer with 3' phosphate, which can be removed by PNKP (Fig. 8A, lane 3). Thus, Tdp1 is able to remove the 3′ PUA that allows to realize the APE1-independent pathway of BER where AP sites are cleaved by bifunctional DNA glycosylases via the β-elimination mechanism.

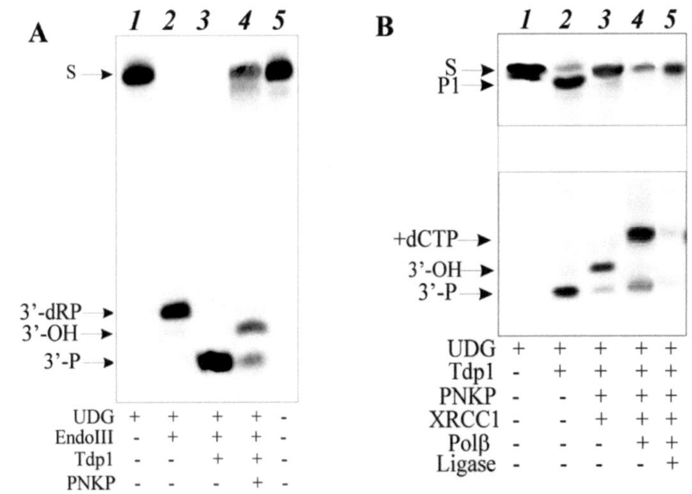


Fig. 8. Tdp1 activity on DNA substrate with 3'-dRP moiety in the single strand break (A) and reconstitution of the AP-DNA substrate repair initiated by Tdp1 (B) (From Lebedeva et al., 2011). **(A)** The 15-mer with 3'-dRP was generated by incubation of AP DNA with EndoIII (lane 2). Following incubation of this product with Tdp1 results in 15-mer with 3'-P (lane 3). Lane 4 shows the 15-mer product with 3'-OH after adding PNKP in the reaction mixture. Lane 1 corresponds to the AP-DNA substrate incubated with UDG. Lane 5 - control. (B) 5'-end labeled AP-DNA substrate was subsequently incubated with the UDG (lane 1), Tdp1 (lane 2), PNKP and XRCC1 (lane 3), Pol β (lane 4), DNA ligase III (lane 5). The components present in different reaction mixtures are indicated.

We tested an ability of Tdp1 to process AP sites (natural or mimicked by THF residue) and found that Tdp1 cleaves both types of AP sites generating the product identical to the product of β,δ-elimination (data not shown). Finally, the repair of AP site was analyzed in a

minimal reconstituted BER system consisting of purified proteins (Fig. 8B). The 5′ $^{32}P$-labeled 32-mer DNA duplex containing uridine at the position 16 was incubated with the purified recombinant UDG, Tdp1, PNKP, Pol β, DNA ligase III, and XRCC1 to mimic DNA repair system. The reaction mixture containing Tdp1 but lacking PNKP (lane 2) generated a product with a 3′-phosphate, which is identical to that produced by NEIL1. Addition of PNKP resulted in a 15-mer product with the 3′-OH termini (lane 3). XRCC1, a scaffold protein, stimulates the activity of BER proteins, such as DNA polymerase β, PNKP, DNA ligase III (Mani et al., 2004; Caldecott, 2003; Whitehouse et al., 2001).
Lastly, DNA polymerase β replaces the missing DNA segment (lane 4) and DNA ligase reseals the DNA (lane 5). So, the repair of AP site initiated by Tdp1 fully restored the intact DNA and generated the products of the expected lengths at each intermediate stage. In summary, human Tdp1 protein can initiate APE1-independent repair of AP sites and 3′ PUA termini that expands the ability of the BER process.

### 2.3.9 XRCC1 interactions with base excision repair DNA intermediates

XRCC1 is known to play a crucial role in the coordination of two overlapping repair pathways, SSBR and BER (Caldecott, 2003). Although the main role of XRCC1 during BER has been attributed to its participation in the post-incision steps (Wong et al., 2005), which are shared with SSBR, the physical and functional interactions with proteins involved in the initiation of modified bases or abasic sites repair (Marsin et al., 2003, Campalans et al., 2005, Vidal et al., 2001, Wiederhold et al., 2004) suggest that XRCC1 presence at the early steps of BER could be important for assuring a correct repair process. One possible role of XRCC1 could be to optimize the passage of DNA substrates from one enzyme to the next one in the pathway by holding the proteins together through its different interacting domains (Caldecott, 2003).
Investigating the interactions of with different BER DNA intermediates generated either by DNA glycosylase hOGG1 or AP endonuclease APE1 we have found that XRCC1 is able to interact with AP sites via formation of the Schiff base intermediate (Nazarkina et al., 2007). Because hOGG1 possesses both, DNA glycosylase and AP lyase activities, either of two DNA intermediates can be produced: DNA duplex containing an intact AP site or a nick with a 3′ PUA moiety (See Fig. 1). By competition experiments using the THF-containing or regular DNA duplex it was demonstrated that XRCC1 binds DNA with an AP site, or its synthetic analogue, with considerably higher affinity than regular DNA duplex.
XRCC1 is known to bind DNA with single-strand breaks with higher affinity that regular DNA duplex (Mani et al., 2004). We then investigated the relative affinities of XRCC1 to different DNA structures that could be BER intermediates in the repair of single or double DNA lesions. The efficiency of cross-linking is maximal with an incised AP site 3′ PUA (Fig. 9A, lane 3). Interestingly, the presence of a strand interruption on the complementary oligonucleotide strongly stimulated the cross-linking of XRCC1 to the AP site. These results suggest that XRCC1 could be important to hold the DNA together during the repair of clustered DNA damage. XRCC1 is also able to cross-link to a 5′ dRP residue downstream of a nick (Fig. 9A, lane 6). Comparative analysis of the patterns of protein cross-linking to AP DNA in cell extracts deficient (EM9) and proficient in XRCC1 (EM9-X) (Fig. 9B, lanes 3–6) revealed the product that can be related with XRCC1 (lane 6). Interestingly, that the band is observed with DNA containing interruption opposite AP site (Fig. 9B, lanes 4 and 6).

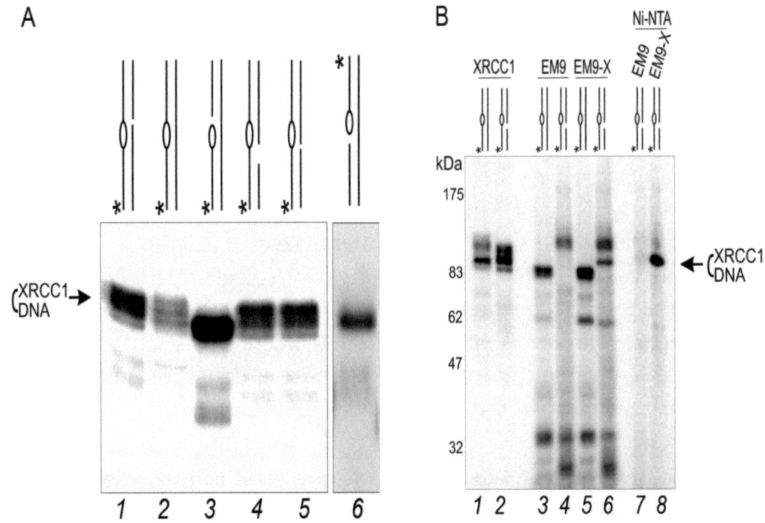


Fig. 9. Interactions of XRCC1 with BER DNA intermediates (From Nazarkina et al., 2007). (A) Cross-linking of XRCC1 to different 5′-$^{32}$P-labeled AP DNA. DNA containing intact AP sites (lanes 1, 2, 4, and 5) and cleaved AP site (3′ PUA) (lane 3) were 5′ end labeled, while DNA containing hydrolyzed AP site (5′ dRP) (lane 6) was 3′ end labeled. (B) Cross-linking of XRCC1 with AP DNA in CHO cell extracts deficient in XRCC1 (EM9) or EM9 expressing His-tagged human XRCC1 (EM9-9). Position of radioactive label in DNA is designated by the asterisk.

To confirm that this product corresponds to the XRCC1 containing conjugate, after trapping with $NaBH_4$, His-tagged XRCC1 was recovered by pull-down using a Ni-NTA resin. After this purification step, the product was recovered from the EM9-X extract (lane 8) but not the EM9 one (lane 7).

Taken together, these results demonstrate XRCC1 ability to interact with intact and cleaved AP sites, including cell extracts, e.g. in the presence of cellular proteins that can interfere with XRCC1 binding to AP DNA.

Thus, using the Schiff-base-mediated cross-linking, we show that XRCC1 displays a specific affinity for AP containing substrates. Although at this time we cannot evaluate the in vivo relevance of covalent complexes between XRCC1 and DNA, considering the Schiff base reversibility, it is tempting to speculate that its formation during BER of AP sites could be a physiological response to situations where a reactive intermediate needs to be protected until the next enzyme recruited by XRCC1 is able to process it.

## 3. Conclusion

Combination of affinity based cross-linking of proteins with specific DNA probes containing intact or cleaved AP sites and MS analysis allowed to identify new players in recognition/processing of these ubiquitous lesions. Some identified proteins are known as regulatory proteins of specific DNA repair processes, not necessarily involved in repair of AP sites, but all these proteins are related to cell radiosensitivity. Two of them—XRCC1 and PARP1—belong to the base excision repair system, but have been previously considered as participants of later stages of the BER process. By virtue of its interaction with AP sites,

PARP1 and XRCC1 can regulate initial stage of BER persisting at AP sites until APE1 could come and initiate AP sites cleavage. The PARP1 activation upon interaction with AP sites and resultant automodification appear to facilitate the BER factor recruitment to stimulate the repair process. In the absence or deficiency of APE1, PARP1 can provide temporal protection of AP sites. Ku antigen can temporarily protect AP sites situated within 1-2 turns of DNA helix from double-strand breaks or displays AP/dRP lyase activity near double-strand ends. The last activity has no analogues and is indispensable for proper repair of DS breaks with particular blocking groups at the ends, which can result from action of ionizing radiation.

In other case of revealed AP/dRP lyase activities, they appear to function under particular physiologic or stressful conditions modulating the capacity of the BER system or providing the appropriate functions of the repair machinery when some participants are missed or inactive. Interestingly, that structural chromatin proteins -HMGB1 and HMGA - were found to interact with AP sites displaying an enzymatic activity. Although being a relative weak, this activity may be biologically significant due to high abundance of these proteins.

## 4. Acknowledgments

This work was supported in part by the Russian Foundation for Basic Research (Project No 10-04-01083) and Program of the Russian Academy of Sciences "Molecular and Cellular Biology".

## 5. References

Abe, N.; Watanabe, T.; Suzuki, Y.; Matsumoto, N.; Masaki, T.; Mori, T.; Sugiyama, M.; Chiappetta, G.; Fusco, A.; & Atomi, Y. (2003). An increased high-mobility group A2 expression level is associated with malignant phenotype in pancreatic exocrine tissue. *Br J Cancer* 89, 2104.

Allinson, S.L.; Dianova, I.I.; & Dianov, G.L. (2001). DNA polymerase β is the major dRP lyase involved in repair of oxidative base lesions in DNA by mammalian cell extracts. *EMBO J* 20, 6919.

Almeida, K.H. & Sobol, R.W. (2007). A unified view of base excision repair: lesion-dependent protein complexes regulated by post-translational modification. *DNA Repair* 6, 695.

Atamna, H.; Cheung, I.; & Ames, B.N. (2000). A method for detecting abasic sites in living cells: age-dependent changes in base excision repair. *Proc Natl Acad Sci USA* 97, 686.

Berner, J.M.; Meza-Zepeda, L.A.; Kools, P.F.; Forus, A.; Schoenmakers, E.F.; Van de Ven, W.J.; Fodstad, O.; & Myklebost, O. (1997). HMGIC, the gene for an architectural transcription factor, is amplified and rearranged in a subset of human sarcomas. *Oncogene* 14, 2935.

Breen, A.P.; & Murphy, J.A. (1995). Reactions of oxyl radicals with DNA. *Free Rad Biol Med* 18, 1033.

Burrows, C.J.; & Muller, J.G. (1998). Oxidative nucleobase modifications leading to strand scission. *Chem Rev* 98, 1109.

Bustin, M. & Reeves, R. (1996) High-mobility-group chromosomal proteins: architectural components that facilitate chromatin function. *Prog Nucleic Acid Res Mol Biol* 54, 35.

Caldecott, K.W. (2003). XRCC1 and DNA strand break repair. *DNA Repair* 2, 955.

Campalans, A.; Marsin, S.; Nakabeppu, Y.; O'connor, T.R; Boiteux, S.; & Radicella, J.P. (2005). XRCC1 interactions with multiple DNA glycosylases: a model for its recruitment to base excision repair. *DNA Repair* 4, 826.

Cleynen, I.; & van de Ven, W.J. (2008). The HMGA proteins: a myriad of functions *Int J Oncol* 32, 289.

Das, A; Wiederhold, L.; Leppard, J.B, Kedar, P.; Prasad, R.; Wang, X.; Boldogh, I.; Karimi-Busheri, F.; Weinfeld, M.; Tomkinson, A.E.; Wilson, S.H., Mitra, S.; & Hazra, T.K. (2006). NEIL2-initiated, APE-independent repair of oxidized bases in DNA: Evidence for a repair complex in human cells *DNA Repair* 5, 1439.

David, S.S. & Williams, S.D. (1998). Chemistry of glycosylases and endonucleases involved in base-excision repair. *Chem Rev* 98, 1221.

Dawson, T.L.; Gores, G.J.; Nieminen, A.L.; Herman, B.; & Lemasters, J.J. (1993). Mitochondria as a source of reactive oxygen species during reductive stress in rat hepatocytes. *Am J Physiol* 264, C961.

de Los Santos, C.; El-Khateeb, M.; Rege, P.; Tian, K.; & Johnson, F. (2004). Impact of the C1' configuration of abasic sites on DNA duplex structure. *Biochemistry* 43, 15349.

Demple, B & Harrison, L. (1994). Repair of oxidative damage to DNA: enzymology and biology. *Annu Rev Biochem* 63, 915.

Demple, B. & DeMott, M.S. (2002). Dynamics and diversions in base excision DNA repair of oxidized abasic lesions. *Oncogene* 21, 8926.

Demple, B; Herman, T; & Chen, D.S. (1991). Cloning and expression of APE, the cDNA encoding the major human apurinic endonuclease: definition of a family of DNA repair enzymes. *Proc Natl Acad Sci U S A* 88, 11450.

Dexheimer, T.S., Antony, S., Marchand, C. & Pommier, Y. (2008). Tyrosyl-DNA phosphodiesterase as a target for anticancer therapy.phosphodiesterase as a target for anticancer therapy. *Anticancer Agents Med Chem* 8, 381.

Downs, J.A.; & Jackson, S.P. (2004) A means to a DNA end: the many roles of Ku. Nat Rev *Mol Cell Biol* 5, 367.

Duncan, T.; Trewick, S.C.; Koivisto, P.; Bates, P.A.; Lindahl, T.; & Sedgwick, B. (2002). Reversal of DNA alkylation damage by two human dioxygenases. *Proc Natl Acad Sci USA* 99, 16660.

Fan, J.; & Wilson, D.M. 3rd. (2005). Protein-protein interactions and posttranslational modifications in mammalian base excision repair, *Free Radic Biol Med* 38, 1121. Frosina, G.; Fortini, P.; Rossi, O.; Carrozzino, F.; Raspaglio, G.; Cox, L.S.; Lane, D.P.; Abbondandolo, A.; & Dogliotti, E. (1996). Two pathways for base excision repair in mammalian cells. *J Biol Chem* 271, 9573.

Grin, I.R.; Khodyreva, S.N.; Nevinsky, G.A.; & Zharkov, D.O. (2006). Deoxyribophosphate lyase activity of mammalian endonuclease VIII-like proteins. *FEBS Lett* 580, 4916.

Gullo, C.; Au, M.; Feng, G.; & Teoh, G. (2006) The biology of Ku and its potential oncogenic role in cancer. *Biochim Biophys Acta* 1765 223-234

Hazra, T.K.; Izumi, T.; Boldogh, I.; Imhoff, B.; Kow, Y.W.; Jaruga, P.; Dizdaroglu, M.; & Mitra, S. (2002). Identification and characterization of a human DNA glycosylase for repair of modified bases in oxidatively damaged DNA. *Proc Natl Acad Sci USA* 99, 3523.

Hegde, M.L.; Hazra, T.K.; & Mitra, S. (2008). Early steps in the DNA base excision/single-strand interruption repair pathway in mammalian cells. *Cell Research* 18, 27.

Hegde, V.; Wang, M.; & Deutsch, W.A. (2004). Human ribosomal protein S3 interacts with DNA base excision repair proteins hAPE/Ref-1 and hOGG1. *Biochemistry* 43, 14211.

Horton, J.K.; Prasad, R.; Hou, E.; & Wilson, S.H. (2000). Protection against methylation-induced cytotoxicity by DNA polymerase β-dependent long patch base excision repair. *J Biol Chem* 275, 2211.

Ilina, E.S.; Lavrik, O.I.; & Khodyreva, S.N. (2008). Ku antigen interacts with abasic sites. *Biochim Biophys Acta* 1784, 1777-1785.

Interthal, H.; Chen, H.J. & Champoux, J.J. (2005). Human Tdp1 cleaves a broad spectrum of substrates, including phosphoamide linkages. *J Biol Chem* 280, 36518.

Jiao Y., Wang, H.C., and Fan, S.J., Growth suppression and radiosensitivity increase by HMGB1 in breast cancer. *Acta Pharmacol. Sin.*, 2007, vol. 28, pp. 1957–1967.

Khodyreva, S.N.; Ilina, E.S.; Sukhanova, M.V.; Kutuzov, M.M. & Lavrik, O.I. (2010a). Poly(ADP-ribose) polymerase 1 interaction with apurinic/apyrimidinic sites. *Dokl Biochem Biophys* 431, 69.

Khodyreva, S.N.; Prasad, R.; Ilina, E.S.; Sukhanova, M.V.; Kutuzov, M.M.; Liu, Y.; Hou, E.W.; Wilson, S.H.; & Lavrik, O.I. (2010b). Apurinic/apyrimidinic (AP) site recognition by the 5′-dRP/AP lyase in poly(ADP-ribose) polymerase-1 (PARP-1) *Proc Natl Acad Sci USA* 107, 22090.

Klungland, A & Lindahl, T. (1997). Second pathway for completion of human DNA base excision-repair: reconstitution with purified proteins and requirement for DNase IV (FEN1). *EMBO J* 16, 3341.

Kurowski, M.A.; Bhagwat, A.S.; Papaj, G.; & Bujnicki, J.M. (2003). Phylogenomic identification of five new human homologs of the DNA repair enzyme AlkB. *BMC Genomics* 4, 48.

Kutuzov, M.M.; Ilina, E.S.; Sukhanova, M.V.; Pyshnaya, I.A.; Pyshnyi, D.V.; Lavrik, O.I.; & Khodyreva, S.N. (2011). Interaction of poly(ADP-ribose) polymerase 1 with apurinic/apyrimidinic sites within clustered DNA damage. *Biochemistry (Moscow)* 76, 147.

Laemmli, U.K. (1970). Cleavage of structural proteins during the assembly of the head of bacteriophage T4. *Nature* 277, 680.

Lan, L.; Nakajima, S.; Oohata, Y.; Takao, M.; Okano, S.; Masutani, M.; Wilson, S.H.; & Yasui, A. (2004). In situ analysis of repair processes for oxidative DNA damage in mammalian cells. *Proc Natl Acad Sci USA* 101, 13738.

Lebedeva, N.A.; Rechkunova, N.I.; and Lavrik, O.I. (2011). AP-site cleavage activity of tyrosyl-DNA phosphodiesterase 1. *FEBS Lett* 585, 683.

Liau, S.S. & Whang, E. (2008). HMGA1 is a molecular determinant of chemoresistance to gemcitabine in pancreatic adenocarcinoma. *Clin Cancer Res* 14, 1470.

Lindahl, T. (1993). Instability and decay of the primary structure of DNA. *Nature* 362, 709.

Lindahl, T.; Satoh, M.S.; Poirier, G.G.; & Klungland, A. (1995). Post-translational modification of poly(ADP-ribose) polymerase induced by DNA strand breaks. *Trends Biochem Sci* 20, 405.

Liu, Y.; Prasad, R.; & Wilson, S.H. (2010). HMGB1: roles in base excision repair and related function. *Biochim Biophys Acta* 1799, 119.

Loeb, L.A. & Preston, B.D. (1986). Mutagenesis by apurinic/apyrimidinic sites. *Annu Rev Genet* 20, 201.

Mani, R.S.; Karimi-Busheri, F.; Fanta, M.; Caldecott, K.W.; Cass, M.; & Weinfeld, C.E. (2004) Biophysical characterization of human XRCC1 and its binding to damaged and undamaged DNA. *Biochemistry* 43, 16505.

Marsin, S. Vidal, A.E.; Sossou, M.; Menissier-de Murcia, J.; Le Page, F.; Boiteux, S.; de Murcia, G.; & Radicella, J.P., (2003). Role of XRCC1 in the coordination and stimulation of oxidative DNA damage repair initiated by the DNA glycosylase hOGG1. *J Biol Chem* 278, 44068.

Matsumoto, Y. & Kim, K. (1995). Excision of deoxyribose phosphate residues by DNA polymerase β during DNA repair. *Science* 269, 699.

McCullough, A.K.; Dodson, M.L.; & Lloyd, R.S. (1999). Initiation of base excision repair: glycosylase mechanisms and structures. *Annu Rev Biochem* 68, 255.

Meyer, B.; Loeschke, S.; Schultze, A.; Weigel, T.; Sandkamp, M.; Goldmann, T.; Vollmer, E.; & Bullerdiek, J. (2007). HMGA2 overexpression in non-small cell lung cancer. *Mol Carcinog* 46, 503.

Miyazawa, J.; Mitoro, A.; Kawashiri, S.; Chada, K.K.; & Imai, K. (2004). Expression of mesenchyme-specific gene HMGA2 in squamous cell carcinomas of the oral cavity. *Cancer Res* 64, 2024.

Mohsin Ali, M.; Kurisu, S.; Yoshioka, Y.; Terato, H.; Ohyama, Y.; Kubo, K.; & Ide, H. (2004). Detection of endonuclease III- and 8-oxoguanine glycosylase-sensitive base modifications in gamma-irradiated DNA and cells by the aldehyde reactive probe (ARP) assay. *J Radiation Res* 45, 229.

Müller, T.A.; Meek, K.; & Hausinger, R.P. (2010). Human AlkB homologue 1 (ABH1) exhibits DNA lyase activity at abasic sites. *DNA Repair* 9, 58.

Nazarkina, Z.K.; Khodyreva, S.N.; Marsin, S.; Lavrik, O.I.; & Radicella, J.P. (2007). XRCC1 interactions with base excision repair DNA intermediates. *DNA Repair* 6, 254.

Ougland, R.; Zhang, C.M.; Liiv, A.; Johansen, R.F.; Seeberg, E.; Hou, Y.M.; Remme, J.; & Falnes, P.Ø. (2004). AlkB restores the biological function of mRNA and tRNA inactivated by chemical methylation. *Molec Cell* 16, 107.

Pascucci, B.; Maga, G.; Hübscher, U.; Bjoras, M.; Seeberg, E.; Hickson, I.D.; Villani, G.; Giordano, C.; Cellai, L.; & Dogliotti, E. (2002). Reconstitution of the base excision repair pathway for 7,8-dihydro-8-oxoguanine with purified human proteins. *Nucleic Acids Res* 30, 2124.

Piersen, C.E.; McCullough, A.K.; & Lloyd, R.S. (2000). AP lyases and dRPases: commonality of mechanism. *Mutat Res* 459, 43.

Piersen, C.E.; Prasad, R.; Wilson, S.H.; & Lloyd, R.S. (1996). Evidence for an imino intermediate in the DNA polymerase β deoxyribose phosphate excision reaction. *J Biol Chem* 271, 17811.

Pinz, K.G., & Bogenhagen, D. (2000). Characterization of a catalytically slow AP lyase activity in DNA polymerase γ and other family A DNA polymerases. *J Biol Chem* 275, 12509.

Podlutsky, A.J.; Dianova, I.I.; Wilson, S.H.; Bohr, V.A.; & Dianov, G.L. (2001). DNA synthesis and dRPase activities of polymerase β are both essential for single-nucleotide patch base excision repair in mammalian cell extracts. *Biochemistry* 40, 809.

Postel, E.H.; Abramczyk, B.M.; Levit, M.N.; & Kyin, S. (2000). Catalysis of DNA cleavage and nucleoside triphosphate synthesis by NM23-H2/NDP kinase share an active site that implies a DNA repair function. *Proc Natl Acad Sci USA* 97, 14194.

Prasad, R.; Liu, Y.; Deterding, L.J.; Poltoratsky, V.P.; Kedar, P.S.; Horton, J.K.; Kanno, S.; Asagoshi, K.; Hou, E.W.; Khodyreva, S.N.; Lavrik, O.I.; Tomer, K.B.; Yasui, A.; & Wilson, S.H. (2007). HMGB1 is a cofactor in mammalian base excision repair. *Mol Cell* 27, 829.

Reeves, R. (2001). Molecular biology of HMGA proteins: hubs of nuclear function. *Gene* 277, 63.

Rieger, R.A.; Zaika, V.; Xie, W.; Johnson, F.; Grollman, A.P.; Iden, C.R.; & Zharkov, D.O. (2006). Proteomic approach to identification of proteins reactive for abasic sites in DNA. *Mol Cell Proteomics* 5, 858.

Roberts, S.A.; Strande, N.; Burkhalter, M.D.; Strom, C.; Havener, J.M.; Hasty, P.; & Ramsden, D.A. (2010). Ku is a 5'-dRP/AP lyase that excises nucleotide damage near broken ends. *Nature* 464, 1214.

Sakano, K.; Oikawa, S.; Hasegawa, K.; & Kawanishi, S. (2001). Hydroxyurea induces site-specific DNA damage via formation of hydrogen peroxide and nitric oxide. *Jpn J Cancer Res* 92, 1166.

Schärer, O.D. (2003). Chemistry and biology of DNA repair. *Angew Chem Int Ed* 42, 2946.

Schulte-Uentrop, L.; El-Awady, R.A.; Schliecker, L.; Willers, H.; & Dahm-Daphi, J. (2008) Distinct roles of XRCC4 and Ku80 in non-homologous end-joining of endonuclease- and ionizing radiation-induced DNA double-strand breaks. *Nucleic Acids Res.* 36, 2561.

Sedgwick, B.; Bates, P.A.; Paik, J.; Jacobs, S.C.; & Lindahl, T. (2006). Repair of alkylated DNA: recent advances. *DNA repair* 6, 429.

Sgarra, R.; Furlan, C.; Zammitti, S.; Lo Sardo, A.; Maurizio, E.; Di Bernardo, J.; Giancotti, V.; & Manfioletti, G. (2008). Interaction proteomics of the HMGA chromatin architectural factors. *Proteomics* 8, 4721.

Sgarra, R.; Zammitti, S; Lo Sardo, A.; Maurizio, E.; Arnoldo, L., Pegoraro, S.; Giancotti, V.; & Manfioletti, G. (2010). HMGA molecular network: From transcriptional regulation to chromatin remodeling. *Biochim Biophys Acta* 1799, 37.

Snowden, A.; Kow, Y.W.; & Van Houten, B. (1990). Damage repertoire of the *Escherichia coli* UvrABC nuclease complex includes abasic sites, base-damage analogues, and lesions containing adjacent 5' or 3' nicks. *Biochemistry* 29, 7251.

Sobol, R.W.; Prasad, R.; Evenski, A.; Baker, A.; Yang, X.-P.; Horton, J.K.; & Wilson, S.H. (2000). The lyase activity of the DNA repair protein β-polymerase protects from DNA-damage-induced cytotoxicity. *Nature* 405, 807.

Srivastava, D.K.; Vande Berg, B.J.; Prasad, R.; Molina, J.T.; Beard, W.A.; Tomkinson, A.E.; & Wilson, S.H. (1998). Mammalian abasic site base excision repair. Identification of the reaction sequence and rate-determining steps. *J Biol Chem* 273, 21203.

Stros, M. (2010) HMGB proteins: interactions with DNA and chromatin. *Biochim Biophys Acta* 1799, 101.

Summer, H.; Li, O.; Bao, Q.; Zhan, L.; Peter, S.; Sathiyanathan, P.; Henderson, D.; Klonisch, T.; Goodman, S.D.; & Droge, P. (2009). HMGA2 exhibits dRP/AP site cleavage activity and protects cancer cells from DNA-damage-induced cytotoxicity during chemotherapy. *Nucleic Acids Res* 37, 4371.

Takao, M.; Kanno, S.; Kobayashi, K.; Zhang, Q.M.; Yonei, S.; van der Horst, G.T.; & and Yasui, A. (2002). A back-up glycosylase in Nth1 knock-out mice is a functional Nei (endonuclease VIII) homologue. *J Biol Chem* 277, 42205.

Tang, D.; Kang, R.; Zeh, H.J. 3rd; & Lotze, M.T. (2010). High-mobility group box 1 and cancer. *Biochim Biophys Acta* 1799, 131.

Vidal, A.E.; Boiteux, S.; Hickson, I.D.;& Radicella, J.P. (2001). XRCC1 coordinates the initial and late stages of DNA abasic site repair through protein–protein interactions, *EMBO J* 20, 6530.

Westbye, M.P.; Feyzi, E.; Aas, P.A.; Vagbo, C.B.; Talstad, V.A.; Kavli, B.; Hagen, L.; Sundheim, O.; Akbari, M.; Liabakk, N.B.; Slupphaug, G.; Otterlei, M.; & Krokan, H.E. (2008). Human AlkB homolog 1 is a mitochondrial protein that demethylates 3-methylcytosine in DNA and RNA. *J Biol Chem* 283, 25046.

Whitehouse, C.J.; Taylor, R.M.; Thistlethwaite, A.; Zhang, H.; Karimi-Busheri, F.; Lasko, D.D.; Weinfeld, M.; & Caldecott, K.W. (2001). XRCC1 stimulates human polynucleotide kinase activity at damaged DNA termini and accelerates DNA single-strand break repair. *Cell* 104, 107.

Wiederhold, L.; Leppard, J.B.; Kedar, P.; Karimi-Busheri, F.; Rasouli-Nia, A.; Weinfeld, M. ; Tomkinson, A.E.; Izumi, T.; Prasad, R.; Wilson, S.H.; Mitra, S. & Hazra, T.K. (2004). AP endonuclease-independent DNA base excision repair in human cells. *Mol Cell* 15, 209.

Wilson 3rd, D.M. & Barsky, D. (2001). The major human abasic endonuclease: formation, consequences and repair of abasic lesions in DNA. *Mutat Res* 485, 283.

Wilson, D.M. 3rd & Thompson, L.H. (1997). Life without DNA repair. *Proc Natl Acad Sci USA* 94, 12754.

Wong, H.; Kim, D.; Hogue, B.A.; McNeill, D.R.; & Wilson, D.M. III. (2005). DNA damage levels and biochemical repair capacities associated with XRCC1 deficiency, *Biochemistry* 44, 14335.

Yang, N.; Galick, H.; & Wallace, S.S. (2004). Attempted base excision repair of ionizing radiation damage in human lymphoblastoid cells produces lethal and mutagenic double-strand breaks. *DNA Repair* 3, 1323.

Yang, S.W.; Burgin, A.B. Jr.; Huizenga, B.N.; Robertson, C.A.; Yao, K.C.; & Nash, H.A. (1996). A eukaryotic enzyme that can disjoin dead-end covalent complexes between DNA and type I topoisomerases. *Proc Natl Acad Sci USA* 93, 11534.

Zharkov, D.O. & Grollman, A.P. (1998). MutY DNA glycosylase: base release and intermediate complex formation. *Biochemistry* 37, 12384.

# Part 3

# Methods in DNA Repair

15

# SiDNA and Other Tools for the Indirect Induction of DNA Damage Responses

Maria Quanz[1,2], Amélie Croset[1,2] and Marie Dutreix[1]
[1]*Institut Curie, Centre National de Recherche Scientifique (CNRS) UMR3347, Institut National de la Santé et de Recherche Médicale (INSERM) U1021, Université Paris-Sud 11, Centre Universitaire, 91405 Orsay*
[2]*DNA Therapeutics SA, 91058 Evry*
*France*

## 1. Introduction

Cells respond to DNA damage by activating an intricate signaling network leading to DNA repair, cell cycle arrest or apoptosis. In recent years, progress has been made in the discovery and characterization of a number of DNA repair pathways, and it has become apparent that the inhibition of specific components of these pathways could offer new targets for combating the resistance of tumors to chemotherapy or radiotherapy. A thorough understanding of the various DNA repair pathways and their regulation is therefore essential. The DNA damage response (DDR) is of great importance in determining cell fate decisions. It includes many signal amplification steps and several steps that are partly redundant due to the ability of different kinases to phosphorylate the same target. Furthermore, the timing and origin of the damage play an important role in determining the DNA repair pathway activated. All this makes it difficult to study the role of one particular protein in DNA damage signaling. In addition, the available tools for activating DNA repair pathways are mostly agents that systematically produce more than one type of DNA damage. Even if the damage caused is initially of one predominant type (as for topoisomerase inhibitors, alkylators or the I-SceI endonuclease system), the damage may rapidly be transformed by normal cellular processes, such as DNA replication, or specific nuclease activities. Studies of the DDR become even more complicated if the agent used to create DNA lesions also damages other cellular components, as is the case for ionizing radiation (IR), alkylators and hydrogen peroxide. Furthermore, the damage is transient, as DNA damage signaling is rapid and lesions are quickly repaired. The signal induced by the damage therefore disappears rapidly, soon after the induction of damage. In some cells, the DNA may not be successfully repaired, leading to apoptosis or senescence. These aspects make it difficult to study the signaling network induced by a given type of damage.

In this chapter, we will provide an overview of the response of the cell to DNA damage and possible ways of inducing a DDR in cells without actually damaging chromatin. We will focus on stabilized short interfering DNA molecules (siDNA), which mimic different types of damage and induce a pure damage-specific response.

## 2. DNA-damaging treatments induce multiple and dynamic responses

DNA is a stable material, as required for the storage of genetic information, but it is also susceptible to spontaneous changes under normal cellular conditions. It has been estimated that each cell spontaneously loses about 5000 purine bases (depurination) every day (Friedberg, 1995). The deamination of cytosine to uracil also occurs spontaneously. In addition to this inherent instability, our genomes are exposed to numerous endogenous or environmental agents, including reactive metabolites, environmental chemicals and ultraviolet radiation, capable of inducing a wide diversity of DNA lesions (Figure 1). The large number of different lesions possible – more than 100 different oxidative modifications

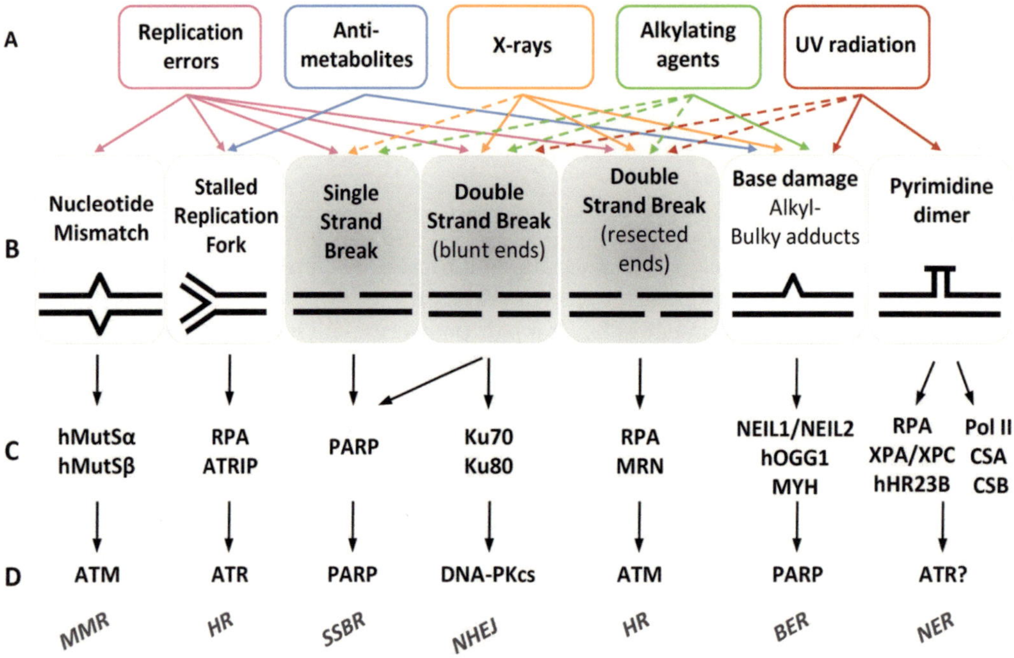


Fig. 1. DNA-damaging treatments induce multiple and dynamic responses mediated by DNA damage sensors and transducers. Common DNA-damaging agents (A) induce several types of DNA damage (B) directly (solid line) or indirectly (dotted line). Single- and double-strand breaks (highlighted in gray) are the most frequent end products of unrepaired damage. DNA damage is recognized by sensor proteins (C) that recruit and/or activate transducers (D), initiating a signal transduction cascade (not shown). Abbreviations: ATM, ataxia telangiectasia mutated; ATR, ataxia and rad3-related; ATRIP, ATR-interacting protein; BER, base excision repair; CSA or CSB, Cockayne Syndrome A or B; DNA-PKcs, DNA-dependent protein kinase catalytic subunit; hOGG1, human 8-hydroxyguanine DNA-glycosylase; HR, homologous recombination repair; hHR23B, human Rad23 homolog B; MMR, mismatch repair; MRN, Mre11-RAD50-Nbs1; MYH, MutY glycosylase homologue; NEIL1, nei endonuclease VIII-like 1; NER, nucleotide excision repair; NHEJ, non-homologous end joining; PARP, poly(ADP-ribose) polymerase; RPA, replication protein A; SSBR, single-strand break repair; UV, ultraviolet; XPC, xeroderma pigmentosum group C.

alone have been identified in DNA (Cadet et al., 1997) – has led to the evolution of many different repair pathways for sensing and repairing the various types of damage.

The complete signaling network for each damage type and its individual contribution to the cellular damage response are not fully understood, but the essential repair mechanisms have been elucidated (reviewed for example by Fortini & Dogliotti (2007); Friedberg (1995; 2001); Helleday et al. (2008); Li (2008); Wyman & Kanaar (2006)). Figure 1 summarizes the main pathways and highlights the sensors (DNA binding proteins that recognize specific DNA lesions) and transducers (enzymes that amplify the damage signal by posttranslational modification of downstream targets) involved in repair and signaling for particular types of damage. The main DNA damage transducers are the phosphoinositide 3-kinase-like kinase (PIKK) family members ATM (ataxia telangiectasia mutated), ATR (ataxia telangiectasia and Rad3-related) and DNA-PK (DNA-dependent protein kinase). A DNA break signal can also be transduced by poly(ADP-ribose) polymerases 1 or 2 (here both designated PARP), which use $NAD^+$ to catalyze the modification of their targets with negatively charged, long and branched ADP-ribose polymers. We provide below a brief description of the DNA repair pathways, the subsets of damage they repair and the transducers that are activated.

### 2.1 Repair processes that do not directly activate transducers

The direct repair of certain alkylation adducts and other uncomplicated base modifications by specialized single enzymes is probably the simplest repair mechanism. O6-alkylguanine DNA alkyltransferase (AGT) is a major enzyme involved in direct repair. It is encoded by the O6-methylguanine-DNA-methyltransferase (MGMT) gene and transfers the alkyl adducts produced by alkylating agents, such as temozolomide, dacarbazine or nitrosourea compounds, from O6-methylguanine, O4-methylthymine, O6-ethylguanine or O6-chloroethylguanine to a cysteine residue within the active site of the enzyme, thereby inactivating the enzyme (Gerson, 2004). Other direct repair enzymes include the DNA dioxygenases ABH2 and ABH3, which can convert 1-methyladenine and 3-methylcytosine back into adenine and cytosine, respectively (Duncan et al., 2002). The repair of alkylated lesions is a rapid process, with most alkylated sites successfully repaired within an hour (Zhu et al., 2009). The types of damage targeted by direct repair processes do not seem to be associated with the activation of damage signaling kinases, probably due to the rapid repair kinetics and the absence of intermediate strand break generation during the repair process.

### 2.2 Repair mechanisms that activate mainly PARP as a transducer

The base excision repair (BER) pathway recognizes and removes bases carrying non-bulky modifications that have been damaged by nonenzymatic alkylation, oxidation, ring saturation, or IR (Chan et al., 2006). BER also eliminates deaminated bases and DNA single-strand breaks (SSBs). As a first step in BER, a damage-specific DNA glycosylase (e.g. hOOG1, NEIL1 or NEIL2) recognizes and excises the damaged base, leading to the formation of a potentially cytotoxic intermediate apurinic or apyrimidinic site (AP site) (Bandaru et al., 2002; Boiteux & Radicella, 2000). The abasic sugar is cleaved by an AP endonuclease (APE1), which generates a strand break that is further processed by PARP, DNA polymerase $\beta$ and ligase III in either short-patch or long-patch pathways (Fortini & Dogliotti, 2007). PARP not only recognizes the intermediate SSB but also acts as a damage transducer amplifying the damage signal by linking poly(ADP-ribose) (PAR) chains to its substrates, including itself. These polymers bind specific proteins, including XRCC1, DNA ligase III, p53 and DNA-PK, affecting the repair process as well as downstream responses to DNA damage (Malanga & Althaus, 2005).

### 2.3 Repair pathways that lead to PIKK activation

Most repair pathways involve the activation of PIKKs as transducers, especially if DNA breaks persist. Since PARPs can also sense DNA breaks, an implication of these enzymes in the pathways described in the following cannot be excluded.

#### 2.3.1 Nucleotide excision repair

The nucleotide excision repair (NER) pathway senses and repairs various bulky, helix-distorting lesions that block DNA replication and transcription (Hanawalt, 2002). These lesions may arise, for example, following exposure to genotoxic compounds, such as polycyclic aromatic hydrocarbons or cisplatin. Two major repair mechanisms are known to be involved in this pathway: transcription-coupled repair, which specifically targets lesions blocking RNA polymerase II, and global genome repair, which deals with lesions in the rest of the genome (Cleaver, 2005). The damage sensors involved in transcription-coupled repair include, in addition to RNA polymerase II, Cockayne Syndrome A and B proteins. By contrast, XPA, Rpa and the XPC-hHR23B complex recognize lesions during global genome NER (Brown et al., 2010; Reardon & Sancar, 2005). NER is a complex multistep process involving the recognition of disrupted base pairing followed by unwinding of the DNA helix around the lesion and dual incision. The oligonucleotide patch carrying the lesion is excised, and the remaining gap is filled by regular DNA replication, using the intact complementary strand as a template. The main transducer kinase activated by the NER pathway is probably ATR, in response to UV-induced DNA damage in particular (Shell et al., 2009).

#### 2.3.2 Mismatch repair

Mismatch repair (MMR) targets mispaired bases and nucleotides and insertion-deletion loops that arise through errors in DNA replication. The mechanisms by which eukaryotic cells distinguish mismatched from correctly matched bases in non replicating DNA remain unclear, but it is thought that recognition involves the contact of MMR proteins with the replication machinery. The eukaryotic mismatch sensors are the heterodimeric hMutS$\alpha$ (MSH2-MSH6) and hMutS$\beta$ (MSH2-MSH3) complexes. Whereas hMutS$\alpha$ preferentially recognizes base-base mismatches and insertion/deletion mispairs of one or two nucleotides, hMutS$\beta$ recognizes larger insertion/deletion mispairs (Li, 2008). The removal of mismatched bases and the restoration of strand integrity resemble the processes occurring in BER and NER. MMR proteins can interact with proteins in other repair pathways, such as BER, NER and homologous recombination, suggesting coordinated crosstalk between these processes (Kunkel & Erie, 2005). hMutS$\alpha$ and hMutS$\beta$ may directly activate DNA damage signaling by physical interaction with ATM, ATR-ATRIP, c-Abl, and the p53-related transcription factor p73 (Kim et al., 2007; Shimodaira et al., 2003; Yoshioka et al., 2006). Consistently, hMutS$\alpha$ and hMutS$\beta$-deficient cells are defective in cell cycle arrest in response to multiple types of DNA damaging agents (Li, 2008). Another model proposes that a DDR could be activated by DNA breaks that are produced during "futile" DNA repair cycles. This model suggests that strand-specific MMR, which targets only newly replicated DNA, engages in repetitive repair cycles when it encounters a DNA lesion in the template strand, and this futile cycling activates ATR and/or ATM signaling leading to cell cycle arrest and apoptosis (Li, 1999; 2008).

### 2.3.3 Double-strand break repair pathways

It is generally accepted that the DNA double-strand break (DSB) is one of the most toxic and mutagenic DNA lesions occurring in human cells. A single DSB can, if left unrepaired, lead to the loss of a chromosome fragment and, thus, the death of the cell. However, despite the potential danger posed by DSBs, eukaryotic cells have evolved ways of improving biological processes based on the controlled induction of a DSB. Examples of this include the generation of variation during meiosis (Inagaki et al., 2010) and in the immune system (Fugmann et al., 2000), and the relaxation of supercoiled DNA by topoisomerases. Another endogenous source of DSBs are reactive oxygen species (ROS) produced by normal cellular processes, such as oxidative respiration, cytochrome P450 metabolism, peroxisomes and inflammatory responses. Examples of exogenous sources of DSBs will be described below.

DSB repair occurs via two main pathways: non homologous end-joining (NHEJ) and homologous recombination (HR) repair (Wyman & Kanaar, 2006). In mammalian cells, NHEJ is the major pathway for repairing breaks not associated with replication. This process may occur in all phases of the cell cycle, but predominantly in G1 phase. NHEJ involves the direct rejoining of two damaged DNA ends in a sequence-independent manner (Helleday et al., 2007; Weterings & van Gent, 2004). This end-joining mechanism is very precise for blunt ends and other simple end structures (van Heemst et al., 2004). However, the processing of incompatible ends may result in sequence alterations, such as deletions, occurring at "complicated" breaks. DNA double-strand breaks are first sensed by the ring-shaped Ku70/80 heterodimer. This DNA-Ku70/80 complex then attracts and activates the serine/threonine kinase activity of the DNA-PK catalytic subunit (DNA-PKcs). Following correct end alignment, DNA-PKcs is autophosphorylated (Weterings & Chen, 2007) and makes the ends available for ligation by ligase IV/XRCC4. Another essential NHEJ factor involved in the ligation of DSBs is XLF/Cernunnos (Ahnesorg et al., 2006; Buck et al., 2006). The MRN (Mre11 (Meiotic recombination 11)-Rad50-Nbs1 (Nijmegen breakage syndrome 1)) complex may facilitate the alignment of the two DNA ends, particularly when end processing is required (de Jager et al., 2001; Moreno-Herrero et al., 2005). The processing of "complex" lesions, such as hairpins, damaged backbone sugar residues, damaged bases, aberrant 5′ hydroxyl groups or 3′ phosphate groups, may involve polynucleotide kinase (Chappell et al., 2002; Koch et al., 2004), the RecQ helicase WRN (Perry et al., 2006), DNA polymerases $\mu$ and $\lambda$ (Nick McElhinny et al., 2005) and the structure-specific nuclease Artemis (Ma et al., 2002; Moshous et al., 2001).

It has recently been suggested that there is an alternative or "backup"-NHEJ (B-NHEJ) pathway that functions in conditions in which the NHEJ pathway is compromised (Iliakis, 2009). The B-NHEJ pathway seems to be dependent principally on histone H1 (Rosidi et al., 2008), PARP, which binds to DSBs with an even greater affinity than that with which it binds SSBs (D'Silva et al., 1999), and DNA ligase III/XRCC1 (Audebert et al., 2004).

Whereas NHEJ repairs DNA in a template-independent fashion by rejoining two broken ends, HR can accurately resynthesize damaged or missing sequence information at the break site, using homologous sequences as a template, preferably the adjacent sister chromatid in S or G2 phase. Several mechanisms of HR have been identified (reviewed for example by Helleday et al. (2007) and Hartlerode & Scully (2009)). All are initiated by 5′→3′ resection at the DSB end, facilitated by the MRN complex (Paull & Gellert, 1998), which plays a critical role in the sensing of DSBs for HR. The MRN complex also recruits and helps to activate ATM (Lee & Paull, 2004; 2005). In addition to MRN, other factors, including CtIP (CTBP-interacting protein), Exo1 and BLM (Bloom's syndrome protein), are required for 5'-end resection in mammalian cells (Hartlerode & Scully, 2009; Sartori et al., 2007; Yun & Hiom, 2009). After resection, single-stranded DNA (ssDNA) rapidly binds the ssDNA-binding protein RPA, which is then replaced by multimers of the Rad51 recombinase, forming a nucleoprotein filament at the end of the ssDNA. Rad51 loading involves direct interaction with BRCA2 (Pellegrini et al., 2002) and other factors (Hartlerode & Scully, 2009; Sy et al., 2009). The Rad51 nucleoprotein filament then captures double-stranded DNA (dsDNA) and scans it for homology (Bianco et al., 1998). When a homologous region is encountered, the 3'-end of the invading strand is extended by a polymerase, using the duplex DNA as a template. From this stage on, the repair pathway may diverge. The DSBR (DNA double-strand break repair pathway, also known as the double Holliday junction model) pathway mostly results in chromosomal crossover, whereas the SDSA (synthesis-dependent strand annealing) pathway ends with non crossover products (Johnson & Jasin, 2000; Liu & West, 2004; Van Dyck et al., 2001).

### 2.4 Dynamics and heterogeneity of DNA damage

One challenge in the study of the cellular response to DNA damage is the multitude of lesions introduced by most genotoxic agents. For instance, the exposure of cells to IR results in damage to all components of the cell, including lipids, proteins and nucleic acids. IR acts directly on the DNA, causing breaks in its phosphodiester backbone. This process accounts for about 30% of the DNA damage induced by IR (Chapman et al., 1973). The radicals produced by the indirect effects of radiation may account for as much as 70% of the DNA damage induced by IR (Chapman et al., 1973). These radicals damage DNA, resulting in a wide diversity of DNA lesions, such as damage to bases and the backbone sugar (oxidation, rearrangement, adducts), intrastrand crosslinks, the formation of abasic sites, single- and double-strand breaks and DNA-protein crosslinks (Jeggo & Lavin, 2009). Complex lesions, such as clustered DSBs and LMDS (locally multiply damaged sites) may also occur. After these complex lesions, DSBs are the most harmful lesions to the cell (Ward, 1975). It has been shown, in rodent cells, that the extent of cell death is directly correlated with the yield of DSB under various X-ray irradiation conditions (Radford, 1985). IR is therefore often used in investigations of the cellular response to DSBs. However, DSBs are not the most frequent type of lesion induced by IR. A dose of 1 Gy, for example, induces about 1000 SSBs and 150 protein-DNA crosslinks, but only 40 DSBs (Friedberg, 1995).

The reaction of various alkylating agents with DNA leads to the formation of highly heterogeneous products. Some agents may preferentially produce certain alkylation products, but the DNA damage generated is never limited to a single type (De Bont & van Larebeke, 2004). Furthermore, as for IR, other cell components, including proteins and ribonucleic acids, may be modified. Cellular responses to these modifications, such as activation of the proteasomal degradation pathway, may interfere with DDR pathways, or be involved in crosstalk with these pathways.

One type of damage can be transformed into another by inefficient repair and DNA replication or transcription (Figure 2). As described above, DNA repair pathways, such as BER, MMR and NER, generate intermediate SSBs. These SSBs may result in DSBs, if the repair is incomplete and the lesion persists (Bonner et al., 2008). The transformation of SSBs into DSBs occurs, for example, when replication forks encounter a SSB on the template and collapse (Strumberg et al., 2000) (Figure 2). Common types of DNA damage interfering with replication fork

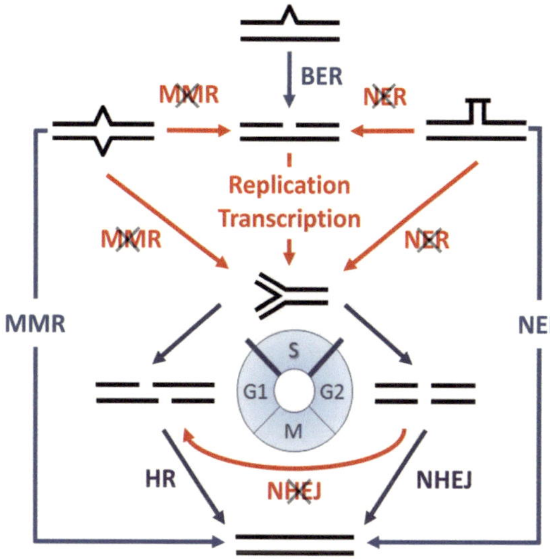


Fig. 2. Transformation of DNA damage. DNA lesions are normally repaired by the corresponding repair pathways. However, deficient repair may result in SSBs or DSBs. If a lesion persists during S-Phase (blue circle), stalled replication forks may arise. The collapse of a stalled replication fork results frequently in DSBs. DNA damage symbols and abbreviations are as for Figure 1.

progression are adducts of DNA bases (Helleday et al., 2008). By the same mechanism, inhibitors of DNA synthesis may also indirectly cause DSBs, as they impair replication fork progression (Lundin et al., 2002). Such inhibitors include aphidicolin, which inhibits DNA polymerases (Ikegami et al., 1978) and hydroxyurea, an inhibitor of ribonucleotide reductase (Bianchi et al., 1986). Topoisomerase inhibitors induce DSBs by exploiting the natural activity of topoisomerases during DNA replication. Topoisomerases resolve the DNA torsions induced during replication, by introducing a transient break in the DNA. Inhibitors of topoisomerases prevent the resealing of the break, by trapping the enzyme in a complex with the DNA (Hsiang et al., 1989; Kohn et al., 1987).

Thus, DSBs are the final outcome of unrepaired damage at the end of all these transformation processes (Figure 2). It is therefore not surprising that redundant and well regulated mechanisms have evolved for detecting, in particular, the presence of this toxic lesion and for activating DDR. DSBs can activate DNA-PK directly and they also activate ATM and ATR after end resection (Lopez-Contreras & Fernandez-Capetillo, 2010; Smith et al., 2010). Under certain conditions, PARP may also signal the presence of a DSB (Iliakis, 2009). The direct precursors of DSBs – SSBs and stalled replication forks – may themselves induce DDR, but there is less redundancy in the detection of these structures. SSBs are probably recognized and signaled to damage checkpoints mostly by PARP (Bouchard et al., 2003) and aberrant replication forks induce ATR activity through the recognition of RPA-coated stretches of ssDNA (Lopez-Contreras & Fernandez-Capetillo, 2010). The lack of redundancy in the signaling of these structures may account for their frequent transformation into DSBs.

### 2.5 Cellular DNA damage response

DNA breaks, including DSBs in particular, induce a highly coordinated DDR process leading to signal amplification, enhanced repair functions, cell cycle arrest or apoptosis. Many proteins are implicated in the DDR, which involves complex spatial and temporal coordination and many dynamic interactions between repair proteins and DNA.

#### 2.5.1 Spatiotemporal organization of the DNA damage response

The components of the DDR pathway may be classified roughly as DNA-damage sensors, mediators, transducers and effectors (Figure 3A). After the sensing of a DNA break, mediator and repair proteins rapidly accumulate on the chromatin surrounding the lesion, to form subnuclear repair foci (Fernandez-Capetillo et al., 2003) (Figure 3B). Protein recruitment to DSBs normally occurs in a hierarchical manner and involves multiple posttranslational modifications, such as phosphorylation, ubiquitination, PARylation or acetylation (Essers et al., 2002; Lukas et al., 2004; Polo & Jackson, 2011). The massive accumulation of DNA repair and signaling factors may lead to structural stabilization of the break. The amplification and maintenance of the DNA-damage signal through the recruitment of multiple copies of transducer kinases to sites of damage is probably an even more important function (Misteli & Soutoglou, 2009).

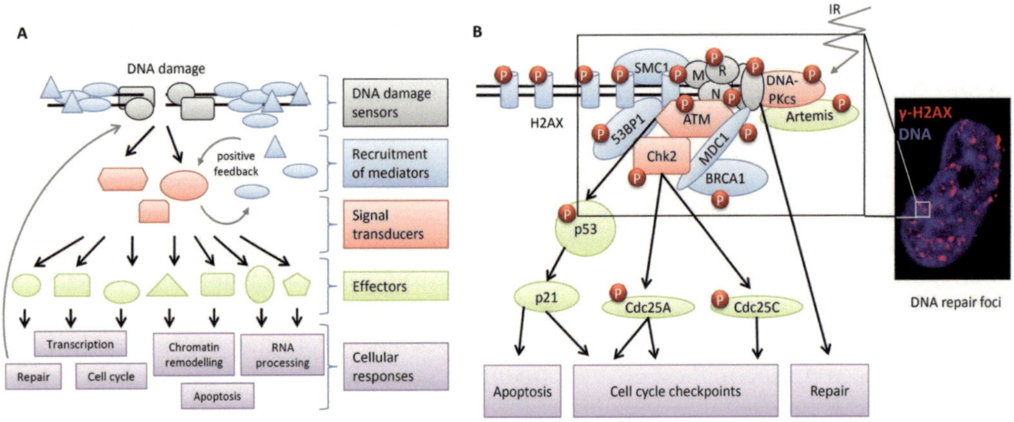


Fig. 3. The DDR signal transduction cascade. (A) DNA damage is first physically recognized by sensor proteins (gray). Mediator proteins (blue) facilitate the recruitment and activation of transducer kinases (red). A positive feedback loop between mediators and transducers leads to the maintenance and amplification of the signal. The transducer kinases then phosphorylate various effector proteins (green), including kinases, transcription factors and repair proteins. Depending on the severity of the damage, this can lead to various cellular responses (purple). (B) Formation of multiprotein complexes at the sites of DSBs (Ward & Chen, 2004) and microscopic visualization of the formation of $\gamma$-H2AX foci in response to IR. The exposure of cells to IR results in the rapid recruitment of numerous proteins to the sites of DNA lesions. The signal transducing kinases ATM and the related DNA-PK initiate a cascade of phosphorylation events (P), amplifying the signal to activate, if necessary, cell cycle checkpoint pathways or apoptosis, in situations in which the damage is too great to be repaired.

DNA break sensors include the MRN complex (Rupnik et al., 2008), Ku70/80, PARP and RPA. Break recognition by these sensors leads to the activation of transducer kinases, such as the PIKKs ATM, ATR and DNA-PK as well as PARP (Iliakis, 2009; Stiff et al., 2004; Ward & Chen, 2001). ATM, DNA-PK and ATR can phosphorylate the serine 139 residue of the histone variant H2AX (yielding $\gamma$-H2AX), at nucleosomes around the lesion. H2AX phosphorylation is probably the earliest posttranslational modification in DDR and may be considered the initial signal amplification step. $\gamma$-H2AX formation is followed by binding of the mediator protein MDC1 (mediator of DNA damage checkpoint 1) to the DSB-flanking chromatin (Jungmichel & Stucki, 2010). Mediator or adaptor proteins help to transmit, enhance and sustain the signaling between sensors and transducers, leading to the spread of the repair machinery along the chromosome. Other mediators include 53BP1 (p53-binding protein 1) and BRCA1 (Li & Zou, 2005; Misteli & Soutoglou, 2009). The recruitment of 53BP1 and BRCA1 to the DSB is indirect, requiring the activity of the E3 ubiquitin ligases RNF8 (Huen et al., 2007; Kolas et al., 2007) and RNF168 (Doil et al., 2009; Stewart et al., 2009). ssDNA compartments may be bound by RPA, which subsequently recruits ATR (Lobrich & Jeggo, 2007) and Rad51. Foci of Rad51 binding colocalize with Rad52 (Liu & Maizels, 2000), Rad54 (Essers et al., 2002), RPA (Raderschall et al., 1999), BRCA1 (Scully et al., 1997) and BRCA2 (Chen et al., 1998). Sustained activation of the transducers results in the transmission of the damage signal to effectors, which relay the signal to downstream pathways with endpoints in different cellular processes, such as checkpoint arrest or apoptosis (Kastan & Bartek, 2004) (Figure 3).

Not all the actors in DNA damage signaling and repair form characteristic foci. Unlike ATM, MDC1, 53BP1, BRCA1/BARD1 and MRN, the central NHEJ proteins Ku70/80 and DNA-PK do not spread to the adjacent chromatin upon recruitment to the break, presumably because they are required at low copy number at sites of damage (Bekker-Jensen et al., 2006; Lukas et al., 2003). The same is true for the effector kinases Chk1 and Chk2, and for p53, which interact only transiently with damage sites, subsequently diffusing rapidly to relay the signal to their soluble downstream targets.

One endpoint of the described signaling cascade in response to DNA damage is the activation of checkpoints to provide the cell with more time for DNA repair. DDR checkpoints have been identified at the G1/S and G2/M boundaries, and during S phase and, potentially, in mitosis (reviewed by Lukas et al. (2004)). After activation, the transducer kinases ATM, ATR or DNA-PK phosphorylate p53 either directly or via ATM-induced activation of the effector kinase Chk (checkpoint kinase) 2. Phosphorylated p53 then induces transcription of the gene encoding the Cdk inhibitor p21, which ultimately prevents transition from G1 to S-phase. Both Chk 1 and 2 activate the G2/M and intra-S checkpoints (Smith et al., 2010). It was long thought that ATM principally phosphorylated Chk1 and that ATR preferentially phosphorylated Chk2. However, this view has been modified by the discovery of various crosstalk between these kinases (Bartek & Lukas, 2003). The precise role of DNA-PK in this regulation remains unclear. PARP may contribute to checkpoint signaling by activation of p53. p53 exhibits high affinity for automodified PARP (Malanga et al., 1998) and p53 functions are impaired in PARP-deficient cells (Wang et al., 1998; Wieler et al., 2003). Furthermore, PARP activation in response to excessive DNA damage leads to extensive $NAD^+$ consumption. The cellular $NAD^+$ depletion can induce cell death through several mechanisms, depending on the cellular context (reviewed by Rouleau et al. (2010)).

### 2.5.2 Complexity of DNA damage response regulation

The outcomes of DNA damage signaling are, literally, a matter of life or death. Depending on the severity of DNA damage, the cell will either repair the damage to enable it to continue dividing or enter apoptosis. Complex, redundant signaling pathways converging on several central node proteins have emerged to ensure that this signaling remains under tight control. These node proteins must obtain input signals from several sources, in the form of protein modifications, before they can relay the signal to downstream effectors. This has a protective effect, greatly reducing the risk of important cell fate decisions, such as entry into apoptosis, occurring in response to a single erroneous input signal (Yarosh, 2001). The nodes in DDR include checkpoint proteins, such as Chk1 and Chk2, which control cell cycling and require input signals from several sources for full activation (McAdams & Arkin, 1999). Another prominent example for a node protein in DNA damage signaling is p53 (Kohn, 1999). The p53 protein has 11 sites for phosphorylation and acetylation, and can theoretically assume about 2000 modification states, if all the possible independent combinations are taken into account. Twelve different kinases can phosphorylate p53, and activated p53 can interact with at least 15 downstream proteins (Yarosh, 2001). The kinases that phosphorylate p53 in response to DNA damage include DNA-PK, ATM and ATR. Full p53 activity requires phosphorylation by both DNA-PK and ATM, at least (Wang et al., 2000). It is therefore now thought that p53 plays a key role in determining the degree of damage, through the assessment of input signals, on which the decision as to whether apoptosis is necessary is based (Kohn, 1999). There is a need to determine the specific conditions under which individual PIKKs become activated. Which (genotoxic) stresses lead to the activation of all transducer kinases? Is it possible to activate a single PIKK specifically, without affecting the others, and what are the cellular consequences of this?

There is also direct interplay between the transducer kinases (Chen et al., 2007). PIKKs can phosphorylate each other in response to DNA damage, resulting in mutual control of their activities. In addition to mediating posttranslational modifications, the kinases seem to regulate each other, either directly or indirectly (Peng et al., 2005). Studies on mutants and siRNA experiments have shown that a decrease in the amount of one of these kinases often leads to a decrease in the amounts of the PIKK sister kinases. The location of the kinases also seems to play an important role. For ATM, for example, the concentration of multiple copies in repair foci plays an important role in kinase activation, whereas DNA-PK does not need such an accumulation of multiple copies for full activation.

Another layer of complexity is added by the partially overlapping substrate specificities of the transducers ATM, DNA-PK and ATR (reviewed by Durocher & Jackson (2001) and Yang et al. (2003)). These transducers signal different types of DNA damage, but it was recently shown that the PIKK-mediated signaling network is highly extensive, with hundreds of phosphorylation events at ATR, ATM and DNA-PK consensus target sites induced by IR (Matsuoka et al., 2007). As discussed above, the plethora of types of damage induced by IR results in the activation of all three PIKKs. It remains to be determined which substrates are specific or overlapping for which transducer kinases in this long list of potential PIKK targets. Further insight into the contributions of individual repair signaling pathways has been provided by studies of the responses induced by damage signals in the absence of chromatin damage. This aspect will be discussed below.

## 3. Methods and mechanisms for inducing a damage response in the absence of chromatin damage

The induction of DNA damage repair pathways by exogenous DNA was first reported in bacteria, into which UV-irradiated lambda bacteriophages (D'Ari & Huisman, 1982; George et al., 1974) or plasmids (Bailone et al., 1984) were introduced. This indirect response is controlled by activation at the sites of exogenous DNA damage of the RecA protein, the key enzyme of the bacterial damage signaling response known as the "SOS response" (see Schlacher & Goodman (2007)). No such mechanism was initially found in mammals, despite a few publications reporting that UV-irradiated H-1 parvovirus or SV40 simian virus induced an "SOS-like" repair pathway in infected mammalian cells (Cornelis et al., 1982). Elucidation of the mechanisms underlying the response to damaged DNA or RNA in the cell took much longer in mammals. We review here the mammalian cell response to oligonucleotides, viral and immunostimulatory DNA and the insight into DDR gained from the analysis of artificial repair foci.

### 3.1 Cellular response to DNA oligonucleotides

In bacteria, ssDNA has been identified as the signal triggering the bacterial SOS repair response. The RecA protein (Rad51 in humans) is directly stimulated by ssDNA, inactivating the LexA repressor and triggering the repair response (Craig & Roberts, 1981). It has been suggested that ssDNA (at SSBs, stalled replication forks or resected DSBs) acts also as the major stimulatory signal for DNA damage responses in eukaryotic cells (Li & Deshaies, 1993; Nur et al., 2003). Several studies based on transfection or the microinjection of synthetic DNA oligonucleotides have analyzed the response of the cell to ssDNA. Studies by Nur et al. (2003) have shown that ssDNA acts upstream from ATM/p53 in DNA damage signaling. The transfection of cells with short (as few as 5 bases) ssDNA molecules with random sequences induced ATM activation and apoptosis, whereas very short (8 bp) dsDNA molecules did not (Nur et al., 2003). The induction of apoptosis by ssDNA is consistent with earlier studies, in which transfection with randomly fragmented DNA (Schiavone et al., 2000) or the nuclear injection of linearized plasmid DNA, circular DNA containing a gap, or single-stranded circular phagemids induced cell cycle arrest or apoptosis (Huang et al., 1996). The activation of ATM by fragmented DNA requires the MRN-assisted assembly of short, linear ssDNA fragments into high-molecular weight complexes, as shown by experiments in *Xenopus laevis* extracts (Costanzo et al., 2004).

So, if ssDNA can activate ATM directly, how is ATM activated in response to DNA double-strand breaks? When DNA double-strand breaks are sensed by the MRN complex, MRN partially unwinds the ends to expose ssDNA (Lee & Paull, 2005). It has been shown in *Xenopus laevis* egg extracts that 70 bp synthetic double-stranded molecules are rapidly resected in an MRN-dependent manner to generate ssDNA oligonucleotides, which activate ATM (Jazayeri et al., 2008). Consistent with these findings, the injection of small synthetic ssDNA oligomers into undamaged cells also induces ATM activation, and the elimination of ssDNA oligomers results in the rapid extinction of ATM activity. In summary, the results obtained from experiments with single-stranded or long double-stranded DNA fragments suggest that short ssDNA molecules are the essential signal for the induction of ATM-dependent cell cycle arrest and apoptosis.

The cellular response to single-stranded oligonucleotides may also have consequences for targeted gene repair with synthetic oligonucleotides. In gene targeting processes, ssDNA molecules are transported to the nucleus, where they align with their complementary sequence in the target gene, facilitating nucleotide exchange (Brachman & Kmiec, 2002). However, the introduction of large amounts of oligonucleotides into cells may induce cell cycle arrest and stalled DNA replication in the corrected cells, due to the ATM activation by the mechanism described above. Ferrara & Kmiec (2006) showed that the transfection of human colorectal cancer cells with 47-mer single-stranded oligonucleotides mostly activated Chk1 and Chk2 in corrected cells. As a consequence, uncorrected cells may outgrow corrected cells. The uncorrected cells probably contain fewer oligonucleotides, too few indeed to generate a local ssDNA concentration high enough to activate ATM. This may account for previous reports of the decline of corrected populations over time (Igoucheva et al., 2004).

### 3.2 Synthetic interstrand crosslinks

The cytotoxic activity of many chemotherapeutic agents, including cisplatin, nitrogen mustards and mitomycin C, is due to the induction of interstrand crosslinks (ICLs) in DNA. These lesions block the strand separation necessary for essential DNA functions, such as transcription and replication. ICLs affect both strands of the chromosome, and their repair is particularly complex. It involves factors from multiple repair pathways and the mechanisms may differ at different stages of the cell cycle. Nucleotide-excision repair, homologous recombination repair, the Fanconi anemia repair pathway, MMR and translesion synthesis have all been shown to participate in ICL repair.

Oligonucleotides containing synthetic ICLs are a valuable tool for the study of ICL repair (Guainazzi & Scharer, 2010). The advantage of such molecules over cell treatment with a cross-linking agent is that it is possible to study the components involved in the repair of specific interstrand crosslink products one at a time. This has mostly involved the ligation of the synthetic ICL-containing DNA fragments into plasmids, followed by analysis of their repair in cell-free extracts or cells (Orelli et al., 2010; Raschle et al., 2008; Wang et al., 2001). The repair of the specific ICL can be analyzed with reporter genes or by enzymatic digestion followed by Southern blotting. Studies with synthetic DNA ICLs have contributed to our understanding of the mechanism of replication-coupled DNA ICL repair (Wang et al., 2001) and the role of the Fanconi anemia pathway in this repair process (Knipscheer et al., 2009).

### 3.3 Viral infection

The highly organized cellular response to DNA damage may be disorganized or hijacked during viral infection (Lilley et al., 2007; Weitzman et al., 2004). Viruses often produce large amounts of exogenous DNA during infection, and generate proteins that interfere with DNA repair pathways and cell cycle checkpoints. Recent studies have suggested that the cellular DNA repair machinery can recognize viral nucleic acids as damage (Lilley et al., 2007). In some cases, the host DNA repair response is inactivated by viruses, whereas in others, the maintenance of a functional host DNA repair machinery seems to increase viral replication. Studies of the interaction of viruses with the host cell DNA repair machinery have improved our understanding of normal cellular DNA repair functions, and viruses may be useful model systems for studying certain aspects of DNA repair (Weitzman & Ornelles, 2005). In this section, we provide an overview of the ways in which viral infection can activate the DDR in cells, thereby focusing on the response to viral genomic material. For a detailed description of the ways in which viral proteins can manipulate the host DNA repair machinery and cell cycle checkpoints, we refer the reader to Chaurushiya & Weitzman (2009), Davy & Doorbar (2007) and Weitzman et al. (2004).

### 3.3.1 DDR induction by DNA viruses

Adenoviruses (Ad), which belong to the parvovirus family, are probably the most thoroughly investigated DNA viruses. Their genome consists of a linear, 36 kb dsDNA molecule, with inverted terminal repeats (ITRs) at each end and origins for DNA replication (Weitzman & Ornelles, 2005). Viral proteins synthesized before viral DNA replication prevent the recognition of the Ad genome by host DNA repair factors. This may involve the targeting, by these proteins, of cellular damage sensors and repair effectors, such as the MRN complex or DNA ligase IV, for degradation and relocalization (Carson et al., 2003; Stracker et al., 2002). Infection with Ad lacking the proteins required for blockade of the host DNA repair machinery results in partial DDR activation. DNA damage mediator proteins accumulate at sites of viral replication (Stracker et al., 2002) and $\gamma$-H2AX is formed at the periphery of viral centers, in a process dependent on host cell PIKK activity (Carson et al., 2003). Despite the interference of viral proteins with the cellular DNA repair system during infection with wild-type Ad, the cellular DDR does not seem to be completely abolished. The foreign DNA induces H2AX phosphorylation during later stages of infection, after the onset of viral DNA replication (Nichols et al., 2009). H2AX phosphorylation follows a pan-nuclear pattern, suggesting that all the H2AX on the host chromatin is phosphorylated by ectopic kinase activation, contrasting with the localized $\gamma$-H2AX formation observed in response to DSBs in the chromatin. Viral replication seems to be required for this phosphorylation, because infection with a nonreplicating virus does not induce $\gamma$-H2AX (Nichols et al., 2009) production. ATR may be the principal kinase phosphorylating H2AX in these conditions, although ATM and DNA-PK also seem to be involved (Nichols et al., 2009).

Pan-nuclear H2AX phosphorylation has also been observed in cells infected with the adeno-associated virus (AAV) (Collaco et al., 2009; Fragkos et al., 2008; Schwartz et al., 2009). The AAV genome, like that of Ad, consists of an ssDNA molecule with ITRs at both ends, resulting in the formation of double-hairpin structures (Brown, 2010). AAV infection requires helper functions, which may be supplied by Ad or other viruses (Geoffroy & Salvetti, 2005), and components of the host cell DNA replication machinery (Nash et al., 2009). Viral replication takes place in the nucleus, where cellular proteins, including RPA, colocalize with viral proteins in replication centers (Stracker et al., 2004). AAV replication in the presence of minimal Ad helper proteins induces a robust DDR-like response. This response is independent of the MRN complex and seems to be mediated principally by DNA-PKcs and, to a lesser extent, by ATM (Collaco et al., 2009; Schwartz et al., 2009). The response involves the accumulation of DNA-PK in compartments in which viral replication is occurring, and the pan-nuclear phosphorylation, not only of H2AX, but also of Smc1 and ATM (Schwartz et al., 2009). In another study, the phosphorylation of RPA, Nbs1 and Chk1/2 was observed, but the phosphorylation pattern was not investigated (Collaco et al., 2009).

In addition to the DNA-PK-dependent DDR induced by AAV replication, studies on recombinant AAV (rAAV) vectors (Carter, 2004), have demonstrated the existence of a requirement for DNA-PKcs and Ku70/80 for viral DNA replication (Choi et al., 2010). The inactivation of DNA-PK by a DNA-PK inhibitor or siRNA significantly decreases the replication of rAAV, and any rAAV DNA that is replicated forms head-to-head or tail-to-tail junctions. Moreover, AAV-ITRs interact directly with Ku proteins, suggesting that viral DNA is recognized directly by cellular NHEJ factors (Choi et al., 2010). Furthermore, DNA-PKcs and Artemis have been shown to open the ITR hairpin loops of rAAV *in vivo*, in a tissue-dependent manner. In the absence of either of these factors, double-stranded linear rAAV genomes capped with covalently closed hairpins at their termini accumulate in cells (Inagaki et al., 2007), confirming the importance of host cell NHEJ proteins for viral DNA end processing. By contrast to the "hyperactivation" of DNA-PK observed in response to replicating AAV, the DNA of UV-inactivated AAV particles activates a DDR involving ATM and ATR, leading to the inhibition of cell cycle progression (Jurvansuu et al., 2005). It has been suggested that the UV-treated DNA mimics stalled replication forks (Jurvansuu et al., 2005), whereas DNA-PK activation is consistent with the presence of DSBs as intermediate products during AAV replication.

DNA-PKcs and Ku70/80 as well as other cellular repair or replication factors including Topoisomerases I and II, MSH2-MSH6, RecQL, PARP and scaffold attachment factor A (SAF-A) are involved in Kaposi's sarcoma-associated herpesvirus (KSHV) lytic replication (Wang et al., 2008). KSHV is a large dsDNA virus and the etiologic agent of several AIDS-associated cancers, including Kaposi's sarcoma (Antman & Chang, 2000). The lytic replication of KSHV and the continuous primary infection of fresh cells are responsible for viral tumorigenicity and pathogenesis, by contrast to what has been reported for other oncogenic viruses (Grundhoff & Ganem, 2004). The proteins listed above bind to KSHV DNA fragments and accumulate in viral replication compartments in the nucleus, suggesting a possible role for these host replication and repair proteins in the viral lytic replication process (Wang et al., 2008).

In the case of infection with herpes simplex virus type 1 (HSV-1), which contains a linear dsDNA molecule, a DNA damage signaling is induced which depends principally on ATR (Lilley et al., 2005; Wilkinson & Weller, 2006). Several members of the cellular DNA damage-sensing machinery, including RPA, RAD51 and Nbs1, are activated and redistributed during viral DNA replication, indicating that infection induces the host response to DNA damage. H2AX is phosphorylated but the $\gamma$-H2AX signal is marginalized to the periphery of viral replication centers (Wilkinson & Weller, 2006). HSV-1 sequesters hyperphosphorylated RPA away from viral replication compartments, thus preventing a normal ATR-signaling response. The partial and mislocalized activation of the cellular DDR leads ultimately to its disorganization.

ATR is also activated during viral replication of the dsDNA virus human cytomegalovirus (HCMV), leading to an induction of $\gamma$-H2AX (Luo et al., 2007). Contrary to what has been observed for HSV-1, $\gamma$-H2AX co-localizes with viral replication compartments during late-stage infections with HCMV. Only a subset of proteins in addition to $\gamma$-H2AX was specifically sequestered in viral replication centers, with other proteins excluded from these centers, impeding both the efficient repair of viral DNA and checkpoint activation (Luo et al., 2007).

ATM-dependent checkpoint signaling takes place during induction of Epstein Barr virus lytic replication (Kudoh et al., 2005) or polyomavirus replication (Dahl et al., 2005). This is accompanied by the phosphorylation of a number of DNA damage markers including H2AX. The cellular ATM activation in response to both viruses leads to a prolonged S-phase advantageous for viral lytic replication. However, both viruses have developed efficient strategies to block ATM-induced p53 downstream signaling that would eventually lead to apoptosis (Dahl et al., 2005; Kudoh et al., 2005). By contrast, the autonomous minute virus of canines (MVC), a member of the parvovirus family, induces apoptosis and G(2)/M-phase arrest in infected canine cells (Chen et al., 2010). This seems to be the result of the induction of an ATM/p53-mediated DDR (Luo et al., 2011). Infected cells display phosphorylation of H2AX, RPA, ATM and ATR. The inhibition or knockdown of ATM decreased cell death and reduced MVC DNA replication.

In summary, studies of the response of the cell to viral genomic material have demonstrated that the activation of a damage response involving ATM (e.g. in the case of MVC) or ATR (UV-inactivated rAAV) leads to cell cycle arrest or p53-dependent cell death, unless downstream effectors are inactivated or sequestered by viral proteins (HSV-1, HCMV). By contrast, DNA-PK activation (Ad, AAV) leads to pan-nuclear H2AX phosphorylation, which does not seem to be detrimental to the cell. These findings have possible consequences for the choice of viral vectors for gene targeting. It remains to be determined whether the "ectopic" phosphorylation of DNA-PK downstream targets affects the stability of the host cell genome or impairs DNA repair in infected cells. It has also been shown that the specific recruitment of a subset of cellular DNA repair factors is essential for viral DNA replication, suggesting that inhibitors targeting these proteins may have antiviral activity.

### 3.3.2 DNA damage signals induced by retroviruses

Interaction with the cellular DNA damage sensing machinery is not limited to DNA viruses. Retroviruses, which contain a single-stranded RNA genome, use a viral-encoded reverse transcriptase to generate a cDNA that is then integrated into the host genome. The preintegration complex contains the cDNA and the viral-encoded integrase enzyme. This enzyme then mediates strand transfer to integrate the viral DNA into the host DNA in a non site-specific fashion (Weitzman et al., 2004). The interaction of retroviruses with the cellular DNA repair machinery has been studied in detail (Lilley et al., 2007; Sakurai et al., 2009; Skalka & Katz, 2005). The NHEJ pathway has been implicated in the sensing and processing of the linear cDNA, although the exact step of the viral life-cycle affected by the cellular DNA repair machinery remains unclear Ariumi et al. (2005). It is possible that the viral cDNA acts directly as a substrate for NHEJ, which circularizes the DNA by end ligation (Li et al., 2001). The circularization of unintegrated DNA in this context may protect the viral DNA from degradation and the cell from apoptosis (Kilzer et al., 2003). Consistent with this hypothesis, the infection with retrovirus of cells lacking NHEJ factors results in apoptosis, suggesting that DNA-PKcs and Ku70/80 may protect against the cellular toxicity of high levels of retroviral cDNA (Li et al., 2001).

Another interaction of retroviruses with the DNA repair machinery is constituted by the role of cellular repair and damage signaling factors in the integration of viral DNA into the host genome (Daniel et al., 1999). During retroviral integration, DSBs are created as an intermediate that may be detected as DNA damage by the host cell (Sakurai et al., 2009). Transient phosphorylation of histone H2AX occurs at retroviral integration sites, and it has been suggested that the completion of the integration process is dependent on DNA-PK (Daniel et al., 1999; 2004). DNA-PK-deficient mouse scid cells infected with three different retroviruses display much lower levels of DNA integration than wild-type cells and die by apoptosis. Furthermore, it has been reported that DNA-PKcs is required for efficient transduction by retroviral vectors (Daniel et al., 1999). Other PIKKs have since been shown to be activated after HIV-1 infection and to play a potential role in provirus integration. The use of caffeine or a small-molecule inhibitor to block the ATM activity results in the inhibition of HIV transduction and replication (Daniel et al., 2005; Lau et al., 2005).

DNA-PK and ATM also seem to be important for correct end processing at the junctions between HIV-1 provirus and host DNA (Sakurai et al., 2009). Large numbers of abnormal junctions are observed in Mre11- and DNA-PKcs-deficient cells, and Artemis-deficient cells also display such abnormalities, suggesting a role for NHEJ processing factors in correct viral integration. Another study has reported a role for Ku70/80 in the targeting of retroviral elements to chromatin domains prone to gene silencing. Higher levels of viral DNA expression are observed in the absence of Ku70/80, with no effect on viral transduction (Masson et al., 2007).

The importance of cellular components of the DDR for the replication of some viruses could be exploited for therapeutic purposes. For instance, a small-molecule ATM-inhibitor displayed antiviral activity in a proof-of-concept study with HIV-1, in which ATM deficiency sensitized cells to retrovirus-induced cell death (Lau et al., 2005).

### 3.4 Tethering of repair factors

Recent studies in yeast and mammals have demonstrated that it is not the DNA lesion that triggers the DDR, leading to the activation of transducer kinases, but the local concentration of signaling factors at repair foci. Soutoglou & Misteli (2008) demonstrated that a DDR can be triggered in the absence of DNA lesions. The artificial localized tethering of repair factors was found to be sufficient to trigger a full DDR response, including cell-cycle arrest, in the absence of DNA breaks. Tethering was achieved by fusing repair proteins to the *Escherichia coli lac* repressor and expressing the resulting constructs in mouse NIH-3T3 cells containing multiple *lacR* binding sites, stably integrated into the genome (Soutoglou & Misteli, 2008). The immobilization of Nbs1, Mre11 or MDC1 alone led to DDR activation. In addition, the tethering of ATM was sufficient to induce ATM kinase activity and autophosphorylation. Consistent with its function downstream from the MRN complex, the induction of ATM activity was not affected by an absence of Mre11 or Nbs1. As similar results were obtained in analogous experiments in *Saccharomyces cerevisiae* (Bonilla et al., 2008), the concentration of key factors on the chromatin may be considered a universal characteristic of DDR initiation and amplification in eukaryotes (Misteli & Soutoglou, 2009). The tethering experiments may be seen as complementary to the experiments with siDNA described below, as the DNA break-mimicking DNA molecules are (i) too short for the formation of repair foci and (ii) not in a chromatin context.

### 3.5 DDR induction by cofactors, oxidative stress or changes in chromatin state

ATM, and consequently the DDR, can be activated in the absence of DNA breaks, by changes in chromatin structure. Bakkenist & Kastan (2003) showed that ATM is rapidly activated by the exposure of cells to chromatin-active agents, such as mild hypotonic buffers, or treatment with chloroquine. Furthermore, histone deacetylase (HDAC) inhibitors, such as TSA, which induces the global decondensation of chromatin, can also induce ATM activity (Jang et al., 2010; Mazumdar et al., 2006). Consistent with its role as a sensor of chromatin structure, ATM can interact with the chromatin via the nucleosome-binding protein HMGN1 before DNA damage occurs. The loss of this interaction in the absence of HMGN1 compromises ATM activation in response to IR (Kim et al., 2009).

ATM-dependent phosphorylation of H2AX during M-phase has been reported to occur in the absence of DNA damage (Ichijima et al., 2005; Mazumdar et al., 2006). The high degree of compaction of mitotic chromosomes may be the signal responsible for activating DNA damage signaling kinases in the absence of apparent DNA lesions (Ichijima et al., 2005).
Another recent study showed that DNA-damage signaling pathways and ATM could be activated directly by hypoxia, apparently in the absence of lesions (Bencokova et al., 2009). The direct mechanism involved is unknown, but the hypoxia-induced activation of ATM is independent of the MRN complex, and active, autophosphorylated ATM has a pan-nuclear rather than focal distribution. The activation of ATM signaling in response to hypoxia may account for the cessation of replication when oxygen levels are low.
ATM is a also a direct sensor of oxidative stress, in the absence of DNA lesions. Oxidation by ROS results in the formation of an active, disulfide-cross-linked, ATM dimer (Guo et al., 2010). The activation of ATM in response to oxidative stress is independent of the MRN complex and leads to the phosphorylation of DDR effectors including p53 and Chk2, but not the chromatin-associated proteins H2AX or Kap1. This confirms that ATM activation through oxidation may occur without the involvement of the DNA damage recognition machinery.
Consistent with ATM activation, the transducer kinase ATR can also be activated in the absence of DNA damage. Toledo et al. (2008) reported the ectopic activation of ATR following overproduction of a fragment of TopBP1 containing a domain known to stimulate ATR kinase activity (Kumagai et al., 2006). ATR activation was sufficient to drive cell cycle arrest and senescence.

### 3.6 Systemic response to foreign DNA

DNA fragments trigger a DDR at the cellular level, but the detection of foreign DNA by specific sensors can trigger an innate immune response at the systemic level (for review see Vilaysane & Muruve (2009), Yanai et al. (2009) and Rathinam & Fitzgerald (2011)). The innate immune system is an integral part of the host response to viral and bacterial intrusion. Its activation leads to diverse cellular responses, including the induction of interferon regulatory factors (IRF) 3 and 7, which regulate the production of type I interferon. Furthermore, NF$\kappa$B is induced, and regulates the expression of pro-inflammatory cytokines (Vilaysane & Muruve, 2009). We provide here a brief overview of the principal sensors of foreign DNA found in humans.
Bacterial DNA differs from mammalian DNA principally in terms of its high CpG dinucleotide content. Furthermore, most of the small number of CpG dinucleotides present in mammalian DNA are methylated, whereas the CpG dinucleotides in bacterial DNA are generally unmethylated (Hemmi et al., 2000). The activation of innate immune responses by nucleic acids is mediated by transmembrane Toll-like receptors (TLRs) and cytosolic receptors. The best understood sensor of microbial DNA is TLR9, which is found principally in plasmacytoid dendritic cells (pDCs) in humans (Hemmi et al., 2000; Wagner, 2004). The endosomal uptake of CpG DNA activates TLR9, which binds MyD88, IRAK4 and IRAK1 that are required for the activation of NF$\kappa$B and the induction of type I interferons via IRF7 (Akira et al., 2006; Vilaysane & Muruve, 2009). Several studies have also shown that, in addition to responding to bacterial DNA, TLR9 plays an important role in host defense against viruses, including DNA viruses such as herpes simplex virus and murine cytomegalovirus (Delale et al., 2005; Lund et al., 2003).

In addition to the membrane-bound TLR9, cytosolic DNA sensors have recently been identified (Yanai et al., 2009). These sensors include TREX1, DNA-dependent activator of interferon regulatory factors (DAI) and a DNA-sensing inflammasome containing absent in melanoma 2 (AIM2). This protein belongs to the HIN-200 family and is a cytoplasmic sensor mediating caspase 1 activation in response to cytoplasmic dsDNA (Burckstummer et al., 2009; Fernandes-Alnemri et al., 2009; Hornung et al., 2009). Another cytosolic DNA sensor and activator of innate immune responses, DAI (also known as DLM-1 and Z-DNA binding protein 1), has also recently been identified (Takaoka et al., 2007). DAI binds dsDNA, leading to its association with the IRF3 transcription factor and the TBK1 serine/threonine kinase, resulting in a signaling cascade that culminates in NF$\kappa$B activation. The activation of interferon responses is restricted by the length of the DNA, with little activation observed in response to DNA molecules of less than 100 bp in length, suggesting that DAI activation requires the formation of a multimeric complex over long stretches of DNA (Takaoka & Taniguchi, 2008).

Several studies have identified the 3′→5′ DNA exonuclease DNaseIII/TREX1 as associated with autoimmune and inflammatory diseases in humans (Crow et al., 2006; Lee-Kirsch et al., 2007). TREX1 is a regulator of DNA homeostasis in the cell and has been reported to counteract the activation of ATM by small ssDNA fragments (section 3.1). Indeed, in the absence of TREX1, 60-65 bp ssDNA polynucleotides accumulate, leading to chronic ATM-dependent DNA damage checkpoint signaling (Yang et al., 2007). Thus, TREX1 is not itself a DNA sensor. Instead, it regulates the accumulation of the ssDNA that can trigger an innate immune response. In addition to linking a DDR factor to the immune response, these findings demonstrate that immune responses may be triggered not only by foreign DNA, but also by self-derived DNA.

The most prominent protein involved in both the DDR and the immune response, in addition to TREX1, is DNA-PKcs. In addition to its long known role in V(D)J recombination in developing lymphocytes (Jeggo et al., 1995), DNA-PKcs has also been reported to phosphorylate IFN regulatory factor-3 (IRF-3) directly (Karpova et al., 2002). IRF-3 plays a key role in the host response to viral infection, and its phosphorylation by DNA-PK after viral infection results in its nuclear retention and delayed proteolysis. Another study has suggested that DNA-PKcs mediates Akt activation in response to CpG-DNA in bone marrow-derived macrophages (BMDMs) (Dragoi et al., 2005). In BMDMs, DNA-PKcs associates with Akt upon CpG-DNA stimulation, thereby triggering the nuclear translocation of Akt. It has been suggested that TLR9 is involved in this pathway, but its possible role remains a matter of debate (Dragoi et al., 2005; Sester et al., 2006). The CpG-DNA/DNAPKcs/Akt pathway may account for the induction, by CpG-DNA and synthetic CpG oligonucleotides, of prosurvival signals delivered to the immune system (Dragoi et al., 2005; Park et al., 2002).

## 4. Signal interfering DNA (siDNA)

As summarized in Figures 1 and 2, difficulties attributing the activation of a specific transducer to a specific type of damage *in vivo* result principally from the multiple type of damage induced by a single treatment, through the mechanism of action of the treatment and metabolism of the initial damage through replication and repair. Moreover, the large DNA molecules sometimes used to induce a damage response (see section 3.1) probably contain sequences recognized by specific proteins that may interfere with DNA damage recognition and repair. We recently tried to overcome these problems by proposing the use of a new class of small molecules (siDNA, for small interfering DNA) each mimicking one particular type of damage and are not degraded, replicated or repaired in the cell.

### 4.1 SiDNA: principle and properties

We initially designed and tested only a few classes of siDNA molecules, to provide proof-of-concept for this approach. However, this concept can be extended to any specific type of damage. An siDNA is a small nucleic acid molecule carrying a modification recognized as a lesion by the sensor and transducer proteins. In addition to mimicking a specific type of damage, siDNA molecules must (i) be resistant to the action of nucleases, (ii) be as small as possible, to minimize the formation of secondary structures or degradation products, (iii) have no specific sequence likely to be recognized by DNA-binding proteins, such as transcription factors, (iv) mimic one single type of damage, ideally one that cannot be processed and (v) be recognized by at least one molecule involved in the DDR. SiDNAs are oligonucleotides chemically synthesized on solid support, by cycles of nucleotide addition. They are protected from exonuclease degradation by three phosphorothioate groups at the free 3′ and 5′ ends. Most siDNA molecules are double-stranded and have a specific modification characteristic of one type of damage. Dissociation of the short duplex is prevented by a linker tethering the two complementary strands at one or both ends of the molecule. The linker molecule

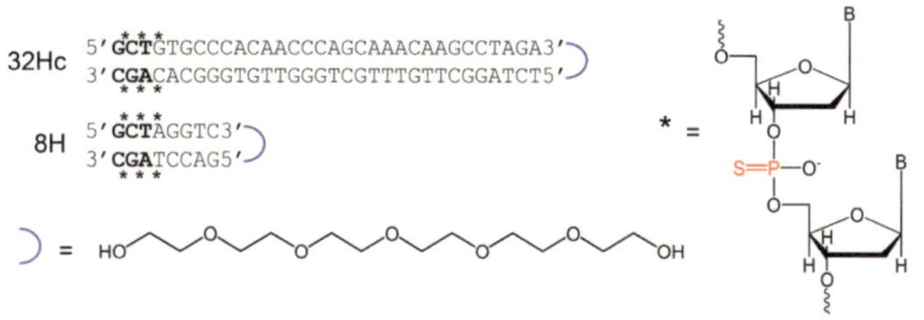


Fig. 4. Structure of the DSB-mimicking Dbait. Dbait 32Hc is a 32 bp DNA molecule tethered to its complementary sequence by a hexaethylene glycol loop (blue half circle) at one end and protected against exonuclease by phosphorothioate nucleotides (asterisks, phosphorothioate bond highlighted in red) at the other end. In the name 32Hc, H stands for hexaethylene glycol and c refers to the sequence. The sequence is not important for recognition as a DSB. The corresponding negative control, 8H, has the same basic structural features as 32Hc, but is too short to bind the central NHEJ components. B, base.

consists of a polyethylene glycol chain that is inert and stable in living systems. The resulting molecules are very stable, with melting temperatures of about 85 to 90°C, despite their small size (between 16 and 64 bp). They are resistant to incubation for six hours with serum or cell extract (unpublished data). Like most nucleic acid-based molecules, siDNAs penetrate cells poorly and complexing with transfection agents (Patil et al., 2005) or lipophilic molecules (Rossi, 2004) is required for efficient entry. Three classes of molecules have already been tested: molecules mimicking double-strand breaks (Dbait), molecules mimicking single-strand breaks (Pbait) and molecules mimicking single-strand DNA stretches (Sbait). An example of the structure of a Dbait molecule is provided in Figure 4. Every siDNA is recognized by specific sensors and triggers a corresponding partial DDR.

### 4.2 SiDNAs induce specific, stable and persistent damage responses

PIKKs and PARP enzymes are thought to be the first transducers activated by DNA damage. We threfore monitored the cellular response induced by siDNAs by detecting the modification of the downstream targets of these enzymes in cells. Using mutant cells defective in the various enzymes, we showed that Dbait activated DNA-PK and PARP, Pbait activated only PARP and Sbait activated only ATM ((Quanz et al., 2009b); to be published). These transducer activations resulted in the posttranslational modification of all known targets of these enzymes investigated. For example, Dbait induces the phosphorylation of H2AX, RPA, p53, Nbs1, Chk1, Chk2, DNA-PK, ATM, Hsp90$\alpha$, and the PARylation of a broad number of proteins. Interestingly, ATM which is also thought to be activated by DSBs, was not activated by Dbait or Pbait, but exclusively by Sbait molecules, which are single-stranded. This is consistent with the model in which DSBs must be partially degraded to activate ATM, as described above. The association of Mre11 with Rad50 and Nbs1 stimulates its endonuclease and exonuclease activities, resulting in the processing of DSB ends, leading to the generation of overhanging ssDNA regions (Paull & Gellert, 1998; 1999). Our results show that DSBs do not directly activate ATM if they remain unprocessed.

The posttranslational modifications induced by the siDNA-mediated activation of transducers persist for more than 24 hours in the cells. Phosphorylated or PARylated effectors have been detected more than one day after treatment and their persistence in cells depends on the turnover rate of the modified protein and the rate of cell division (Quanz et al., 2009b). Phosphorylated histone H2AX, for instance, was detected up to five days after treatment with Dbait, when Dbait molecules were no longer present in the cell. Similar results were obtained for other effectors, suggesting that siDNAs do not induce feedback control mechanisms ensuring the rapid return of cells to an "unactivated" state when repair is completed. At least three phosphatases, protein phosphatase 2A (PP2A), wild-type p53-induced phosphatase (Wip1) and protein phosphatase 5 (PP5), are involved in the DDR. It remains unclear how these phosphatases are activated during DDR, but they are instrumental in ATM activation (Ali et al., 2004; Goodarzi et al., 2004; Shreeram et al., 2006). The results of studies of unrepairable siDNAs suggest that the phosphatases or the proteasome must be activated by a "successful repair" signal instead, rather than simply removing phosphates or the modified proteins as a part of an equilibrium.

### 4.3 Transducer activation by siDNA is not sufficient to induce complete DDR

Although transducers are fully activated and all their molecular targets seem to be modified, the siDNAs Dbait and Pbait do not trigger the major end-points of the DDR response: cell-cycle arrest and apoptosis. In the absence of genotoxic or other stresses, cells with strong siDNA responses continue to divide at the same rate as untreated cells and do not enter apoptosis (Quanz et al., 2009b). This suggests that the DDR requires a correct spatio-temporal organization and/or more than a single damage signaling input for full execution. This is consistent with the model described above, in which redundant pathways may control the risk of erroneous signaling in cells (Yarosh, 2001). According to this hypothesis, the signal resulting from one siDNA treatment would not be sufficient to trigger a complete DDR response.

SiDNAs also differ from chromosomal DNA damage in their location and the timing of the different activation processes. SiDNAs constitute an artificial form of damage outside the context of chromatin and able to cross the cytoplasm, which contains a subset of effectors and transducers, such as DNA-PK and PARP. These signaling enzymes are therefore activated in the cytoplasm and modify the targets present in this compartment (Quanz et al., submitted, Figure 5). The lack of coordination of target modifications at the site of DNA damage prevents

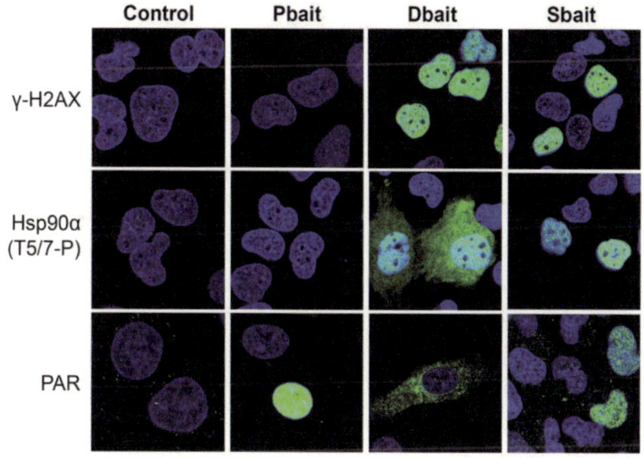


Fig. 5. Differential cytoplasmic and nuclear transducer activation by different siDNAs. Both Dbait and Sbait treatment lead to the phosphorylation of H2AX (green, top) and Hsp90$\alpha$ (green, middle) and induce a PARylation signal (green, bottom). Unlike Sbait, Dbait is already recognized in the cytoplasm, inducing cytoplasmic Hsp90$\alpha$ phosphorylation and a cytoplasmic PARylation signal. Pbait, which activates only PARP, induces PARylation but not the phosphorylation of H2AX or Hsp90$\alpha$. The negative control is an siDNA molecule that is too short to recruit and activate DNA damage transducers. The cell nuclei are shown in blue.

the further accumulation of DNA repair proteins at repair foci at these sites (Quanz et al., 2009b). For example, in cells treated with Dbait, DNA-PK autophosphorylation is detected in both the cytoplasm and the nucleus and H2AX is phosphorylated along the length of the chromosome. After the irradiation of Dbait-treated cells, repair proteins, such as Nbs1, 53BP1, Rad51, do not relocate to sites of damage or form repair foci. However, despite their incapacity to form repair foci, irradiated siDNA-treated cells display a complete DDR response, with the induction of apoptosis (Quanz et al., 2009b).

#### 4.4 SiDNAs inhibit DNA repair

The disturbance of the spatiotemporal organization of the DDR by siDNA leads to inhibition of the formation of repair foci after irradiation. Cells treated with Dbait or Pbait are therefore sensitive to IR or other DNA damaging agents. Irradiated DNA is repaired with two-component kinetics. Most of the damage is repaired rapidly, with no significant effect of Dbait treatment. By contrast, the repair of the residual damage (15-20%), which takes longer, is strongly affected by Dbait treatment (Quanz et al., Figure 6). The slowly repaired damage is thought to correspond to DSBs with complex ends (Riballo et al., 2004) and/or to be predominantly located at the periphery of genomic heterochromatin, in regions of condensed chromatin (Goodarzi et al., 2010; Mosesso et al., 2010). As a consequence of the inhibition of repair, cells treated with Dbait are highly sensitive to irradiation. This property has been used *in vivo* in the development of new drugs for treating radioresistant tumors. DT01, a clinical product from the Dbait class of siDNAs, increases the survival of nude mice xenografted with radioresistant melanoma (Quanz et al., 2009a). DT01 efficacy is strictly dependent on the dose

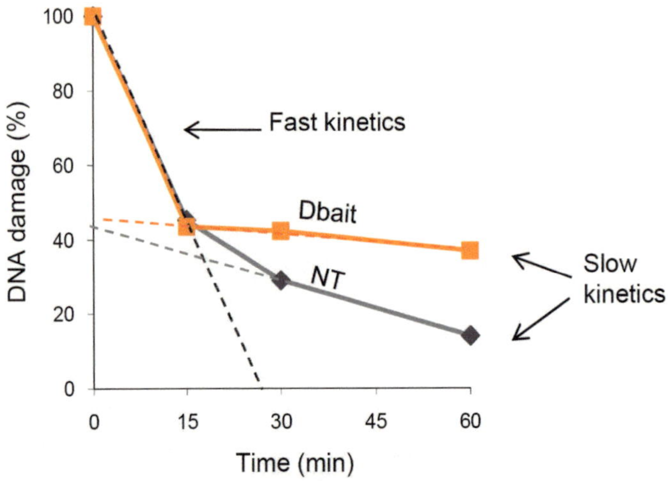


Fig. 6. Dbait inhibits slow DNA repair. MRC5 cells transfected or not transfected with Dbait were irradiated with 8 Gy. DNA damage repair was followed by alkaline comet assays over a period of 60 min.

administered (Figure 7) and is independent of the associated radiotherapy protocol. A phase I/II clinical trial will be initiated in 2011, to assess the efficacy of a treatment combining DT01 and radiotherapy for the treatment of local metastases of melanoma.

## 5. Conclusion

The study of DNA repair is a complicated task, due to the diversity of damage induced by DNA-damaging agents and the subsequent conversion of the damage by repair pathways or the DNA replication machinery. Furthermore, the damage may be repaired by different repair pathways, depending on the phase of the cell cycle at the time of damage. Finally, if the damage to the chromosome is too extensive, the cell undergoes apoptosis or senescence. The use of different techniques to induce a specific type of damage in the absence of chromosomal DNA damage within the cell has greatly contributed to our understandings of individual repair pathways. The tethering of repair proteins has demonstrated that the local concentration of damage signaling factors is sufficient to trigger a full damage response, independently of the presence of actual cellular damage. Consistent with this, agents modifying chromatin topology can induce DNA damage transducer activity in the absence of DNA lesions. Studies of the recognition of viral genomic material have contributed to our understanding of the cellular DDR. For example, studies of adenovirus interference with damage signaling through degradation of the MRN complex have suggested that MRN plays an upstream role in damage detection. Synthetic ICL constructs, introduced into cells on plasmids, have proved a useful tool for investigating this specific type of DNA damage. This approach made it possible to demonstrate the contribution of the Fanconi anemia pathway to the repair of ICLs. Studies based on the use of DNA fragments have identified ssDNA as the universal signal of the ATM-induced DDR. The introduction into cells of small double-stranded siDNA molecules, which are resistant to exonuclease attack and repair , has made it possible to demonstrate that DSBs alone activate DNA-PK only, leading to the phosphorylation of a multitude of downstream targets. However, unlike

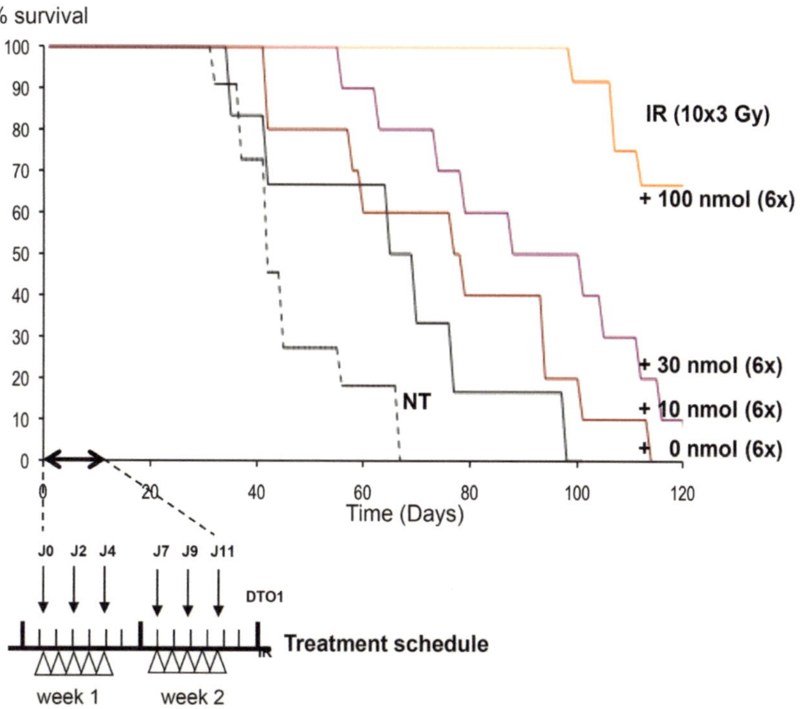


Fig. 7. The survival of xenografted animals is dependent on DT01 dose. Kaplan-Meier representation of the survival of nude mice with xenografted SK28 melanoma tumors. After two weeks of treatment, consisting of six injections of DT01 injections (arrows) at various doses and the administration of 3 Gy in 10 fractions (triangles, tumor volume was assessed. The ethical limit for tumor volume was 2000 mm$^3$. NT: untreated control group.

ATM activation by ssDNA, DNA-PK activation has a much smaller impact on the cell cycle and apoptosis induction. Thus, siDNA can be used as a tool for the specific activation of individual repair signaling enzymes, making it possible to investigate specific branches of the damage response, which is not possible with conventional DNA damaging agents that induce a plethora of different lesions. A similar approach could now be used for other kinds of DNA damage, to check for activation of the corresponding downstream repair pathways in cells. This should make it possible to answer currently unresolved questions, concerning the impact of PARP-signaling or mismatch-signaling on cell fate, for example. This should not only deepen our understanding of the specific pathways activated in response to a particular type of damage, but should also be useful in cancer treatment. The "jamming" of specific repair signaling pathways may help to overcome resistance to treatment and to enhance the response to cancer treatments targeting DNA.

## 6. Acknowledgments

We apologize to the many groups whose primary research papers could not be cited owing to space constraints. Work in the authors' laboratory was supported by Institut Curie, CNRS, INSERM, and ANR grant ANR-08-Biot-009-02.

## 7. References


Ahnesorg, P., Smith, P. & Jackson, S. P. (2006). XLF interacts with the XRCC4-DNA ligase iv complex to promote DNA nonhomologous end-joining, *Cell* 124(2): 301–13.

Akira, S., Uematsu, S. & Takeuchi, O. (2006). Pathogen recognition and innate immunity, *Cell* 124(4): 783–801.

Ali, A., Zhang, J., Bao, S., Liu, I., Otterness, D., Dean, N. M., Abraham, R. T. & Wang, X. F. (2004). Requirement of protein phosphatase 5 in DNA-damage-induced ATM activation, *Genes Dev* 18(3): 249–54.

Antman, K. & Chang, Y. (2000). Kaposi's sarcoma, *N Engl J Med* 342(14): 1027–38.

Ariumi, Y., Turelli, P., Masutani, M. & Trono, D. (2005). DNA damage sensors ATM, ATR, DNA-pkcs, and parp-1 are dispensable for human immunodeficiency virus type 1 integration, *J Virol* 79(5): 2973–8.

Audebert, M., Salles, B. & Calsou, P. (2004). Involvement of poly(adp-ribose) polymerase-1 and xrcc1/DNA ligase iii in an alternative route for DNA double-strand breaks rejoining, *J Biol Chem* 279(53): 55117–26.

Bailone, A., Brandenburger, A., Levine, A., Pierre, M., Dutreix, M. & Devoret, R. (1984). Indirect sos induction is promoted by ultraviolet light-damaged minif and requires the minif lyna locus, *J Mol Biol* 179(3): 367–90.

Bakkenist, C. J. & Kastan, M. B. (2003). DNA damage activates ATM through intermolecular autophosphorylation and dimer dissociation, *Nature* 421(6922): 499–506.

Bandaru, V., Sunkara, S., Wallace, S. S. & Bond, J. P. (2002). A novel human DNA glycosylase that removes oxidative DNA damage and is homologous to escherichia coli endonuclease viii, *DNA Repair (Amst)* 1(7): 517–29.

Bartek, J. & Lukas, J. (2003). Chk1 and chk2 kinases in checkpoint control and cancer, *Cancer Cell* 3(5): 421–9.

Bekker-Jensen, S., Lukas, C., Kitagawa, R., Melander, F., Kastan, M. B., Bartek, J. & Lukas, J. (2006). Spatial organization of the mammalian genome surveillance machinery in response to DNA strand breaks, *J Cell Biol* 173(2): 195–206.

Bencokova, Z., Kaufmann, M. R., Pires, I. M., Lecane, P. S., Giaccia, A. J. & Hammond, E. M. (2009). ATM activation and signaling under hypoxic conditions, *Mol Cell Biol* 29(2): 526–37.

Bianchi, V., Pontis, E. & Reichard, P. (1986). Changes of deoxyribonucleoside triphosphate pools induced by hydroxyurea and their relation to DNA synthesis, *J Biol Chem* 261(34): 16037–42.

Bianco, P. R., Tracy, R. B. & Kowalczykowski, S. C. (1998). DNA strand exchange proteins: a biochemical and physical comparison, *Front Biosci* 3: D570–603.

Boiteux, S. & Radicella, J. P. (2000). The human ogg1 gene: structure, functions, and its implication in the process of carcinogenesis, *Arch Biochem Biophys* 377(1): 1–8.

Bonilla, C. Y., Melo, J. A. & Toczyski, D. P. (2008). Colocalization of sensors is sufficient to activate the DNA damage checkpoint in the absence of damage, *Mol Cell* 30(3): 267–76.

Bonner, W. M., Redon, C. E., Dickey, J. S., Nakamura, A. J., Sedelnikova, O. A., Solier, S. & Pommier, Y. (2008). Gammah2ax and cancer, *Nat Rev Cancer* 8(12): 957–67.

Bouchard, V. J., Rouleau, M. & Poirier, G. G. (2003). Parp-1, a determinant of cell survival in response to DNA damage, *Exp Hematol* 31(6): 446–54.

Brachman, E. E. & Kmiec, E. B. (2002). The 'biased' evolution of targeted gene repair, *Curr Opin Mol Ther* 4(2): 171–6.
Brown, K. E. (2010). The expanding range of parvoviruses which infect humans, *Rev Med Virol* 20(4): 231–44.
Brown, K. L., Roginskaya, M., Zou, Y., Altamirano, A., Basu, A. K. & Stone, M. P. (2010). Binding of the human nucleotide excision repair proteins xpa and xpc/hr23b to the 5r-thymine glycol lesion and structure of the cis-(5r,6s) thymine glycol epimer in the 5'-gtgg-3' sequence: destabilization of two base pairs at the lesion site, *Nucleic Acids Res* 38(2): 428–40.
Buck, D., Malivert, L., de Chasseval, R., Barraud, A., Fondaneche, M. C., Sanal, O., Plebani, A., Stephan, J. L., Hufnagel, M., le Deist, F., Fischer, A., Durandy, A., de Villartay, J. P. & Revy, P. (2006). Cernunnos, a novel nonhomologous end-joining factor, is mutated in human immunodeficiency with microcephaly, *Cell* 124(2): 287–99.
Burckstummer, T., Baumann, C., Bluml, S., Dixit, E., Durnberger, G., Jahn, H., Planyavsky, M., Bilban, M., Colinge, J., Bennett, K. L. & Superti-Furga, G. (2009). An orthogonal proteomic-genomic screen identifies aim2 as a cytoplasmic DNA sensor for the inflammasome, *Nat Immunol* 10(3): 266–72.
Cadet, J., Berger, M., Douki, T. & Ravanat, J. L. (1997). Oxidative damage to DNA: formation, measurement, and biological significance, *Rev Physiol Biochem Pharmacol* 131: 1–87.
Carson, C. T., Schwartz, R. A., Stracker, T. H., Lilley, C. E., Lee, D. V. & Weitzman, M. D. (2003). The mre11 complex is required for ATM activation and the g2/m checkpoint, *EMBO J* 22(24): 6610–20.
Carter, B. J. (2004). Adeno-associated virus and the development of adeno-associated virus vectors: a historical perspective, *Mol Ther* 10(6): 981–9.
Chan, K. K., Zhang, Q. M. & Dianov, G. L. (2006). Base excision repair fidelity in normal and cancer cells, *Mutagenesis* 21(3): 173–8.
Chapman, J. D., Reuvers, A. P., Borsa, J. & Greenstock, C. L. (1973). Chemical radioprotection and radiosensitization of mammalian cells growing in vitro, *Radiat Res* 56(2): 291–306.
Chappell, C., Hanakahi, L. A., Karimi-Busheri, F., Weinfeld, M. & West, S. C. (2002). Involvement of human polynucleotide kinase in double-strand break repair by non-homologous end joining, *EMBO J* 21(11): 2827–32.
Chaurushiya, M. S. & Weitzman, M. D. (2009). Viral manipulation of DNA repair and cell cycle checkpoints, *DNA Repair (Amst)* 8(9): 1166–76.
Chen, A. Y., Luo, Y., Cheng, F., Sun, Y. & Qiu, J. (2010). Bocavirus infection induces mitochondrion-mediated apoptosis and cell cycle arrest at g2/m phase, *J Virol* 84(11): 5615–26.
Chen, B. P., Uematsu, N., Kobayashi, J., Lerenthal, Y., Krempler, A., Yajima, H., Lobrich, M., Shiloh, Y. & Chen, D. J. (2007). Ataxia telangiectasia mutated (ATM) is essential for DNA-pkcs phosphorylations at the thr-2609 cluster upon DNA double strand break, *J Biol Chem* 282(9): 6582–7.
Chen, J., Silver, D. P., Walpita, D., Cantor, S. B., Gazdar, A. F., Tomlinson, G., Couch, F. J., Weber, B. L., Ashley, T., Livingston, D. M. & Scully, R. (1998). Stable interaction between the products of the BRCA1 and BRCA2 tumor suppressor genes in mitotic and meiotic cells, *Mol Cell* 2(3): 317–28.

Choi, Y. K., Nash, K., Byrne, B. J., Muzyczka, N. & Song, S. (2010). The effect of DNA-dependent protein kinase on adeno-associated virus replication, *PLoS One* 5(12): e15073.

Cleaver, J. E. (2005). Cancer in xeroderma pigmentosum and related disorders of DNA repair, *Nat Rev Cancer* 5(7): 564–73.

Collaco, R. F., Bevington, J. M., Bhrigu, V., Kalman-Maltese, V. & Trempe, J. P. (2009). Adeno-associated virus and adenovirus coinfection induces a cellular DNA damage and repair response via redundant phosphatidylinositol 3-like kinase pathways, *Virology* 392(1): 24–33.

Cornelis, J. J., Su, Z. Z. & Rommelaere, J. (1982). Direct and indirect effects of ultraviolet light on the mutagenesis of parvovirus h-1 in human cells, *EMBO J* 1(6): 693–9.

Costanzo, V., Paull, T., Gottesman, M. & Gautier, J. (2004). Mre11 assembles linear DNA fragments into DNA damage signaling complexes, *PLoS Biol* 2(5): E110.

Craig, N. L. & Roberts, J. W. (1981). Function of nucleoside triphosphate and polynucleotide in escherichia coli reca protein-directed cleavage of phage lambda repressor, *J Biol Chem* 256(15): 8039–44.

Crow, Y. J., Hayward, B. E., Parmar, R., Robins, P., Leitch, A., Ali, M., Black, D. N., van Bokhoven, H., Brunner, H. G., Hamel, B. C., Corry, P. C., Cowan, F. M., Frints, S. G., Klepper, J., Livingston, J. H., Lynch, S. A., Massey, R. F., Meritet, J. F., Michaud, J. L., Ponsot, G., Voit, T., Lebon, P., Bonthron, D. T., Jackson, A. P., Barnes, D. E. & Lindahl, T. (2006). Mutations in the gene encoding the 3'-5' DNA exonuclease trex1 cause aicardi-goutieres syndrome at the ags1 locus, *Nat Genet* 38(8): 917–20.

Dahl, J., You, J. & Benjamin, T. L. (2005). Induction and utilization of an ATM signaling pathway by polyomavirus, *J Virol* 79(20): 13007–17.

Daniel, R., Katz, R. A. & Skalka, A. M. (1999). A role for DNA-PK in retroviral DNA integration, *Science* 284(5414): 644–7. Daniel, R Katz, R A Skalka, A M AI40721/AI/NIAID NIH HHS/United States AI40835/AI/NIAID NIH HHS/United States CA71515/CA/NCI NIH HHS/United States etc. Research Support, Non-U.S. Gov't Research Support, U.S. Gov't, P.H.S. United states Science (New York, N.Y.) Science. 1999 Apr 23;284(5414):644-7.

Daniel, R., Marusich, E., Argyris, E., Zhao, R. Y., Skalka, A. M. & Pomerantz, R. J. (2005). Caffeine inhibits human immunodeficiency virus type 1 transduction of nondividing cells, *J Virol* 79(4): 2058–65.

Daniel, R., Ramcharan, J., Rogakou, E., Taganov, K. D., Greger, J. G., Bonner, W., Nussenzweig, A., Katz, R. A. & Skalka, A. M. (2004). Histone H2AX is phosphorylated at sites of retroviral DNA integration but is dispensable for postintegration repair, *J Biol Chem* 279(44): 45810–4.

D'Ari, R. & Huisman, O. (1982). DNA replication and indirect induction of the sos response in escherichia coli, *Biochimie* 64(8-9): 623–7.

Davy, C. & Doorbar, J. (2007). G2/m cell cycle arrest in the life cycle of viruses, *Virology* 368(2): 219–26.

De Bont, R. & van Larebeke, N. (2004). Endogenous DNA damage in humans: a review of quantitative data, *Mutagenesis* 19(3): 169–85.

de Jager, M., van Noort, J., van Gent, D. C., Dekker, C., Kanaar, R. & Wyman, C. (2001). Human rad50/mre11 is a flexible complex that can tether DNA ends, *Mol Cell* 8(5): 1129–35.

Delale, T., Paquin, A., Asselin-Paturel, C., Dalod, M., Brizard, G., Bates, E. E., Kastner, P., Chan, S., Akira, S., Vicari, A., Biron, C. A., Trinchieri, G. & Briere, F. (2005). Myd88-dependent and -independent murine cytomegalovirus sensing for ifn-alpha release and initiation of immune responses in vivo, *J Immunol* 175(10): 6723–32.

Doil, C., Mailand, N., Bekker-Jensen, S., Menard, P., Larsen, D. H., Pepperkok, R., Ellenberg, J., Panier, S., Durocher, D., Bartek, J., Lukas, J. & Lukas, C. (2009). Rnf168 binds and amplifies ubiquitin conjugates on damaged chromosomes to allow accumulation of repair proteins, *Cell* 136(3): 435–46.

Dragoi, A. M., Fu, X., Ivanov, S., Zhang, P., Sheng, L., Wu, D., Li, G. C. & Chu, W. M. (2005). DNA-pkcs, but not tlr9, is required for activation of akt by cpg-DNA, *EMBO J* 24(4): 779–89.

D'Silva, I., Pelletier, J. D., Lagueux, J., D'Amours, D., Chaudhry, M. A., Weinfeld, M., Lees-Miller, S. P. & Poirier, G. G. (1999). Relative affinities of poly(adp-ribose) polymerase and DNA-dependent protein kinase for DNA strand interruptions, *Biochim Biophys Acta* 1430(1): 119–26.

Duncan, T., Trewick, S. C., Koivisto, P., Bates, P. A., Lindahl, T. & Sedgwick, B. (2002). Reversal of DNA alkylation damage by two human dioxygenases, *Proc Natl Acad Sci U S A* 99(26): 16660–5.

Durocher, D. & Jackson, S. P. (2001). DNA-PK, ATM and ATR as sensors of DNA damage: variations on a theme?, *Curr Opin Cell Biol* 13(2): 225–31.

Essers, J., Houtsmuller, A. B., van Veelen, L., Paulusma, C., Nigg, A. L., Pastink, A., Vermeulen, W., Hoeijmakers, J. H. & Kanaar, R. (2002). Nuclear dynamics of rad52 group homologous recombination proteins in response to DNA damage, *EMBO J* 21(8): 2030–7.

Fernandes-Alnemri, T., Yu, J. W., Datta, P., Wu, J. & Alnemri, E. S. (2009). Aim2 activates the inflammasome and cell death in response to cytoplasmic DNA, *Nature* 458(7237): 509–13.

Fernandez-Capetillo, O., Celeste, A. & Nussenzweig, A. (2003). Focusing on foci: H2AX and the recruitment of DNA-damage response factors, *Cell Cycle* 2(5): 426–7.

Ferrara, L. & Kmiec, E. B. (2006). Targeted gene repair activates chk1 and chk2 and stalls replication in corrected cells, *DNA Repair (Amst)* 5(4): 422–31.

Fortini, P. & Dogliotti, E. (2007). Base damage and single-strand break repair: mechanisms and functional significance of short- and long-patch repair subpathways, *DNA Repair (Amst)* 6(4): 398–409.

Fragkos, M., Breuleux, M., Clement, N. & Beard, P. (2008). Recombinant adeno-associated viral vectors are deficient in provoking a DNA damage response, *J Virol* 82(15): 7379–87.

Friedberg, E. C. (1995). *DNA repair and mutagenesis*, American Society for Microbiology, Washington, DC.

Friedberg, E. C. (2001). How nucleotide excision repair protects against cancer, *Nat Rev Cancer* 1(1): 22–33.

Fugmann, S. D., Lee, A. I., Shockett, P. E., Villey, I. J. & Schatz, D. G. (2000). The rag proteins and v(d)j recombination: complexes, ends, and transposition, *Annu Rev Immunol* 18: 495–527.

Geoffroy, M. C. & Salvetti, A. (2005). Helper functions required for wild type and recombinant adeno-associated virus growth, *Curr Gene Ther* 5(3): 265–71.

George, J., Devoret, R. & Radman, M. (1974). Indirect ultraviolet-reactivation of phage lambda, *Proc Natl Acad Sci U S A* 71(1): 144–7.

Gerson, S. L. (2004). Mgmt: its role in cancer aetiology and cancer therapeutics, *Nat Rev Cancer* 4(4): 296–307.

Goodarzi, A. A., Jeggo, P. & Lobrich, M. (2010). The influence of heterochromatin on DNA double strand break repair: Getting the strong, silent type to relax, *DNA Repair (Amst)* 9(12): 1273–82.

Goodarzi, A. A., Jonnalagadda, J. C., Douglas, P., Young, D., Ye, R., Moorhead, G. B., Lees-Miller, S. P. & Khanna, K. K. (2004). Autophosphorylation of ataxia-telangiectasia mutated is regulated by protein phosphatase 2a, *EMBO J* 23(22): 4451–61.

Grundhoff, A. & Ganem, D. (2004). Inefficient establishment of kshv latency suggests an additional role for continued lytic replication in kaposi sarcoma pathogenesis, *J Clin Invest* 113(1): 124–36.

Guainazzi, A. & Scharer, O. D. (2010). Using synthetic DNA interstrand crosslinks to elucidate repair pathways and identify new therapeutic targets for cancer chemotherapy, *Cell Mol Life Sci* 67(21): 3683–97.

Guo, Z., Kozlov, S., Lavin, M. F., Person, M. D. & Paull, T. T. (2010). ATM activation by oxidative stress, *Science* 330(6003): 517–21.

Hanawalt, P. C. (2002). Subpathways of nucleotide excision repair and their regulation, *Oncogene* 21(58): 8949–56.

Hartlerode, A. J. & Scully, R. (2009). Mechanisms of double-strand break repair in somatic mammalian cells, *Biochem J* 423(2): 157–68.

Helleday, T., Lo, J., van Gent, D. C. & Engelward, B. P. (2007). DNA double-strand break repair: from mechanistic understanding to cancer treatment, *DNA Repair (Amst)* 6(7): 923–35.

Helleday, T., Petermann, E., Lundin, C., Hodgson, B. & Sharma, R. A. (2008). DNA repair pathways as targets for cancer therapy, *Nat Rev Cancer* 8(3): 193–204.

Hemmi, H., Takeuchi, O., Kawai, T., Kaisho, T., Sato, S., Sanjo, H., Matsumoto, M., Hoshino, K., Wagner, H., Takeda, K. & Akira, S. (2000). A toll-like receptor recognizes bacterial DNA, *Nature* 408(6813): 740–5.

Hornung, V., Ablasser, A., Charrel-Dennis, M., Bauernfeind, F., Horvath, G., Caffrey, D. R., Latz, E. & Fitzgerald, K. A. (2009). Aim2 recognizes cytosolic dsdna and forms a caspase-1-activating inflammasome with asc, *Nature* 458(7237): 514–8. Hornung, Veit Ablasser, Andrea Charrel-Dennis, Marie Bauernfeind, Franz Horvath, Gabor Caffrey, Daniel R Latz, Eicke Fitzgerald, Katherine A AI-065483/AI/NIAID NIH HHS/United States AI-067497/AI/NIAID NIH HHS/United States R01 AI067497-03/AI/NIAID NIH HHS/United States R01 AI067497-04/AI/NIAID NIH HHS/United States Research Support, N.I.H., Extramural Research Support, Non-U.S. Gov't England Nature Nature. 2009 Mar 26;458(7237):514-8. Epub 2009 Jan 21.

Hsiang, Y. H., Lihou, M. G. & Liu, L. F. (1989). Arrest of replication forks by drug-stabilized topoisomerase i-DNA cleavable complexes as a mechanism of cell killing by camptothecin, *Cancer Res* 49(18): 5077–82.

Huang, L. C., Clarkin, K. C. & Wahl, G. M. (1996). Sensitivity and selectivity of the DNA damage sensor responsible for activating p53-dependent g1 arrest, *Proc Natl Acad Sci U S A* 93(10): 4827–32.

Huen, M. S., Grant, R., Manke, I., Minn, K., Yu, X., Yaffe, M. B. & Chen, J. (2007). Rnf8 transduces the DNA-damage signal via histone ubiquitylation and checkpoint protein assembly, *Cell* 131(5): 901–14.

Ichijima, Y., Sakasai, R., Okita, N., Asahina, K., Mizutani, S. & Teraoka, H. (2005). Phosphorylation of histone H2AX at m phase in human cells without DNA damage response, *Biochem Biophys Res Commun* 336(3): 807–12.

Igoucheva, O., Alexeev, V. & Yoon, K. (2004). Oligonucleotide-directed mutagenesis and targeted gene correction: a mechanistic point of view, *Curr Mol Med* 4(5): 445–63.

Ikegami, S., Taguchi, T., Ohashi, M., Oguro, M., Nagano, H. & Mano, Y. (1978). Aphidicolin prevents mitotic cell division by interfering with the activity of DNA polymerase-alpha, *Nature* 275(5679): 458–60.

Iliakis, G. (2009). Backup pathways of nhej in cells of higher eukaryotes: cell cycle dependence, *Radiother Oncol* 92(3): 310–5.

Inagaki, A., Schoenmakers, S. & Baarends, W. M. (2010). DNA double strand break repair, chromosome synapsis and transcriptional silencing in meiosis, *Epigenetics* 5(4).

Inagaki, K., Ma, C., Storm, T. A., Kay, M. A. & Nakai, H. (2007). The role of DNA-pkcs and artemis in opening viral DNA hairpin termini in various tissues in mice, *J Virol* 81(20): 11304–21.

Jang, E. R., Choi, J. D., Park, M. A., Jeong, G., Cho, H. & Lee, J. S. (2010). ATM modulates transcription in response to histone deacetylase inhibition as part of its DNA damage response, *Exp Mol Med* 42(3): 195–204.

Jazayeri, A., Balestrini, A., Garner, E., Haber, J. E. & Costanzo, V. (2008). Mre11-rad50-nbs1-dependent processing of DNA breaks generates oligonucleotides that stimulate ATM activity, *Embo J* 27(14): 1953–62.

Jeggo, P. A., Taccioli, G. E. & Jackson, S. P. (1995). Menage a trois: double strand break repair, v(d)j recombination and DNA-PK, *Bioessays* 17(11): 949–57. Bioessays. 1995 Nov;17(11):949-57.

Jeggo, P. & Lavin, M. F. (2009). Cellular radiosensitivity: how much better do we understand it?, *Int J Radiat Biol* 85(12): 1061–81.

Johnson, R. D. & Jasin, M. (2000). Sister chromatid gene conversion is a prominent double-strand break repair pathway in mammalian cells, *EMBO J* 19(13): 3398–407.

Jungmichel, S. & Stucki, M. (2010). Mdc1: The art of keeping things in focus, *Chromosoma* .

Jurvansuu, J., Raj, K., Stasiak, A. & Beard, P. (2005). Viral transport of DNA damage that mimics a stalled replication fork, *J Virol* 79(1): 569–80.

Karpova, A. Y., Trost, M., Murray, J. M., Cantley, L. C. & Howley, P. M. (2002). Interferon regulatory factor-3 is an in vivo target of DNA-PK, *Proc Natl Acad Sci U S A* 99(5): 2818–23.

Kastan, M. B. & Bartek, J. (2004). Cell-cycle checkpoints and cancer, *Nature* 432(7015): 316–23.

Kilzer, J. M., Stracker, T., Beitzel, B., Meek, K., Weitzman, M. & Bushman, F. D. (2003). Roles of host cell factors in circularization of retroviral DNA, *Virology* 314(1): 460–7.

Kim, W. J., Rajasekaran, B. & Brown, K. D. (2007). Mlh1- and ATM-dependent mapk signaling is activated through c-abl in response to the alkylator n-methyl-n′-nitro-n′-nitrosoguanidine, *J Biol Chem* 282(44): 32021–31.

Kim, Y. C., Gerlitz, G., Furusawa, T., Catez, F., Nussenzweig, A., Oh, K. S., Kraemer, K. H., Shiloh, Y. & Bustin, M. (2009). Activation of ATM depends on chromatin interactions occurring before induction of DNA damage, *Nat Cell Biol* 11(1): 92–6.

Knipscheer, P., Raschle, M., Smogorzewska, A., Enoiu, M., Ho, T. V., Scharer, O. D., Elledge, S. J. & Walter, J. C. (2009). The fanconi anemia pathway promotes replication-dependent DNA interstrand cross-link repair, *Science* 326(5960): 1698–701.

Koch, C. A., Agyei, R., Galicia, S., Metalnikov, P., O'Donnell, P., Starostine, A., Weinfeld, M. & Durocher, D. (2004). XRCC4 physically links DNA end processing by polynucleotide kinase to DNA ligation by DNA ligase iv, *EMBO J* 23(19): 3874–85.

Kohn, K. W. (1999). Molecular interaction map of the mammalian cell cycle control and DNA repair systems, *Mol Biol Cell* 10(8): 2703–34.

Kohn, K. W., Pommier, Y., Kerrigan, D., Markovits, J. & Covey, J. M. (1987). Topoisomerase ii as a target of anticancer drug action in mammalian cells, *NCI Monogr* (4): 61–71.

Kolas, N. K., Chapman, J. R., Nakada, S., Ylanko, J., Chahwan, R., Sweeney, F. D., Panier, S., Mendez, M., Wildenhain, J., Thomson, T. M., Pelletier, L., Jackson, S. P. & Durocher, D. (2007). Orchestration of the DNA-damage response by the rnf8 ubiquitin ligase, *Science* 318(5856): 1637–40.

Kudoh, A., Fujita, M., Zhang, L., Shirata, N., Daikoku, T., Sugaya, Y., Isomura, H., Nishiyama, Y. & Tsurumi, T. (2005). Epstein-barr virus lytic replication elicits ATM checkpoint signal transduction while providing an s-phase-like cellular environment, *J Biol Chem* 280(9): 8156–63.

Kumagai, A., Lee, J., Yoo, H. Y. & Dunphy, W. G. (2006). Topbp1 activates the ATR-atrip complex, *Cell* 124(5): 943–55.

Kunkel, T. A. & Erie, D. A. (2005). DNA mismatch repair, *Annu Rev Biochem* 74: 681–710.

Lau, A., Swinbank, K. M., Ahmed, P. S., Taylor, D. L., Jackson, S. P., Smith, G. C. & O'Connor, M. J. (2005). Suppression of hiv-1 infection by a small molecule inhibitor of the ATM kinase, *Nat Cell Biol* 7(5): 493–500.

Lee, J. H. & Paull, T. T. (2004). Direct activation of the ATM protein kinase by the mre11/rad50/nbs1 complex, *Science* 304(5667): 93–6.

Lee, J. H. & Paull, T. T. (2005). ATM activation by DNA double-strand breaks through the mre11-rad50-nbs1 complex, *Science* 308(5721): 551–4.

Lee-Kirsch, M. A., Gong, M., Chowdhury, D., Senenko, L., Engel, K., Lee, Y. A., de Silva, U., Bailey, S. L., Witte, T., Vyse, T. J., Kere, J., Pfeiffer, C., Harvey, S., Wong, A., Koskenmies, S., Hummel, O., Rohde, K., Schmidt, R. E., Dominiczak, A. F., Gahr, M., Hollis, T., Perrino, F. W., Lieberman, J. & Hubner, N. (2007). Mutations in the gene encoding the 3'-5' DNA exonuclease trex1 are associated with systemic lupus erythematosus, *Nat Genet* 39(9): 1065–7.

Li, G. M. (1999). The role of mismatch repair in DNA damage-induced apoptosis, *Oncol Res* 11(9): 393–400.

Li, G. M. (2008). Mechanisms and functions of DNA mismatch repair, *Cell Res* 18(1): 85–98.

Li, J. J. & Deshaies, R. J. (1993). Exercising self-restraint: discouraging illicit acts of s and m in eukaryotes, *Cell* 74(2): 223–6.

Li, L., Olvera, J. M., Yoder, K. E., Mitchell, R. S., Butler, S. L., Lieber, M., Martin, S. L. & Bushman, F. D. (2001). Role of the non-homologous DNA end joining pathway in the early steps of retroviral infection, *EMBO J* 20(12): 3272–81.

Li, L. & Zou, L. (2005). Sensing, signaling, and responding to DNA damage: organization of the checkpoint pathways in mammalian cells, *J Cell Biochem* 94(2): 298–306.

Lilley, C. E., Carson, C. T., Muotri, A. R., Gage, F. H. & Weitzman, M. D. (2005). DNA repair proteins affect the lifecycle of herpes simplex virus 1, *Proc Natl Acad Sci U S A* 102(16): 5844–9.

Lilley, C. E., Schwartz, R. A. & Weitzman, M. D. (2007). Using or abusing: viruses and the cellular DNA damage response, *Trends Microbiol* 15(3): 119–26.

Liu, Y. & Maizels, N. (2000). Coordinated response of mammalian rad51 and rad52 to DNA damage, *EMBO Rep* 1(1): 85–90.

Liu, Y. & West, S. C. (2004). Happy hollidays: 40th anniversary of the holliday junction, *Nat Rev Mol Cell Biol* 5(11): 937–44.

Lobrich, M. & Jeggo, P. A. (2007). The impact of a negligent g2/m checkpoint on genomic instability and cancer induction, *Nat Rev Cancer* 7(11): 861–9.

Lopez-Contreras, A. J. & Fernandez-Capetillo, O. (2010). The ATR barrier to replication-born DNA damage, *DNA Repair (Amst)* 9(12): 1249–55.

Lukas, C., Falck, J., Bartkova, J., Bartek, J. & Lukas, J. (2003). Distinct spatiotemporal dynamics of mammalian checkpoint regulators induced by DNA damage, *Nat Cell Biol* 5(3): 255–60.

Lukas, J., Lukas, C. & Bartek, J. (2004). Mammalian cell cycle checkpoints: signalling pathways and their organization in space and time, *DNA Repair (Amst)* 3(8-9): 997–1007.

Lund, J., Sato, A., Akira, S., Medzhitov, R. & Iwasaki, A. (2003). Toll-like receptor 9-mediated recognition of herpes simplex virus-2 by plasmacytoid dendritic cells, *J Exp Med* 198(3): 513–20.

Lundin, C., Erixon, K., Arnaudeau, C., Schultz, N., Jenssen, D., Meuth, M. & Helleday, T. (2002). Different roles for nonhomologous end joining and homologous recombination following replication arrest in mammalian cells, *Mol Cell Biol* 22(16): 5869–78.

Luo, M. H., Rosenke, K., Czornak, K. & Fortunato, E. A. (2007). Human cytomegalovirus disrupts both ataxia telangiectasia mutated protein (ATM)- and ATM-rad3-related kinase-mediated DNA damage responses during lytic infection, *J Virol* 81(4): 1934–50.

Luo, Y., Chen, A. Y. & Qiu, J. (2011). Bocavirus infection induces a DNA damage response that facilitates viral DNA replication and mediates cell death, *J Virol* 85(1): 133–45.

Ma, Y., Pannicke, U., Schwarz, K. & Lieber, M. R. (2002). Hairpin opening and overhang processing by an artemis/DNA-dependent protein kinase complex in nonhomologous end joining and v(d)j recombination, *Cell* 108(6): 781–94.

Malanga, M. & Althaus, F. R. (2005). The role of poly(adp-ribose) in the DNA damage signaling network, *Biochem Cell Biol* 83(3): 354–64.

Malanga, M., Pleschke, J. M., Kleczkowska, H. E. & Althaus, F. R. (1998). Poly(adp-ribose) binds to specific domains of p53 and alters its DNA binding functions, *J Biol Chem* 273(19): 11839–43.

Masson, C., Bury-Mone, S., Guiot, E., Saez-Cirion, A., Schoevaert-Brossault, D., Brachet-Ducos, C., Delelis, O., Subra, F., Jeanson-Leh, L. & Mouscadet, J. F. (2007). Ku80 participates in the targeting of retroviral transgenes to the chromatin of cho cells, *J Virol* 81(15): 7924–32.

Matsuoka, S., Ballif, B. A., Smogorzewska, A., McDonald, E. R., r., Hurov, K. E., Luo, J., Bakalarski, C. E., Zhao, Z., Solimini, N., Lerenthal, Y., Shiloh, Y., Gygi, S. P. & Elledge, S. J. (2007). ATM and ATR substrate analysis reveals extensive protein networks responsive to DNA damage, *Science* 316(5828): 1160–6.

Mazumdar, M., Lee, J. H., Sengupta, K., Ried, T., Rane, S. & Misteli, T. (2006). Tumor formation via loss of a molecular motor protein, *Curr Biol* 16(15): 1559–64.

McAdams, H. H. & Arkin, A. (1999). It's a noisy business! genetic regulation at the nanomolar scale, *Trends Genet* 15(2): 65–9.

Misteli, T. & Soutoglou, E. (2009). The emerging role of nuclear architecture in DNA repair and genome maintenance, *Nat Rev Mol Cell Biol* 10(4): 243–54.

Moreno-Herrero, F., de Jager, M., Dekker, N. H., Kanaar, R., Wyman, C. & Dekker, C. (2005). Mesoscale conformational changes in the DNA-repair complex rad50/mre11/nbs1 upon binding DNA, *Nature* 437(7057): 440–3.

Mosesso, P., Palitti, F., Pepe, G., Pinero, J., Bellacima, R., Ahnstrom, G. & Natarajan, A. T. (2010). Relationship between chromatin structure, DNA damage and repair following x-irradiation of human lymphocytes, *Mutat Res* 701(1): 86–91.

Moshous, D., Callebaut, I., de Chasseval, R., Corneo, B., Cavazzana-Calvo, M., Le Deist, F., Tezcan, I., Sanal, O., Bertrand, Y., Philippe, N., Fischer, A. & de Villartay, J. P. (2001). Artemis, a novel DNA double-strand break repair/v(d)j recombination protein, is mutated in human severe combined immune deficiency, *Cell* 105(2): 177–86.

Nash, K., Chen, W., Salganik, M. & Muzyczka, N. (2009). Identification of cellular proteins that interact with the adeno-associated virus rep protein, *J Virol* 83(1): 454–69.

Nichols, G. J., Schaack, J. & Ornelles, D. A. (2009). Widespread phosphorylation of histone H2AX by species c adenovirus infection requires viral DNA replication, *J Virol* 83(12): 5987–98.

Nick McElhinny, S. A., Havener, J. M., Garcia-Diaz, M., Juarez, R., Bebenek, K., Kee, B. L., Blanco, L., Kunkel, T. A. & Ramsden, D. A. (2005). A gradient of template dependence defines distinct biological roles for family x polymerases in nonhomologous end joining, *Mol Cell* 19(3): 357–66.

Nur, E. K. A., Li, T. K., Zhang, A., Qi, H., Hars, E. S. & Liu, L. F. (2003). Single-stranded DNA induces ataxia telangiectasia mutant (ATM)/p53-dependent DNA damage and apoptotic signals, *J Biol Chem* 278(14): 12475–81.

Orelli, B., McClendon, T. B., Tsodikov, O. V., Ellenberger, T., Niedernhofer, L. J. & Scharer, O. D. (2010). The xpa-binding domain of ercc1 is required for nucleotide excision repair but not other DNA repair pathways, *J Biol Chem* 285(6): 3705–12.

Park, Y., Lee, S. W. & Sung, Y. C. (2002). Cutting edge: Cpg DNA inhibits dendritic cell apoptosis by up-regulating cellular inhibitor of apoptosis proteins through the phosphatidylinositide-3'-oh kinase pathway, *J Immunol* 168(1): 5–8.

Patil, S. D., Rhodes, D. G. & Burgess, D. J. (2005). DNA-based therapeutics and DNA delivery systems: a comprehensive review, *Aaps J* 7(1): E61–77.

Paull, T. T. & Gellert, M. (1998). The 3' to 5' exonuclease activity of mre 11 facilitates repair of DNA double-strand breaks, *Mol Cell* 1(7): 969–79.

Paull, T. T. & Gellert, M. (1999). Nbs1 potentiates atp-driven DNA unwinding and endonuclease cleavage by the mre11/rad50 complex, *Genes Dev* 13(10): 1276–88.

Pellegrini, L., Yu, D. S., Lo, T., Anand, S., Lee, M., Blundell, T. L. & Venkitaraman, A. R. (2002). Insights into DNA recombination from the structure of a rad51-BRCA2 complex, *Nature* 420(6913): 287–93.

Peng, Y., Woods, R. G., Beamish, H., Ye, R., Lees-Miller, S. P., Lavin, M. F. & Bedford, J. S. (2005). Deficiency in the catalytic subunit of DNA-dependent protein kinase causes down-regulation of ATM, *Cancer Res* 65(5): 1670–7.

Perry, J. J., Yannone, S. M., Holden, L. G., Hitomi, C., Asaithamby, A., Han, S., Cooper, P. K., Chen, D. J. & Tainer, J. A. (2006). Wrn exonuclease structure and molecular mechanism imply an editing role in DNA end processing, *Nat Struct Mol Biol* 13(5): 414–22.

Polo, S. E. & Jackson, S. P. (2011). Dynamics of DNA damage response proteins at DNA breaks: a focus on protein modifications, *Genes Dev* 25(5): 409–33.

Quanz, M., Berthault, N., Roulin, C., Roy, M., Herbette, A., Agrario, C., Alberti, C., Josserand, V., Coll, J. L., Sastre-Garau, X., Cosset, J. M., Larue, L., Sun, J. S. & Dutreix, M. (2009). Small-molecule drugs mimicking DNA damage: a new strategy for sensitizing tumors to radiotherapy, *Clin Cancer Res* 15(4): 1308–16.

Quanz, M., Chassoux, D., Berthault, N., Agrario, C., Sun, J. S. & Dutreix, M. (2009). Hyperactivation of DNA-PK by double-strand break mimicking molecules disorganizes DNA damage response, *PLoS One* 4(7): e6298.

Raderschall, E., Golub, E. I. & Haaf, T. (1999). Nuclear foci of mammalian recombination proteins are located at single-stranded DNA regions formed after DNA damage, *Proc Natl Acad Sci U S A* 96(5): 1921–6.

Radford, I. R. (1985). The level of induced DNA double-strand breakage correlates with cell killing after x-irradiation, *Int J Radiat Biol Relat Stud Phys Chem Med* 48(1): 45–54.

Raschle, M., Knipscheer, P., Enoiu, M., Angelov, T., Sun, J., Griffith, J. D., Ellenberger, T. E., Scharer, O. D. & Walter, J. C. (2008). Mechanism of replication-coupled DNA interstrand crosslink repair, *Cell* 134(6): 969–80.

Rathinam, V. A. & Fitzgerald, K. A. (2011). Innate immune sensing of DNA viruses, *Virology* 411(2): 153–62.

Reardon, J. T. & Sancar, A. (2005). Nucleotide excision repair, *Prog Nucleic Acid Res Mol Biol* 79: 183–235.

Riballo, E., Kuhne, M., Rief, N., Doherty, A., Smith, G. C., Recio, M. J., Reis, C., Dahm, K., Fricke, A., Krempler, A., Parker, A. R., Jackson, S. P., Gennery, A., Jeggo, P. A. & Lobrich, M. (2004). A pathway of double-strand break rejoining dependent upon ATM, artemis, and proteins locating to gamma-H2AX foci, *Mol Cell* 16(5): 715–24.

Rosidi, B., Wang, M., Wu, W., Sharma, A., Wang, H. & Iliakis, G. (2008). Histone h1 functions as a stimulatory factor in backup pathways of nhej, *Nucleic Acids Res* 36(5): 1610–23.

Rossi, J. J. (2004). Medicine: a cholesterol connection in rnai, *Nature* 432(7014): 155–6.

Rouleau, M., Patel, A., Hendzel, M. J., Kaufmann, S. H. & Poirier, G. G. (2010). Parp inhibition: Parp1 and beyond, *Nat Rev Cancer* 10(4): 293–301.

Rupnik, A., Grenon, M. & Lowndes, N. (2008). The mrn complex, *Curr Biol* 18(11): R455–7.

Sakurai, Y., Komatsu, K., Agematsu, K. & Matsuoka, M. (2009). DNA double strand break repair enzymes function at multiple steps in retroviral infection, *Retrovirology* 6: 114.

Sartori, A. A., Lukas, C., Coates, J., Mistrik, M., Fu, S., Bartek, J., Baer, R., Lukas, J. & Jackson, S. P. (2007). Human ctip promotes DNA end resection, *Nature* 450(7169): 509–14.

Schiavone, N., Papucci, L., Luciani, P., Lapucci, A., Donnini, M. & Capaccioli, S. (2000). Induction of apoptosis and mitosis inhibition by degraded DNA lipotransfection mimicking genotoxic drug effects, *Biochem Biophys Res Commun* 270(2): 406–14.

Schlacher, K. & Goodman, M. F. (2007). Lessons from 50 years of sos DNA-damage-induced mutagenesis, *Nat Rev Mol Cell Biol* 8(7): 587–94.

Schwartz, R. A., Carson, C. T., Schuberth, C. & Weitzman, M. D. (2009). Adeno-associated virus replication induces a DNA damage response coordinated by DNA-dependent protein kinase, *J Virol* 83(12): 6269–78.

Scully, R., Chen, J., Ochs, R. L., Keegan, K., Hoekstra, M., Feunteun, J. & Livingston, D. M. (1997). Dynamic changes of BRCA1 subnuclear location and phosphorylation state are initiated by DNA damage, *Cell* 90(3): 425–35.

Sester, D. P., Brion, K., Trieu, A., Goodridge, H. S., Roberts, T. L., Dunn, J., Hume, D. A., Stacey, K. J. & Sweet, M. J. (2006). Cpg DNA activates survival in murine macrophages through tlr9 and the phosphatidylinositol 3-kinase-akt pathway, *J Immunol* 177(7): 4473–80.

Shell, S. M., Li, Z., Shkriabai, N., Kvaratskhelia, M., Brosey, C., Serrano, M. A., Chazin, W. J., Musich, P. R. & Zou, Y. (2009). Checkpoint kinase ATR promotes nucleotide excision repair of uv-induced DNA damage via physical interaction with xeroderma pigmentosum group a, *J Biol Chem* 284(36): 24213–22.

Shimodaira, H., Yoshioka-Yamashita, A., Kolodner, R. D. & Wang, J. Y. (2003). Interaction of mismatch repair protein pms2 and the p53-related transcription factor p73 in apoptosis response to cisplatin, *Proc Natl Acad Sci U S A* 100(5): 2420–5.

Shreeram, S., Hee, W. K., Demidov, O. N., Kek, C., Yamaguchi, H., Fornace, A. J., J., Anderson, C. W., Appella, E. & Bulavin, D. V. (2006). Regulation of ATM/p53-dependent suppression of myc-induced lymphomas by wip1 phosphatase, *J Exp Med* 203(13): 2793–9.

Skalka, A. M. & Katz, R. A. (2005). Retroviral DNA integration and the DNA damage response, *Cell Death Differ* 12 Suppl 1: 971–8.

Smith, J., Tho, L. M., Xu, N. & Gillespie, D. A. (2010). The ATM-chk2 and ATR-chk1 pathways in DNA damage signaling and cancer, *Adv Cancer Res* 108: 73–112.

Soutoglou, E. & Misteli, T. (2008). Activation of the cellular DNA damage response in the absence of DNA lesions, *Science* 320(5882): 1507–10.

Stewart, G. S., Panier, S., Townsend, K., Al-Hakim, A. K., Kolas, N. K., Miller, E. S., Nakada, S., Ylanko, J., Olivarius, S., Mendez, M., Oldreive, C., Wildenhain, J., Tagliaferro, A., Pelletier, L., Taubenheim, N., Durandy, A., Byrd, P. J., Stankovic, T., Taylor, A. M. & Durocher, D. (2009). The riddle syndrome protein mediates a ubiquitin-dependent signaling cascade at sites of DNA damage, *Cell* 136(3): 420–34.

Stiff, T., O'Driscoll, M., Rief, N., Iwabuchi, K., Lobrich, M. & Jeggo, P. A. (2004). ATM and DNA-PK function redundantly to phosphorylate H2AX after exposure to ionizing radiation, *Cancer Res* 64(7): 2390–6.

Stracker, T. H., Carson, C. T. & Weitzman, M. D. (2002). Adenovirus oncoproteins inactivate the mre11-rad50-nbs1 DNA repair complex, *Nature* 418(6895): 348–52.

Stracker, T. H., Cassell, G. D., Ward, P., Loo, Y. M., van Breukelen, B., Carrington-Lawrence, S. D., Hamatake, R. K., van der Vliet, P. C., Weller, S. K., Melendy, T. & Weitzman, M. D. (2004). The rep protein of adeno-associated virus type 2 interacts with single-stranded DNA-binding proteins that enhance viral replication, *J Virol* 78(1): 441–53.

Strumberg, D., Pilon, A. A., Smith, M., Hickey, R., Malkas, L. & Pommier, Y. (2000). Conversion of topoisomerase i cleavage complexes on the leading strand of ribosomal DNA into 5'-phosphorylated DNA double-strand breaks by replication runoff, *Mol Cell Biol* 20(11): 3977–87.

Sy, S. M., Huen, M. S. & Chen, J. (2009). Palb2 is an integral component of the BRCA complex required for homologous recombination repair, *Proc Natl Acad Sci U S A* 106(17): 7155–60.

Takaoka, A. & Taniguchi, T. (2008). Cytosolic DNA recognition for triggering innate immune responses, *Adv Drug Deliv Rev* 60(7): 847–57.

Takaoka, A., Wang, Z., Choi, M. K., Yanai, H., Negishi, H., Ban, T., Lu, Y., Miyagishi, M., Kodama, T., Honda, K., Ohba, Y. & Taniguchi, T. (2007). Dai (dlm-1/zbp1) is a cytosolic DNA sensor and an activator of innate immune response, *Nature* 448(7152): 501–5.

Toledo, L. I., Murga, M., Gutierrez-Martinez, P., Soria, R. & Fernandez-Capetillo, O. (2008). ATR signaling can drive cells into senescence in the absence of DNA breaks, *Genes Dev* 22(3): 297–302.

Van Dyck, E., Stasiak, A. Z., Stasiak, A. & West, S. C. (2001). Visualization of recombination intermediates produced by rad52-mediated single-strand annealing, *EMBO Rep* 2(10): 905–9.

van Heemst, D., Brugmans, L., Verkaik, N. S. & van Gent, D. C. (2004). End-joining of blunt DNA double-strand breaks in mammalian fibroblasts is precise and requires DNA-PK and XRCC4, *DNA Repair (Amst)* 3(1): 43–50.

Vilaysane, A. & Muruve, D. A. (2009). The innate immune response to DNA, *Semin Immunol* 21(4): 208–14.

Wagner, H. (2004). The immunobiology of the tlr9 subfamily, *Trends Immunol* 25(7): 381–6.

Wang, S., Guo, M., Ouyang, H., Li, X., Cordon-Cardo, C., Kurimasa, A., Chen, D. J., Fuks, Z., Ling, C. C. & Li, G. C. (2000). The catalytic subunit of DNA-dependent protein kinase selectively regulates p53-dependent apoptosis but not cell-cycle arrest, *Proc Natl Acad Sci U S A* 97(4): 1584–8.

Wang, X., Ohnishi, K., Takahashi, A. & Ohnishi, T. (1998). Poly(adp-ribosyl)ation is required for p53-dependent signal transduction induced by radiation, *Oncogene* 17(22): 2819–25.

Wang, X., Peterson, C. A., Zheng, H., Nairn, R. S., Legerski, R. J. & Li, L. (2001). Involvement of nucleotide excision repair in a recombination-independent and error-prone pathway of DNA interstrand cross-link repair, *Mol Cell Biol* 21(3): 713–20.

Wang, Y., Li, H., Tang, Q., Maul, G. G. & Yuan, Y. (2008). Kaposi's sarcoma-associated herpesvirus ori-lyt-dependent DNA replication: involvement of host cellular factors, *J Virol* 82(6): 2867–82.

Ward, I. & Chen, J. (2004). Early events in the DNA damage response, *Curr Top Dev Biol* 63: 1–35.

Ward, I. M. & Chen, J. (2001). Histone H2AX is phosphorylated in an ATR-dependent manner in response to replicational stress, *J Biol Chem* 276(51): 47759–62.

Ward, J. F. (1975). Radiation-induced strand breakage in DNA, *Basic Life Sci* 5B: 471–2.

Weitzman, M. D., Carson, C. T., Schwartz, R. A. & Lilley, C. E. (2004). Interactions of viruses with the cellular DNA repair machinery, *DNA Repair (Amst)* 3(8-9): 1165–73.

Weitzman, M. D. & Ornelles, D. A. (2005). Inactivating intracellular antiviral responses during adenovirus infection, *Oncogene* 24(52): 7686–96.

Weterings, E. & Chen, D. J. (2007). DNA-dependent protein kinase in nonhomologous end joining: a lock with multiple keys?, *J Cell Biol* 179(2): 183–6.

Weterings, E. & van Gent, D. C. (2004). The mechanism of non-homologous end-joining: a synopsis of synapsis, *DNA Repair (Amst)* 3(11): 1425–35.

Wieler, S., Gagne, J. P., Vaziri, H., Poirier, G. G. & Benchimol, S. (2003). Poly(adp-ribose) polymerase-1 is a positive regulator of the p53-mediated g1 arrest response following ionizing radiation, *J Biol Chem* 278(21): 18914–21.

Wilkinson, D. E. & Weller, S. K. (2006). Herpes simplex virus type i disrupts the ATR-dependent DNA-damage response during lytic infection, *J Cell Sci* 119(Pt 13): 2695–703.

Wyman, C. & Kanaar, R. (2006). DNA double-strand break repair: all's well that ends well, *Annu Rev Genet* 40: 363–83.

Yanai, H., Savitsky, D., Tamura, T. & Taniguchi, T. (2009). Regulation of the cytosolic DNA-sensing system in innate immunity: a current view, *Curr Opin Immunol* 21(1): 17–22.

Yang, J., Yu, Y., Hamrick, H. E. & Duerksen-Hughes, P. J. (2003). ATM, ATR and DNA-PK: initiators of the cellular genotoxic stress responses, *Carcinogenesis* 24(10): 1571–80.

Yang, Y. G., Lindahl, T. & Barnes, D. E. (2007). Trex1 exonuclease degrades ssdna to prevent chronic checkpoint activation and autoimmune disease, *Cell* 131(5): 873–86.

Yarosh, D. B. (2001). Why is DNA damage signaling so complicated? chaos and molecular signaling, *Environ Mol Mutagen* 38(2-3): 132–4.

Yoshioka, K., Yoshioka, Y. & Hsieh, P. (2006). ATR kinase activation mediated by mutsalpha and mutlalpha in response to cytotoxic o6-methylguanine adducts, *Mol Cell* 22(4): 501–10.

Yun, M. H. & Hiom, K. (2009). Ctip-BRCA1 modulates the choice of DNA double-strand-break repair pathway throughout the cell cycle, *Nature* 459(7245): 460–3.

Zhu, Y., Hu, J., Hu, Y. & Liu, W. (2009). Targeting DNA repair pathways: a novel approach to reduce cancer therapeutic resistance, *Cancer Treat Rev* 35(7): 590–6.

16

# DNA Repair in Pathogenic Eukaryotic Cells: Insights from Comparative Genomics of Parasitic Protozoan

Laurence A. Marchat[1,2], Mavil López-Casamichana[3], Esther Orozco[3] and César López-Camarillo[3]
*[1]Escuela Nacional de Medicina y Homeopatía-IPN, Programa Institucional de Biomedicina Molecular*
*[2]Programa de Doctorado en Biotecnología en Red-IPN*
*[3]Universidad Autónoma de la Ciudad de México, Posgrado en Ciencias Genómicas*
*México*

## 1. Introduction

Numerous external and internal DNA damaging agents can affect genetic material to produce single-strand breaks (SSB), double strand breaks (DSB), inter- and intra-strand cross-links in the form of cyclobutane pyrimidine dimers and (6-4)-photoproducts, oxidation and alkylation of bases, or formation of bulky chemical adducts. Cells possess several biological processes that act in a coordinated way to supervise DNA molecules and properly repair DNA lesions to minimize genetic information loss. This DNA repair system, which has been conserved throughout eukaryotes and prokaryotes evolution, includes various pathways that can be classified according to the type of DNA lesion they can restore: i) DSB, the most detrimental lesions of DNA, can be repaired by homologous recombination (HRR) and non-homologous end joining (NHEJ) pathways [Fleck & Nielsen, 2004]; ii) aberrant bases or nucleotides from a single strand DNA can be repaired by base excision repair (BER), nucleotide excision repair (NER) and mismatch repair (MMR) pathways using the complementary strand as template for DNA synthesis. BER mainly restores non-bulky lesions that result from bases alkylation, oxidation or deamination [Krokan et al., 1997]. The main task of NER pathway, which consists in two subpathways: global genome repair (GGR) to remove damage in the overall genome and transcription-coupled repair (TCR) to specifically repair the transcribed strand of active genes, is to eliminate photoproducts produced by ultraviolet (UV) light and other bulky lesions, such as inter- and intra-strand crosslinks [Prakash &Prakash, 2000]. MMR allows the removal of base mismatches and small insertion/deletion loops (IDL) that are formed during the replication process [Marti et al., 2002].

The genome of protozoan parasites is continuously subjected to the effects of antiparasitic drugs and host immune system attacks, which can affect its stability and therefore parasite survival. Thus, efficient DNA maintenance mechanisms are necessary to detect and accurately repair damaged nucleotides. The fully sequenced genome of the four major human pathogens described here provides new insights into parasite biology, including molecular features of

DNA repair mechanisms, and genome evolution. *Entamoeba histolytica* and *Giardia lamblia* (syn. *G. intestinalis, G. duodenalis*) are intestinal parasites that cause diarrheal diseases. *E. histolytica* is responsible for fulminating dysentery, bloody diarrhea, weight loss, fatigue, abdominal pain, which affect 50 million people and provoke 100,000 deaths in developing countries each year. In some cases, *E. histolytica* trophozoites can cross the intestinal wall and use the blood stream to reach different vital organs of the human body, usually the liver (but also the lungs, brain or spleen) to provoke liver abscesses, which can be fatal if untreated [Guo et al., 2007]. *G. lamblia* is another contributor to the enormous burden of diarrheal diseases with over 250 million symptomatic human infections per year worldwide. This anaerobic flagellated protozoa colonises and reproduces in the small intestine of several vertebrates, including human, causing giardiasis, commonly known as Beaver fever, which is characterized by diarrhea, excess gas, stomach or abdominal cramps, upset stomach, and nausea. Additionally, *Giardia* infection has an adverse impact on child linear growth and psychomotor development since the parasite causes iron-deficiency anemia, micronutrient deficiencies and growth retardation associated with diarrhea and malabsorption syndrome [Ankarklev et al., 2010]. Individuals become infected by *E. histolytica* and *G. lamblia* through ingesting or coming into contact with food, soil, or water that have been contaminated by the feces of an infected human or animal. *Plasmodium falciparum* is the protozoan parasite responsible for human malaria, which is one of the most severe infectious diseases with 240 million cases in 2009 and more than 1 million deaths in children each year in Africa alone. The presence of the parasite in red blood cells lead them to stick to blood vessels through a process called cytoadherence, which produce the obstruction of the microcirculation and dysfunction of multiple organs, typically the brain in cerebral malaria. Symptoms usually include fever and headache, in severe cases progressing to coma, and death (Kokwaro, 2009). Trichomoniasis caused by *Trichomonas vaginalis* is the most common nonviral sexually transmitted disease (STD) in the world [WHO, 1995]. It has long been recognized as a frequent cause of vaginitis in women and urethritis in men, but data now link it to cervical cancer and bad pregnancy outcomes [Cotch et al., 1997], as well as to an enhanced risk for human immunodeficiency virus transmission [Sorvillo & Kerndt , 1998]. Here, we combined the use of genomic approaches based on bioinformatic analysis of parasite genome sequence with the review of published reports to perform a comparative description of DNA repair machineries from *E. histolytica, G. lamblia, P. falciparum* and *T. vaginalis,* which cause high morbidity and mortality in many developed and developing countries.

## 2. DNA repair machineries in pathogenic eukaryotic cells

### 2.1 Identification of DNA repair machineries

In order to identify amino acids sequences of *E. histolytica, G. lamblia, P. falciparum* and *T. vaginalis* proteins related to DNA repair factors, we performed similarity searches in the Eupath database (http://eupathdb.org/eupathdb/) using the *Saccharomyces cerevisiae* DNA repair proteins from HRR, NHEJ, BER, NER and MMR machineries as probes [reviewed in Lopez-Camarillo et al., 2009]. Putative gene products were selected from BLAST analysis against each parasite database using the Blosum 62 scoring matrix and the following criteria: (i) at least 20% identity and 35% homology to the query sequence and (ii) e-value lower than 0.002, unless a portion of the protein showed a very strong similarity. All sequences, as well as the *E. histolytica* sequences obtained from previous work [López-Camarillo et al., 2009], were then verified by BLAST against *S. cerevisiae* and *Homo sapiens* databases to confirm their identity. Additionally, we also retrieved data from published reports about *G. lamblia,*

*P. falciparum* and *T. vaginalis* (**Table 1**). The absence of a given sequence in the table indicates that the corresponding gene was not identified in the parasite genome or that the sequence was too divergent to be detected by our *in silico* strategy.

None of the protozoan parasites studied here has the complete DNA repair pathways reported in yeast. HRR is the most conserved pathway suggesting that it is the mayor DSB repair pathway in these protozoan parasites. *E. histolytica, G. lamblia, P. falciparum* and *T. vaginalis* genomes contain most of the RAD52 epistasis group genes, although their functional relevance remains to be determined. Homologs for RAD50, RAD51, MRE11, RAD54 and RPA (lacking the RAD52 interacting domain) have been previously reported in *P. falciparum* [Voss et al., 2002; Malik et al., 2008]. In agreement with its participation in DNA repair, the *PfRad51* gene is overexpressed in the mitotically active schizont stage and in response to methyl methane sulfonate [Bhattacharyya & Kumar, 2003]. In. *T. vaginalis*, RAD50 y MRE11 were previously published as components of the meiotic recombination machinery, although meiosis has not been observed in this organism [Malik et al., 2008]. Ramesh et al. [2005] and Malik et al. [2008] identified the *Rad50/Mre11*, *Rad52* and *Dmc1 genes* involved in meiotic recombination machinery by HRR in *Giardia*. Intriguingly, *G. lamblia* and *P. falciparum* lack the *nsb1* homologue (*xrs2* in Yeast) that is a component of the MRN complex involved in DSB detection and 3´ ssDNA tails conversion. Recently, we published the *E. histolytica* RAD52 epistasis group involved in HRR [Lopez-Casamichana et al., 2007, 2008]. Interestingly, RT-PCR assays evidenced that some genes were down-regulated, whereas others were up-regulated when DSB were induced by UV-C irradiation, which revealed an intricate transcriptional modulation of *E. histolytica* RAD52 epistasis group related genes in response to DNA damage. Particularly, *Ehrad51* mRNA expression was 16-, 11- and 4-fold increased at 30 min, 3 h and 12 h, respectively. DNA microarrays assays confirmed the activation of *EhMre11, EhRad50*, and *EhRad54* genes at 5 min after DSB induction, suggesting that they represent early sensors of damage in HRR pathway [Weber et al., 2009]. Additionally, the molecular characterization of EhRAD51 showed that the presence of all the functional domains reported in yeast and human homologues. EhRAD51 was upregulated and redistributed from cytoplasm to the nucleus of trophozoites at 3 h after DNA damage and it was able to catalyze specific single-strand DNA (ssDNA) transfer to homologous double strand DNA (dsDNA) forming the three-stranded pairing molecule called D-loop structure, confirming that it is a *bonafide* recombinase in *E. histolytica* [Lopez-Casamichana et al., 2008].

*G. lamblia* and P. *falciparum* only have three of the eight factors of the NHEJ pathway (including the MNR complex also involved in HRR), which strongly suggest that they preferably use HRR to repair DSB. In contrast, almost all NEHJ pathway factors have been identified in *E. histolytica* and *T. vaginalis*, including the LIF1 ligase, RAD27 nuclease and MRE11/RAD50/NSB1 proteins. However, *E. histolytica* genome does not contain a homologous gene for KU80 subunit [López-Camarillo et al., 2009] and *T. vaginalis* lacks both *ku70* and *ku80* genes [Carlton et al., 2007]. As these proteins form a single KU complex that recognizes DSB sites and recruits other DNA repair factors, our findings could appear contradictory. The absence of conserved KU proteins has also been reported in *Encephalitozoon cunili* [Gill & Fast, 2007] and yeast [Hefferin & Tomkinson, 2005], thus it is possible that these organisms use highly divergent KU proteins to perform the NHEJ pathway.

The other key DNA repair mechanisms represented by BER, NER and MMR pathways operate to repair aberrant bases or nucleotides from a ssDNA using the complementary strand as template for DNA synthesis. As in *E. histolytica* [Lopez-Camarillo et al., 2009], the *G. lamblia* BER pathway appears to be largely incomplete, lacking *apn1, mag1, ogg1, rad10, mus81* and *mms4* genes. Both parasites live under oxygen-limiting conditions and have a highly reduced form of mitocondria called mitosomes [Tovar et al., 1999, 2003]. Then the absence of OGG1 could indicate that they do not suffer oxidative damage to mitochondrial DNA. In contrast, *Plasmodium* Flap endonuclease-1 (PfFEN-1) and Pf DNA Ligase I (PfLigI) have enzymatic activities similar to other species [Gardner et al., 2002; Casta et al., 2008], indicating that BER pathway should be functional in this parasite although several components are lacking.

Most genes involved in NER pathway are represented in *E. histolytica* [Lopez-Camarillo et al., 2009], *G. lamblia, P. falciparum and T. vaginalis* genomes suggesting that this mechanism could be potentially active in these eukaryotic parasites. PfXPB/RAD25, PfXPG/RAD2 and PfXPD/RAD3 have been previously reported in *P. falciparum* [Gardner et al., 2002; Bethke et al., 2007; Casta et al., 2008]. Additionally, the overexpression of *EhDdb1, EhRad23* and *EhRad54* genes after UV-induced DNA damage in *E. histolytica* [Weber et al., 2009] suggested that these genes could be involved in chromatin remodeling complexes as their homologues in human and yeast. *E. histolytica, G. lamblia* and *T. vaginalis* have various *rad3* genes to form the NEF3 complex (RAD2, RAD3, RAD25) of the BER pathway. Particularly, we identified six *rad3* genes and an additional truncated gene in *T. vaginalis*. On the other hand, all the parasites studied here lack almost one of the components of the TFIIH complex subunits (TFB1, TFB2 or TFB3).

As in bacteria, *Drosophila melanogaster, H. sapiens* and many other organisms [Lisby & Rothstein, 2005], *E. histolytica, G. lamblia* [Ramesh et al., 2005], *P. falciparum* [Bethke et al., 2007] and *T. vaginalis* [Malik et al., 2008] have almost all *S. cerevisiae* MMR genes, including the components of the MUTSα (MSH2/MSH6) heterodimer, which strongly suggest that MMR could be an active DNA repair pathway in these parasites. Notably, *E. histolytica* and *P. falciparum* have two *msh2* genes. However, neither *E. histolytica* nor *P. falciparum* present the *msh3* gene that is required for the formation of the MUTSβ (MSH2/MSH3) heterodimer. PfMSH2-1, PfMSH2-2, PfMSH6, PfMLH1 and PfPMS1 proteins potentially participating in MMR have been previously reported in *P. falciparum*. Inhibition of *PfMSH2-2* gene increased mutation rate and microsatellite polymorphism, indirectly demonstrating its relevance in MMR and microsatellite slippage prevention. Moreover, antimalarial drug resistance has been recently related to a defective DNA mismatch repair, mainly in PfMutLα content [Castellini et al., 2011], which demonstrated the relevance of this mechanism for the parasite biology.

| **Gene name** | *E. histolytica* | *G. lamblia* | *P. falciparum* | *T. vaginalis* | *S. cerevisiae* |
|---|---|---|---|---|---|
| **Homologous recombination repair (HRR) pathway** | | | | | |
| *rad50* | C4M2L7 | Q6WD96 | C6KSQ6 | A2FAD3 | P12753 |
| *mre11* | Q86C23<br>C4LVX7<br>C4M8N7* | Q86CI9<br>A8BR27* | PFA0390w** | A2ECB0 | P32829 |
| *nbs1* | C4M874 | - | - | A2DHF7 | P33301 |
| *rad51* | C4M4K4 | Q86C21 | Q8IIS8<br>Pf11_0087** | A2FXT7 | P25454 |
| *rad52* | C4M197 | Q6WD95 | - | - | P06778 |
| *rad54*<br>*rad54b* | C4LVM6<br>C4M7S7 | - | Q8IAN4 | A2FNE0 | P32863 |
| *rad51c*<br>*rad57* | C4M5L7 | - | - | A2GIB8 | P38953<br>P25301 |

| **Gene name** | *E. histolytica* | *G. lamblia* | *P. falciparum* | *T. vaginalis* | *S. cerevisiae* |
|---|---|---|---|---|---|
| *rad59* | - | - | - | - | Q12223 |
| *exo1* | C4MBM5 | A8BQ11 | Q8IBK1 | A2E2N7 | P39975 |
| *rpa1* | C4M8G6 | - | Q9U0J0<br>Q8I3A1 | A2G5D0 | P22336 |
| *rpa2* | C4LT79 | - | - | - | P26754 |
| *sgs1* | C4M4V5 | A8BAJ1<br>A8B9Y0 | Q8I2W7<br>Q8ILG5 | A2DYY2 | P35187 |
| *rad24* | C4M5T7 | - | - | A2D9F4 | P32641 |
| *hpr5* | - | - | Q8I3W6 | A2F783 | P12954 |
| rad17<br>ddc1<br>mec3 | -<br>-<br>- | -<br>-<br>- | -<br>-<br>- | -<br>A2F0Q2<br>- | P48581<br>Q08949<br>Q02574 |
| **Non homologous end joining (NHEJ) pathway** | | | | | |
| *ku80*<br>*ku70* | C4MBG9<br>- | -<br>- | -<br>- | -<br>- | P32807<br>Q04437 |
| *lif1* | - | - | - | - | P53150 |
| *dnl4* | C4M5H3 | - | - | A2DFX6 | Q08387 |
| *rad27* | C4M6G8 | A8B672<br>D3KG58 | Q7K734<br>Q8IJW1 | A2GNP0 | P26793 |
| **Base excision repair (BER) pathway** | | | | | |
| *apn1* | - | - | Q9BMG7 | - | P22936 |
| *apn21* | - | A8BGE2 | O97240 | - | P38207 |
| *mag1* | - | - | - | - | P22134 |
| *ogg1* | - | - | Q8I2Y2 | - | P53397 |
| *ntg1* | C4M764<br>C4LYM7 | - | Q8II68 | A2DS55 | P31378 |
| *ung1* | C4LUV5 | A8B632 | Q8ILU6 | A2GFQ7 | P12887 |
| *pcna* | C4M9R9 | A8BIU1 | P61074<br>Q7KQJ9 | A2DQV2 | P15873 |
| *rad1* | C4LT01 | D3KH96 | Q8ID22 | A2DS24 | P06777 |
| *rad10* | C4LW01 | - | O96136 | A2DBF5 | P06838 |
| *cdc9* | C4M5H3 | A8BWV4 | Q8IES4 | A2DFX6 | P04819 |
| *mus81* | - | - | - | A2FKU9 | Q04149 |
| *mms4* | - | - | - | A2DHF7 | P38257 |
| **Nucleotide excision repair (NER) pathway** | | | | | |
| *rad2* | C4M0V9 | - | O96154 | A2GNP0 | P07276 |
| *rad3* | C4M8K7<br>C4M8Q4<br>C4M6T8 | A8BYS3<br>A8B495 | Q8I2H7 | A2G2G8<br>A2E4I6<br>A2F1W2<br>A2DDD4<br>A2E1B9<br>A2ELX1<br>A2G2G9* | P06839 |

| Gene name | *E. histolytica* | *G. lamblia* | *P. falciparum* | *T. vaginalis* | *S. cerevisiae* |
|---|---|---|---|---|---|
| *rad4* | - | - | - | - | P14736 |
| *rad7* | - | - | - | - | P06779 |
| *rad14* | - | - | - | - | P28519 |
| *rad16* | - | A8BL62 | Q8I4S6 | A2D9P9 | P31244 |
| *rad23* | C4MAR5 | D3KF29* | Q8IJS8 | A2FM19 | P32628 |
| *rad25* | C4MA19 | A8BMI7 | Q8IJ31 | A2DEA8 | Q00578 |
| *rad26* | C4MAR8 | A8BK31 | - | A2EXQ4 | P40352 |
| *rad28* | - | - | Q8IJ73 | A2DZ24 | Q12021 |
| *ssl1* | C4LV67 | A8BA50 | Q8IEG6 | A2ENQ3 | Q04673 |
| *tfb1* | C4LWV8 | - | - | - | P32776 |
| *tfb2* | C4MIG0 | - | Q8I4Y8 | A2E2N2 | Q02939 |
| *tfb3* | - | D3KH94 | Q8I3Y3 | - | Q03290 |
| *tfb4* | C4M9E2 | A8B6C2 | Q8IDG5 | A2EYI3 | Q12004 |
| **Mismatch repair (MMR) pathway** | | | | | |
| *mlh1* | C4M5R1 | - | Q8IIJ0 | A2EGR5 | P38920 |
| *msh2* | C4M9J9<br>B1N4L6 | Q6WD97 | Q8ILI9<br>C0H4L8 | A2EP54 | P25847 |
| *msh3* | - | - | - | - | P25336 |
| *msh6* | C4M4T8 | A8BC61 | Q8I447 | A2EA54 | Q03834 |
| *pms1* | C4LW71 | A8B4I6 | Q8IBJ3 | A2G2B4 | P14242 |

Table 1. Comparison of DNA repair machineries from *E. histolytica, G. lamblia, P. falciparum, T. vaginalis* and *S. cerevisiae*. * fragment, ** PlasmoDB database.

### 2.2 Conservation of DNA repair pathways

To investigate the degree of conservation of DNA repair pathways in protozoan parasites, we next determined the values of Smith-Waterman identity scores between *E. histolytica* proteins and their corresponding orthologues in *G. lamblia, P. falciparum* and *T. vaginalis* by BLAST analysis based in pairwaise sequence alignments and calculated the mean value for each DNA repair machinery (**Fig. 1**). Data of the MNR complex which participate in HRR and NHEJ pathways were included in both mechanisms. DSB repair pathways were generally more conserved than Excision Repair mechanisms. Considering amino acids identity, mean values for HRR and NHEJ pathways were higher in *E. histolytica/P. falciparum* comparison, suggesting that *E. histolytica* machinery was closer to *P. falciparum* than to *G. lamblia* and *T. vaginalis* machineries. The comparison *E. histolytica/G. lamblia* evidenced that HRR is highly conserved between both parasites, whereas components of the other pathways were more divergent. In the case of *E. histolytica/P. falciparum* comparison, NHEJ appeared to be more conserved that HRR, while the identity of HRR and NHEJ factors was very similar in *E. histolytica/T. vaginalis*. In all the parasites, the RAD51 recombinase is the most conserved protein (51%, 58% and 64% when *E. histolytica* protein sequence was compared with *G. lamblia, P. faciparum* and *T. vaginalis* orthologues, respectively), which is consistent with its relevant role in HRR mechanism.

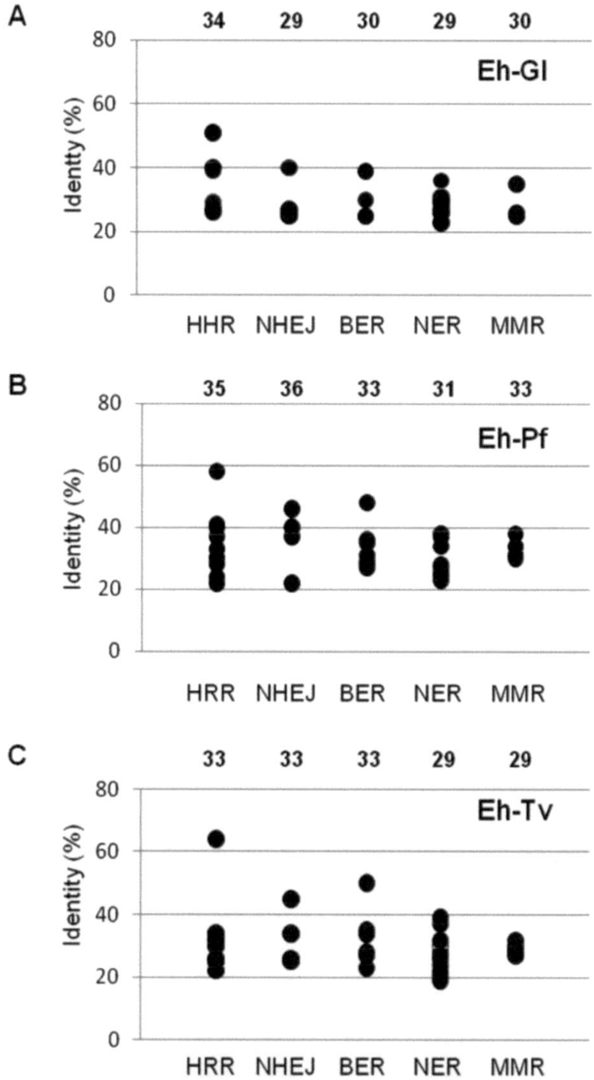


Fig. 1. **Conservation of DNA repair pathways between** *E. histolytica* **and** *G. lamblia* **(A),** *P. falciparium* **(B) and** *T. vaginalis* **(C).** Amino acids sequences from orthologous proteins were compared by Blast and the percentage of identity was determined through pair wise alignment of the most conserved region. Average identity of all pathways is indicated above each graph.

### 2.3 DNA repair activity in cell free lysates evidences the functionality of DNA repair proteins

Although insights about the activity of DNA repair proteins in protozoa have been mainly obtained from experimental evidence based in heterologous expression and characterization of recombinant proteins, some reports showed that DNA repair activity could be detected in whole cell extracts, supporting the notion that DNA repair pathways already operates *in vivo*. For instance, Haltiwanger et al., (2000) reported the characterization of an AP endonuclease activity in a *P. falciparum* cell free lysate. Authors provide evidence for the presence of class II, $Mg^{2+}$–dependent and independent AP endonucleases in the extracts. Moreover, they detected that *Plasmodium* AP endonuclease(s) possessed a 3′-phosphodiesterase activity similar to those described in other class II AP endonucleases [Demple et al., 1986]. In a related study, it was reported that a *P. falciparum* lysate contained uracil DNA glycosylase, AP endonuclease, DNA polymerase, flap endonuclease, and DNA ligase activities [Haltiwanger et al., 2000]. In contrast, DNA repair activities in cell lysates have not been detected in *Entamoeba, Giardia* and *Trichomonas* parasites. These data remark the utility of cell free lysates to understand DNA repair pathways, and pointed out to the urgency to investigate endogenous DNA repair activities using whole cell extracts in parasites where no data is available.

## 3. Functional categorization of *Entamoeba histolytica* DNA repair genes

To define the putative functions of *E. histolytica* DNA repair genes in unrelated DNA repair processes, we investigated the functional diversity of genomic maintenance pathways using Gene Ontology (GO) annotations. Functional related gene groups were predicted by the David bioinformatic resources (http://david.abcc.ncifcrf.gov/gene2gene.jsp), using a functional classification tool which generates a gene-to-gene similarity matrix based in shared functional annotation using over 75,000 terms from 14 functional annotation sources, allowing the classification of highly related genes in functionally related groups. Results from this analysis revealed that a large number of DNA repair genes were miss-annotated in parasites genome databases (43%). However, our analysis clearly showed that the majority of these genes seems to participate in DNA repair related processes. Besides, 57% of genes were predicted to function in DNA repair related process. 11% of genes participates in DNA damage repair, and 18% and 8% have helicase and endonuclease functions, respectively (**Fig. 2**).

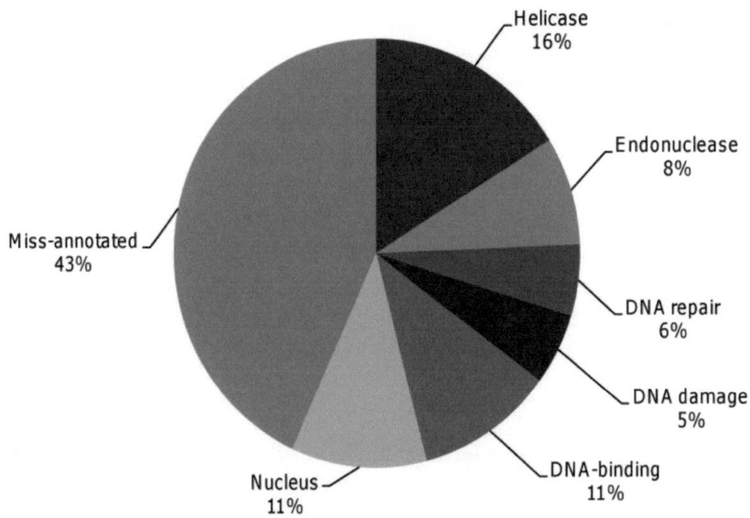


Fig. 2. **Functional categorizations of** *E. histolytica* **DNA repair genes.** Biological processes and molecular functions were determined using David software (http://david.abcc.ncifcrf.gov/gene2gene.jsp). Percentage of genes included in individual categories is given.

## 4. Duplicated genes: The case of *rad3*

Gene duplicates represent for 8-20% of the genes in eukaryotic cells, and the rates of gene duplication are estimated at between 0.2% and 2% per gene per million years. Gene duplications are one of the major motors in the evolution of genetic systems and may occur in homologous recombination, retrotransposition event, or duplication of an entire chromosome [Zhang, 2003]. Duplicated genes are believed to be a main system for the establishment of new gene functions generating evolutionary novelty [Long & Langley, 1993; Gilbert et al., 1997].

A detailed examination of **Table 1** revealed that several DNA repair genes are duplicated in protozoan parasites, while there is only one gene in yeast. For example, the HRR machinery includes two *rad51* genes in *P. falciparum*, two *rad54* and *mre11* genes in *E. histolytica* [Lopez-Casamichana et al., 2008], two *rpa1* genes in *T. vaginalis*, and two *sgs1* genes in *G. lamblia* and *P. falciparum*. We also identified two *rad27* genes in *P. falciparum* and *G. lamblia* NHEJ pathway, two *E. histolylica ntg1* and *P. falciparum pcna* genes in the BER pathway, as well as two *msh2* genes for the MMR pathway in *E. histolytica* and *P. falciparum*. But the most duplicated gene was the *rad3* gene from the NER mechanism, since there are three genes in *E. histolytica*, two in *G. lamblia* and six in *T. vaginalis*, whereas *P. falciparum* has only one *rad3* gene, alike yeast. Remarkably, gene duplication is evident for many other genes in *T. vaginalis* and reflexes the massive gene expansion inside the large genome of this pathogen [Hartl & Wirth, 2006]. In yeast, the RAD3 protein is involved in mitotic recombination and spontaneous mutagenesis, becoming essential for cell viability in the absence of DNA injury. Furthermore, this protein participates in the repair of UV-irradiated DNA via NER, and constitutes a subunit of RNA polII initiation factor TFIIH [Moriel-Carretero & Aguilera, 2010]. *S. cerevisiae* RAD3 is related to the *H. sapiens* XPD, also known as ERCC2. Defects in human XPD result in a wide range of diseases, including Xeroderma pigmentosum (XP), Cockayne's syndrome, and Trichothiodystrophy characterized by a wide spectrum of symptoms ranging from cancer susceptibility to neurological and developmental defects [Liu et al., 2008].

In order to describe the inferred evolutionary relationships among the most abundant duplicated gene found through the analysis of DNA repair machineries from the human pathogens studied here, we have undertaken a phylogenetic analysis of RAD3 helicase orthologues in *S. cerevisiae*, *E. histolytica*, *T. vaginalis*, *G. lamblia* and *P. falciparum*. We evaluated the minimum evolution of RAD3 proteins through the construction of Neighbor-Joining phylogenetic tree using the *MEGA* version 5.05 [Tamura et al., 2011]. The robustness was established by bootstrapping test, involving 500 replications of the data based on the criteria of 50% majority-rule consensus (**Fig. 3**). Two main branches that came from a common ancestor can be observed. On one branch, *T. vaginalis* RAD3 parologues are clustered into two sister proteins pairs (A2E1B9 and A2ELX1, A2E4I6 and A2DDD4), that have each evolved from the same ancestor. Besides, *E. histolytica* C4M6T8 is closer to *T. vaginalis* A2E4I6 and A2DDD4, than to its own paralogues. The other branch supports *T. vaginalis* A2G2G8 that is closely related to yeast and *P. falciparum* RAD3 proteins that came off the same node. Interestingly, these two organisms only have one *rad3* gene. This branch also includes *E. histolytica* C4M8K7 and C4M8Q4 sister proteins pair. Intriguingly, the two *Giardia* RAD3 proteins have emerged from different nodes and appeared to be more related to orthologues from other species than to each other; particularly, the branch supporting *Giardia* A8B495 also includes *Trichomonas* A2E1B9 and A2ELX1, while *Giardia* A8BYS3 is on the other branch, isolated from the other proteins, such as *Trichomonas* A2F1W2, which suggested that these proteins have evolved early.

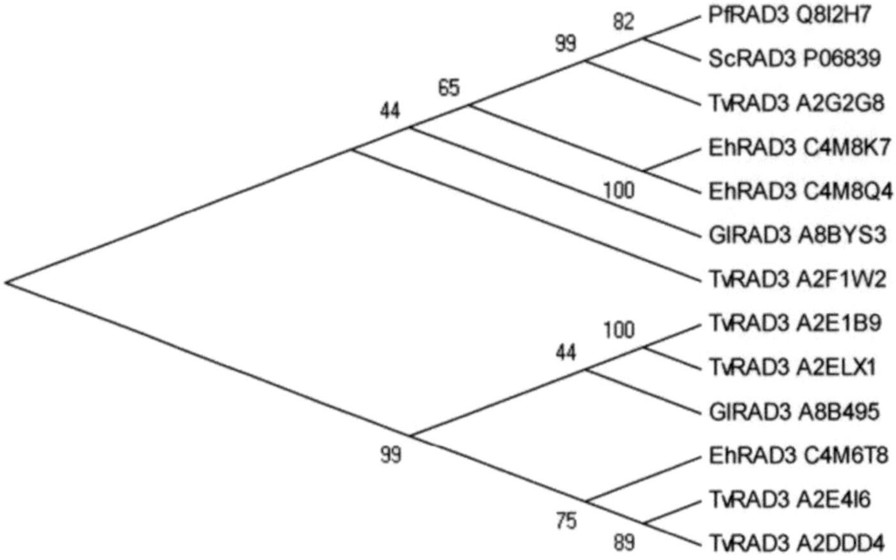


Fig. 3. **Phylogenetic relationships between RAD3 from** *S. cerevisiae***,** *E. histolytica***,** *T. vaginalis***,** *G. lamblia* **and** *P. falciparum***.** The unrooted tree was created with the MEGA 5.05 program using the Neighbor Joining algorithm based on ClustalW. Numbers above the tree nodes indicate the percentage of times that the branch was recovered in 500 replications.

## 5. Molecular organization of the MNR complex

The MRE11-RAD50-NBS1 (MRN) complex is considered to have an imperative function in DSB repair. This protein complex operates as DSB sensor, co-activator of DSB-induced cell cycle checkpoint signaling, and as a DSB repairs effector in both the HRR and NHEJ pathways [Taylor et al., 2010; Rass et al., 2009]. Additionally, it has also been found to associate with telomeres maintenance at the ends of linear chromosomes. MRE11 and RAD50 orthologues have been reported in all taxonomic Kingdoms. MRE11, RAD50, and XRS2 (the *S. cerevisiae* homologue of vertebrate-specific NBS1) were initially recognized through yeast resistance to DNA damage induced by UV light and X-rays and meiotic recombination studies [Ogawa et al., 1995]. To efficiently perform these functions, this complex has shown particular enzymatic roles. Biochemical experiments have revealed that the phosphoesterase domain of MRE11 works as both a single-and double-stranded DNA endonuclease, besides as 3′-5′ dsDNA exonuclease [D'Amours & Jackson, 2002]. Furthermore, RAD50 and NBS1/Xrs2 are able to promote the activity of MRE11, in an ATP dependent manner [Paul & Gellert, 1998]. ATP binding by RAD50 stimulates the binding of the MR complex to 3′ overhangs and, also, ATP hydrolysis is required to arouse the cleavage of DNA hairpins, inducing modification of endonuclease specificity via DNA relaxing [Paull & Gellert, 1998; de Jager et al., 2002].

In this chapter, we have identified the presence of *Mre11* and *Rad50* genes in the genome of *E. histolytica, T. vaginalis, G. lamblia* and *P. falciparum.* However, all analyzed pathogenic eukaryotic cells, with the exception *of E. histolytica,* lack the *Xrs2* homologue. The absence of a NBS1/Xrs2 homologous sequence in the other parasites might seem antagonistic to the idea of the existence of an active MRN complex. However we cannot discard the possibility that these microorganisms use a very divergent NBS1 protein, or even that this third component could be unessential. In order to initiate the characterization of components of MRN complex in these parasites, we studied the structural and evolutionary relationships between MRE11, RAD50 and NBS1 through PSI-BLAST analysis in comparison to human and yeast orthologues. This program generates a weighted profile from the sequences detected in the first pass of a gapped-BLAST search and iteratively searches the database using this profile as the query, allowing the inclusion of sequences with e-value cut off higher than 0.01 [Alschult et al., 1997]. Using the e-value threshold as a similarity measure, we evidenced a close relation between putative EhMRE11, HsMRE11, ScMRE11, TvMRE11 and PfMRE11. Conversely, GlMRE11 turned out to be less similar to the others, being closer to *E. histolytica* and *T. vaginalis* proteins (**Fig. 4**). On the other hand, analysis of RAD50 orthologues exposed a great conservation of these proteins, since all e-value threshold were <0.0001. As we have previously reported, EhNBS1 is closer to its human homologue than yeast [Lopez-Casamichana et al., 2007].

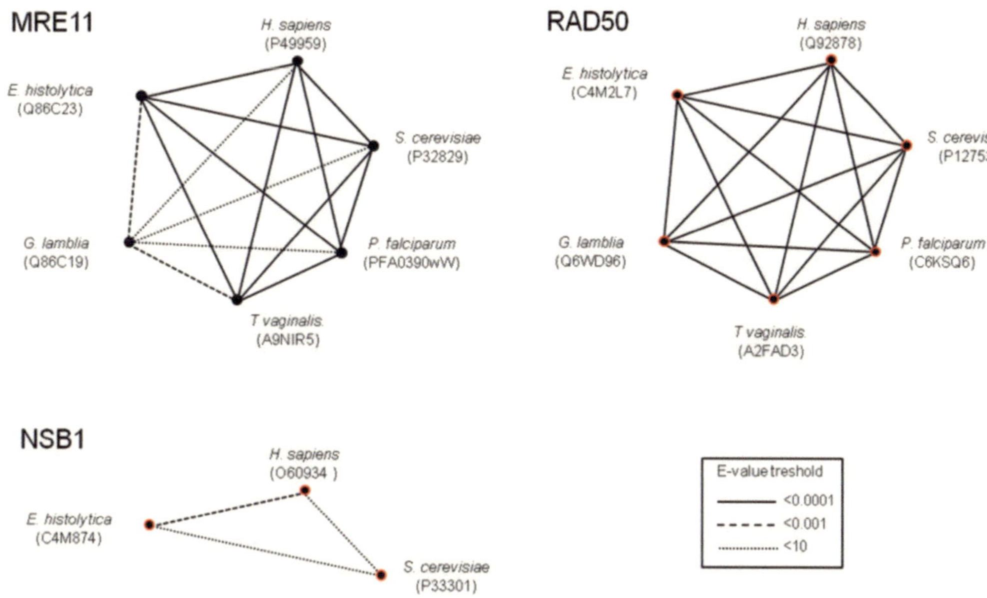


Fig. 4. **Individual protein relationships of MRN complex in pathogenic eukaryotic cells.** Similarity was evaluated through PSI-BLAST analysis. The width of connecting lines indicates similarity level.

To better understand the functionality of MRN complex in these parasites, predicted amino acid sequences of RAD50 and MRE11 were compared through multiple alignment using ClustalW software (http://www.ebi.ac.uk/ clustalw/). Reported functional and structural domains were surveyed using Prosite (http://www.expasy.org/tools/scanprosite/), Pfam (http://www.sanger.ac.uk /Software/Pfam/), SMART (http://smart.emblheidelberg.de/) and Motif Scan (http://myhits.isb-sib.ch/cgi-bin/motifscan) programs. For all studied parasites, our search revealed that the MRE11 orthologues contain the N-terminal Mn2+/Mg2+-dependent nuclease domain including the five conserved phosphoesterase motifs described in yeast protein [Hopkins & Paull, 2008]. Moreover, C-terminal DNA binding domains were also identified [Williams et al., 2007; D'Amours & Jackson, 2002] (**Fig. 5A**).

RAD50 proteins displayed sequence and organizational homology to structural maintenance of chromosome (SMC) family members that control the higher-order structure and dynamics of chromatin. The N-terminal Walker A and C-terminal Walker B nucleotide binding motifs, which associate one with another to form a bipartite ATP-binding cassette (ABC)-type ATPase domain, were predicted [Hopfner et al., 2000; Hopfner et al, 2001]. Furthermore, amino acids flanking Walker motifs form coiled-coil configurations that converge with the cysteine zinc hook (CysXXCys) motif [Hopfner et al., 2002] (**Fig. 5B**). In the interphase of Walker domains, there are two MRE11 binding sites. Formation of the stable MRE11-RAD50 complex is reached by each unit of the MRE11 dimer binding a RAD50 molecule at the intersection of its globular and coiled-coil domains [de Jager et al., 2001a]. Scanning force microscopy experiments have demonstrated that whereas the globular head of the Mre112Rad502 complex links with the ends of linear dsDNA, the two coiled-coil regions of RAD50 are stretchy "arms", and project outward away from the DNA [Hopfner et al., 2002].

The third member of the MRN complex is NBS1 protein that was only detected in *E. histolytica*, but not in *G. lamblia*, *P. falciarum* neither *T. vaginalis*. We have previously reported that EhNBS1 consists of an FHA domain and adjacent BRCT domains at its N-terminus [Lopez-Casamichana et al., 2007]. In *Homo sapiens*, the FHA domain binds phosphorylated threonine residues in Ser-X-Thr motifs present in DNA damage proteins, including CTP1 and MDC1. The BRCT domains in human NBS1 fix Ser-X-Thr motifs when the serine residue is phosphorylated. These phospho-dependent interactions are significant for recruiting repair machineries and checkpoint proteins to DNA DSBs [Lloyd et al., 2009; Williams et al., 2009]. In reconstitution studies, the affinity of MRE11-RAD50 for DNA and its nuclease activity is further enhanced by the addition of NBS1 [Paull & Gellert, 1999].

## 6. Molecular organization of the RAD51 recombinase

RAD51 recombinase is an essential protein in HRR pathway that catalyzes strand transfer between a broken DNA and its undamaged homologous strand, allowing damaged region to be repaired [Thacker, 2005] Strand exchange reaction is initiated by RAD51-coating of ssDNA released from DSBs, to generate a nucleoprotein filament. This active thread binds the intact dsDNA substrate, searching and locating homologous sequences, and promoting DNA strand exchange in an ATP-dependent manner, forming a heteroduplex structure [Paques & Haber, 1999]. After DNA damage, RAD51 protein has been observed in nuclear complexes forming discrete foci, which are considered as the recombinational DNA repair

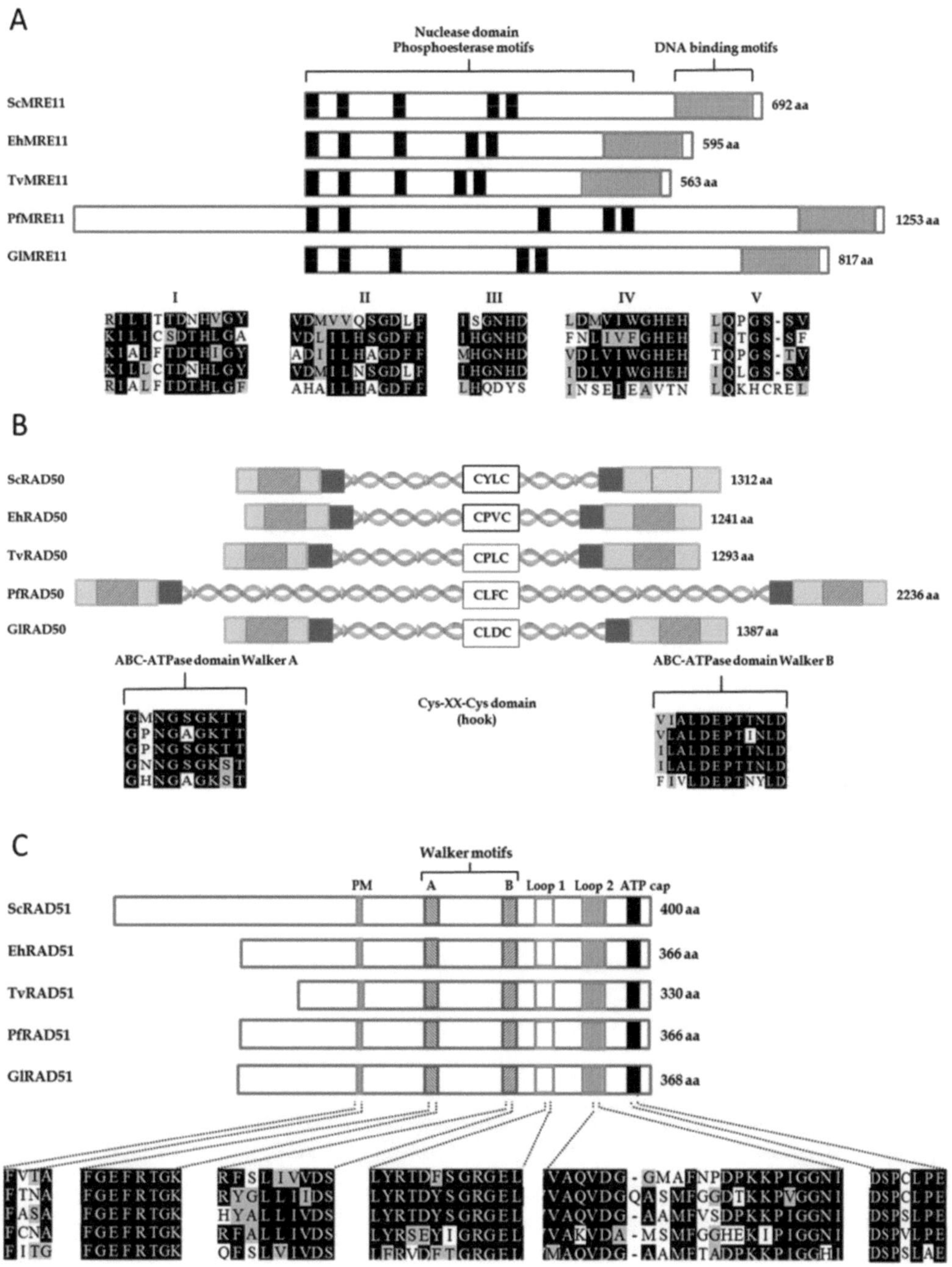


Fig. 5. **Comparison of the amino acids sequence of MRE11, RAD50 and RAD51 proteins of *S. cerevisae E. histolytica, T. vaginalis, P. falciparum* and *G. lamblia*. (A)**. Functional and structural domains of MRE11 proteins. MRE11 phosphoesterase motifs I-V (black

rectangles) and DNA-binding domains (gray rectangles). **(B)**. Functional and structural domains of RAD50 proteins. Walker A (N terminus) and Walker B (C terminus) are marked in the ABC-ATPase domains (gray rectangles), while MRE11-binding sites flank Walker motifs (dark gray rectangles) and the CysXXCys hook domain (white rectangles) are labeled in the coiled-coil central regions. **(C)**. Functional and structural domains of RAD51 proteins. Polymerization motif (PM), as well as Walker A and B motifs, L1 and L2 regions and ATP cap appear as colored rectangles. Boxshade panels: black boxes, identical aa; grey boxes, conserved substitutions.

sites [Tashiro et al., 2000]. RAD51 proteins have been identified in *Trypanosoma brucei* and *Plasmodium falciparum* parasites, which perform HRR to switch the expression of genes encoding surface membrane glycoproteins and generate antigenic variation [Conway et al., 2002; Freitas-Junior et al., 2000]. Furthermore, recombinational rearrangements are responsible for amplification of the multidrug resistance *pfmdr1* gene in *P. falciparum* [Triglia et al., 1991] demonstrating the relevance of HRR to generate genomic versatility and plasticity in protozoan parasites. Molecular analysis and functional assays confirmed that recombinant EhRAD51 is a *bonafide* recombinase that is able to catalyze specific ssDNA transfer to homologous dsDNA forming the three-stranded pairing molecule called D-loop structure. In addition, *E. histolytica RAD51* sequence conserves the typical architecture of RECA/RAD51 family members [Lopez-Casamichana et al., 2008]. Amino acid sequences multiple alignment of RAD51 orthologues from *E. histolytica, S. cerevisae, T. vaginalis, G. lamblia* and *P. falciparum* revealed that all these proteins share functional and structural conserved motifs (**Fig. 5C**). Each of them contains the putative polymerization motif (PM), which tethers individual subunits to form quaternary assemblies in human RAD51 protein [Bell, 2005]. We also identified the ATPase Walker A or phosphate binding loop (P-loop) and Walker B motifs residues, the ssDNA binding loops L1 and L2, as well as the ATP stacking motif or ATP cap at the C terminus, which are essential for nucleofilament assembling and ATP hydrolysis in RAD51/RECA-like recombinases [Shin et al., 2003; Conway et al., 2004].

## 7. Conclusions

Protozoan parasites are continuously subjected to the effects of antiparasitic drugs and host immune system attacks, which can affect their genome stability and therefore, their survival. In order to maintain the integrity of their DNA molecules, parasites have developed several mechanisms that are efficient to detect and accurately repair damaged nucleotides. Bioinformatic analyses of fully sequenced genomes are useful to identify molecular machineries for DNA repair in protozoan parasites of clinical relevance such as *Entamoeba histolyica, Giardia lamblia, Plasmodium falciparum* and *Trichomonas vaginalis,* which have a world-wide distribution with a high prevalence in developing countries. The computational data presented here provide new information on the evolution of DNA repair proteins and their potential relevance for DNA damage response in these major human pathogens. Future directions would include functional assays, as well as protein expression and protein-protein interactions analysis for the most relevant proteins, in order to contribute to the further elucidation of mechanisms regulating genome integrity in these organisms.

## 8. Acknowledgments

Genes and predicted protein sequences were obtained from the Eupath database (http://eupathdb.org/eupathdb/) and Uniprot Knowledgebase (http://www.uniprot.org/). This work was supported by UACM (México), CONACyT (México), COFAA-IPN (Mexico), SIP-IPN (Mexico) and European Community grants.

## 9. References

Alschult, S.F., Madden, T.L., Schaffer, A.A., Zang, J., Zang, Z., Miller, W., Lipman, D.J. (1997). Gapped BLAST and PSI-BLAST: a new generation of protein database search programs. *Nucleic Acid Research*, (September 1997), Vol.25, pp. 3389-3402, ISSN 0305-1048

Ankarklev, J., Jerlstrom-Hultqvist, J., Ringqvist, E., Troell, K., Svard, S.G. (2010). Behind the smile: cell biology and disease mechanisms of Giardia species. *Nature Reviews Microbiology*, Vol.8, (June 2010), pp. 413–422. ISSN: 1740-1526

Bethke, L., Thomas, S., Walker, K., Lakhia, R., Rangarajan, R., Wirth, D. (2007). The role of DNA mismatch repair in generating genetic diversity and drug resistance in malaria parasites. *Molecular and Biochemical Parasitology*, Vol. 155, No. 1, (September 2007), pp. 18–25. ISSN 0166-6851

Bell, C.E. (2005). Structure and mechanism of Escherichia coli RecA ATPase. Molecular Microbiology, Vol.58, No.2, (October 2005, pp.358-366, ISSN 0950-382X

Bhattacharyya, M.K., Kumar, N. (2003). Identification and molecular characterisation of DNA damaging agent induced expression of Plasmodium falciparum recombination protein PfRad51. *International Journal* for *Parasitology*, Vol.33, (October 2002), pp. 1385–1392. ISSN 0020-7519.

Carlton, J.M., Hirt, R.P., Silva, J.C., Delcher, A.L., Schatz, M., Zhao, Q., Wortman, J.R., Bidwell,S.L., Alsmark, U.C., Besteiro, S., et al. (2007). Draft genome sequence of the sexually transmitted pathogen Trichomonas vaginalis. *Science*, Vol. 315, No. 5809, (January 2007), pp. 207-212. ISSN 0036-8075

Casta, L.J., Buguliskis, J.S., Matsumoto, Y., Taraschi, T.F. (2008). Expression and biochemical characterization of the Plasmodium falciparum DNA repair enzyme, flap endonuclease-1 (PfFEN-1). *Molecular and Biochemical Parasitology*, Vol. 157, No. 1, (January 2008), pp. 1-12. ISSN 0166-6851

Castellini, M.A., Buguliskis, J.S., Casta, L.J., Butz, C.E., Clark, A.B., Kunkel, T.A., Taraschi, T.F. (2011). Malaria drug resistance is associated with defective DNA mismatch repair Molecular and Biochemical Parasitology, Vol. 177, No. 2 (June 2010), pp. 143-147. ISSN 0166-6851

Conway, C., Proudfoot, C., Burton, P., Barry, J.D., McCulloch, R. (2002). Two pathways of homologous recombination in Trypanosoma brucei. *Molecular Microbiology*, Vol.45, No.6, (September 2002), pp. 1687-1700, ISSN 0950-382X

Conway, A.B., Lynch, T.W., Zhang, Y., Fortin, G.S, Fung, C.W., Symington, L.S., Rice, P.A. (2004). Crystal structure of a Rad51 filament. *Nature structural & molecular biology*, Vol.11, No.8, (August 2004), pp. 791-796, ISSN 1545-9993

Cotch, M.F., Pastorek, J.G., Nugent, R.P., Hillier, S.L., Gibbs, R.S., Martin, D.H. et al. (1997). Trichomonas vaginalis associated with low birth weight and preterm delivery. The Vaginal Infections and Prematurity Study Group. *Sexually transmitted diseases*, Vol. 4, No.6, (July 1997), pp. 353-360. ISSN0148-5717

D'Amours, D., Jackson, S.P. (2002). The Mre11 complex: at the crossroads of DNA repair and checkpoint signalling. *Nature* Reviews *Molecular Cell Biology*, Vol. 3, (May 2002), pp. 317–327, ISSN 1471-0072

de Jager, M., Dronkert, M.L., Modesti, M., Beerens, C.E., Kanaar, R.,van Gent, D.C. (2001). DNA-binding and strand-annealing activities of human Mre11: implications for its roles in DNA double-strand break repair pathways. *Nucleic Acids Research*, Vol.29, (March 2001), pp. 1317–1325, ISSN 0305-1048

de Jager, M., van Noort, J., van Gent, D.C., Dekker, C., Kanaar, R., Wyman, C. (2001a). Human Rad50/Mre11 is a flexible complex that can tether DNA ends. *Molecular Cell,*), Vol.8, (November, 2001 pp. 1129–113, ISSN 1097-2765

Demple B, Johnson A, Fung D. Exonuclease III and endonuclease IV remove 3' blocks from DNA synthesis primers in H2O2-damaged Escherichia coli. 1986 *Proceedings of the National Academy of Sciences of the United States of America*. Voln 83, No.20, (October 1986), pp. 7731-7735, ISSN 0027-8424

Fleck, O., Nielsen, O. (2004) DNA repair. Journal of Cell Science, Vol. 117, Pt. 4, (February), pp. 515–517, ISSN: 0021-9533

Freitas-Junior, L.H., Bottius, E., Pirrit, L.A., Deitsch, K.W., Scheidig, C., Guinet, F., Nehrbass, U., Wellems, T.E., Scherf, A. (2000). Frequent ectopic recombination of virulence factor genes in telomeric chromosome clusters of P. falciparum. *Nature*, Vol.407, No.6807, (October 2000), pp. 1018-1022, ISSN 0028-0836

Gardner, M.J., Hall, N., Fung, E., White, O., Berriman, M., Hyman, R.W. et al. (2002). Genome sequence of the human parasite Plasmodium falciparum. *Nature*, Vol. 419, No. 6906, (October 2002), pp. 498–511. ISSN 0028-0836

Gilbert, W., de Souza, S. J., Long, M. Y. (1997). Origin of genes. *Proceedings of the National Academy of Sciences of the United States of America*, Vol.94, No.15, (July 1997), pp. 7698–7703, ISSN 0027-8424

Gill, E.E., Fast, N.M. (2007). Stripped-down DNA repair in a highly reduced parasite. *BMC Molecular Biology*, Vol. 8, (March), pp. 24. ISSN 1471-2199

Guo, X., Houpt, E., Petri, W.A.Jr. (2007). Crosstalk at the initial encounter: interplay between host defense and ameba survival strategies. *Current Opinion in Immunology*, Vol.19, (August 2007), pp. 376–384, ISSN 0952-7915

Haltiwanger, B.M., Karpinich, N.O, and Taraschi, T.F. (2000) Characterization of class II apurinic/apyrimidinic endonuclease activities in the human malaria parasite, *Plasmodium falciparum*. *Biochemical Journal*, Vol. 345, (January 2000), pp. 85-89, ISSN 0264-6021.

Haltiwanger, B.M, Matsumoto Y., Nicolas E., Dianov G.L., Bohr V.A., Taraschi T.F. (2000) DNA base excision repair in human malaria parasites is predominantly by a long-patch pathway. *Biochemistry*. Voln. 39, No. 4, (February 2000), pp. 763-72, ISSN 0006-2960.

Hartl, D.L., Wirth, D.F. (2006), Duplication, gene conversion, and genetic diversity in the species-specific acyl-CoA synthetase gene family of Plasmodium falciparum. *Molecular and Biochemical Parasitology*, Vol.150, No.1, (November, 2006), pp.10-24, ISSN 0166-6851

Hefferin, M.L., Tomkinson, A.E. (2005). Mechanism of DNA double-strand break repair by non-homologous end joining. *DNA Repair (Amsterdam)*, Vol. 4, No. 6, (June 2005), pp. 639-648. ISNN 1568-7864

Hopfner, K.P., Karcher, A., Shin, D.S., Craig, L., Arthur, L.M., Carney, J.P., Tainer, J.A. (2000) Structural biology of Rad50 ATPase: ATP-driven conformational control in DNA double-strand break repair and the ABCATPase superfamily. *Cell*, Vol.101, No.7, (June 2000), pp. 789-800, ISSN 0092-8674

Hopfner, K.P., Karcher, A., Craig, L., Woo, T.T., Carney, J.P., Tainer, J.A. (2001) Structural biochemistry and interaction architecture of the DNA double-strand break repair Mre11 nuclease and Rad50-ATPase. *Cell*, Vol.105, No.4, (May 2011), pp.473-485, ISSN 0092-8674

Hopfner, K.P., Craig, L., Moncalian, G., Zinkel, R.A., Usui, T., Owen, B.A. et al. (2002). The Rad50 zinc-hook is a structure joining Mre11 complexes in DNA recombination and repair. *Nature*, Vol.418, No. 6897, (August 202), pp. 562-566, ISSN 0028-0836

Hopkins, B.B., Paull, T.T. (2008). The P. furiosus mre11/rad50 complex promotes 5′ strand resection at a DNA double-strand break. *Cell*, Vol.135, (October 2008), pp. 250-260, ISSN 0092-8674

Kokwaro, G. (2009). Ongoing challenges in the management of malaria. *Malaria Journal*, Vol.8, Suppl 1, (October 2009), pp. S2. ISSN 1475-2875

Krokan, H.E., Standal, R., Slupphaug, G. (1997). DNA glycosylases in the base excision repair of DNA. *The Biochemistry Journal*, Vol. 325, No.1, (July 1997), pp. 1-16. ISSN 0264-6021

Lisby, M., Rothstein, R. (2005). Localization of checkpoint and DNA repait proteins in eukaryotes. *Biochimie*, Vol.87, No.7, (July), pp. 579589, ISNN 0300-9084

Liu H, Rudolf J, Johnson KA, McMahon SA, Oke M, Carter L, McRobbie AM, Brown SE, Naismith JH, White MF. (2008), Structure of the DNA repair helicase XPD. *Cell*, Vol.133, No.5, (May 2008), pp.801-12, ISSN 0092-8674

Lloyd, J. et al. (2009) A supramodular FHA/BRCT-repeat architecture mediates Nbs1 adaptor function in response to DNA damage. *Cell*, Vol.139, No. , (October 200), pp. 100-111, ISSN 0092-8674

Long, M. Y., Langley, C. H. (1993). Natural selection and the origin of jingwei, a chimeric processed functional gene in Drosophila. *Science*, Vol.260, No.91, (April 1993), pp.91-5, ISSN 0036-8075

López-Camarillo, C., Lopez-Casamichana, M., Weber, C., Guillen, N., Orozco, E., Marchat, L.A. (2009). DNA repair mechanisms in eukaryotes: Special focus in Entamoeba histolytica and related protozoan parasites. *Infection, Genetics and Evolution*, Vol.9, No.6, (December 2008), pp. 1051-1056. ISSN 1567-1348.

López-Casamichana, M., Orozco, E., Marchat, L.A., Lopez-Camarillo, C., (2007). Insights in DNA repair and homologous recombination in Entamoeba histolytica: in silico characterization of EhMRN complex. *Proceedings of the 5th European Congress on Tropical Medicine and International Health,* Monduzzi Editore s.r.l, pp. 7–11 , Medimond, ISBN: 13602276, Italy

López-Casamichana, M., Orozco, E., Marchat, L.A., López-Camarillo, C. (2008). Transcriptional profile of the homologous recombination machinery and characterization of the EhRAD51 recombinase in response to DNA damage in Entamoeba histolytica. *BMC* Molecular Biology, Vol.9, (April 2008), pp.35. ISSN 1471-2199

Malik, S.B., Pightling, A.W., Stefaniak, L.M., Schurko, A.M., Logsdon, J.M. Jr. (2007). An expanded inventory of conserved meiotic genes provides evidence for sex in Trichomonas vaginalis. *PLoS One,* Vol.3, No.8, (August 2007), e2879. ISSN 1932-6203

Marti, T.M., Kunz, C., Fleck, O. (2002). DNA mismatch repair and mutation avoidance pathways. *Journal of Cellular Physiology,* Vol.191, (April 2002), pp. 28-41. ISSN 0021-9541

Moriel-Carretero M, Aguilera A. (2010). Replication fork breakage and re-start: New insights into Rad3/XPD-associated deficiencies. *Cell Cycle,* Vol.9, No.15, (August 2010), pp.2958-62, ISSN 1538-4101

Ogawa, H., Johzuka, K., Nakagawa, T., Leem, S.H., Hagihara, A.H. (1995). Functions of the yeast meiotic recombination genes, MRE11 and MRE2. *Advances in Biophysics,* Vol.31, pp. 67–76. ISSN 0065-227X

Paques, F., Haber, J.E. (1999). Multiple pathways of recombination induced by double-strand breaks in Saccharomyces cerevisiae. *Microbiology and Molecular Biology Reviews,* Vol.63, No.2, (June 1999), pp. 349-404, ISSN 1092-2172

Paull, T.T., Gellert, M. (1999). Nbs1 potentiates ATP-driven DNA unwinding and endonuclease cleavage by the Mre11/Rad50 complex. *Genes & Development,* Vol.13, No.10, (May 1999). pp. 1276-1288. ISSN 0890-9369

Paull, T.T., Gellert, M. (1998). The 30 to 50 exonuclease activity of Mre11 facilitates repair of DNA double-strand breaks. *Molecular Cell,* Vol. 1, (June 1998), pp. 969–979, ISSN 1097-2765

Prakash, S., Prakash, L. (2000). Nucleotide excision repair in yeast. *Mutation Research,* Vol.451, No.1-2, (June 2000), pp. 13-24. ISSN 1383-5742

Ramesh, M.A., Malik, S.B., Logsdon, J.M.Jr. (2005). A phylogenomic inventory of meiotic genes: evidence for sex in Giardia and an early eukaryotic origin of meiosis. *Current Biology,* Vol.15, (January 2005), pp. 185-191. ISSN 0960-9822

Rass, E., Grabarz, A., Plo, I., Gautier, J., Bertrand, P. , Lopez, B.S. (2009). Role of Mre11 in chromosomal nonhomologous end joining in mammalian cells. *Nature Structural & Molecular Biology,* Vol.16, (August 2009), pp. 819–824, ISSN 1545-9985

Shin, D.S., Pellegrini, L., Daniels, D.S., Yelent, B., Craig, L., Bates, D. et al. (2003). Full-length archaeal Rad51 structure and mutants: mechanisms for RAD51 assembly and control by BRCA2. *EMBO Journal,* Vol.22, (September 2003), pp. 4566-4576, ISSN 0261-4189

Sorvillo, F., Kerndt, P. (1998). Trichomonas vaginalis and amplification of HIV-1 transmission. *The Lancet*, Vol.351, (January 1998), pp. 213-214. ISSN 0140-6736

Tamura, K., Peterson, D., Peterson, N., Stecher, G., Nei, M., Kumar, S. (2011). MEGA5: Molecular Evolutionary Genetics Analysis using Maximum Likelihood, Evolutionary Distance, and Maximum Parsimony Methods. *Molecular Biology and Evolution* (submitted), *ISSN 0737-4038*

Tashiro, S., Walter, J., Shinohara, A., Kamada, N., Cremer, T. (2000). Rad51 accumulation at sites of DNA damage and in postreplicative chromatin. *Journal of Cell Biology*, Vol.150, No.2, (July 2000), pp. 283-291, INSS 1540-8140

Taylor, E.M., Cecillon, S.M., Bonis, A., Chapman, J.R., Povirk, L.F., Lindsay,H.D. (2010). The Mre11/Rad50/Nbs1 complex functions in resection-basedDNA end joining in Xenopus laevis. *Nucleic Acids Research*, Vol.38, (November 2009), pp. 441–454, ISSN 0305-1048

Thacker, J. (2005). The RAD51 gene family, genetic instability and cancer. *Cancer Letters*, 2005 Mar 10;Vol. 219, No. 2, (March 2005), pp. 125-135, ISSN 0304-3835

Tovar, J., Leon-Avila, G., Sanchez, L.B., Sutak, R., Tachezy, J., et al. (2003). Mitochondrial remnant organelles of Giardia function in iron-sulphur protein maturation. *Nature*, Vol. 426, No. 6963, (November 2003), pp. 172-176; ISSN 0028-0836

Tovar J, Fischer A, Clark CG. (1999). The mitosome, a novel organelle related to mitochondria in the amitochondrial parasite Entamoeba histolytica. *Molecular Microbiology*, Vol. 32, No. 5, (June 1999), pp. 1013-1021. ISSN: 0950-382X

Triglia, T., Foote, S.J., Kemp, D.J., Cowman, A.F. (1991). Amplification of the multidrug resistance gene pfmdr1 in Plasmodium falciparum has arisen as multiple independent events. *Molecular and Cellular Biology*, Vol.11, No.10, (October 2010), pp. 5244-5250, ISSN 0270-7306

Voss, T.S., Mini, T., Jenoe, P., Beck, H.P. (2002). Plasmodium falciparum possesses a cell cycle-regulated short type replication protein A large subunit encoded by an unusual transcript. *The* Journal *of Biological* Chemistry, Vol.277, No.20, (May 2002), pp. 17493-17501. ; ISSN 0021-9258

Weber, C., Marchat, L.A., Guillen, N., López-Camarillo, C. (2009). Effects of DNA damage induced by UV irradiation on gene expression in the protozoan parasite Entamoeba histolytica. *Molecular* & Biochemical *Parasitology*, Vol. 164, No. 2, (April 2009), pp. 165-169. ISSN 0166-6851

World Health Organization (WHO). (1995). Global Programme on AIDS Report 1995. Geneva: WHO; 1995. An overview of selected curable sexually transmitted diseases

Williams, R.S., Dodson, G.E., Limbo, O., Yamada, Y., Williams, J.S., Guenther, G. et al. (2009). Nbs1 flexibly tethers Ctp1 and Mre11-Rad50 to coordinate DNA double-strand break processing and repair. *Cell*, Vol.139, No.1, (October 2009), pp. 87-99, ISSN 0092-8674

Williams, R.S., Williams, J.S., Tainer, J.A. (2007). Mre11-Rad50-Nbs1 is a keystone complex connecting DNA repair machinery, double-strand break signaling, and the chromatin template. *Biochemistry and Cell Biology*, Vol.85, (August 2007), pp. 509–520, ISSN 0829-8211

Zhang, J. (2003). Evolution by gene duplication: an update. *Trends in Ecology & Evolution*, (June 2003) Vol. 18, No. 6, pp.292-298, ISSN 0169-5347

# 17

# Mechanisms of Mutagenic DNA Nucleobase Damages and Their Chemical and Enzymatic Repairs Investigated by Quantum Chemical Methods

Eric A. C. Bushnell[1], Jorge Llano[2], Leif A. Eriksson[3] and James W. Gauld[1]
[1]*University of Windsor, Department of Chemistry and Biochemistry, Windsor, Ontario*
[2]*Grant MacEwan University, Department of Physical Sciences, Edmonton, Alberta*
[3]*School of Chemistry, National University of Ireland, Galway*
[1,2]*Canada*
[3]*Ireland*

## 1. Introduction

A cells genetic information, its 'blueprint of life', is contained within its DNA. This biologically important molecule, however, can be attacked by high-energy ionizing radiation and oxidizing agents resulting in a range of possible damage. For instance, nucleobases can undergo chemical modifications or degradation such as oxidation, deamination, alkylation or be cleaved from the sugar-phosphate backbone. (De Bont & van Larebeke 2004; Friedberg et al. 2004; Hecht 1999; Kamiya et al. 1998; Labet et al. 2008a; Lindahl 1993; Lysetska et al. 2002; Neeley & Essigmann 2006; Rydberg & Lindahl 1982; Taylor 1994; Wang 2008) Similarly, the deoxyribose sugar moieties may also undergo various chemical modifications. These events can lead further to the formation of DNA-DNA or DNA-protein cross-links or DNA-strand breaks. (Kumar & Sevilla 2010; Lipfert et al. 2004) Importantly, damage to DNA can significantly affect its replication and transcription. This can ultimately result in cell apoptosis or protein mutations and pathological diseases such as cancer. (Pages & Fuchs 2002)

Experimentally, there have been numerous detailed *in vivo* and *in vitro* investigations into the processes and pathways involved in the damage of DNA. (See, for instance, Kumar & Sevilla 2010; Mishina et al. 2006, Wetmore et al. 2001) Radiolysis experiments with photometric, electrochemical and electron paramagnetic resonance detection, enzymatic inhibition and mutagenesis studies have identified a large number of reaction intermediates and rate constants for many damage and repair processes. For more in-depth reviews of experimental investigations on DNA damage processes the reader is also directed to relevant chapters in this present book. Unfortunately, however, many uncertainties and questions still remain about DNA damage and repair.

Computational chemistry provides an alternate and also complementary approach for obtaining a deeper understanding of chemical processes. This is in part because it can not only be applied to systems that are amenable to experimental investigation but also to those systems or reactions that may be too challenging or even impossible to study using such experimental techniques. Furthermore, it is nowadays possible to apply highly accurate and reliable computational methods to larger, more complete biochemical models. Thus, using such approaches one can not only reconcile theory with experiment but, for example, compare the feasibility of differing proposed reaction mechanisms or identify new pathways.

There have been numerous computational investigations on or related to DNA damage and repair. In this chapter the application of Computational Chemistry to the study of DNA damage and repair is illustrated through a review of a number of relevant computational investigations that we have performed. More specifically, we have applied high accuracy density functional theory (DFT)-based methods to the study of several important primary and secondary nucleobase damage pathways and repair mechanisms. The chapter is divided into sections, each of which focuses on select results concerning a damage and/or repair process involving either the nucleobase or phosphate components of DNA:

2. **Nucleobase oxidation via ionizing radiation**: describes primary redox damage in nucleobases. In particular, the Gibbs Free Energies of solution-phase electron (ET), proton (PT) and proton-coupled electron (PTET) transfers for all DNA bases are examined. In addition, the potential of alkylthiols to act as repair agents of such damage is considered.
3. **8-Oxopurine formation in purine, adenine and guanine**: focuses on secondary damage of purine nucleobases. Specifically, the mechanisms of •OH attack leading to formation of 8-oxopurine derivatives are discussed as well as the Gibbs Free Energy changes of possible associated ET, PT and PTET processes.
4. **Deamination of oxidized cytosine**: examines the thermochemistry of several possible mechanisms by which oxidized cytosine, a pyrimidine nucleobase, may undergo deamination.
5. **Oxidation of serine phosphate: Implications for DNA**: investigates radicals formed from radiation-induced damage of serine phosphate.
6. **Oxidative repair of alkylated nucleobases: The catalytic mechanism of AlkB**: describes key results of our studies on the enzymatic mechanism of AlkB, a member of the family of α-ketoglutarate-Fe(II)-dependent dioxygenase enzymes that catalyse the oxidative repair of alkylated nucleobases.

### 1.1 Methods

For the detailed study of electronic properties of biochemical systems the current computational chemistry methods of choice for investigators are those of density functional theory (DFT). The principle reasons for this is that they inherently include electron correlation effects via their basis upon the electron density of the chemical system. Such effects are often important, for example, in accurately describing bond making and breaking processes, or weakly bound systems such as reaction transition structures. Furthermore, regardless of the number of electrons in the chemical system, the electron density is only ever a function of the three Cartesian coordinates. Thus, with such methods one can use larger and more complete chemical models consisting of 150 or more atoms. In addition, they are usually highly reliable and accurate.(See, for example, Llano 2010) For biochemical systems, the currently most widely used DFT functional is B3LYP,(Becke 1993a; Becke 1993b; Lee et al. 1988) and it has been used throughout this chapter.

Many biochemical processes occur within a polar environment, in particular an enzyme active site or aqueous medium. This can influence the properties and reactions of a biomolecule. Hence, it can be important to include such effects in the computational model. Each study described in this chapter has used a polarizable continuum (PCM)-based approach(Cammi & Tomasi 1995; Miertus et al. 1981) in the integral equation formulism (IEF).(Cances & Mennucci 1998; Cances et al. 1997; Mennucci et al. 1997) In this method the chemical system is effectively 'wrapped' in a density-fitting polar dielectric medium. Within this chapter a dielectric constant ($\varepsilon$) value of 4.0 has been used when modeling reactions within a protein active site, while the standard value for water at 298 K has been used for reactions modeled in aqueous environments. The specific computational details of each investigation are outlined in their respective section and in the appropriate article.
In order to determine relative free energies of reactions in which protons and electrons act as independent ions, it can be necessary to use 'fundamental values' such as the chemical potential of an electron or proton in a vacuum or aqueous solution under standard conditions. The values used in this chapter are given in **Table 1.** These have been obtained by means of a first principles quantum and statistical mechanics approach, the details of which are provided in a recent paper by Llano and Eriksson.(Llano & Eriksson 2002)

| Quantity | eV | kcal mol$^{-1}$ |
|---|---|---|
| $\mu_{0K}^{vac}(e^-)$ | 0.0 | 0.0 |
| $\mu_{298K,1atm}^{\Theta,SHE}(e^-)$ | -4.34 ± 0.02 | -100.03 ± 0.5 |
| $\mu_{298K,1atm}^{\Theta,aq}(e^-)$ | -1.6638 ± 0.04 | -38.37 ± 0.5 |
| $\mu_{298K,1atm}^{\Theta,aq}(H^+)$ | -11.6511 ± 0.02 | -268.68 ± 0.5 |

Table 1. Chemical potentials of an electron in vacuum and an electron and proton in aqueous reference states.(Llano & Eriksson 2002).

## 2. Nucleobase oxidation via ionizing radiation

Ionizing radiation can potentially be absorbed by any of the three nucleotide components of DNA (i.e., phosphate, sugar or nucleobase) or its surrounding waters; also an essential part of DNA structure.(Kumar & Sevilla 2010) Primary damage of, for example, nucleobases, is caused by their direct absorption of radiation. Secondary damage (such as that described later in this chapter) can also occur, for instance, when the radiation is absorbed by the solvent, thus generating radicals or solvated electrons which then attack the nucleobase.(von Sonntag 1987; von Sonntag 1996)
Direct absorption (primary damage) can cause the formation of a radical-cationic base via the loss of an electron, i.e., generation of an electron hole. Due to the stacking of nucleobases within DNA charge transfer (transfer of the hole) can then occur along the strand. Consequently, this enables 'primary damage related' reactions to occur distant from the site of initial damage. The potential for charge transfer due to the $\pi$-orbital interactions between bases was proposed as early as 1962. (Eley & Spivey 1962) Alternatively, however, it may enable charge recombination to occur further along the chain. This is because radical-anionic bases can be formed by the capture of the free electrons, where the resulting damage to the nucleobase also constitutes primary damage. Guanine has the lowest ionization potential of

the four DNA nucleobases, followed by adenine.(Hush & Cheung 1975; Kumar & Sevilla 2010; Steenken & Jovanovic 1997; Yang et al. 2004) Consequently, they are in general oxidized to give their radical-cations while thymine and cytosine act as electron sinks and form their radical-anions. However, vice versa, in the transfer of electron holes guanine typically acts as a sink for DNA radiative oxidation.(Cadet et al. 2008; Kumar & Sevilla 2010) Reduction/oxidation of a nucleobase can significantly affect its properties. In particular, it has been shown that their oxidation greatly increases their acidity (lowers their $pK_a$).(Kumar & Sevilla 2010) Indeed, the formation of a radical base is often associated with proton transfer reactions that can lead to further nucleobase damage. However, as has also been noted, these same proton transfers can result in nucleobase repair.(Llano & Eriksson 2004b)

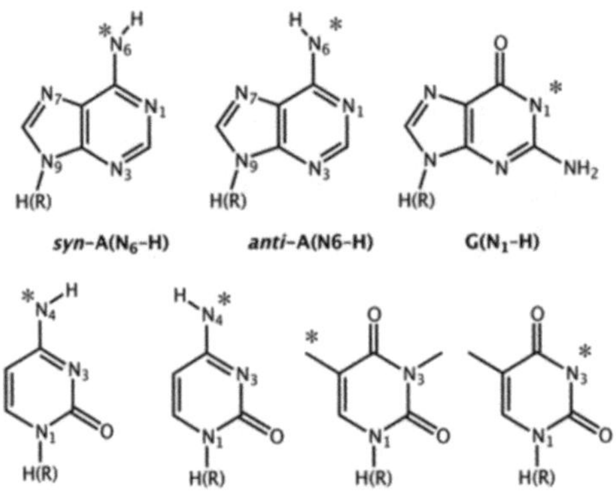


Fig. 1. Structures of the dehydrogenated nucleobases for both the cations and anions. The position of the missing hydrogen is marked by the asterisk.

Unfortunately, our understanding of these important electron- (ET) and proton-transfer (PT) reactions is incomplete.(Llano & Eriksson 2004a) This is not only due to the highly transient and reactive nature of key species involved, but also because experimental measurements of free energies for such processes can only be obtained indirectly.(Llano & Eriksson 2004a) Moreover, at times, the available experimental techniques (photoelectron spectroscopy, mass spectroscopy, pulse radiolysis and electrochemical techniques) appear to give contradictory results.(Seidel et al. 1996) Using computational methods we have investigated the processes involved in the oxidation and reduction of DNA nucleobases.(Llano & Eriksson 2004a) In particular, the nature of the ET process, the effect of PT on such processes, and vice versa, was examined using the chemical models shown in **Figure 1**.

All optimizations were performed at the B3LYP/6-31(+)G(d,p) level of theory; diffuse functions only being included for anionic species'. Harmonic vibrational frequencies and zero-point vibrational energies (ZPVE) were calculated at this same level of theory. Relative energies and absolute chemical potentials were then obtained via single point calculations at the IEF-PCM/B3LYP/6-311+G(2df,p) level of theory, in aqueous solvent, based on the above optimized structures with inclusion of the appropriate Gibbs corrections. In combination with the values listed in **Table 1**, the free energies for oxidation of the four neutral DNA bases and the corresponding anions was determined. Specifically, the free energies were calculated for the three different reference states used to define the absolute chemical potential of the electron: in vacuum, aqueous or the SHE reference state.

| $B^{\bullet -}_{(aq)}$ | ⟶ | | | $B_{(aq)}$ | ⟶ | | | $B^{\bullet +}_{(aq)}$ |
|---|---|---|---|---|---|---|---|---|
| | $-e^-_{(vac)}$ | $-e^-_{(aq)}$ | $-e^-_{(SHE)}$ | | $-e^-_{(vac)}$ | $-e^-_{(aq)}$ | $-e^-_{(SHE)}$ | |
| $A^{\bullet -}$ | 40.7 | 2.3 | -59.3 (-56.0)[a] | A | 136.7 | 98.3 | 36.7 (32.7)[c] | $A^{\bullet +}$ |
| $G^{\bullet -}$ | 37.9 | -0.5 | -62.1 (-63.2)[a] | G | 125.9 | 87.5 | 25.9 (29.7)[c] | $G^{\bullet +}$ |
| $T^{\bullet -}$ | 51.9 | 13.5 | -48.1 (-25.6)[b] | T | 145.2 | 106.8 | 45.2 (39.2)[c] | $T^{\bullet +}$ |
| $C^{\bullet -}$ | 43.3 | 9.9 | -51.7 (-25.8)[b] | C | 147.6 | 109.2 | 47.6 (36.9)[c] | $C^{\bullet +}$ |

Table 2. Calculated (see text) standard free energies (in kcal mol$^{-1}$) of primary ionizations of the four nucleobases in aqueous solution. Experimental values are in parenthesis and taken from references: [a] (Seidel et al. 1996), [b] (Steenken et al. 1992), [c] (Steenken & Jovanovic 1997).

ET is a common process that occurs upon absorption of radiation by nucleobases. Using a first principles approach the free energy changes involved with such a process for all four DNA nucleobases were calculated and are shown in **Table 2.**(Llano & Eriksson 2002) It can be seen that the ionization of each of the anionic bases ($B^{\bullet -}_{(aq)}$) can be either endothermic or exothermic depending on the reference state of the electron. For example, in the vacuum or aqueous state the oxidation of the anionic bases is generally an endothermic process. The only exception occurs for guanine in the aqueous state in which the process is marginally exothermic (-0.5 kcal mol$^{-1}$). In contrast, in the case of the SHE reference state, oxidation of each base is markedly exothermic. For $A^{\bullet -}$ and $G^{\bullet -}$ the values calculated are in close agreement to those obtained experimentally.(Seidel et al. 1996; Steenken & Jovanovic 1997; Steenken et al. 1992) In contrast, those calculated for $C^{\bullet -}$ and $T^{\bullet -}$ are not in as good agreement, being almost twice the corresponding experimental values. However, the overall trends are consistent; the oxidation of $C^{\bullet -}$ or $T^{\bullet -}$ is thermodynamically less favorable than that of $A^{\bullet -}$ or $G^{\bullet -}$. Conversely, the reverse process, capture of a solvated electron by C or T (i.e., $C/T_{(aq)} + e^-_{(aq)} \rightarrow C/T^{\bullet -}_{(aq)}$) is thermodynamically preferred (-9.9 kcal mol$^{-1}$ and -13.5 kcal mol$^{-1}$, respectively) compared to that involving A or G (-2.3 kcal mol$^{-1}$ and 0.5 kcal mol$^{-1}$, respectively).

Oxidation of the neutral bases is calculated to be endothermic for each reference state of the electron (**Table 2**). The degree of endothermicity, however, depends on the reference state being most endothermic in vacuum and least for the SHE reference state. Unlike that observed for the radical anion bases, the SHE calculated values for the neutral bases are all in good agreement with experiment. The largest difference occurs for C and is now only 10.7 kcal mol$^{-1}$ compared to the 25.9 kcal mol$^{-1}$ difference for $C^{\bullet -}$, while the smallest difference (-3.8 kcal mol$^{-1}$) is observed for guanine. In addition, neutral G is calculated to have the lowest free energy of oxidation and is thus the easiest of the four DNA nucleobases to be ionized, in agreement with experimental observations.

The free energies associated with the loss of a proton from the resulting radical-cationic bases to solution were calculated and are given in **Table 3**. For $A/G^{\bullet +}$ the energy changes associated with deprotonations to form *syn*-A($N_6$-H), *anti*-A($N_6$-H), and G($N_1$-H) were determined to be quite small at just -0.6, -0.7 and -0.3 kcal mol$^{-1}$ respectively.(Llano & Eriksson 2004a) In contrast, the energy changes associated with deprotonation of $C/T^{\bullet +}$ to give *syn*-C($N_4$-H) or *anti*-C(N4-H) and T($C_5$-H) are larger at -5.2, -4.5 and -22.3 kcal mol$^{-1}$, respectively.(Llano & Eriksson 2004a) It is noted that T($C_5$-H) has only been observed in the solid state and not in solution,(Steenken 1989) and thus will not be discussed herein. Unlike the other deprotonation processes, formation of T($N_3$-H) was found to be endothermic and

| Cationic Radical Base | ΔG (kcal $mol^{-1}$) | Deprotonated Radical Base |
|---|---|---|
| $A^{\bullet+}$ | -0.7 (≤ 1.4)[a] | *syn*-A($N_6$-H), |
| $A^{\bullet+}$ | -0.6 (≤ 1.4)[a] | *anti*-A($N_6$-H) |
| $G^{\bullet+}$ | -0.3 (5.3)[a] | G($N_1$-H) |
| $T^{\bullet+}$ | -22.3 | T($C_5$-H) |
| $T^{\bullet+}$ | 9.9 (4.9)[a] | T($N_3$-H) |
| $C^{\bullet+}$ | -5.2 (~5.4)[a] | *syn*-C($N_4$-H), |
| $C^{\bullet+}$ | -4.5 (~5.4)[a] | *anti*-C($N_4$-H) |

Table 3. Calculated (see text) standard Gibbs energies (in kcal $mol^{-1}$) of the decay of the radical cations. Experimental values included in parenthesis taken from references: [a] (Steenken 1989; Steenken 1992).

had the largest absolute free energy change (9.9 kcal $mol^{-1}$).(Llano & Eriksson 2004a) Thus, the loss of a proton in aqueous conditions is thermodynamically favorable for the radical-cationic bases except for proton loss from $N_3$—H in thymine. The unfavourable decay of $T^{\bullet+}$ via deprotonation of $N_3$-H suggests that the ion may have a long enough lifetime such that it may instead obtain an electron, a thermodynamically favourable process (**Table 2**). Thus, $T^{\bullet+}$ may instead preferably react to regenerate the neutral base T rather than decay.(Llano & Eriksson 2004a)

Having established an understanding of the energies associated with oxidation of the anionic and neutral bases, energy changes associated with possible repair mechanisms of this damage were then investigated. For the deprotonated neutral radical bases ($B(-H)^{\bullet}_{(aq)}$) regeneration can occur via three possible pathways: (i) ET followed by PT (**Table 4**); (ii) a proton-coupled electron transfer (PTET) (**Table 5**) or (iii) direct transfer of a hydrogen atom. From **Table 4** it can be seen that reduction of the deprotonated bases is exothermic under all reference states with the exception of T($N_3$-H)$^{\bullet}$ in the SHE reference state. However, the energy change for protonating all of the reduced bases ($B(-H)^{-}_{(aq)}$) is favorable. Protonation of G($N_1$-H)$^-$ has the smallest free energy change suggesting that the conjugate acid is relatively stronger than the other neutral bases. Importantly, the more acidic a molecule, the more powerful it is as a reducing agent. Thus, as G has the smallest energy cost of deprotonation of any of the DNA bases it is more likely to reduce the other bases and thereby act as an electron hole sink, as observed experimentally.

| $B(-H)^{\bullet}_{(aq)}$ | → | | | $B(-H)^{-}_{(aq)}$ | → | $B_{(aq)}$ |
|---|---|---|---|---|---|---|
| | $+e^{-}_{(vac)}$ | $+e^{-}_{(aq)}$ | $+e^{-}_{(SHE)}$ | | $+H^{+}_{(aq)}$ | |
| *syn*-A($N_6$-H)$^{\bullet}$ | -113.2 | -74.9 | -13.2 | *syn*-A($N_6$-H)$^-$ | -22.7 (≥ -19.1)[a] | A |
| *anti*-A($N_6$-H)$^{\bullet}$ | -113.9 | -75.6 | -13.9 | *anti*-A($N_6$-H)$^-$ | -22.2 (≥ -19.1)[a] | A |
| G($N_1$-H)$^{\bullet}$ | -111.5 | -73.2 | -11.5 | G($N_1$-H)$^-$ | -14.4 (-13.0)[a] | G |
| T($N_3$-H)$^{\bullet}$ | -72.3 | -34.0 | 27.7 | T($N_3$-H)$^-$ | -50.6 | T |
| *syn*-C($N_4$-H)$^{\bullet}$ | -123.0 | -84.6 | -23.0 | *syn*-C($N_4$-H)$^-$ | -19.4 (-17.7)[a] | C |
| *anti*-C($N_4$-H)$^{\bullet}$ | -123.4 | -85.0 | -23.4 | *anti*-C($N_4$-H)$^-$ | -19.6 (-17.7)[a] | C |

Table 4. Calculated (see text) standard Gibbs energies (in kcal $mol^{-1}$) of the regeneration of the nucleobases via a ET then PT process. Experimental values included in parenthesis taken from references: [a] (Steenken 1989; Steenken 1992).

Under alkaline conditions it is expected that ET would occur prior to PT, as seen in **Table 4**. However, under acidic conditions a PTET process may occur. The associated calculated energy values are given in **Table 5**. As can be seen, the free energy changes for ET are exothermic for all reference states when it occurs simultaneously with a PT. Importantly, the free energies associated with electron addition are decidedly more favorable in the case of a PTET process compared to that observed in the previous ET process (cf. **Table 4**).

| $B(-H)^{\bullet}_{(aq)}$ | → | | | $B_{(aq)}$ |
|---|---|---|---|---|
| | $+e^{-}_{(vac)}$ | $+e^{-}_{(aq)}$ | $+e^{-}_{(SHE)}$ | |
| *syn*-A($N_6$-H)• | -136.0 | -97.6 | -36.0 (-46.8)[a] | A |
| *anti*-A($N_6$-H)• | -136.1 | -97.7 | -36.1 (-46.8)[a] | A |
| G($N_1$-H)• | -125.6 | -87.3 | -26.5 (-19.7)[a] | G |
| T($N_3$-H)• | -155.1 | -116.7 | -55.1 | T |
| *syn*-C($N_4$-H)• | -142.4 | -104.0 | -42.4 | C |
| *anti*-C($N_4$-H)• | -143.0 | -104.6 | -43.0 | C |

Table 5. Calculated (see text) standard Gibbs energies of the regeneration of the nucleobases via a PTET process. Experimental values included in parenthesis taken from references: [a] (Steenken & Jovanovic 1997).

The aqueous state reduction of the neutral radical bases ($B(-H)^{\bullet}_{(aq)}$) by addition of $H^{\bullet}_{(aq)}$ was calculated to be exothermic for all DNA bases. More specifically, the free energy changes for reduction of *syn* / *anti*-A($N_6$-H)• and -C($N_4$-H)• are -85.0, -85.1, -91.4 and -92.0 kcal $mol^{-1}$, respectively while for G($N_1$-H)• and T($N_3$-H)• they are -74.6 and -104.1 kcal $mol^{-1}$, respectively. It is likely that this process is important under low pH conditions where the free protons would scavenge the hydrated electrons to yield $H^{\bullet}$. These free energy changes are less exothermic than those seen in the PTET process (cf. **Table 5**; $e^{-}_{(aq)}$ results). However, under acidic conditions the PTET and $H^{\bullet}$ processes would likely compete as they both react at diffusion-limited rates. Of all possible three reduction mechanisms for B(-H)•, PTET processes show the greatest change in free energy.

| Deprotonated Radical Base | $\Delta_{ET}G^{\ominus}$ | $\Delta_{PTET}G^{\ominus}$ |
|---|---|---|
| *syn*-A($N_6$-H)• | -5.1 | -13.5 |
| *anti*-A($N_6$-H)• | -5.8 | -13.6 |
| G($N_1$-H)• | -3.4 | -3.1 |
| T($N_3$-H)• | -32.6 | -32.6 |
| *syn*-C($N_4$-H)• | -14.9 | -19.9 |
| *anti*-C($N_4$-H)• | -15.3 | -20.5 |

Table 6. Calculated (see text) standard Gibbs energies (in kcal $mol^{-1}$) of the regeneration of the nucleobases by methylthiol. $\Delta_{ET}G^{\ominus}$ is the free energy change for $B(-H)^{\bullet}_{(aq)} + MeS^{-}_{(aq)} = B(-H)^{-}_{(aq)} + MeS^{\bullet}_{(aq)}$ while $\Delta_{PTET}G^{\ominus}$ is the free energy change for $B(-H)^{\bullet}_{(aq)} + MeSH_{(aq)} = B_{(aq)} + MeS^{\bullet}_{(aq)}$.

Clearly, the possible processes by which the neutral bases may be regenerated are inherently favorable regardless of whether the electrons originate from vacuum, dilute aqueous solutions or SHE reference states. However, they still require that there be a suitable reductant. It has been noted that in solution a free thiol could be a likely reductant for transfer of a H• to a radical-cationic DNA base, thereby repairing the lesion.(von Sonntag 1987; von Sonntag 1996). Hence, the applicability of thiols to act as such a reductant was also investigated. It should be noted that although the process of repairing the nucleobase can occur via enzymatic or other chemical processes, only the latter involving methylthiol is discussed here. The calculated free energy costs associated with regeneration of the deprotonated radical bases by methylthiol ($CH_3SH$) are given in **Table 6**.

Two possible reduction pathways exist:

i. $B(-H)^{\bullet}_{(aq)} + MeS^{-}_{(aq)} \rightarrow B(-H)^{-}_{(aq)} + MeS^{\bullet}_{(aq)}$

ii. $B(-H)^{\bullet}_{(aq)} + MeSH_{(aq)} \rightarrow B_{(aq)} + MeS^{\bullet}_{(aq)}$

**Pathway i** most likely only occurs under basic conditions. However, as can be seen from **Table 6**, for *syn*– / *anti*–A($N_6$–H)• and –C($N_4$–H)• an initial loss of the –SH proton markedly lowers the reductive ability of the thiol. That is, the overall free energy change associated with regeneration of the nucleobases is reduced, i.e., $\Delta_{ET}G^{\ominus}$ is less exothermic than $\Delta_{PTET}G^{\ominus}$. However, for G($N_1$–H)• and T($N_3$–H)• the free energy changes are quite close for both possible regeneration pathways. The markedly larger values of $\Delta_{PTET}G^{\ominus}$ compared to $\Delta_{ET}G^{\ominus}$ for all adenine and cytosine species considered suggests that PTET is the favoured process at any pH for these nucleobases. However, the negligible difference observed for guanine and thymine suggest that the preferred path will depend on the reaction conditions, e.g., pH. Importantly, regardless of the preferred pathway the calculated free energies indicate they are both favorable, exothermic processes.

## 3. 8-Oxopurine formation in purine, adenine and guanine

A major type of secondary DNA damage is that caused by the attack of hydroxyl radicals.(Llano & Eriksson 2004a; von Sonntag 1987; von Sonntag 1996) Such radicals can be formed when metals or hydrogen peroxide are present.(Burrows & Muller 1998) In addition, however, the absorption of radiation by water can lead to not only the formation of solvated electrons but also of reactive oxygen species such as •OH. Furthermore, related modifications of nucleobases can occur via the reaction of their radical cation with water. For instance, reaction of $G^{\bullet+}$ with $H_2O$ has been suggested to be an important alternative pathway in DNA modification.(Candeias & Steenken 2000) Unfortunately, due to the high reactivity of these radicals where the rates of reaction are typically diffusion controlled,(Llano & Eriksson 2004a) it is impossible for radical scavengers to prevent them from damaging DNA. It has been suggested that approximately half of the damage done by •OH occurs at the nucleobases. In the purine bases the hydroxyl has been observed to attack at their double bonds to form the $C_4$, $C_5$ and $C_8$ adducts with the latter (i.e., **B8OH**$^{\bullet}_{(aq)}$) being the major product of oxidation and radiolysis.(Hagen 1986; Hatahet 1998; Kasai et al. 1986; Llano & Eriksson 2004b; Teoule 1987)

The subsequent oxidation of **B8OH**$^{\bullet}_{(aq)}$ to give **8–OHB**$_{(aq)}$ may occur via either of the two pathways shown in **Figure 2**: (i) a PT followed by an ET(Cullis et al. 1996) or (ii) a PTET mechanism(Candeias & Steenken 2000). The resulting common **8–OHB**$_{(aq)}$ product of both pathways can then undergo tautomerization to yield the corresponding 8–oxo derivative (**8–oxoB**$_{(aq)}$). It is noted that the barrier for tautomerization of 8–hydroxy–purine (**8–OHPu**$_{(aq)}$) has been calculated to be quite low at only 7.0 kcal mol$^{-1}$ with the keto form (**8–oxoPu**$_{(aq)}$) being favoured over the enol form by 10.6 kcal mol$^{-1}$. (Llano & Eriksson 2004b)

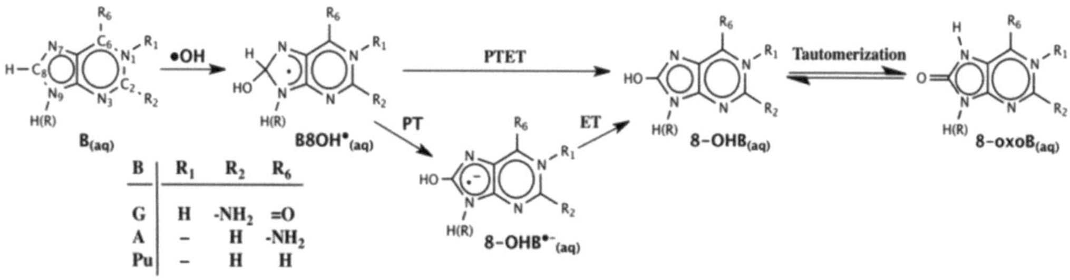

Fig. 2. Two proposed pathways for •OH attack at the C8 position of a purine base and subsequent oxidation to generate the 8-oxo purine derivative.

The **8–oxoG/A** products are in fact major stable DNA purine oxidation products produced via the radiolysis of water.(Hagen 1986; Hatahet 1998; Kasai et al. 1986; Teoule 1987) However, it is been observed that the adenine derivative (**8-oxoA**) is formed only about one–third of the time compared to the guanine derivative (**8-oxoG**).(Burrows & Muller 1998; Llano & Eriksson 2004b) Importantly, however, the formation of either **8–oxoB** species promotes the formation of mutagenic lesions that can cause mispairings resulting in G:C and T:A transversions.(Cheng et al. 1992; Cullis et al. 1996; Llano & Eriksson 2004b; Newcomb 1998; Pavlov et al. 1994) Such lesions are in fact caused by the further oxidation of **8–oxoB** to their corresponding **8–oxoB•(–H7)** derivatives. Moreover, it has been shown that depending on the reaction conditions both spiroiminodi- and guanidino-hydantoin are also major products formed by further oxidation of **8–oxoG**.(Munk et al. 2008) It has been suggested that these further reactions occur because the **8–oxoB** species' have lower ionization potentials than any other native base.(Cadet & Vigny 1990; Chatgilialoglu et al. 2000) Hence, they could act as a trap for a migrating electron hole.(Sponer et al. 2004; Yao et al. 2005) Unfortunately, however, despite detailed experimental study, the exact route by which such species' (**8–oxoB** and **8–oxoB•(–H7)**) may be formed remains unclear.(Llano & Eriksson 2004b)

We performed a computational investigation on the processes by which **8–OHB$_{(aq)}$** may be formed for purine, adenine and guanine.(Llano & Eriksson 2004b) In addition, the subsequent oxidations by which **8–oxoB** and **8–oxoB•(–H7)** may be formed were also examined using a first principles approach.(Llano & Eriksson 2002) Optimized structures, harmonic vibrational frequencies and ZPVEs were calculated at the B3LYP/6–31(+)G(d,p) level theory; diffuse functions only being included for anionic species'. Relative Gibbs Free energies were obtained by performing single point calculations at the IEF-PCM/B3LYP/6-311+G(2df,p) level of theory, in aqueous solvent, based on the above structures with inclusion of the appropriate Gibbs corrections.

Attack of •OH at the $C_8$ position in purine, adenine or guanine results in formation of the corresponding radical hydroxylated intermediates **B8OH•** (**Figure 3**). Notably, they are stabilized relative to the isolated reactants by -13.4, -14.9 and -15.8 kcal mol$^{-1}$ for purine, adenine and guanine respectively.

The oxidation of **B8OH•$_{(aq)}$** may then be initiated via PT from its -$C_8$—H moiety (**Figure 3**). This step, resulting in formation of the corresponding radical-anionic derivatives **8–OHB•–$_{(aq)}$** was calculated to be significantly endothermic for all three purine bases considered with a minimum free energy cost of ~28 kcal mol$^{-1}$. Notably, the largest costs of 35.4 and 47.4 kcal mol$^{-1}$ are observed for adenine and guanine, respectively. This suggests that a strong base is

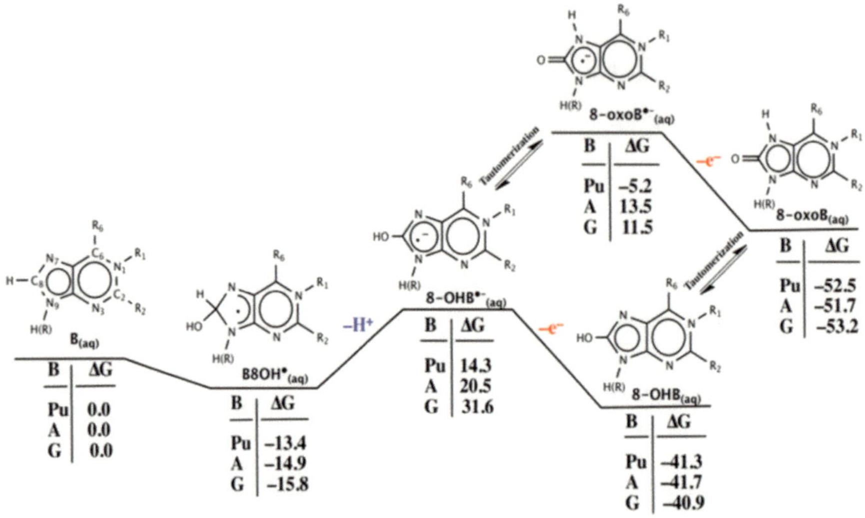


Fig. 3. Calculated (see text) standard Gibbs energies (kcal mol-1) for PT initiated oxidation of **B8OH•.**

required for deprotonation of $C_8$ in **B8OH•(aq)** and is unlikely to occur under neutral or acidic conditions. The resulting **8-OHB•−(aq)** ions can then either oxidize further via loss of an electron to give **8-OHB(aq)** or tautomerize to give **8-oxoB•−(aq)**. As can be seen in **Figure 3**, both possible processes are thermodynamically preferred. Importantly, however, these latter two species can subsequently undergo tautomerization and electron loss, respectively to give the same **8-oxoB(aq)** product species. The barriers for tautomerization of the radical-anionic (**8-OHPu•−(aq)**) and neutral purine (**8-OHPu(aq)**) are both low at just 5.2 and 7.1 kcal mol-1, respectively. (Llano & Eriksson 2004b) Thus, the choice of pathway from **8-OHB•−(aq)** to **8-oxoB(aq)** may in fact be controlled by the thermodynamics of the loss of an electron. From **Figure 3** it can be seen that for purine and guanine the largest decreases in free energy observed for electron loss along either of these two paths occurs for the oxidation of the enol radical anion **8-OHB•−(aq)** to give **8-OHB(aq)** with decreases of 55.6 and 72.5 kcal mol-1 respectively. In contrast, for adenine the largest decrease (65.2 kcal mol-1) is observed for loss of an electron from the keto radical anion **8-oxoB•−(aq)** to give **8-oxoB(aq)**. Thus for purine and guanine it is likely that formation of **8-oxoB(aq)** occurs via tautomerization of **8-OHB(aq)**, while for adenine it involves oxidation of **8-oxoB•−(aq)**.

As shown in **Figure 4**, oxidation of **B8OH•(aq)** may alternatively be initiated by ET, giving rise to **B8OH+(aq)** ions. Similar to that observed for an initial PT from **B8OH•(aq)** (cf. **Figure 3**), this process is also found to be endothermic for all three purine nucleobases. However, with the exception of purine, the energy costs incurred are now significantly less. Indeed, for **A/G8OH•(aq)** ET is thermodynamically preferred to PT by 24.1 and 47.2 kcal mol-1 respectively. It is further noted that for guanine, the reactant **G8OH•(aq)** is essentially thermoneutral with the **G8OH+(aq)** intermediate. Furthermore, the subsequent PT from **B8OH+(aq)** to give **8-OHB(aq)** is highly exothermic for all bases by 57.1, 45.3 and 25.3 kcal mol-1 for purine, adenine and guanine, respectively. This is in contrast to the highly endothermic initial PT observed in **B8OH•(aq)** (cf. **Figure 3**). For the ET initiated oxidation pathway tautomerization can only happen once PT has occurred, that is, once **8-OHB(aq)** has been formed. This rearrangement, which results directly in formation of **8-oxoB(aq)**, is exothermic for all bases considered by 10.0 – 12.3 kcal mol-1. It should be noted that in addition to the possible ET and PT initiated processes, a PTET (i.e., the concerted loss of electron and proton) process may also occur. However, the overall free energy change for formation of **8–OHB** via this alternate path is -27.9, -26.8 and -25.1 kcal mol-1 relative to **B8OH$^{\bullet}$$_{(aq)}$** for purine, adenine and guanine, respectively.

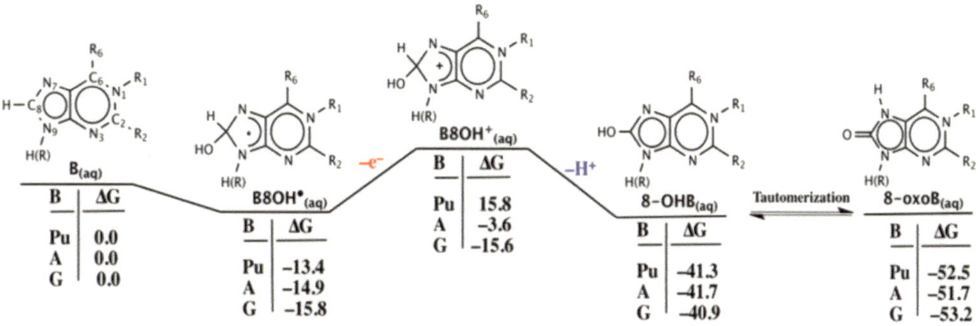


Fig. 4. Calculated (see text) standard Gibbs energies (kcal mol-1) for the ET initiated oxidation pathway in **B8OH$^{\bullet}$**.

The formation of **8–oxoB$^{\bullet}$(-H7)$_{(aq)}$** can potentially be achieved by further oxidation of the neutral tautomers **8–oxoB$_{(aq)}$** and **8–OHB$_{(aq)}$**, initiated by loss of an electron (**Figure 5**). For both species', however, this ET process is endothermic. For purine and adenine the lowest associated energy costs (46.1 and 30.5 kcal mol-1 respectively) are incurred for ET from **8–oxoB$_{(aq)}$** while for guanine it is incurred from **8–OHB$_{(aq)}$** with a cost of 20.1 kcal mol-1. Notably, for both **8–oxoB$_{(aq)}$** and **8–OHB$_{(aq)}$** the loss of an electron from the guanine-derivative (**8–oxoG$_{(aq)}$** and **8–OHG$_{(aq)}$**) is preferred to that from the corresponding adenine or purine-derivatives. Regardless, however, a suitable oxidant is required in order to oxidize either **8–oxoB$_{(aq)}$** or **8–OHB$_{(aq)}$**. The barriers for tautomerization for both the neutral **8–oxoB$_{(aq)}$/8–OHB$_{(aq)}$** and radical-cationic **8–OHB$^{\bullet+}$$_{(aq)}$/8–oxoB$^{\bullet+}$$_{(aq)}$** species' are quite low at

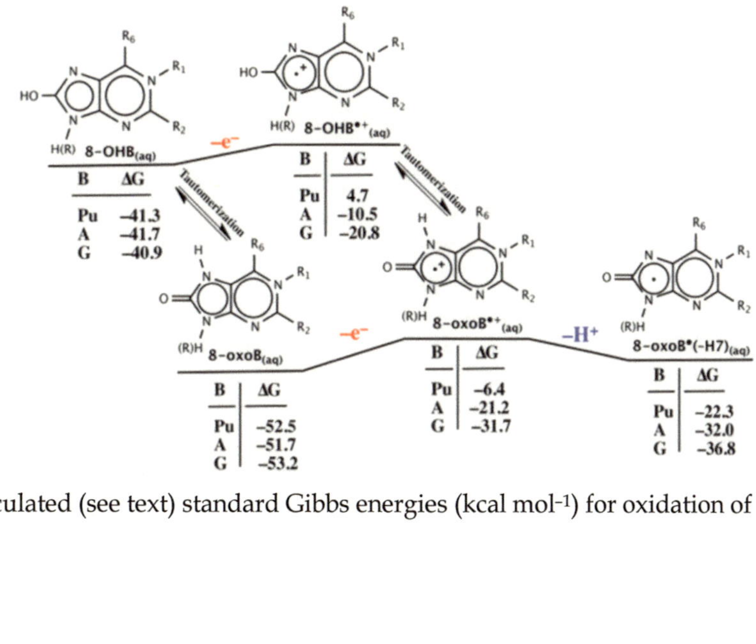


Fig. 5. Calculated (see text) standard Gibbs energies (kcal mol-1) for oxidation of **8–OHB** and **8–oxoB.**

just 7.0 and 9.2 kcal mol$^{-1}$, respectively.(Llano & Eriksson 2004b) Thus, once formed, such species are expected to be able to easily interconvert between their enol and keto forms with equilibrium favouring the latter. However, once the **8–oxoB$^{\bullet+}$$_{(aq)}$** species is formed, loss of a proton ($H^+$) from N7 to give **8–oxoB$^{\bullet}$(–H7)$_{(aq)}$** is exothermic for all bases (**Figure 5**). Notably, **8–oxoG$^{\bullet}$(–H7)$_{(aq)}$** is calculated to lie 4.8 kcal mol$^{-1}$ lower in energy than the corresponding adenine derivative **8–oxoA$^{\bullet}$(–H7)$_{(aq)}$** and may thus help explain the preference of its formation over that of **8–oxoA**.

## 4. Deamination of oxidized cytosine

In addition to damage by ionizing radiation it has been found that nucleobases are susceptible to oxidation by one–electron oxidants, e.g., nitrosoperoxycarbonate present during inflammatory processes.(Cadet et al. 2006; Lee et al. 2007) The purine base guanine, despite having the lowest ionization potential, is not the sole target for oxidants. In particular it has been observed that the pyrimidine bases are also susceptible to oxidation.(Decarroz et al. 1986; Douki & Cadet 1999; Wagner et al. 1990) Importantly, this oxidation leads to degradation via two possible competing pathways that are initiated by deprotonation of: (i) the methylene carbon of the sugar moiety ($C_1$') attached to the pyrimidine nitrogen ($N_1$) or (ii) the exocyclic amine attached to $C_4$ of the ring. Notably, the latter path has been suggested to lead to hydrolytic deamination of the pyrimidine ring.(Decarroz et al. 1987)
Previous computational investigations have investigated the deamination of non-oxidized cytosine, in particular via the attack of water or an hydroxyl anion ($^-$OH) at its $C_4$ centre and via NO$^{\bullet}$ attack at $N_4$.(Almatarneh et al. 2006; Labet et al. 2009) While the lowest barrier was obtained for the nucleophilic attack of $OH^-$ at $C_4$, the calculated value was 9.6 kcal mol$^{-1}$ higher than that obtained experimentally. However, the susceptibility of cytosine to one–electron oxidation suggests that possible mechanisms for deamination of $C^{\bullet+}$ should also be taken into consideration. The importance of considering such reactions is further underlined by the fact that the product of oxidation and deamination of cytosine is the highly mutagenic uracil residue.
We used computational chemistry methods to investigate the deamination of cytosine via the oxidized cytosine intermediate $C^{\bullet+}$ and via a deprotonated cytosine. Optimized structures and their corresponding harmonic vibrational frequencies were obtained at the IEF–PCM/B3LYP/6–311G(d,p) level of theory in aqueous solvent. Relative free energies were obtained at the same level of theory with inclusion of the appropriate Gibbs energy corrections.
In **section 2** it was shown that the one–electron oxidation of cytosine with the loss of the electron and proton in aqueous solution (i.e. $C \rightarrow e^-_{(aq)} + H^+_{(aq)} + C(–N_4)^{\bullet}_{(aq)}$) occurs with a sizeable free energy cost of approximately 104 kcal mol$^{-1}$ (**Table 4**). The optimized structure of the oxidized $C(–N_4)^{\bullet}_{(aq)}$ ring (not shown) is similar to that of neutral cytosine being planar with similar bond lengths, in agreement with other theoretical studies.(Cauet et al. 2006; Wetmore et al. 2000; Wetmore et al. 1998) The calculated spin densities and Mulliken charges showed that the positive charge is delocalized over the ring with the greatest change in partial charges occurring at $C_5$ (+0.24e) while for spin densities they occur at $C_5$ (0.64) and $N_1$ (0.30).
The loss of a proton from $N_4$ in $C^{\bullet+}$ can result in the formation of either *syn–* or *anti–*C($N_4$–H)$^{\bullet}$ with the former being slightly more stable (**Table 4**). However, in the resulting *anti–* form it was found that when $H_2O$ is added, analogous to spontaneous deamination of the

neutral base,(Labet et al. 2008a) it forms a hydrogen-bond bridge between $N_3$ and $N_4$ (**RC**: **Figure 6**). Thus, only the *anti–* form is discussed herein. It is noted that the addition of $H_2O$ has negligible effect on the Mulliken charges and spin densities of *anti*–C($N_4$–H)$^\bullet$ and with no delocalization onto the water itself.

Deamination is then initiated by transfer of a $H^\bullet$ from the water onto the $N_3$ ring centre (**Figure 6**). This process proceeds via **TS1** with a barrier of 16.8 kcal mol$^{-1}$ to give intermediate **I1**, lying 11.5 kcal mol$^{-1}$ higher in free energy than **RC** and is thus endergonic. Intermediate **I1** resembles a complex between a cytosine tautomer and a hydroxyl radical. Interestingly, upon $H^\bullet$ transfer the partial charge on $C_4$ has increased by +0.29e to 0.38e close to that observed on $C_4$ (0.37e) in neutral cytosine. Thus, in **I1** $C_4$ has the same electrophilicity as in the neutral base. Indeed, the next step is nucleophilic attack of the $^\bullet$OH moiety at the $C_4$ centre. This occurs via **TS2** with a barrier of 8.6 kcal mol$^{-1}$ relative to **I1**; 20.1 kcal mol$^{-1}$ with respect to **RC**. It should be noted that for spontaneous deamination of cytosine in water the analogous hydroxylation also occurs via attack of water at the $C_4$ position with simultaneous transfer of a proton from the $H_2O$ moiety onto the amino $N_4$ centre with concomitant cleavage of the $C_4$—$N_4$ bond. However, it proceeds with a barrier four to five times larger than that observed above for reaction via **TS2**.(Labet et al. 2008b) In the resulting intermediate **I2**, lying just 4.2 kcal mol$^{-1}$ higher in energy than the initial complex **RC**, the $C_4$ centre is now tetrahedral with a $C_4$—OH bond length of 1.432 Å. There are then five possible pathways by which deamination of **I2** may occur, hereafter referred to as **Path A, B, C, D,** and **E**. The free energy changes associated with each are summarized in **Table 7**.

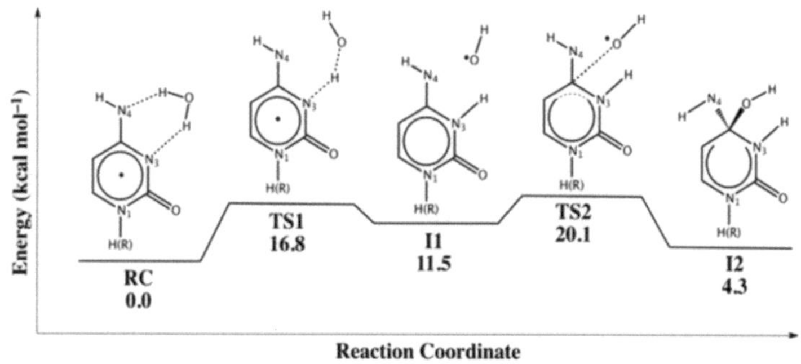


Fig. 6. Calculated (see text) relative free energies for initial abstraction of $H^\bullet$ from $H_2O$ by *anti*–C($N_4$–H)$^\bullet$ with subsequent attack of $^\bullet$OH at the $C_4$ centre.

| Path A | ΔG | Path B | ΔG | Path C | ΔG | Path D | ΔG | Path E | ΔG |
|---|---|---|---|---|---|---|---|---|---|
| **I2** | 4.3 | **I2** | 4.3 | **I2** | 4.3 | **I2** | 4.3 | **I2** | 4.3 |
| $^{A}$**I3** | -9.0 | $^{B}$**TS3** | 38.3 | $^{A}$**I3** | -9.0 | $^{D}$**TS3** | 31.1 | $^{A}$**I3** | -9.0 |
| $^{A}$**I4** | -0.2 | $^{B}$**I3** | 13.1 | $^{C}$**TS3** | 30.4 | $^{D}$**I3** | 6.5 | $^{E}$**TS3** | 24.9 |
| $^{A}$**TS3** | 7.1 | $^{B}$**I4** | 7.5 | $^{B}$**I4** | 7.5 | $^{D}$**I4** | 0.1 | $^{D}$**I4** | 0.1 |
| $^{A}$**P** | -7.5 | $^{B}$**TS4** | 9.4 | $^{B}$**TS4** | 9.4 | $^{D}$**TS4** | 2.2 | $^{D}$**TS4** | 2.2 |
| | | $^{B}$**P** | 11.4 | $^{B}$**P** | 11.4 | $^{D}$**P** | -22.0 | $^{D}$**P** | -22.0 |

Table 7. Calculated (see text) relative free energies for stationary points along **Path A, B, C, D** and **E** for deamination of **I2** in aqueous solution.

**Path A** begins with protonation of the $N_4$ centre in **I2** where the proton originates from the surrounding dilute aqueous solvent. The resulting intermediate $^{A}$**I3** lies 13.3 kcal mol$^{-1}$ lower in energy than **I2**. This is followed by a second protonation of $N_4$ with the proton again originating from the surrounding dilute aqueous solvent. In contrast to the first, this second protonation is endergonic by 8.8 kcal mol$^{-1}$. However, the resulting intermediate $^{A}$**I4** still lies lower in energy than **I2** by 4.5 kcal mol$^{-1}$. In $^{A}$**I4** the initial -$N_4H$ group in **I2** has now formally become an -$N_4H_3^+$ group. Consequently, the next step is the loss of $NH_3$ by simple cleavage of the C—N bond. This occurs with a barrier of 7.3 kcal mol$^{-1}$ relative to $^{A}$**I4** (**Table 7**). It should be noted that the resulting product complex of $^{A}$**P** lies 11.8 kcal mol$^{-1}$ lower in energy than **I2** and resembles a complex between $NH_3^{\bullet+}$ and protonated uracil.(Labet et al. 2008b)

In contrast, in **Path B** the initial 'protonation' of $N_4$ is achieved via an intramolecular rearrangement from the $N_3$—H group and does not originate from solution. This reaction proceeds via the four-membered ring TS $^{B}$**TS3** at a significant cost of 34.0 kcal mol$^{-1}$ to give intermediate $^{B}$**I3**, lying 8.8 kcal mol$^{-1}$ higher in energy than **I2** (**Table 7**). However, similar to **Path A** the second step is protonation of $N_4$ with the proton originating from solution. This process is exergonic with the resulting intermediate $^{B}$**I4** lying 5.6 kcal mol$^{-1}$ lower in free energy than $^{B}$**I3**. The subsequent cleavage of the $C_4$—$N_4H_3^+$ bond occurs via $^{B}$**TS4** to give the product complex $^{B}$**P**. However, unlike for **Path A**, $^{B}$**P** is higher in energy than **I2** by 7.1 kcal mol$^{-1}$ and instead resembles a complex between $NH_3$ and the oxidized enol form of Uracil.

Like **Path A**, the alternate **Path C** begins with the exothermic protonation of $N_4$ by a proton originating from solution to give $^{A}$**I3** (**Table 7**). Now, however, the second proton is obtained via the intramolecular proton transfer that initiated **Path B**, i.e., by transfer from the $N_3$—H group. This reaction proceeds via $^{C}$**TS3** with a considerable barrier of 39.4 kcal mol$^{-1}$, even higher than that observed in **Path B**, to give intermediate $^{B}$**I4**. The remaining step, cleavage of the $C_4$—$N_4$ bond, is then identical to that of **Path B** as is the product formed.

**Path D**, unlike the previous paths, involves an initial intramolecular proton transfer from the $C_4$—OH hydroxyl onto the $N_4$ centre (**Table 7**). This reaction proceeds via $^{D}$**TS3** at a cost of 26.8 kcal mol$^{-1}$. While this barrier is still quite high, it is 7.2 and 12.6 kcal mol$^{-1}$ lower than the analogous intramolecular rearrangements in **Paths B** and **C** and is thus kinetically favoured. The resulting intermediate formed $^{D}$**I3** lies only 2.2 kcal mol$^{-1}$ higher in energy than **I2**. This is then followed by protonation of the $N_4$ centre by a proton originating from solution, similar to **Paths A** and **B**. This step is exothermic with the intermediate formed, $^{D}$**I4**, lying 6.4 kcal mol$^{-1}$ lower in energy than $^{D}$**I3**. The next and final step is the loss of $NH_3$ and occurs via $^{D}$**TS4** with a quite small barrier of just 2.1 kcal mol$^{-1}$. The resulting product $^{D}$**P**, resembling a complex between $NH_3$ and oxidized uracil, is markedly lower in energy than **I2** by 26.3 kcal mol$^{-1}$. Importantly, it is in fact the lowest energy product complex obtained of all those considered herein.

The final path considered, **Path E**, begins with the same exothermic intermolecular protonation of $N_4$ as in **Paths A** and **C** and again leads to formation of $^{A}$**I3**. The next step, however, is intramolecular proton transfer from the $C_4$—OH group to $N_4$ as occurs in **Path D**. Importantly, it proceeds via $^{E}$**TS3** with a higher barrier (33.9 kcal mol$^{-1}$) than observed in **Path D** (26.8 kcal mol$^{-1}$) to give $^{D}$**I4**. The final step is then cleavage of the $C_4$—$N_4$ bond as in **Path D** to give $^{D}$**P**.

Thus, while deamination via donation of both protons from the aqueous solution (**Path A**) may have the lowest associated barriers, the resulting product is not the most thermodynamically favoured. In contrast, in those cases in which only one proton originates from solution (**Paths B - E**), only those involving intramolecular rearrangement of a proton from $C_4-OH$ (**Paths D** and **E**) are exothermic and lead to formation of the most thermodynamically preferred product (**$^D$P**). Furthermore, the barrier for this rearrangement is lowest when it occurs prior to proton donation from the solvent. Lastly in the case where both protonations occur via intermolecular processes, $NH_3^{\bullet+}$ is formed (**$^A$P**) while $NH_3$ is formed when only a single proton originates from exogenous sources (**$^B$P** and **$^D$P**).

## 5. Oxidation of serine phosphate: Implications for DNA

As mentioned in **section 2**, the exposure of DNA to high-energy radiation can also cause damage at its phosphate backbone. In particular, it can cause strand breaks via cleavage of the phosphoester bonds.(Lipfert et al. 2004) When the absorption of radiation causes the ionization of the phosphate it has been shown that it then abstracts a $H^\bullet$ from the deoxyribose ring at either its $C_{4'}$ or $C_{5'}$ position. This is then followed by heterolytic cleavage of the phosphoester bond.(Lipfert et al. 2004; Steenken & Goldbergerova 1998) Alternatively, the strand break may be preceded by chemical modification of the nucleobase or deoxyribose ring or the phosphoester bond may simply undergo a direct cleavage.(Lipfert et al. 2004)

Experimentally it can be difficult to clearly observe and characterize damage within DNA due to its size. Thus, it is common to either use short fragments or model compounds that can reproduce or mimic the damage and associated processes that may occur. For example, serine phosphate contains a phosphate bond as well as a carboxylate that can act as an electron scavenger much like the bases within DNA itself. Thus, it is often used in experimental studies on the processes of DNA damage at its phosphate and subsequent bond cleavage reactions and in fact has led to a deeper understanding of those processes involved.

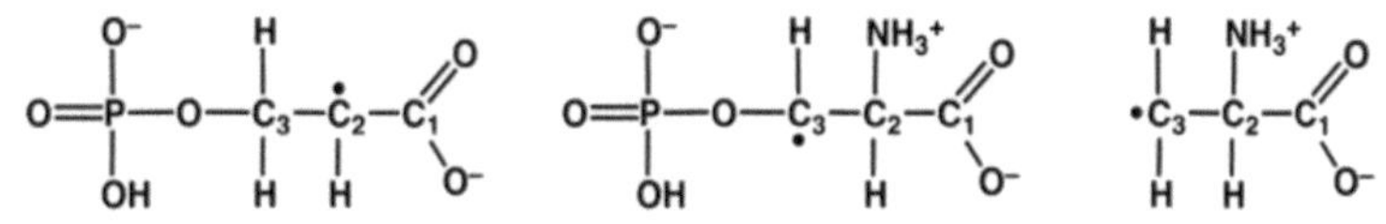

(I) (II) (III)

Fig. 7. The $C_2$-centered radical **I** and $C_3$-centered radicals **II** and **III** proposed to be formed upon the irradiation of non- and partially-deuterated single crystals of L-*O*-serine phosphate. (Sanderud & Sagstuen 1996)

In particular, evidence has been obtained suggesting the formation of several different radical species. Specifically, the irradiation of non- and partially-deuterated single crystals of L-*O*-serine phosphate has been suggested to produce the three radicals **I, II** and **III** shown in **Figure 7**.(Sanderud & Sagstuen 1996) In particular, it is thought that upon irradiation serine phosphate can take up a now free electron to form a $C_1$-centered radical anion. This may then undergo deamination to form the $C_2$-centered radical anion **I**. Alternatively, a serine phosphate may lose an electron to form a neutral $C_1$-centered radical which then undergoes decarboxylation to give a $C_2$-centered radical. This latter radical may then abstract a $H^\bullet$ from the $C_3$ position of another serine phosphate to generate the $C_3$-centered radical anion **II**. In contrast, the neutral $C_3$-centered radical **III** is proposed to be formed via the uptake of a free electron by serine phosphate to give a P-centered radical anion which then simply undergoes loss of the phosphate group.

We investigated the nature of radicals **I**, **II** and **III** by obtaining optimized structures at the B3LYP/6-31G(d) level of theory. Hyperfine coupling constants (HFCCs) were then calculated via single point calculations at the B3LYP/6-311+G(2df,p) level of theory on the above structures and are listed for all three radicals in **Table 8**.(Lipfert et al. 2004)

In the optimized structure of radical **I** the largest spin density is located on $C_2$ (0.71) while the carbonylic oxygen of the carboxylate group also has significant spin density (0.18). This delocalization of spin density is due to conjugation between the singly occupied molecular orbital (SOMO) on $C_2$ and the $C_1$=O $\pi$-bond. In addition, it is noted that near planarity was observed for $C_1$ and $C_2$ and their substituents, in agreement with experiment.(Sanderud & Sagstuen 1996) With respect to its calculated HFCCs, as can be seen in **Table 8** the values calculated for the α-hydrogen are in good agreement with experiment. The slight deviation in $A_{iso}$ from experiment is possibly due to the fact that the calculations are performed in the gas-phase on an isolated molecule and hence effects due to crystal packing are ignored. The calculated HFCCs for the two β-hydrogens are also in good agreement with the experiment. However, a rotational scan was performed in order to obtain the dihedral angle between the β-hydrogens and SOMO that gave HFCCs in best agreement between theory and experiment. It was found that this occurred for dihedral angles of -1.7° and 117.2°.

| Radical | Atom | $A_{iso}$ | $T_{xx}$ | $T_{yy}$ | $T_{zz}$ |
|---|---|---|---|---|---|
| I | $\alpha$-$H_{(calcd)}$ | -43.1 | 28.2 | -1.2 | -29.5 |
| | $\alpha$-$H_{(exp)}$ | -54.2 | 32.3 | 3.3 | -29.0 |
| | $\beta$-$H_{1(calcd)}$ | 105.6 | 8.7 | -2.4 | -6.3 |
| | $\beta$-$H_{1(exp)}$ | 104.3 | 7.2 | -2.0 | -5.3 |
| | $\beta$-$H_{2(calcd)}$ | 57.8 | 8.3 | -3.6 | -4.7 |
| | $\beta$-$H_{2(exp)}$ | 57.4 | 8.1 | -3.9 | -4.2 |
| II | $\alpha$-$H_{(calcd)}$ | -53.3 | -36.1 | -1.4 | 37.5 |
| | $\alpha$-$H_{(exp)}$ | -51.0 | -34.5 | 3.8 | 30.7 |
| | $\beta$-$H_{(calcd)}$ | 15.4 | 10.8 | -4.0 | -6.8 |
| | $\beta$-$H_{(exp)}$ | 25.0 | 14.0 | -7.0 | -8.0 |
| | $\beta$-$N_{(calcd)}$ | 12.7 | 2.1 | -0.9 | -1.2 |
| | $\beta$-$N_{(exp)}$ | 15.9 | 2.1 | -0.3 | -1.8 |
| | $\gamma$-$H_{(calcd)}$ | 1.9 | 4.3 | -1.5 | -2.8 |
| | $\gamma$-$H_{(exp)}$ | 5.9 | 10.1 | -4.1 | -5.8 |
| III | $\alpha$-$H_{1(calcd)}$ | -48.8 | -37.3 | -1.7 | 39.0 |
| | $\alpha$-$H_{1(exp)}$ | -47.1 | -22.0 | -1.5 | 23.6 |
| | $\alpha$-$H_{2(calcd)}$ | -59.3 | -37.4 | -1.5 | 38.8 |
| | $\alpha$-$H_{2(exp)}$ | -50.8 | -24.6 | 0.5 | 24.2 |
| | $\beta$-$H_{(calcd)}$ | 73.0 | 8.9 | -2.2 | -6.7 |
| | $\beta$-$H_{(exp)}$ | 73.0 | (13.3) | (-6.6) | (-6.6) |

Table 8. Comparison of calculated (see text) and experimental (Sanderud & Sagstuen 1996) isotropic and anisotropic components (MHz) of the hyperfine coupling tensor of radicals **I**, **II**, and **III**.

In contrast to radical **I**, the best agreement between computational and experimental HFCCs for radicals **II** and **III** was not obtained for their proposed structures shown in **Figure 7**. Rather, the structures that gave best agreement were found to be the radical-cationic forms of **II** and **III**; that is, structures in which their phosphate and carboxylic acid groups are neutral while the amino group is protonated. Hence, these latter structures were used in all HFCC studies on radicals **II** and **III**.

For radical-cationic **II** the calculated HFCCs for the α-hydrogen are generally in good agreement with the experimental values with $A_{iso}$ differing by just 2.3 MHz (**Table 8**). However, for both β-hydrogens, less satisfactory agreement between theory and experiment is observed. Specifically, the calculated $A_{iso}$ values of 15.4 and 12.7 MHz differ from their corresponding experimental values by 9.6 and 3.2 MHz, respectively. As noted for the α-hydrogen in **I**, these differences are likely due to bulk crystal effects not being modeled in the calculations. Similarly, for the γ-hydrogens on the amino group, a difference of 4.0 MHz is seen between the calculated and experimental values. However, it has been stated that the given experimental value is associated with a degree of uncertainty.(Sanderud & Sagstuen 1996) In the optimized structure of **II** the $C_3$ centre is not completely planar where an angle between the hydrogen on $C_3$ and the plane defined by $C_3$-$C_2$-O was found to be 22.0°.(Lipfert et al. 2004) This is in good agreement with the corresponding experimentally determined value of 19.5°.(Sanderud & Sagstuen 1996) It is noted that the $C_3$ centre and adjacent oxygen have spin densities of 0.84 and 0.11 respectively, suggesting slight delocalization of the SOMO. Dobbs et al.(Dobbs et al. 1971; Dobbs et al. 1972) have suggested that this is due to incomplete rehybridization of the carbon-centered radical and is common when the carbon is bonded to an oxygen.

Indeed, in radical-cationic **III** in which the phosphate group on $C_3$ has been lost, i.e., there is no $C_3-O$ bond, the radical is now fully localized on $C_3$. Furthermore, from **Table 8** it can be seen that quite good agreement is obtained for α-$H_1$ and the β-hydrogen with differences of 1.7 and 0.0 MHz respectively, while α-$H_2$ differs slightly more by 8.5 MHz. It should be noted that in order to obtain the best agreement for the HFCCs of the α-hydrogens they had to be tilted out of the plane by 5°. That is, the planarity of the $C_3$ centre had to be reduced. This is similar to that observed need in related studies on the methyl radical ($^{\bullet}CH_3$) to slightly pyramidalize the carbon centre in order to obtain best agreement between the calculated and experimentally measured HFCCs.(Eriksson et al. 1994)

## 6. Oxidative repair of alkylated nucleobases: the catalytic mechanism of AlkB

A common type of DNA damage is the alkylation of nucleobases at one or more of their oxygen and nitrogen centres.(Liu et al. 2009) This can be caused by endo- or exogenous agents such as S-adenosylmethionine or tobacco smoke, respectively.(Hecht 1999; Rydberg & Lindahl 1982) Consequently, cells have developed several methods by which to mediate or repair such damage. One approach is to use enzymes known as DNA glycolsylases to simply excise the damaged nucleobase via an acid-base cleavage of its N-glycosidic bond.(Mishina et al. 2006; Sedgwick et al. 2007) Alternatively, repair enzymes may use a non-redox mechanism to remove only the alkyl group. For example, $O^6$-methylguanine-DNA methyltransferase transfers the methyl of $O^6$-methylguanine onto an active site cysteinyl residue.(Lindahl et al. 1988) However, a third approach is alkyl group removal using a redox mechanism catalysed by the AlkB family of enzymes.

Although included in the α-ketoglutarate-Fe(II)-dependant dioxygenase superfamily, the AlkB family is the only one known to oxidatively dealkylate nucleobases.(Falnes et al. 2002; Trewick et al. 2002) Specifically, under physiological conditions they oxidatively repair the methylated nucleobases 1-meA, 1-meG, 3-meC and 3-meT (**Figure 8**).(Yang et al. 2008) It is noted, however, that they have been demonstrated to also be able to remove longer alkyl chains.(Delaney et al. 2005; Duncan et al. 2002; Koivisto et al. 2003; Mishina et al. 2005)

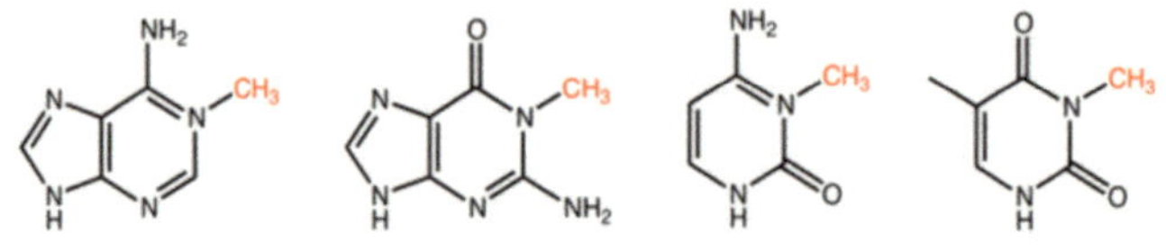


Fig. 8. Examples of methylated substrates that are dealkylated by the AlkB family of enzymes. The methyl groups to be removed have been colored in red.

Several X-ray crystal structures have been obtained of AlkB complexed with, for instance, cosubstrate or coproducts.(Yang et al. 2008; Yu et al. 2006) From these structures it was concluded that the active site of AlkB contains an Fe(II) ion ligated via two histidyl ($His_{131}$, $His_{187}$) and an aspartyl ($Asp_{133}$) residue. Furthermore, the α-ketoglutarate (α-KG) co-substrate bidentately ligates to the Fe(II) centre via carboxyl and ketone oxygens,(Falnes et al. 2002; Mishina et al. 2005; Trewick et al. 2002) while the methylated nucleobase sits adjacent to the Fe(II) centre. Based on these structures it was proposed that the mechanism of AlkB begins with activation of $O_2$: on binding to the Fe(II) centre the $O_2$ moiety is reduced to $O_2^{\bullet -}$ while the Fe centre is oxidized to Fe(III).(Berglund et al. 2002; Nakajima & Yamazaki 1987) The $O_2^{\bullet -}$ moiety formed then attacks the α-KG cosubstrate converting it to succinate with concomitant formation of an oxo-ferryl Fe(IV)=O species, a strong oxidizing agent.(Clifton et al. 2006; Kovaleva & Lipscomb 2008; Liu et al. 2009) However, the =O group of the oxo-ferryl sits in the apical position and thus is not ideally situated to react with the methylated nucleobase. Hence, it reorients to an equatorial position.(Yu et al. 2006)

An X-ray crystal structure (PDB: 2FD8) has been obtained under anaerobic conditions of AlkB with the single-strand trinucleotide dT-(1-me-dA)-dT bound within its active site.(Yu et al. 2006) Based on this experimental structure we obtained an appropriate chemical model for our computational studies. In particular, key active site residues, the Fe(II) centre, and α-KG modeled by pyruvate were included. A crystal structure water observed to be ligated to the Fe(II) centre in the apical position was replaced by $O_2$ while the substrate 1-methyladenine was modeled as 3-methyl-4-amino pyrimidinyl cation ($3me4amPym^+$). Calculations were then performed at the IEF-PCM($\varepsilon$=4.0)-B3LYP/LACV3P+(d,p)//B3LYP/LACVP(d) level of theory. For complete details on the model and methods used please refer to Liu et al. 2009.(Liu et al. 2009)

In this chapter we focus on key findings of the oxidative demethylation stage of the mechanism, shown schematically in **Figure 9**. However, it should be noted that the initial $O_2$ activation process preferentially occurs in the quintet spin state with a rate-limiting barrier of just 9.1 kcal $mol^{-1}$. The lowest energy pathway for the subsequent reorientation of the Fe(IV)=O species was also found to occur for the quintet spin state. Furthermore, it was found to proceed via a concerted mechanism with a barrier of 11.3 kcal $mol^{-1}$. For the oxidative demethylation itself, the lowest energy pathway also occurred on the quintet surface; the next lowest spin state, the triplet, at all times being higher in energy. Thus, herein, only the results for the quintet spin state are discussed. However, the energies for the triplet surface have been included in **Figure 9** for purposes of comparison.

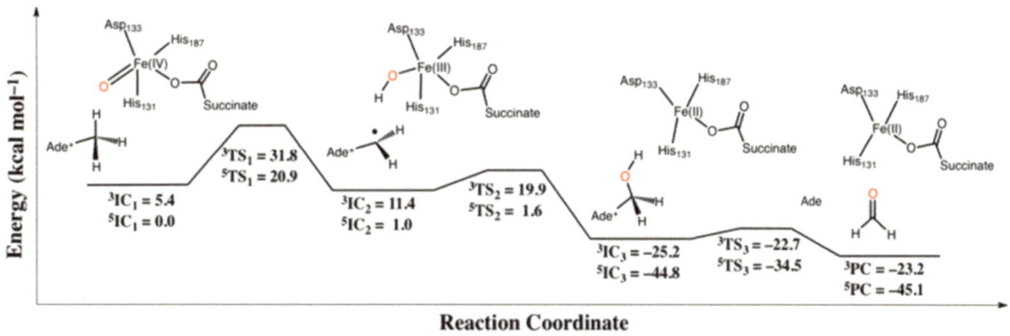


Fig. 9. Potential energy surface for the dealkylation of the methylated adenine nucleobase model 3me4amPym$^+$ in the triplet and quintet spin states.

In the apical position, the Fe(IV)=O oxygen is approximately 4.12 Å from the nearest target methyl hydrogen of the 3me4amPym$^+$ substrate. However, in $^5$**IC**$_1$, where it now lies in the equatorial position trans to His$_{187}$, this distance has been reduced dramatically to 2.68 Å. Demethylation is initiated by abstraction of a hydrogen (H$^\bullet$) from the target methyl group of the substrate by the Fe(IV)=O oxygen. This step proceeds via the transition structure $^5$**TS**$_1$ at a cost of 20.9 kcal mol$^{-1}$ to give intermediate $^5$**IC**$_2$ lying just 1.0 kcal mol$^{-1}$ higher in energy than $^5$**IC**$_1$. In $^5$**TS**$_1$ the cleaving -CH$_2$—H bond has lengthened to 1.30 Å while the corresponding FeO···H$^\bullet$ distance is quite short at 1.22 Å.(Liu et al. 2009)

This step is not only the rate limiting step in the actual demethylation of 3me4amPym$^+$, but is also the highest reaction barrier obtained in the overall mechanism of AlkB.(Liu et al. 2009) In the related α-KG-Fe(II) non-heme enzyme TauD, which catalyses hydroxylation of propene, abstraction of a methyl hydrogen by the Fe(IV)=O species was also calculated to be the rate limiting step.(de Visser 2006) The barrier in AlkB, however, is significantly higher. It has been observed that in C—H activating heme enzymes the barrier for such an abstraction is linearly related to the BDE of the substrates C—H bond being cleaved.(de Visser et al. 2004; Kaizer et al. 2004) Thus, the significantly higher barrier observed in AlkB compared to TauD is likely due to the 14.3 kcal mol$^{-1}$ greater -CH$_2$—H bond energy in its substrate, 3me4amPym$^+$. It should be noted that experimentally $k_{cat}$ for AlkB has been measured to be 4.5 min$^{-1}$,(Koivisto et al. 2003; Yu et al. 2006) corresponding to a rate-limiting barrier of 19.8 kcal mol$^{-1}$; in good agreement with the present calculated barrier height for $^5$**TS**$_1$.

In $^5$**IC**$_2$ the Fe(IV)=O has been reduced to Fe(III)—OH while the substrate now contains a methylene-carbon centered radical (see **Figure 9**). The next step is a 'rebound', transfer, of the hydroxyl group from the Fe-OH moiety to the substrate's radical centre. This reaction is almost barrierless proceeding via $^5$**TS**$_2$ with a cost of only 0.6 kcal mol$^{-1}$. Significantly, the resulting intermediate $^5$**IC**$_3$ lies markedly lower in energy than $^5$**IC**$_1$ by -44.8 kcal mol$^{-1}$. Thus, effectively, the result of the first two steps in demethylation are exothermic insertion of an oxygen into a C—H bond of the substrates methyl group with reduction of the Fe(IV) centre to Fe(II). The much lower relative energy of $^5$**IC**$_3$ may also reflect the structural rearrangement that occurs at the Fe centre which has gone from penta- to tetra-coordinate.

The final step in the demethylation of 3me4amPym$^+$ is decomposition of the hydroxylated intermediate to give 4–amino pyrimidine, the model for the demethylated nucleobase, and formaldehyde (**Figure 9**). In this step an active site $Glu_{136}$ residue acts as a general base and deprotonates the Ade-$CH_2OH$ hydroxyl with concomitant cleavage of the $_{Ade}N-CH_2OH$ bond.(Liu et al. 2009) This reaction proceeds via $^5$**TS$_3$** at the modest cost of 10.3 kcal mol$^{-1}$. It is noted that in $^5$**TS$_3$** the $_{Ade}N\cdots CH_2OH$ and Ade-$CH_2O-H$ bonds have lengthened to 1.58 and 1.22 Å, respectively, highlighting their concomitant cleavage. The product-bound complex $^5$**PC** lies 45.1 kcal mol$^{-1}$ lower in relative energy than the initial reactant complex $^5$**IC$_1$**. Thus, demethylation of 1-methyladenine is calculated to be a quite exothermic process.

## 7. Conclusion

In this chapter the application of density functional theory (DFT)-based methods to the study of DNA damage and repair mechanisms has been illustrated.
In particular, it was shown how they may be used to provide accurate detailed insights into the thermochemistry of fundamental chemical processes such as electron and proton transfers and thus, help to explain a number of experimental observations. Furthermore, through such studies they were able to show differences in the preferred oxidation pathways for the various DNA nucleobases. Similarly, by the careful examination of calculated hyperfine coupling constants, the nature *and* structure of radicals that may be formed upon exposure of DNA to radiation were deduced. Such an understanding also aids in determining the mechanism by which they may be formed. Finally, their versatility for the investigation of damage and repair mechanisms was highlighted. Indeed, by examining several pathways using seemingly quite simple chemical models, we have been able to deduce the preferred mechanism by which the deamination of cytosine radical may occur including (i) the preferred proton source(s), (ii) the order in which they are added to the leaving nitrogen centre, and (iii) the thermodynamically preferred products. Finally, similar methods in combination with much larger chemical models were used to also elucidate the oxidative dealkylation repair mechanism of AlkB. Together, these studies highlight the versatility and accuracy of DFT methods when used in combination with well-chosen chemical models for the study of DNA damage and repair.

## 8. Acknowledgements

JWG, JL and EACB acknowledge the Natural Sciences and Engineering Research Council (NSERC, Canada) for funding and CGS & PGSD scholarships (EACB) and JL and LAE thank the Swedish Science Research Council (VR) for funding. LAE also acknowledges the National University of Ireland (Galway) for financial support. SHARCNET (Canada) and the National Supercomputing Centre (Linköping, Sweden) are acknowledged for additional computational resources.

## 9. References

Almatarneh, M. H., Flinn, C. G., Poirier, R. A., & Sokalski, W. A. (2006). "Computational study of the deamination reaction of cytosine with $H_2O$ and OH." *J. Phys. Chem. A*, 110(26), 8227-8234.

Becke, A. D. (1993a). "A Mixing of Hartree-Fock and Local Density-Functional Theories." *J. Chem. Phys.*, 98, 1372.

Becke, A. D. (1993b). "Density-Functional Thermochemistry .3. The Role of Exact Exchange." *J. Chem. Phys.*, 98(7), 5648-5652.

Berglund, G. I., Carlsson, G. H., Smith, A. T., Szoke, H., Henriksen, A., & Hajdu, J. (2002). "The catalytic pathway of horseradish peroxidase at high resolution." *Nature*, 417(6887), 463-468.

Burrows, C. J., & Muller, J. G. (1998). "Oxidative nucleobase modifications leading to strand scission." *Chem. Rev.*, 98(3), 1109-1151.

Cadet, J., Douki, T., & Ravanat, J. L. (2006). "One-electron oxidation of DNA and inflammation processes." *Nat. Chem. Biol.*, 2(7), 348-349.

Cadet, J., Douki, T., & Ravanat, J. L. (2008). "Oxidatively generated damage to the guanine moiety of DNA: Mechanistic aspects and formation in cells." *Accounts Chem. Res.*, 41(8), 1075-1083.

Cadet, J., & Vigny, P. (1990). Bioorganic Photochemistry. Photochemistry and the Nucleic Acids, H. Morrison, ed., Wiley, New York, 1-272.

Cammi, R., & Tomasi, J. (1995). "Remarks on the use of the apparent surface-charges (ASC) methods in solvation problems - Iterative versus matrix-inversion procedures and the renormalization of the apparent charges." *J. Comput. Chem.*, 16(12), 1449-1458.

Cances, E., & Mennucci, B. (1998). "New applications of integral equations methods for solvation continuum models: ionic solutions and liquid crystals." *J. Math. Chem.*, 23(3-4), 309-326.

Cances, E., Mennucci, B., & Tomasi, J. (1997). "A new integral equation formalism for the polarizable continuum model: Theoretical background and applications to isotropic and anisotropic dielectrics." *J. Chem. Phys.*, 107(8), 3032-3041.

Candeias, L. P., & Steenken, S. (2000). "Reaction of HO center dot with guanine derivatives in aqueous solution: Formation of two different redox-active OH-Adduct radicals and their unimolecular transformation reactions. Properties of G(-H)(center dot)." *Chem.-Eur. J.*, 6(3), 475-484.

Cauet, E., Dehareng, D., & Lievin, J. (2006). "Ab initio study of the ionization of the DNA bases: Ionization potentials and excited states of the cations." *J. Phys. Chem. A*, 110(29), 9200-9211.

Chatgilialoglu, C., Ferreri, C., Bazzanini, R., Guerra, M., Choi, S. Y., Emanuel, C. J., Horner, J. H., & Newcomb, M. (2000). "Models of DNA C1 ' radicals. Structural, spectral, and chemical properties of the thyminylmethyl radical and the 2 '-deoxyuridin-1 '-yl radical." *J. Am. Chem. Soc.*, 122(39), 9525-9533.

Cheng, K. C., Cahill, D. S., Kasai, H., Nishimura, S., & Loeb, L. A. (1992). "8-hydroxyguanine, an abundant form of oxidative dna damage, causes g -> t and a -> c substitutions." *J. Biol. Chem.*, 267(1), 166-172.

Clifton, I. J., McDonough, M. A., Ehrismann, D., Kershaw, N. J., Granatino, N., & Schofield, C. J. (2006). "Structural studies on 2-oxoglutarate oxygenases and related double-stranded beta-helix fold proteins." *J. Inorg. Biochem.*, 100(4), 644-669.

Cullis, P. M., Malone, M. E., & MersonDavies, L. A. (1996). "Guanine radical cations are precursors of 7,8-dihydro-8-oxo-2'-deoxyguanosine but are not precursors of immediate strand breaks in DNA." *J. Am. Chem. Soc.*, 118(12), 2775-2781.

De Bont, R., & van Larebeke, N. (2004). "Endogenous DNA damage in humans: a review of quantitative data." *Mutagenesis*, 19(3), 169-185.

de Visser, S. P. (2006). "Propene activation by the oxo-iron active species of taurine/alpha-ketoglutarate dioxygenase (TauD) enzyme. How does the catalysis compare to heme-enzymes?" *J. Am. Chem. Soc.*, 128(30), 9813-9824.

de Visser, S. P., Kumar, D., Cohen, S., Shacham, R., & Shaik, S. (2004). "A predictive pattern of computed barriers for C-H hydroxylation by compound I of cytochrome P450." *J. Am. Chem. Soc.*, 126(27), 8362-8363.

Decarroz, C., Wagner, J. R., & Cadet, J. (1987). *Free Radical Res. Commun.*(2), 295-301.

Decarroz, C., Wagner, J. R., Vanlier, J. E., Krishna, C. M., Riesz, P., & Cadet, J. (1986). "Sensitized photooxidation of thymidine by 2-methyl-1-1,4-naphthoquinone - characterization of the stable photoproducts." *Int. J. Radiat. Biol.*, 50(3), 491-505.

Delaney, J. C., Smeester, L., Wong, C. Y., Frick, L. E., Taghizadeh, K., Wishnok, J. S., Drennan, C. L., Samson, L. D., & Essigmann, J. M. (2005). "AlkB reverses etheno DNA lesions caused by lipid oxidation in vitro and in vivo." *Nat. Struct. Mol. Biol.*, 12(10), 855-860.

Dobbs, A. J., Gilbert, B. C., & Norman, R. O. C. (1971). "Electron spin resonance studies .27. geometry of oxygen-substituted alkyl radicals." *J. Chem. Soc. A*(1), 124-&.

Dobbs, A. J., Gilbert, B. C., & Norman, R. O. C. (1972). "Electron-spin resonance studies .32. information from hyperfine splittings for aliphatic radicals about shape and conformation." *J. Chem. Soc.-Perkin Trans. 2*(6), 786-&.

Douki, T., & Cadet, J. (1999). "Modification of DNA bases by photosensitized one-electron oxidation." *Int. J. Radiat. Biol.*, 75(5), 571-581.

Duncan, T., Trewick, S. C., Koivisto, P., Bates, P. A., Lindahl, T., & Sedgwick, B. (2002). "Reversal of DNA alkylation damage by two human dioxygenases." *Proc. Natl. Acad. Sci. U. S. A.*, 99(26), 16660-16665.

Eley, D. D., & Spivey, D. I. (1962). "Semiconductivity of organic substances .9. Nucleic acid in dry state." *Trans. Faraday Soc.*, 58, 411.

Eriksson, L. A., Malkin, V. G., Malkina, O. L., & Salahub, D. R. (1994). "The effects of nonlocal gradient corrections in density-functional calculations of hydrocarbon radical hyperfine structures." *Int. J. Quantum Chem.*, 52(4), 879-901.

Falnes, P. O., Johansen, R. F., & Seeberg, E. (2002). "AlkB-mediated oxidative demethylation reverses DNA damage in Escherichia coli." *Nature*, 419(6903), 178-182.

Friedberg, E. C., McDaniel, L. D., & Schultz, R. A. (2004). "The role of endogenous and exogenous DNA damage and mutagenesis." *Curr. Opin. Genet. Dev.*, 14(1), 5-10.

Hagen, U. (1986). "Current aspects on the radiation-induced base damage in dna." *Radiat. Environ. Biophys.*, 25(4), 261-271.

Hatahet, A., & Wallace, Z.Z. (1998). DNA Damage and Repair, DNA Repair in Prokaryotes and Lower Eukaryotes, J. A. Nickoloff, Hoekstra, M.F., ed., Humana Press, New Jersey.

Hecht, S. S. (1999). "DNA adduct formation from tobacco-specific N-nitrosamines." *Mutat. Res.-Fundam. Mol. Mech. Mutagen.*, 424(1-2), 127-142.

Hush, N. S., & Cheung, A. S. (1975). "Ionization-potentials and donor properties of nucleic-acid bases and related compounds." *Chem. Phys. Lett.*, 34(1), 11-13.

Kaizer, J., Klinker, E. J., Oh, N. Y., Rohde, J. U., Song, W. J., Stubna, A., Kim, J., Munck, E., Nam, W., & Que, L. (2004). "Nonheme (FeO)-O-IV complexes that can oxidize the C-H bonds of cyclohexane at room temperature." *J. Am. Chem. Soc.*, 126(2), 472-473.

Kamiya, H., Iwai, S., & Kasai, H. (1998). "The (6-4) photoproduct of thymine-thymine induces targeted substitution mutations in mammalian cells." *Nucleic Acids Res.*, 26(11), 2611-2617.

Kasai, H., Crain, P. F., Kuchino, Y., Nishimura, S., Ootsuyama, A., & Tanooka, H. (1986). "Formation of 8-hydroxyguanine moiety in cellular dna by agents producing oxygen radicals and evidence for its repair." *Carcinogenesis*, 7(11), 1849-1851.

Koivisto, P., Duncan, T., Lindahl, T., & Sedgwick, B. (2003). "Minimal methylated substrate and extended substrate range of Escherichia coli AlkB protein, a 1-methyladenine-DNA dioxygenase." *J. Biol. Chem.*, 278(45), 44348-44354.

Kovaleva, E. G., & Lipscomb, J. D. (2008). "Versatility of biological non-heme Fe(II) centers in oxygen activation reactions." *Nat. Chem. Biol.*, 4(3), 186-193.

Kumar, A., & Sevilla, M. D. (2010). "Proton-Coupled Electron Transfer in DNA on Formation of Radiation-Produced Ion Radicals." *Chem. Rev.*, 110(12), 7002-7023.

Labet, V., Grand, A., Cadet, J., & Eriksson, L. A. (2008a). "Deamination of the radical cation of the base moiety of 2 '-deoxycytidine: A theoretical study." *ChemPhysChem*, 9(8), 1195-1203.

Labet, V., Grand, A., Morell, C., Cadet, J., & Eriksson, L. A. (2008b). "Proton catalyzed hydrolytic deamination of cytosine: a computational study." *Theor. Chem. Acc.*, 120(4-6), 429-435.

Labet, V., Grand, A., Morell, C., Cadet, J., & Eriksson, L. A. (2009). "Mechanism of nitric oxide induced deamination of cytosine." *Phys. Chem. Chem. Phys.*, 11, 2379-2386.

Lee, C. T., Yang, W. T., & Parr, R. G. (1988). "Development of the colle-salvetti correlation-energy formula into a functional of the electron-density." *Phys. Rev. B*, 37(2), 785-789.

Lee, Y. A., Yun, B. H., Kim, S. K., Margolin, Y., Dedon, P. C., Geacintov, N. E., & Shafirovich, V. (2007). "Mechanisms of oxidation of guanine in DNA by carbonate radical anion, a decomposition product of nitrosoperoxycarbonate." *Chem.-Eur. J.*, 13(16), 4571-4581.

Lindahl, T. (1993). "Instability and decay of the primary structure of dna." *Nature*, 362(6422), 709-715.

Lindahl, T., Sedgwick, B., Sekiguchi, M., & Nakabeppu, Y. (1988). "Regulation and expression of the adaptive response to alkylating-agents." *Annu. Rev. Biochem.*, 57, 133-157.

Lipfert, J., Llano, J., & Eriksson, L. A. (2004). "Radiation-induced damage in serine phosphate-insights into a mechanism for direct DNA strand breakage." *J. Phys. Chem. B*, 108(23), 8036-8042.

Liu, H. N., Llano, J., & Gauld, J. W. (2009). "A DFT Study of Nucleobase Dealkylation by the DNA Repair Enzyme AlkB." *J. Phys. Chem. B*, 113(14), 4887-4898.

Llano, J., & Eriksson, L. A. (2002). "First principles electrochemistry: Electrons and protons reacting as independent ions." *J. Chem. Phys.*, 117(22), 10193-10206.

Llano, J., & Eriksson, L. A. (2004a). "First principles electrochemical study of redox events in DNA bases and chemical repair in aqueous solution." *Phys. Chem. Chem. Phys.*, 6(9), 2426-2433.

Llano, J., & Eriksson, L. A. (2004b). "Oxidation pathways of adenine and guanine in aqueous solution from first principles electrochemistry." *Phys. Chem. Chem. Phys.*, 6(19), 4707-4713.

Llano, J., & Gauld, J.W. (2010). Mechanistics of Enzyme Catalysis: From Small to Large Active-Site Models, In: *Quantum Biochemistry: Electronic Structure and Biological Activity*, Matta, C. F., 643-666, Wiley-VCH, Weinheim.

Lysetska, M., Knoll, A., Boehringer, D., Hey, T., Krauss, G., & Krausch, G. (2002). "UV light-damaged DNA and its interaction with human replication protein A: an atomic force microscopy study." *Nucleic Acids Res.*, 30(12), 2686-2691.

Mennucci, B., Cances, E., & Tomasi, J. (1997). "Evaluation of solvent effects in isotropic and anisotropic dielectrics and in ionic solutions with a unified integral equation method: Theoretical bases, computational implementation, and numerical applications." *J. Phys. Chem. B*, 101(49), 10506-10517.

Miertus, S., Scrocco, E., & Tomasi, J. (1981). "Electrostatic interaction of a solute with a continuum - a direct utilization of abinitio molecular potentials for the prevision of solvent effects." *Chem. Phys.*, 55(1), 117-129.

Mishina, Y., Duguid, E. M., & He, C. (2006). "Direct reversal of DNA alkylation damage." *Chem. Rev.*, 106(2), 215-232.

Mishina, Y., Yang, C. G., & He, C. (2005). "Direct repair of the exocyclic DNA adduct 1,N-6-ethenoadenine by the DNA repair AlkB proteins." *J. Am. Chem. Soc.*, 127(42), 14594-14595.

Munk, B. H., Burrows, C. J., Schlegel, H. B. (2008). "An Exploration of Mechanisms for the Transformation of 8-Oxoguanine to Guanidinohydantoin and Spiroiminodihydantoin by Density Functional Theory." *J. Am. Chem. Soc.*, 130, 5245-5256

Nakajima, R., & Yamazaki, I. (1987). "The mechanism of oxyperoxidase formation from ferryl peroxidase and hydrogen-peroxide." *J. Biol. Chem.*, 262(6), 2576-2581.

Neeley, W. L., & Essigmann, J. M. (2006). "Mechanisms of formation, genotoxicity, and mutation of guanine oxidation products." *Chem. Res. Toxicol.*, 19(4), 491-505.

Newcomb, T. G., & Loeb, L.A. (1998). DNA Damage and Repair, DNA Repair in Prokaryotes and Lower Eukaryotes, J. A. Nickoloff, Hoekstra, M.F., ed., Humana Press, New Jersey.

Pages, V., & Fuchs, R. P. P. (2002). "How DNA lesions are turned into mutations within cells?" *Oncogene*, 21(58), 8957-8966.

Pavlov, Y. I., Minnick, D. T., Izuta, S., & Kunkel, T. A. (1994). "DNA-replication fidelity with 8-oxodeoxyguanosine triphosphate." *Biochemistry*, 33(15), 4695-4701.

Rydberg, B., & Lindahl, T. (1982). "Non-enzymatic methylation of DNA by the intracellular methyl-group donor s-adenosyl-l-methionine is a potentially mutagenic reaction." *Embo J.*, 1(2), 211-216.

Sanderud, A., & Sagstuen, E. (1996). "EPR and ENDOR studies of H-1 and N-14 hyperfine and quadrupolar couplings in crystals of L-O-serine phosphate after X-irradiation at 295 K." *J. Phys. Chem.*, 100(22), 9545-9555.

Sedgwick, B., Bates, P. A., Paik, J., Jacobs, S. C., & Lindahl, T. (2007). "Repair of alkylated DNA: Recent advances." *DNA Repair*, 6(4), 429-442.

Seidel, C. A. M., Schulz, A., & Sauer, M. H. M. (1996). "Nucleobase-specific quenching of fluorescent dyes .1. Nucleobase one-electron redox potentials and their correlation with static and dynamic quenching efficiencies." *J. Phys. Chem.*, 100(13), 5541-5553.

Sponer, J. E., Miguel, P. J. S., Rodriguez-Santiago, L., Erxleben, A., Krumm, M., Sodupe, M., Sponer, J., & Lippert, B. (2004). "Metal-mediated deamination of cytosine: Experiment and DFT calculations." *Angew. Chem.-Int. Edit.*, 43(40), 5396-5399.

Steenken, S. (1989). "Purine-bases, nucleosides, and nucleotides - aqueous-solution redox chemistry and transformation reactions of their radical cations and e- and OH adducts." *Chem. Rev.*, 89(3), 503-520.

Steenken, S. (1992). "Electron-transfer-induced acidity basicity and reactivity changes of purine and pyrimidine-bases - consequences of redox processes for DNA-base pairs." *Free Radic. Res. Commun.*, 16(6), 349-379.

Steenken, S., & Goldbergerova, L. (1998). "Photoionization of organic phosphates by 193 nm laser light in aqueous solution: Rapid intramolecular H-transfer to the primarily formed phosphate radical. A model for ionization-induced chain-breakage in DNA?" *J. Am. Chem. Soc.*, 120(16), 3928-3934.

Steenken, S., & Jovanovic, S. V. (1997). "How easily oxidizable is DNA? One-electron reduction potentials of adenosine and guanosine radicals in aqueous solution." *J. Am. Chem. Soc.*, 119(3), 617-618.

Steenken, S., Telo, J. P., Novais, H. M., & Candeias, L. P. (1992). "One-electron-reduction potentials of pyrimidine-bases, nucleosides, and nucleotides in aqueous-solution - consequences for DNA redox chemistry." *J. Am. Chem. Soc.*, 114(12), 4701-4709.

Taylor, J. S. (1994). "Unraveling the molecular pathway from sunlight to skin-cancer." *Accounts Chem. Res.*, 27(3), 76-82.

Teoule, R. (1987). "Radiation-induced DNA damage and its repair." *Int. J. Radiat. Biol.*, 51(4), 573-589.

Trewick, S. C., Henshaw, T. F., Hausinger, R. P., Lindahl, T., & Sedgwick, B. (2002). "Oxidative demethylation by Escherichia coli AlkB directly reverts DNA base damage." *Nature*, 419(6903), 174-178.

von Sonntag, C. (1987). *The Chemical Basis of Radiation Biology*, Taylor & Francis, London.

von Sonntag, C., Schuchmann, H.P. (1996). Encyclopedia of Molecular Biology and Molecular Medicine, R. A. Meyers, ed., VCH, Weinheim.

Wagner, J. R., Vanlier, J. E., Decarroz, C., Berger, M., & Cadet, J. (1990). "Photodynamic methods for oxy radical-induced dna-damage." *Method Enzymol.*, 186, 502-511.

Wang, Y. S. (2008). "Bulky DNA lesions induced by reactive oxygen species." *Chem. Res. Toxicol.*, 21(2), 276-281.

Wetmore, S. D., Boyd, R. J., & Eriksson, L. A. (2000). "Electron affinities and ionization potentials of nucleotide bases." *Chem. Phys. Lett.*, 322(1-2), 129-135.

Wetmore, S. D., Eriksson, L. A. & Boyd, R. J., (2001). A Multi-Component Model for Radiation Damage to DNA from its Constituents in Theoretical Biochemistry Processes and Properties of Biological Systems, In: *Theoretical and Computational Chemistry*, Eriksson, L. A., 409-466, Elsevier, Amsterdam.

Wetmore, S. D., Himo, F., Boyd, R. J., & Eriksson, L. A. (1998). "Effects of ionizing radiation on crystalline cytosine monohydrate." *J. Phys. Chem. B*, 102(38), 7484-7491.

Yang, C. G., Yi, C. Q., Duguid, E. M., Sullivan, C. T., Jian, X., Rice, P. A., & He, C. (2008). "Crystal structures of DNA/RNA repair enzymes AlkB and ABH2 bound to dsDNA." *Nature*, 452(7190), 961-U4.

Yang, X., Wang, X. B., Vorpagel, E. R., & Wang, L. S. (2004). "Direct experimental observation of the low ionization potentials of guanine in free oligonucleotides by using photoelectron spectroscopy." *Proc. Natl. Acad. Sci. U. S. A.*, 101(51), 17588-17592.

Yao, L. S., Li, Y., Wu, Y., Liu, A. Z., & Yan, H. G. (2005). "Product release is rate-limiting in the activation of the prodrug 5-fluorocytosine by yeast cytosine deaminase." *Biochemistry*, 44(15), 5940-5947.

Yu, B., Edstrom, W. C., Benach, J., Hamuro, Y., Weber, P. C., Gibney, B. R., & Hunt, J. F. (2006). "Crystal structures of catalytic complexes of the oxidative DNA/RNA repair enzyme AlkB." *Nature*, 439(7078), 879-884.

# Part 4

## Insights into Therapeutic Strategies

18

# DNA Radiosensitization: The Search for Repair Refractive Lesions Including Double Strand Breaks and Interstrand Crosslinks

Tsvetan G. Gantchev[1,2], Marie-Eve Dextraze[1] and Darel J. Hunting[1]
[1]*Department of Nuclear Medicine & Radiobiology, Faculté de medicine, Université de Sherbrooke, Sherbrooke, Québec,*
[2]*Department of Gene Regulations, Institute of Molecular Biology, Bulgarian Academy of Sciences, Sofia,*
[1]*Canada*
[2]*Bulgaria*

## 1. Introduction

More than half of all cancer patients receive radiotherapy (RT) as part of their treatment regimens. The cytotoxicity of ionizing radiation is mainly mediated by the ensuing DNA damage. Double-stranded DNA breaks (DSB) are generally accepted to be the most important lesions for the induction of cell death by ionizing radiation because they are much more difficult to repair than single strand breaks, although their radiation yield is very low, at two orders of magnitude less than that of single strand breaks (SSB) (Hempel & Mildenberger, 1987). The role of other DNA lesions such as base damage and interstrand crosslinks in cell killing has not been yet fully elucidated. Gamma-radiation inflicts DNA damage *via* two separated processes: i) direct interaction with DNA and; ii) indirect damage produced by secondary radicals ($^{\bullet}OH$, $^{\bullet}H$ and $e^{-}_{aq}$) generated after water radiolysis (Michaels & Hunt, 1978). Among the $H_2O$ derived radicals, hydroxyl radicals ($^{\bullet}OH$) are the species primarily responsible for strand break formation and DNA base damage (> 35%). Hydrated electrons, $e^{-}_{aq}$, which are generated at a yield comparable to the $^{\bullet}OH$ (G-values of ~ $2.8 \times 10^{-7}$ mol.J$^{-1}$), participate in only ~ 8% of the total damage and the exact nature of DNA damage formed *in vivo* by $e^{-}_{aq}$ is obscure (Nabben *et al.*, 1982). In vertebrate cells, the majority of RT-induced DSB are repaired by non-homologous end joining (NHEJ) with some contribution from homologous recombination repair (HRR) during the late S and G2 phases of the cell cycle (Jackson, 2002; Takata *et al.*, 1998). The repair of other DNA damages, such as interstrand crosslinks (ICL) is more complicated and less understood (Wang, 2007; Moldovan & D'Andrea, 2009). ICLs can be recognized by the nucleotide excision repair (NER) system and it is accepted that ICL repair involves nucleolytic cleavage at or near the site of ICL to produce a suitable substrate that can subsequently be repaired by homologous recombination (HR) (D'Andrea & Grompe, 2003; Moldovan & D'Andrea, 2009a, Liu *et al.*, 2010).

An approach to improve the effectiveness of RT is either to enhance the formation of lethal DNA lesions, or to use inhibitors of DNA repair pathways (or both) and thus to render tumor cells more sensitive to ionizing radiation. A novel strategy to inhibit radiation-induced double strand break repair was recently promoted by using short modified DNA molecules that mimic double strand breaks (Dbaits) and artificially activate the DNA-PK pathway (Quanz *et al.*, 2009). Likewise, using siRNA screening of genes involved in DNA damage repair, Higgins *et al.* (2010) identified POLQ (DNA polymerase θ) as a potential tumor-specific target whose knockdown led to tumor cell-specific radiosensitization. However, with the exception of oxygen-enhancing or mimetic agents and platinum derivatives such as cis-platinum, which amplify DNA damage, the only direct DNA radiosensitizing agents known to date are halogenated uracils, such as 5-bromodeoxyuridine (BrdU). BrdU administration to cultured cells, animals and humans leads to replacement of isosteric thymine by 5-bromouracil during replication and excision repair of DNA. The basic pathway of BrdU radiolysis and DNA strand break formation in solution was described many years ago (Zimbrick *et al.*, 1969a,b). It involves dissociative $e^-_{aq}$ attachment to BrdU, followed by the formation of a 5-uracil-yl σ-radical (•U) and a bromine ion ($Br^-$, Fig. 1). The reaction is very efficient in air-free solutions, with $k(e^-_{aq} + BrU) = 2.6 \times 10^{10}\ M^{-1}s^{-1}$ and $G(U) = 2.4 \times 10^{-7}\ mol.J^{-1}$, but interactions with •OH may intervene and can lead to somewhat different products. BrdU is also an efficient UV-light absorbing phtotosensitizer; the homolytic Br−C bond cleavage, however, results in two

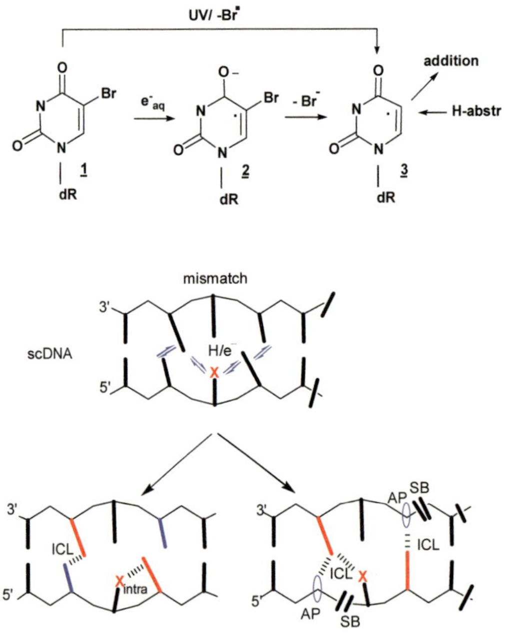


Fig. 1. Primary reaction mechanism of 5-BrdU sensitization and subsequent damages in wobble scDNA. The dynamic structure of scDNA facilitates electron (hydrogen atom) transfer (ET) between the two strands. The ET direction depends on the BrdU local sequence context (e.g. purine *vs.* pyrimidine environment). In the scheme the 5-uracil-yl radical (3) and its products are denoted by X. Modified bases (reduced or oxidized; red and blue), uracil and/or 2'-deoxyribose may further interact between and/or with undamaged bases and oxygen to form various products, including AP-sites, intra- and inter-strand crosslinks (ICL) and strand breaks (SB).

radical species (•U and •Br). It is generally assumed that •U abstracts an H-atom from 2′-deoxyribose to form a strand break or accepts an electron from a neighboring base (inter-base chain $e^-$ transfer (ET), generating an oxidized base), which eventually terminates with the formation of a guanine cation radical, $G^{+\bullet}$ (Nese *et al.*, 1992). •U-radical addition reactions may result in DNA crosslinks (Fig. 1), but this was only recently shown experimentally (Zeng & Wang, 2007). New findings show that electron capture and migration along BrdU-substituted DNA might be contra-thermodynamically selective and, thus far more complicated (Yoshioka *et al.*, 1999; Aflatooni *et al.*, 1998). In cells, radiosensitization by BrdU (typically at ~20-30% thymine replacement) gives about 2-3 fold radiotoxicity enhancement and in most cell types parallels similar increase in the DSB yield, and/or the decreased rate of their repair (Sawada & Okada, 1972). Further characteristics of BrdU-mediated DSB and other DNA damages *in vivo* (*e.g.* DNA crosslinks) are scarcely available.

## 2. DNA-structure/conformation dependent BrdU-sensitized formation of strand breaks

A crucial difference between the radiosensitization of single and double stranded DNA by BrdU was not known until our work with purified *semi*-complementary (mismatched) DNA showing the single stranded specificity of BrdU-induced DNA damage (Cecchini *et al.*, 2004). In parallel experiments, using BrdU-substituted (or not) single-stranded (ssDNA), double-stranded (dsDNA) and mismatched (wobble) semi-complementary (scDNA) DNA we have found that BrdU efficiently sensitizes single stranded BrdU-substituted (brominated) oligonucleotides, but not when these are hybridized to completely complementary oligonucleotides to form normal dsDNA duplexes. We estimate that BrdU radiosensitization efficiency in dsDNA drops up to 20-fold compared to that in ssDNA. Comparative measurements of radiolytic loss of the bromine atom in ssDNA *vs.* dsDNA likewise indicate that this process is greatly suppressed in dsDNA (Cecchini *et al.*, 2004, 2005a). In mismatched, scDNA duplexes, strand brakes are formed in loci encompassing nucleotides surrounding BrdU. However, high efficiency single strand break formation takes place on the brominated strand, or on the opposite, non-brominated strand but have not been detected on both, suggesting that they are mutually exclusive events (Hunting *et al.*, unpublished; Cecchini *et al.*, 2005b). Experiments performed with scDNA bearing variable number of mismatches (from one to five) and containing a single BrdU substitution gave qualitatively similar results. The radiation dose-response for strand break formation was linear for both the brominated and the opposite, non-brominated strand within the single-stranded regions of a standard model scDNA containing a bulge formed by up to five mismatched bases (Dextraze *et al.*, 2007). Interestingly, UVB-irradiation of BrdU-substituted DNA also demonstrated DNA-structure specificity, but in this situation BrdU greatly enhances breakage of only the brominated strand in dsDNA, or either the brominated or the non-brominated strand in the case of scDNA (Cecchini *et al.*, 2005b; Chen *et al.*, 2000). The different effects initiated by radiolysis and photolysis, especially with BrdU-dsDNA, underline the role of DNA structure-conformation properties in solution as a prerequisite for the initial electron-capture by BrdU and/or the propagation of an excess-electron along the polymer after gamma-irradiation.

The importance of DNA structure during sensitization by BrdU is further demonstrated by comparison of the damages induced in A- and B-form DNA. Using brominated 25-mer oligonucleotides hybridized to complementary or semi-complementary ones with five mismatched bases: AAT(orBU)AA, we have shown that strand breaks are specific for B-DNA, whereas A-DNA only undergoes formation of alkali-labile DNA lesions (Dextraze *et al.,* 2007). Piperidine-sensitive lesions are observed exclusively at the site of BrdU substitution. Generally, the cleavage reaction is a confluence of at least three factors: $e^{-}_{aq}$ capture, forward electron transfer and charge recombination. The strand break positions migrate along the DNA strand, however, there is a clear preference for the dA 5′-flanking BrdU. Similarly, 5′-dABrdU-sequence preference has been observed in UV-induced BrdU DNA cleavage (Chen *et al.*, 2000). This is to be expected since in B-DNA the 5′ proximal 2′-deoxyribose would be the ultimate H-atom donor to the uracil-5-yl radical, whereas in A-DNA conformational (spatial) restrictions render the same 5′dA 2′-deoxyribose a less-accessible H-donor. Therefore, in A-DNA the uracil-5-yl radical is more likely to abstract H-atoms from other donors (bases), thus oxidizing proximal to the BrdU-site bases which results in alkali-labile site formation.

Sequence-preferential strand break formation was examined in a series of 25-mer scDNA encompassing a central 1- or 5-mer mismatched site with BrdU incorporated (brominated strand) in a purine 5′d(AABrdUAA), 5′d(GGBrdUGG), or a pyrimidine 5′d(ATBrdUTA) environment, and the semi-complimentary (non-brominated) strand contained any of the sequences: 5′d(AATAA), 5′d(CCCCC), 5′d(GGGGG), or 5′d(ATTTA) (twelve permutations in total) (Dextraze *et al.*, 2007; 2009). While there was no significant change between the strand-break yields in ssDNA and typically there were no changes in strand breaks produced on each strand (*i.e.*, brominated *vs.* nonbrominated), two wobble sequence permutations derived from the above pattern: d(GGBrdUGG)^d(GGGGG) and d(ATBrdUTA)^d(ATTTA) produced more breaks on the brominated strand, whereas the generation of breaks was enhanced in the non-brominated strand in the combinations: d(GGBrdUGG)^d(AATAA), d(GGBrdUGG)^d(ATTTA), and d(AABrdUAA)^d(GGGGG). Similarly irradiation of the same scDNA, gave different patterns of interstrand crosslinks (see below).

## 3. BrdU sensitized formation of interstrand crosslinks (ICL) in mismatched (wobble) DNA duplexes

In addition to increasing strand break generation by ionizing radiation, the presence of bromouracil induces formation of DNA interstrand crosslinks (ICL). This process occurs in single stranded regions within double stranded DNA (*i.e.*, in scDNA) and requires the presence of B-DNA (Dextraze *et al.*, 2007; 2009). Although anticipated, the generation of ICL during radiosensitization with BrdU has not been demonstrated experimentally prior to our work (Cecchini *et al.*, 2005a). Formation of intra-strand crosslinks has been reported in UVB-irradiated BrdU-substituted synthetic DNA (Zeng & Wang, 2006) and in cells (Zeng & Wang, 2007). However, the generation of DNA ICLs by ionizing radiation has been largely ignored in favor to studies on double-strand breaks and their repair. At least part of the problem is technical; it is difficult to detect and quantify ICLs when the same agent forms both strand breaks and ICL, because the analysis of ICL generally involves a denaturing step. Apart from multiple damage events that may cause the disappearance of ICL-products due to DNA backbone cleavage at nucleotides located between the ICL-site and the radiolabel, another factor that obstructs DNA-ICL detection is that ICLs may decompose under prolonged irradiation, especially in the presence of $O_2$ (Ding & Greenberg, 2007).

Therefore, ICL detection and quantitation implies careful selection of the irradiation conditions. In our experience, the presence of a mild •OH-radical scavenger (20 mM EDTA) sufficiently protects against ICL destruction, and even enhances ICL yields up to 1 kGy irradiation dose. A typical ICL- migration pattern observed in agarose denaturing gel electrophoresis of $^{32}P$-labeled scDNA samples containing different mismatched regions and subjected to γ-irradiated (750 Gy) is shown in Fig. 2. The figure exemplifies the fact that, depending on the mismatched-sequence context of the incorporated BrdU, ICL-DNA segments are formed, which differ in their length, structure and yield. Comparative analyses of ICL yields and various electrophoretic-band patterns depending on DNA structure are presented in (Dextraze *et al.*, 2009). Although, no ICL chemical structure identification has been done yet, quantitative data show that d(AABrdUAA)^d(GGGGG) and d(GGBrdUGG)^d(CCCCC) bulge patches are the least prone to crosslink formation in DNA wobbles, while efficient crosslinking takes place in T-enriched bulge structures, *e.g.* d(GGBrdUGG)^d(ATTTA) and d(ATBrdUTA)^d(ATTTA). The calculated total ICL radiation yield (G) in the later sequences (*i.e.* including all ICL bands) is in the range of (1-4) $x10^{-8}$ mol.$J^{-1}$. Taking into account that $G(e^{-}_{aq}) = 2.75x10^{-7}$ mol $J^{-1}$ it follows that the formation of interstrand crosslinks in BrdU-scDNA is an event that occurs at least once with every ten solvated electrons produced. Ding and Greenberg (2007) reported γ-radiolysis production of ICL in unsubstituted dsDNA and identified the structure as T[5m-6n]A (Fig. 6B). Under their irradiation conditions the estimated G-value of the single ICL is ~ (3-4) $x10^{-4}$ nmol.$J^{-1}$. These data underline that BrdU-sensitized ICL formation in mismatched scDNA duplex is much more efficient (> $10^4$ - fold) than in normal dsDNA.

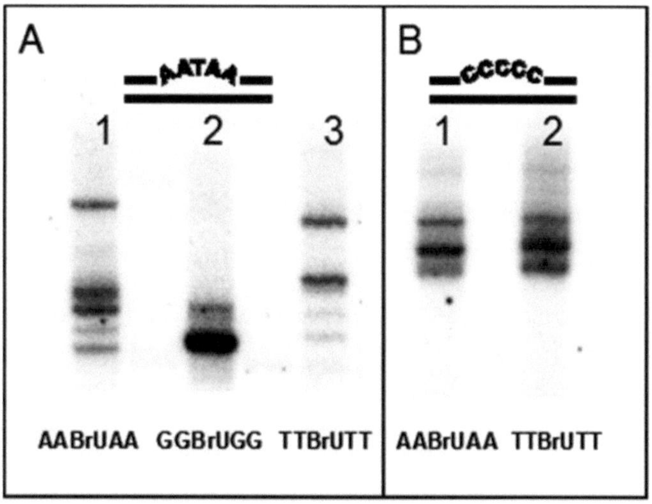


Fig. 2. Sequence-dependent BrdU-radiosensitized formation of ICL in wobble scDNA, as seen by the different electrophoretic mobility of the ICL bands. The central quintet sequence of the brominated strand is shown at the bottom; the opposite strand comprises $d(A_2TA_2)$ or $d(C)_5$ as shown on the top; there is a 5-b.p. central mismatch in all samples, except for lane-3 (panel A) where a single BU^T mismatch is present. The figure exemplifies the role of mismatched sequence (length and composition) on the ICL nature and yields; the individual chemical structures, however have not been yet determined. For a tentative ICL assignment, see Dextraze M.-E., *et al.*, (2009); for recently identified ICL structures, see Fig. 6.

## 4. Peptide nucleic acids (PNA) as sequence targeted radiosensitizers

In searching for new RT approaches to inflict heavy DNA damage (specific, repair-refractive and lethal) we developed the concept of cell radiosensitization by non-covalently bound DNA radiosensitizers. Our original idea was to use *semi*-complementary BrdU-substituted oligonucleotide vectors which would hybridize to specific genomic sequences and create a mismatch at the site of the bromouracil. In theory, the sequences of the BUdR-loaded oligonucleotide vectors could be designed to efficiently form crosslinks with the target DNA upon radiation, since, as discussed above, the crosslinking efficiency is dependent on the target sequence. However, the use of oligonucleotides as vectors to bring BrUdR close to cellular DNA has many pitfalls (similarly to the antisense RNA applications) and instead we focused on peptide nucleic acids (PNA) as vectors, because PNAs are resistant to degradation and are able to invade DNA duplexes under physiological conditions. To our surprise, PNA were found to efficiently form crosslinks with DNA under ionizing radiation even without bearing halogenated bases.

PNA: $R_1$-ATG-CCG-ATC-GTA-$R_2$

DNA: 3'-TAC-GGC-TAG-CAT-5'

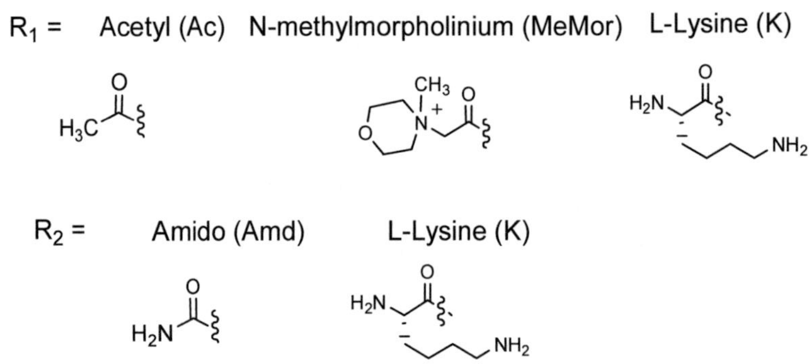


Fig. 3. The 12-mer PNA-DNA heteroduplex sequence (top) used in γ-radiation experiments to induce ICL and the variable N- and C-capping groups ($R_1$ and $R_2$) on PNA.

PNAs are nucleic acid analogues with an uncharged peptide-like backbone (Nielsen, 1995; Porcheddu & Giacomelli, 2005; Pellestor *et al.*, 2008). PNAs bind strongly to complimentary DNA and RNA sequences. Originally designed as ligands for the recognition of double stranded DNA (Egholm *et al.*, 1993; Demidov *et al.*, 1995) their unique physicochemical properties allow them to recognize and invade complimentary sequences in specific genes and to interfere with the transcription of that particular gene (antigene strategy) (Nielsen *et al.*, 1994; Ray & Norden, 2000; Pooga *et al.*, 2001; Cutrona, *et al.*, 2000; Doyle *et al.*, 2001; Romanelli *et al.*, 2001; Kaihatsu *et al.*, 2004). The introduction of a bulky charged amino acid (*e.g.* lysine, Fig. 3) improves binding specificity, solubility and cell uptake (Menchise *et al.*, 2003). PNAs have several advantages over oligo-deoxyribonucleotides including: greater chemical and biochemical stability (PNAs are not substrates for proteases, peptidases and nucleases), greater affinity towards targets (lack of electrostatic repulsion between hybridizing strands, Fig. 4), and more sequence-specific binding.

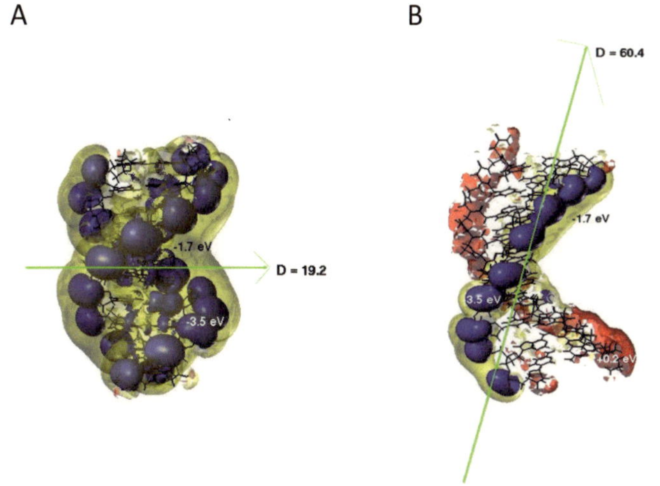


Fig. 4. Electrostatic potentials surrounding 10-mer 3D-models of $(DNA)_2$ and DNA-PNA duplexes, calculated using Sybyl modeling interface and dielectric constant, D = 4. Color-codes as indicated: electronegative potentials -3.5 eV, -1.7 eV (dark blue and yellow) and electropositive +0.2 eV (red). (A) Symmetric electronegative potential surfaces along the two strands of the DNA duplex expand over all backbone atoms (blue) and the two grooves (yellow). (B) Asymmetric isopotential surfaces around PNA-DNA duplex. The electropositive/neutral PNA backbone region (red) extends over the minor and major groove atoms (0 - 0.2 eV at distances ~ 0.1 Å), but the DNA backbone atoms remain enveloped by a negative surface (-3.5 eV). The resultant dipole momenta (green vectors) are 19.2 D and 60.4 D for the DNA-DNA and PNA-DNA duplexes, respectively. In the latter case it is oriented diagonally from PNA to DNA strand and can be a driving force for $e^{-}aq$ interaction with accessible PNA backbone and groove atoms.

We have studied hybridization of DNA oligonucleotides with PNA, where PNA bear (or not) N- or C-terminal amino groups ($-NH_2$, lysine, or methylmorpholinium) (Fig. 3, Gantchev *et al.*, 2009). After γ-irradiation (typically 750 Gy) of PNA-DNA heteroduplexes, those with PNA containing free amino group ends formed ICLs (Fig. 5). The multiple bands in each lane represent different crosslinked products and match the number of available amino groups in each heteroduplex. The ICL-formation efficiency is high, G = (5-8) $x10^{-8}$ $mol.J^{-1}$. This G-value even exceeds the ICL yields observed after irradiation BrdU-substituted wobble DNA under identical conditions. Using selective scavengers it was shown that ICL formation in PNA-DNA heteroduplexes strongly depends on the availability of solvated electrons ($e^{-}_{aq}$), but proceeds only with a concomitant presence of •OH radicals (Gantchev *et al.*, 2009). Thus, it appears that PNA-DNA ICLs arise in a concerted free radical mechanisms resembling those involved in DNA multiply damaged sites (MDS). By hybridizing 12-mer PNAs with shorter (11-mer), or longer (up to 16-mer) complementary oligo-deoxyribonucleotides thus creating unpaired (single-stranded) regions (deletions and overhangs) at one, or both duplex ends we compared sequence effects on the cross-linking reaction (*e.g.* dT vs. dA termini), the susceptibility of duplex ends to radiation damage, *etc.* The 3′- and 5′- DNA terminal dT nucleotides proved to be of most importance for the efficient ICL formation. Since hydrolysis of N-glycosidic bonds in γ-damaged nucleotides and/or direct 2′-deoxiribose oxidation yields AP (apurinic/apyrimidinic) abasic sites as a common DNA lesion; we also assessed the role of AP-sites in the PNA-DNA ICL formation using synthetic AP-containing oligo-deoxyribonucletides. We found that presence of AP-sites at different positions of the DNA strand (3′- or 5′-end, and/or penultimate to the ends) results in ICL formation without radiation, but instead required addition of a strong reductant, *e.g.* $NaCNBH_3$. The electrophoretic gel-mobility of thus formed ICL bands resembled that of γ-radiation generated ones. Therefore, we concluded that AP-sites on the DNA strand are the likely partners of the free $NH_2$, or α- and ε-amino groups of Lys at the PNA ends in the formation of DNA-PNA crosslinks *via* a Schiff-base reaction, followed by imine reduction.

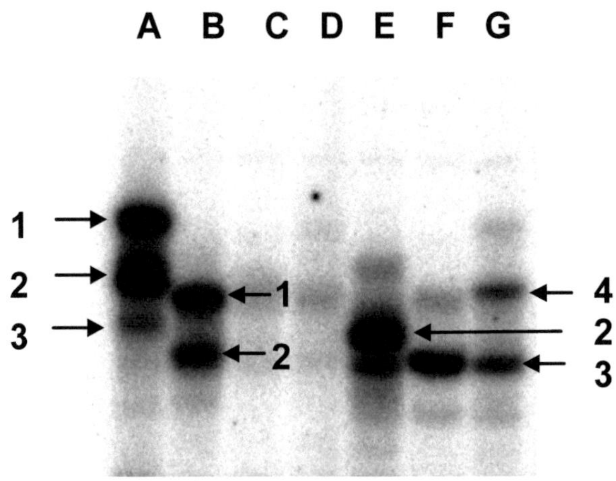


Fig. 5. Electrophoretic migration of bands representing the covalent PNA-DNA dimers (ICL). Aqueous solutions of $^{32}P$-DNA hybridized with various PNA were γ-irradiated (750 Gy) under $N_2$ – atmosphere and in the presence of 25 mM EDTA. Samples differ only by the type of capping groups on PNA ends ($R_1$ and $R_2$, Fig. 3). Lanes from left to right: (A) $NH_2$-K-PNA; (B) $NH_2$-PNA; (C) Ac-PNA; (D) MeMor-K-PNA; (E) $NH_2$-PNA-K; (F) Ac-PNA-K; and (G) MeMor-PNA-K; (1- 4): different crosslinked products involving the different amino groups. No ICL are formed with Ac-PNA (C) and MeMor-K-PNA (D). Adapted from Gantchev *et al.*, (2009).

## 5. Mechanistic and structural aspects of the ICL formation in DNA duplexes and DNA-PNA heteroduplexes

In comparison to inter-strand crosslinks (ICLs), the intra-strand DNA crosslinks have been better studied, mostly as part of locally multiply damage sites (MDS, clustered/tandem DNA lesions). Recently, Wang and co-workers (Lin *et al.*, 2010) found that the exposure of BrdU-substituted telomer G-quadruplex DNA to UVA light results in the formation of G[8-5]U intra-strand crosslink (Fig. 6A). This finding presents evidence that free radical reactions, involving 5-uracil-yl-radical (•U) can also be a source of ICL, albeit not in completely dsDNA duplexes. Thus, Ding & Greenberg (2010) reported radiolytic formation of ICL in anaerobic solutions by BrdU-mimetic iodo-aryl nucleotides incorporated into synthetic dsDNA duplex. Similarly to BrdU-dsDNA irradiation, in these model systems stand breaks and alkali-labile lesions were also induced at the halogenated site and at the flanking nucleotides. The conclusions from this study highlight the importance of the local DNA structure (wobble *vs.* normal duplex) in terms of Watson-Crick pairing restrictions that likely prevent the 5-uracil-yl σ-radical (in contrast to the aryl radical) interaction with the opposite strand bases to produce ICL. The chemical structures of several DNA inter-strand crosslinks have been reported only recently. Several groups have focused on the identification of ICL structures synthesized in model systems using light- and/or oxidation-sensitive precursors (Hong *et al.*, 2006; Weng *et al.*, 2007; Peng *et al.*, 2008; Kim & Hong, 2008; Op de Beeck & Madder, 2011). A few structures have been definitively identified in natural conditions and, to our knowledge, only one in cellular DNA (Regulus *et al.*, 2007) (Fig. 6C). However, the authors in Regulus *et al.*, (2007) failed to present evidence that this crosslink is exclusively an inter-strand crosslink in cells. Mechanistically, the sole ICL-structure that is exclusively generated with the participation of a primary radiation-induced 5-(2′-deoxyuridinyl) methyl free radical, a product of •OH-induced hydrogen-atom abstraction from thymine, is the T[5m-6n]A crosslink (Ding & Greenberg, 2007; Ding *et al.*, 2008) (Fig. 6B).

A common pathway for ICL formation in dsDNA is the condensation reaction between aldehydes (*e.g.* in abasic DNA sites) and exocyclic amines of opposite bases. Under γ-radiation abasic (AP-apurinic/apyrimidinic) sites are generated either *via* direct H-atom abstraction by •OH radicals from 2′-deoxyribose or after oxidative base damage followed by N-glycosidic bond-cleavage. Oxidation of each of the five positions in 2′-deoxyribose in DNA is possible, but under γ-radiation the best known reactions involve H-atom abstraction at C1′-, C2′- and C4′-positions. The 4′-keto abasic site formed after C4′-oxidation (C4′-AP) is generally known as the "native" abasic site (Chen & Stubbe 2004). Subsequent interactions of sugar radicals with oxygen and/or elimination reactions give a variety of closed-cycle/open-chain aldehydic products, accompanied (or not) by DNA strand-cleavage (Dedon, 2008). One of the first reported, and structurally identified DNA-ICL generated by γ-radiation and/or selective 4′-position 2′-deoxyribose oxidation by bleomycin in model systems and in cells (Fig. 6C; Regulus *et al.*, 2007; Cadet *et al.*, 2010) is produced *via* electrophilic interaction between 2′-deoxypentos-4-ulose abasic site (opened C4′-AP) and N4-dC. Formation of this ICL is accompanied by a DNA strand break. In a series of works, Greenberg and collaborators studied the ICL formation with participation of oxidized native C4′-AP (Sczepanski *et al.*, 2008, 2009a) and 5′-(2-phosphoryl-1,4-dioxobutane, DOB) (Guan & Greenberg, 2009) sites. DOB is produced concomitantly with a single-strand break byDNA-damaging agents capable of abstracting an H-atom from the C5′-position. When oxidized C4′-AP was opposed by dA, a single crosslink formation occurred exclusively with an adjacent dA on the 5′-side. The crosslink formation was attributed to condensation of C4′-AP with the N6-amino group of dA and less favorably with N4-amino group of dC, but not with dG or dT. Interestingly, C4′-AP produced ICLs in which both strands are either intact or ICLs, where the C4-AP containing strand was cleaved (3′ to the AP-site), while DOB-ICLs were always accompanied by an adjacent to the AP-site single-strand break, and thus constituting a clustered type (MDS) lesion.

In contrast, following γ-radiation of BrdU-substituted wobble-DNA (scDNA) duplexes multiple crosslinked products were generated which impedes their chemical identification (Cecchini et al., 2005a; Dextraze et al., 2009). However, in DNA-PNA heteroduplexes, because the amino-groups attached to PNA are exogenous and could be omitted/varied,

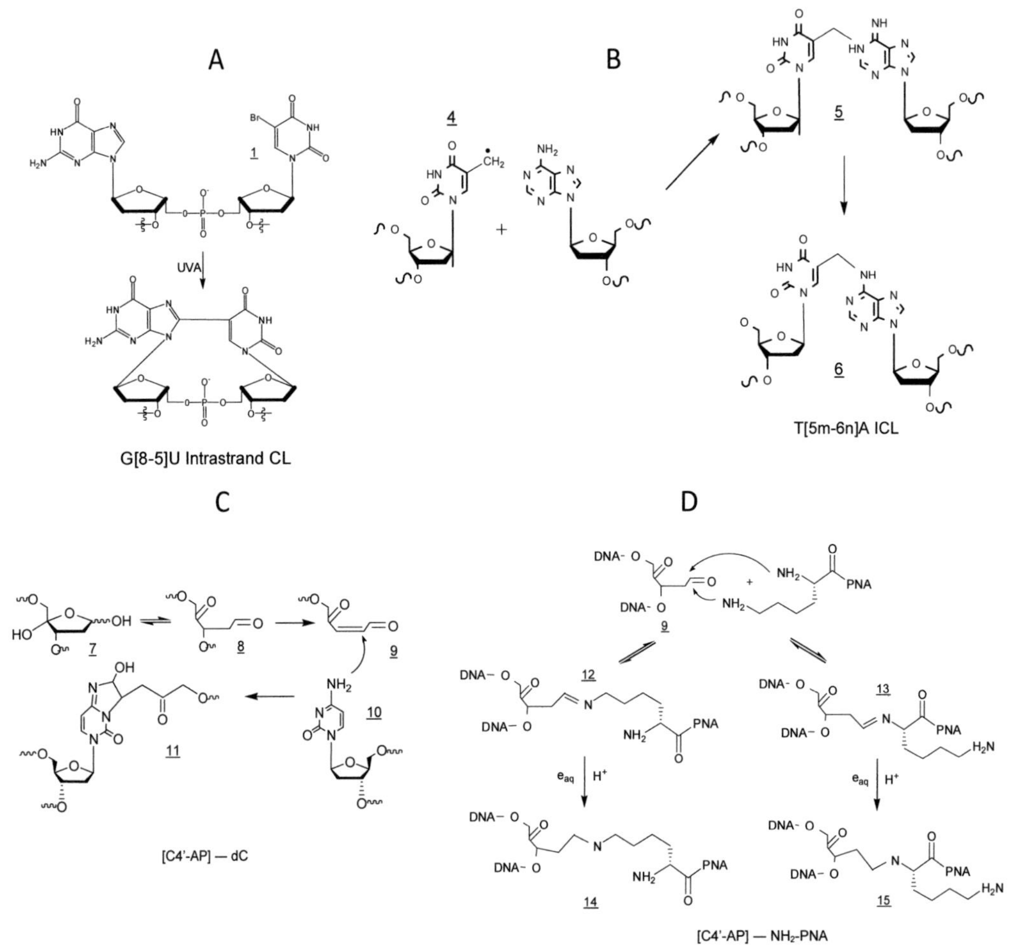


Fig. 6. Chemical structures of known intra- and interstrand crosslinks as generated in model DNA systems, UV and ionizing radiation: (A) The structure of G[8-5]U intrastrand crosslink; the only known crosslink formed *via* direct addition to •U-radical (3). This pathway was not found for ICL formation in normal dsDNA, probably due to steric restrictions, however interstrand crosslinks generated with the participation of 5-uracil-yl radical are possible in wobble scDNA (Fig. 1); (B) The formation of T[5m-6n]A ICL initiated by •OH radical H-abstraction from 5-$CH_3$dT (4); the intermediate product is addition to N1 (5), which is further rearranged to the final product (6), (Ding *et al.*, 2008); (C) The ICL (11) formed *via* condensation reaction of exocyclic $NH_2$-group of dC with β-elimination product (9) of an oxidized C4'-AP abasic site (7 and 8). This ICL is associated with a SSB formation, (Regulus *et al.*, 2007) and; (D) Reaction of C4'-AP native abasic site (9) with L-Lys-capped PNA resulting in the formation of PNA-DNA interstrand crosslinks *via* Schiff base (12 and 13). Two free $NH_2$-groups are equally reactive which can produce two ICLs of different structure (14 and 15). The abasic sites are formed by γ-radiation oxidation of DNA (*e.g.* by •OH radicals). The concomitant solvated electrons, $e_{aq}^-$ are the essential reducing species required to convert Schiff bases in irreversible ICLs, (Gantchev *et al.*, 2009).

together with the synthetically positioned AP-sites on DNA the participation of these two entities in the ICL formation was positively identified (Gantchev *et al.*, 2009). Our data are consistent with a mechanism of ICL formation that involves formation of Schiff bases between PNA-amino functional groups and radiation-damage induced AP-sites on DNA. This type of covalent bonding is widely accepted to take place in the formation of covalent links between $NH_2$-peptide (protein) groups and damaged (aldehydic) DNA sites, albeit in the presence of an exogenous reducing agent (Mazumder *et al.*, 1996). The new finding is that apart from the prerequisite •OH-mediated, or direct γ-damage of DNA (formation of AP-sites), γ-radiation also provides reducing equivalents to transform the initially formed Schiff base linkage into a more stable reduced bond (amine), *i.e.* to produce irreversible ICL (Fig. 6D). This presents a typical case of radiation-induced MDS, where the synergism of the interactions of •OH, $e^-_{aq}$, and possibly even •H radicals on PNA-DNA results in ICL. The 3D-modeling (Gantchev *et al.*, 2009) confirms experimental data that open-chain C4'-AP at several DNA-strand end, or penultimate positions are structurally allowed to form covalent bonds with the ε- and α-amino groups of opposite Lys residues, or PNA $NH_2$-terminal groups and in all cases although, intra-helical ICLs are solvent accessible (*e.g.* the transient Schiff bases are available for interaction with $e^-_{aq}$). Importantly, if dsDNA duplexes are compared, the $e^-_{aq}$ and solvent accessibility holds for the open structures in BrdU-DNA bubbles in scDNA, only (see below).

Solvated electrons ($e^-_{aq}$) are indispensible species for the formation of both strand breaks and interstrand crosslinks sensitized by BrdU in scDNA and crosslinks in DNA-PNA heteroduplexes. The $e^-_{aq}$ interaction rate with oxygen, $k(e^-_{aq} + O_2) = 2x10^{10}\ M^{-1}s^{-1}$ is high, therefore hypoxic experimental conditions are important. The radiosensitization properties of BrdU are based on its ability to undergo dissociative electron transfer (ET) which is initiated by electron capture either from solution, or following excess ET from surrounding DNA bases (Fig. 1). The classical reducibility (electron affinity, EA) trend of nucleobases is BrU>U~T>C>A>G (Aflatooni *et al.*, 1998; Richardson *et al.*, 2004), with BrU being only ~ 40 mV easier to reduce than thymidine (Gaballah *et al.*, 2005). Using the approach described by Michaels & Hunt (1978) and quantitation of BrdU-mediated damage in mismatched duplexes, we calculated a value for $k(e^-_{aq}$ + BrdU-scDNA) of $\sim 2x10^{10}\ M^{-1}s^{-1}$. This value is particularly interesting in that the rate constant for BrdU interaction with $e^-_{aq}$ in mismatched, scDNA (single-stranded regions of the duplex) is practically the same as for the free base BrU in solution (Zimbrick *et al.*, 1969a) (*i.e.* essentially diffusion controlled) and, about two orders of magnitude higher than in normal dsDNA. Based on our results from the irradiation of solutions containing PNA-DNA hybrids, we calculated a rate constant for the formation of PNA-DNA crosslinks, assuming only interactions with hydrated electrons, equal to: $k(e^-_{aq}$ + PNA) ~ $5x10^9\ M^{-1}s^{-1}$, which is also high. While high rate interaction of $e^-_{aq}$ with PNA-DNA hetereoduplexes can be attributed to the lack of electrostatic repulsion (see Fig. 4 and legend), the increased rate of interaction with wobble scDNA is less obvious. We hypothesized that $e^-_{aq}$ may have a restricted access to BrdU when incorporated in a normal DNA duplex, although the Br-atom is partially solvent-exposed in the major groove. To address this issue we applied molecular modeling and nanosecond scale molecular dynamics (MD) simulations, where the excess electron in solution was modeled as a localized $e^-(H_2O)_6$ anionic cluster (Gantchev & Hunting, 2008, 2009). We compared the dynamics and interactions of $e^-_{aq}$ with dsDNA containing a normal BrdU•dA pair in the center of the duplex (dsDNA) with that of a wobble DNA containing a single mismatched

BrdU^dT pair (scDNA), *i.e.* replacing dA with dT. Rather unexpectedly we found that the occupancy of the close-to-DNA space for scDNA and dsDNA at cut-off distance <5 Å was 0.7% vs. 1.6%, respectively (from a total of 4,000 MD configurations). However, the electron interacted with a larger number of individual bases in scDNA. For instance, in dsDNA, the electron moved closely toward only four nucleobases, all from the non-brominated DNA strand, while in scDNA eleven nucleobases from both strands were found to come within reach of $e_{aq}^-$. The different clustering of the electron (occupation of close to DNA sites) in both duplexes is presented graphically in Fig. 7 (see legend for details). Notably, BrU incorporated in the central (sixth) position of both DNA duplexes, was approached by $e_{aq}^-$ several times in scDNA only. Likewise only in scDNA, the $e_{aq}^-$ preferentially occupied close sites and formed contacts with the two most perturbed thymidines (dT5 and dT7) flanking BrdU. At present, there is no explanation for the disparity of $e_{aq}^-$ interactions with dsDNA *vs.* scDNA, other than the different dynamic structure of the isosteric DNA sequences under study, including the dynamics of structured water and Debay-Hückel layers (Gantchev & Hunting, 2008, 2009). The exposure of wobble-pair pyrimidine carbonyl groups into the DNA grooves results in excess solvation of the mismatched pairs (Sherer & Cramer, 2004).

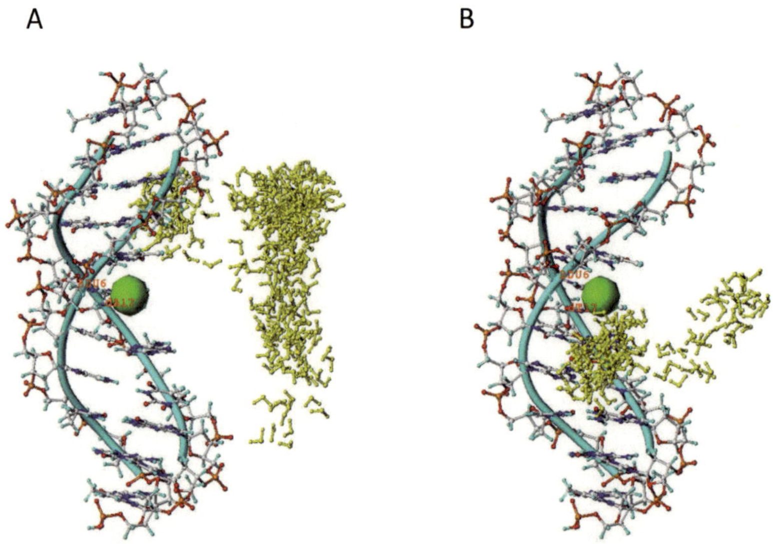


Fig. 7. Superimposed snapshots from ns MD of regular (left) and mismatched (right) 11-mer DNA containing a Watson-Crick BrU6•A17 normal pair, or BrU^T17 wobble pair, respectively. The $e^-_{aq}$ is represented by a $e^-[H_2O]_6$ anionic cluster. The shown dynamic states are selected by the rule, distance $|e^-_{aq}$ – nucleobase$| < 5$ Å. From the total of 59 states for normal DNA, there are no configurations where $e^-_{aq}$ is close to the central BrU6•A17 base pair. In contrast, in the wobble scDNA from the all 22 states obeying the same selection rule, ~ 65% show close approach to the wobble BrU6^T17 pair. The electron resides most often in the vicinity of the flanking T7 base and less frequently approaches BrU6 and T17. Hydration water and counterions are not shown; BrU•A and BrU^T are in the middle and labeled. Color code: Br-vdW sphere (green); DNA backbone (cyan); nucleotide atoms (standard color); $e^-_{aq}$ (yellow). For details see: Gantchev & Hunting, (2008, 2009).

In addition, the incorporated mismatched pairs (T^T or BU^T) alter the dynamics of the neighboring bases due to incomplete 5'-stacking. Together with the narrowing of the minor groove these phenomena bring the two strands closer which creates conditions for cross-strand (cs) stacking and single and multiple cross-strand (cs) H-bonding not only within the mismatched regions, but also encompassing penultimate nucleotides to create extended "zipper-like" motives (Špačková *et al.*, 2000). The properties of single-mismatch scDNA duplexes, including the effect of the nearest sequence context (*e.g.* presence of T-tract DNA) have been discussed elsewhere (Gantchev *et al.*, 2005). A schematic presentation of the most often formed cross-strand inter-base contacts is given in Fig. 8. The close presence of $e_{aq}^{-}$, although causes dynamic instability and fluctuations around the mismatched BrdU^dT pair does not abolish, but in contrast, provokes additional frequent cs-H-bonding interactions (Gantchev & Hunting, 2009). All these findings are important in terms of facilitated charge-transfer along UV-, or γ-activated BrdU-scDNA. The intrahelical electron or hole transfer to BrdU and/or •U-yl radical are the next important factor that is largely expected to control the efficiency (and location) of the ensuing DNA damage; the formation of DSB and ICL. Indeed, recently a more effective electron transfer has been reported for mismatched duplexes than for fully complementary DNA (Ito *et al.*, 2009). Using a two electron acceptor DNA model system with incorporated BrdA, BrdG, BrdU and TT-dimer Fazio *et al.* (Fazio *et al.*, 2011) were able to estimate the absolute electron-hoping rates in DNA and have shown that the electron transfer is more efficient in 5′ → 3′ direction. As mentioned, in unsubstituted DNA pyrimidine rather than purine bases have been considered as trapping sites for excess electrons. This is illustrated by resonant free electron attachment experiments (Stokes *et al.*, 2007) which show that both thymine and cytosine form stable valence anions for low energy electrons, *i.e.* both thymine and cytosine possess positive adiabatic electron affinities. However, recently a stabile anionic state of adenine ($A^-$) has been detected (Haranczyk *et al.*, 2007). Subsequently, this finding has been shown to have a pronounced effect in the ultrafast ET in DNA and on dissociative bond cleavage (Wang *et al.*, 2009), including ET to BrdU from $A^-$ acting as primary trap of radiolysis-generated pre-hydrated electrons (Wang *et al..*, 2010). These new developments in the field add to the existing puzzles of the precise determination of successive chain events leading to multiple BrdU-sensitized damages (DSB and ICL) in wobble scDNA.

Repair of interstrand crosslinks (ICLs) requires multiple strand incisions to separate the two covalently linked DNA strands. It is unclear how these incisions are generated. DNA double-strand breaks (DSBs) have been identified as intermediates in ICL repair, but eukaryotic enzymes responsible for producing these intermediates are not well known (Wang, 2007; Moldovan & D'Andrea, 2009a,b; D'Andrea & Grompe, 2003; Liu *et al.*, 2010; Hanada *et al.*, 2006). Ongoing research shows that in cell free model systems ICLs of different chemical structure exert different effects during repair and some may be difficult to repair. The repair refractive character of a particular ICL resulting from the C4′-AP abasic site and identified to occur as a clustered ICL-SSB lesion (Sczepanski *et al.*, 2008, 2009a) was recently demonstrated to give rise to even more toxic DSBs when subjected to NER (Sczepanski *et al..*, 2009b). Likewise, during UvrABC nucleotide excision repair of the well-defined T[5m-6n]A single-lesion crosslink imbedded in dsDNA (Fig. 6B, Ding *et al.*, 2008), DSB were produced in almost 30% of the excision events (Peng *et al.*, 2010).

DNA packing into chromatin adds to the complexity of DNA damage recognition and removal, because the highly condensed chromatin is, in general, refractory to DNA repair (Hara *et al.*, 2000; Thoma, 2005). In order to grant access to DNA repair machinery, the

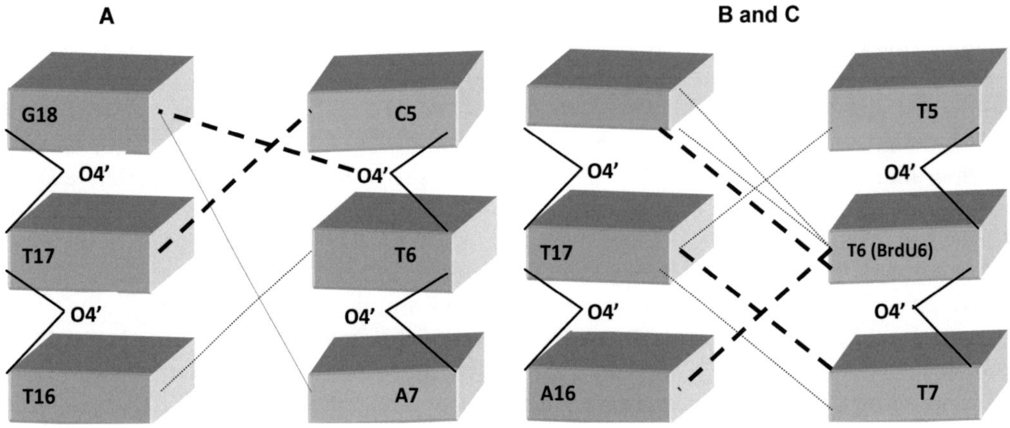


Fig. 8. Nearest-neighbour sequence effects in wobble semi-complementary DNA (scDNA) as observed by MD (adapted from Gantchev *et al.* 2005). Schematic presentation of the frequent cross-strand (cs) inter-base contacts formed in the studied 11-mer DNA duplexes containing a single mismatch: T^T or T^BrU, incorporated in the central triplets: d(CTA)•(TTG) (A), d(TTT)•(ATA) (B) and d(TBrdUT)•(ATA) (C): bold dashed lines (most frequently observed cs H-bons), dotted lines (less frequent cs H-bonds). Note that cs contacts in (C) coincide with those observed also in the presence of $e^-_{aq}$ (Gantchev & Hunting, 2009). These data underline the importance of the wobble DNA dynamic structure for both, interstrand ET and high-frequency opposite-strand atom encounter for the generation of (asymmetric) ICL (Fig. 1).

chromatin response to DNA damage involves activation of ATP-dependent chromatin-remodeling complexes and histone post-translational modification pathways (Peterson & Côte, 2004; Nag & Smerdon, 2009; Méndez-Acuña *et al.*, 2010). Again, DSBs recognition and repair in the context of chromatin rearrangement is better studied and understood at the expense of other DNA damages, such as ICLs. One crucial chromatin modification, the phosphorylation of the histone variant H2AX (γH2AX) is perhaps the best example of a histone modification in response to DSB induction in DNA (Van Attikum & Gasser, 2005). Despite the progress achieved in understanding of the repair of certain UV-induced DNA damages (intra-strand crosslinks), *e.g.* cyclobutane pyrimidine dimers (CPD) and 6-4 pyrimidine photoadducts (6-4 PP), or the acetylaminofluorene-guanine (AAF-G) covalent adduct, little is known about the effects of other bulky DNA lesions (*e.g.* ICLs) on the nucleosome structural dynamics and its interplay with the versatile NER pathway (Smerdon & Lieberman, 1978; Pehrson, 1995; Gaillard et al., 2003; Gospodinov & Herceg, 2011). There is a consensus that NER functionality depends primarily on the damage recognition step, which in turn depends on the degree of DNA helix distortion induced by a particular lesion (Cai *et al.*, 2007). It has been hypothesized that structurally different interstrand crosslinks would affect chromatin remodeling and damage recognition in different ways, and some ICLs might retain their refractive character to recognition/repair, or at least will exert an altered repair efficacy. Thus, a recent *in vivo* study (Hlavin *et al.*, 2010) confirmed that the structure of synthetic interstrand crosslinks between mismatched bases affects the repair rate (in this case, transcription coupled NER). It can be further hypothesized that PNA-patches hybridized to DNA (*e.g.*, > 8-10 b.p.; PNA- invaded DNA strands, PNA-DNA triple helices, and/or DNA-PNA covalent adducts) would be difficult to repair without a loss of DNA information, and/or would require major chromatin remodeling. Indeed, Faruqi *et al.* (1998) designed PNAs that bind to the *sup*FG1 mutation reporter gene and found that 8- or 10- b.p. PNA bound to this site induces mutations at frequencies in the range of 0.1%, well above the *in vivo* background. Later, the same group (Kim *et al.*, 2006) demonstrated that a psoralen-*bis*-PNA conjugate directs the formation of a photoadduct at the 5′-TpA step of the PNA binding site to the same *sup*FG1 gene. In mammalian cells, the UV-generated PNA-targeted psoralen phtoadducts induced mutations as high as 0.46%, *i.e.* 6.5-fold above the background.

## 6. Conclusion

In conclusion, there is a need to better understand the parameters which control the formation and repair of complex DNA lesions, such as interstrand crosslinks. Such complex, repair refractive lesions may offer a means to selectively kill tumor cells by taking advantage of either enhanced formation or reduced repair within the tumor environment.

## 7. References

Aflatooni K., Gallup G. A., Burrow P.D. (1998) Electron Attachment Energies of the DNA Bases. *Journal of Physical Chemistry A*, 102, 6205–6207.

Cadet J., Douki T., Ravanat J.-L. (2010) Oxidatively generated base damage to cellular DNA. *Free Radical Biology & Medicine* 49, 9–21.

Cai Y., Patel D.J., Geacintov N.E., Broyde S. (2007) Dynamics of benzo[a]pyren-derived guanine DNA lesion in TGT and CGC sequence contexts: Enhanced mobility in TGT explains conformational heterogeneity, flexible bending, and greater susceptibility to nucleotide excision repair. *Journal of Molecular Biology* 374, 292-305.

Cecchini S., Girouard S., Huels M.A., Sanche L., Hunting D.J. (2004) Single strand specific radiosensitization of DNA by Bromodeoxyuridine. *Radiation Research* 162, 604-615.

Cecchini S., Girouard S., Huels M.A., Sanche L., Hunting D.J. (2005a) Interstrand crosslinks: a new type of gamma-ray damage in bromodeoxyuridine-substituted DNA. *Biochemistry* 44, 1932–1940.

Cecchini S., Masson C., La Madeleine C., Huels M.A., Sanche L., Wagner J.R., Hunting D.J. (2005b) Interstrand cross-link induction by UV radiation in bromodeoxyuridine-substituted DNA: Dependence on DNA conformation. *Biochemistry*, 44, 16957-16966.

Chen J., Stubbe JA. (2004) Synthesis and Characterization of Oligonucleotides Containing a 4′-Keto Abasic Site. *Biochemistry* 43, 5278–5286.

Chen T., Cook G.P., Koppisch A.T., Greenberg M.M. (2000) Investigation of the Origin of the Sequence Selectivity for the 5-Halo-2′-deoxyuridine Sensitization of DNA to Damage by UV-Irradiation. *Journal of the American Chemical Society* 122, 3861-3866.

Cutrona G., Carpaneto E.M., Ulivi M., Roncella S., Landt O., Ferrarini M., Boffa L.C. (2000) Effects in live cells of a c-*myc* anti-gene PNA linked to a nuclear localization signal. *Nature Biotechnology* 18, 300-303.

D'Andrea A.D., Grompe M. (2003) The Fanconi anaemia/BRCA pathway. *Nature Reviews Cancer* 3, 23-34.

Dedon P.C. (2008) The Chemical Toxycology of 2-Deoxyribose Oxidation in DNA. *Chemical Research in Toxicology* 21, 206-219.

Demidov V.V., Yavnilovich M.V., Belotserkovskii B.P., Frank-Kamenetskii M.D., Nielsen P.E. (1995) Kinetics and mechanism of polyamide ("peptide") nucleic acid binding to duplex DNA. *Proceedings of the National Academy of Sciences USA* 92, 2637-2641.

Dextraze M.-E., Wagner J.R., Hunting D.J. (2007) 5-Bromodeoxyuridine radiosensitization: conformation-dependent DNA damage. *Biochemistry* 46, 9089–9097.

Dextraze M.-E., Cecchini S., Bergeron F., Girouard S., Turcotte K., Wagner J.R., Hunting D.J. (2009) Reaching for the other side: Generating sequence-dependent interstrand crosslinks with 5-bromodeoxyuridine and γ-rays. *Biochemistry* 48, 2005-2011.

Ding H., Greenberg M.M. (2007) γ-Radiolysis and Hydroxyl Radical Produce Interstrand Cross-Links in DNA Involving Thymidine. *Chemical Research in Toxicology* 20, 1623–1628.

Ding H., Majumdar A., Tolman J.R., Greenberg M.M. (2008) Multinuclear NMR and Kinetic Analysis of DNA Interstrand Cross-Link Formation. *Journal of the American Chemical Society*, 130, 17981–17987.

Ding H., Greenberg M.M. (2010) DNA Damage and Interstrand Cross-Link Formation upon Irradiation of Aryl Iodide C-Nucleotide Analogues. *Journal of Organic Chemistry* 75, 535–544.

Doyle D.F., Braasch D.A., Simmons C.G., Janowski B.A., Corey D.R. (2001) Inhibition of gene expression inside cells by peptide nucleic acids: Effect of mRNA target sequence, mismatched bases, and PNA length. *Biochemistry* 40, 53-64.

Egholm M., Buchardt O., Christensen L., Behrens C., Freir S.M., Driver D.A., Berg R.H., Kim S.K., Norden B., Nielsen P.E. (1993) PNA hybridizes to complementary oligonucleotides obeying the Watson-Crick hydrogen-bonding rules. *Nature* 365, 566-568.

Faruqi F.A., Egholm M., Glazer P.M. (1998) Peptide nucleic acid-targeted mutagenesis of a chromosomal gene in mouse cells. *Proceedings of the National Academy of Sciences U.S.A.* 95, 1398-1403.

Fazio D., Trindler C., Heil K., Chatgilialoglu C., Carell T. (2011) Investigation of Excess-Electron Transfer in DNA Double-Duplex Systems Allows Estimation of Absolute Excess-Electron Transfer and CPD Cleavage Rates. *Chemistry A European Journal* 17, 206-212.

Gaballah S.T., Collier G., Netzel T.L. (2005) Charge Transfer Excited-State Dynamics in DNA Duplexes Substituted with an Ethynylpyrenyldeoxyuridine Electron Source and a Fluorodeoxyuridine Electron Trap. *Journal of Physical Chemistry B*, 109, 12175–12181.

Gaillard H., Fitzgerald D.J., Smith C.L., Peterson C.L., Richmond T.J., Thoma F. (2003) Chromatin remodeling activities act on UV-damaged nucleosomes and modulate DNA damage accessibility to photolyase. *Journal of Biological Chemistry* 278, 17655-17663.

Gantchev T.G., Cecchini S., Hunting D.J. (2005) Dynamic conformational states of DNA containing T•T or BrdU•T mispaired bases: wobble H-bond pairing versus cross-strand inter-atomic contacts. *Journal of Molecular Modeling* 11, 141–159.

Gantchev T.G., Hunting D.J. (2008) Probing the interactions of the solvated electron with DNA by molecular dynamics simulations: bromodeoxyuridine substituted DNA. *Journal of Molecular Modeling* 14, 451–464.

Gantchev T.G., Hunting D.J. (2009) Probing the interactions of the solvated electron with DNA by molecular dynamics simulations: II. Bromodeoxyuridine - thymidine mismatched. *Journal of Molecular Modeling* 15, 9 -23.

Gantchev T.G., Girouard S., Dodd D.W., Wojciechowski F., Hudson R.H.E., Hunting D.J. (2009) γ-Radiation Induced Interstrand Cross-Links in PNA:DNA Heteroduplexes. *Biochemistry* 48, 7032–7044.

Gospodinov A., Herceg Z. (2011) Chromatin: The entry to and exit from DNA repair. *Post-translational Modifications in Health and Disease,* C. Vidal (ed.), Protein Reviews, Springer, v. 13, pp. 387-409.

Guan L., Greenberg M.M. (2009) DNA Interstrand Cross-Link Formation by the 1,4-Dioxobutane Abasic Lesion. *Journal of the American Chemical Society,* 131, 15225-15231.

Hanada K., Budzowska M., Modesti M., Maas A., Wyman C., Essers J., Kanaar R. (2006) The structure-specific endonuclease Mus81–Eme1 promotes conversion of interstrand DNA crosslinks into double-strands breaks. *The EMBO Journal* 25, 4921–4932.

Hara R., Mo, J. Sancar, A. (2000) DNA damage in the nucleosome core is refractory to repair by human excision nuclease. *Molecular Cell Biology* 20, 9173-9181.

Haranczyk M., Gutowski M., Li X., Bowen K.H. (2007) Bound anionic states of adenine. *Proceedings of the National Academy of Sciences* 104, 4804–4807.

Hempel K., Mildenberger E. (1987) Determination of G-values for single and double strand break induction in plasmid DNA using agarose gel electrophoresis and a curve-fitting procedure. *International Journal of Radiation Biology* 52, 125-138.

Higgins G.S., Prevo R., Lee Y.-F., Helleday T., Muschel R.J., Taylor S., Yoshimura M., Hickson I.D., Bernhard E.J., McKenna W.G. (2010) A Small Interfering RNA Screen of Genes Involved in DNA Repair Identifies Tumor-Specific Radiosensitization by POLQ Knockdown. *Cancer Research* 70, 2984–2993.

Hlavin E.M., Smeaton M.B., Noronha A.M., Wilds C.J., Miller P.S. (2010) Cross-Link Structure Affects Replication-Independent DNA Interstrand Cross-Link Repair in Mammalian Cells. *Biochemistry* 49, 3977–3988.

Hong I.S., Ding H., Greenberg M.M. (2006) Radiosensitization by a Modified Nucleotide that Produces DNA Interstrand Cross-Links under Hypoxic Conditions. *Journal of the American Chemical Society* 128, 2230–2231.

Hunting D.J. *et al.*, unpublished.

Ito T., Kondo A., Kamashita, T., Tanabe K., Yamada H., Nishimoto S. (2009) Pathways of excess electron transfer in phenothiazine-tethered DNA containing single-base mismatches, *Organic & Biomolecular Chemistry* 7, 2077–2081.

Jackson S.P. (2002) Sensing and repairing DNA double-strand breaks. Carcinogenesis 23, 687-696.

Kaihatsu K., Jonowski B.A., Corey D.R. (2004) Recognition of chromosomal DNA by PNAs. *Chemistry & Biology* 11, 749-758.

Kim Y., Hong I.S. (2008) PNA/DNA interstrand cross-links from a modified PNA base upon photolysis or oxidative conditions. *Bioorganic and Medicinal Chemistry Letters* 18, 5054-5057.

Kim K.-H. Nielsen P.E., Glazer P.M. (2006) Site-specific gene modification by PNAs conjugated to psoralen. *Biochemistry,* 45, 314-323.

Lin G., Zhang J., Zeng Y., Luo H., Wang Y. (2010) Conformation-Dependent Formation of the G[8-5]U Intrastrand Cross-Link in 5-Bromouracil-Containing G-Quadruplex DNA Induced by UVA Irradiation. *Biochemistry* 49, 2346–2350.

Liu T., Ghosal G., Yuan J., Chen J., Huang J. (2010) FAN1 Acts with FANCI-FANCD2 to Promote DNA Interstrand Cross-Link Repair. *Science* 329, 693- 696.

Mazumder A., Neamati N., Pilon A.A., Sunder S., Pommier Y. (1996) Chemical trapping of ternary complexes of human immunodeficiency virus type I integrase, divalent metal, and DNA substrates containing an abasic site. *Journal of Biological Chemistry* 271, 27330-27338.

Menchise V., De Simone G., Tedeschi T., Corradini R., Sforza S., Marchelli R., Capasso D., Saviano M., Pedone C. (2003) Insights into peptide nucleic acid (PNA) structural features: The crystal structure of a D-lysine-based chiral PNA-DNA duplex. *Proceedings of the National Academy of Sciences USA* 100, 12021-12026.

Méndez-Acuña, L., Di Tomaso M.V., Palitti F., Martínez-López W. (2010) Histone post-translational modifications in DNA damage response. *Cytogenetic and Genome Research* 128, 28-36.

Michaels H.B., Hunt J.W. (1978) A model for radiation damage in cells by direct effect and by indirect effect: A radiation chemistry approach. *Radiation Research* 74, 23-34.

Moldovan G.L., D'Andrea A.D. (2009a) FANCD2 Hurdles the DNA Interstrand Crosslink. *Cell* 139, 1222.

Moldovan G.-L., D'Andrea A.D. (2009b) How the Fanconi Anemia Pathway Guards the Genome. *Annual Review of Genetics* 43, 223.

Nabben F.J., Karman J.Pl., Loman H. (1982) Inactivation of biologically active DNA by hydrated electrons. *International Journal of Radiation Biology* 42, 23-30.

Nag R., Smerdon M.J. (2009) Altering the chromatin landscape for nucleotide excision repair. *Mutation Research: Reviews in Mutation Research* 682, 13-20.

Nese C., Yuan Z., Schuchmann M.N., von Sonntag C. (1992) Electron transfer from nucleobase electron adducts to 5-bromouracil. Is guanine an ultimate sink for the electron in irradiated DNA? *International Journal of Radiation Biology* 62, 527-541.

Nielsen P.E. (1995) DNA analogues with nonphosphodiester backbones. *Annual Review of Biophysics and Biomolecular Structure* 24, 167-183.

Nielsen P.E., Egholm M., Buchardt O. (1994) Sequence-specific transcription arrest by peptide nucleic acid bound to the DNA template strand. *Gene* 149, 139-145.

Op de Beeck M., Madder A. (2011) Unprecedented C-Selective Interstrand Cross-Linking through in Situ Oxidation of Furan-Modified Oligodeoxynucleotides. *Journal of the American Chemical Society* 133, 796–807.

Pehrson, J.R. (1995) Probing the conformation of nucleosome linker DNA in situ with pyrimidine dimer formation. *Journal of Biological Chemistry* 270, 22440-22444.

Pellestor F., Paulasova P., Hamamah S. (2008) Peptide nucleic acids (PNAs) as diagnostic devices for genetic and cytogenetic analysis. *Current Pharmaceutical Design* 14, 2439-2444.

Peng X., Ghosh A.K., Van Houten B., Greenberg M.M. (2010) Nucleotide Excision Repair of a DNA Interstrand Cross-Link Produces Single- and Double-Strand Breaks. *Biochemistry* 49, 11-19.

Peng X., Hong I.S., Li H., Seidman M.M., Greenberg M.M. (2008) Interstrand Cross-Link Formation in Duplex and Triplex DNA by Modified Pyrimidines. *Journal of the American Chemical Society* 130, 10299–10306.

Peterson C.L., Côte J. (2004) Cellular machineries for chromosomal DNA repair. *Genes & Development* 18, 602-616.

Pooga M., Land T., Bartfai T., Langel Ü. (2001) PNA oligomers as tools for specific modulation of gene expression. *Biomolecular Engineering* 17, 183-192.

Porcheddu A. and Giacomelli G. (1996) PNA-nucleic acid complexes. Structure, stability and dynamics. *Quarterly Reviews of Biophysics* 29, 369-394.

Porcheddu A., Giacomelli G. (2005) Peptide nucleic acids (PNAs), A chemical Overview. *Current Medicinal Chemistry* 12, 2561-2599.

Quanz M., Berthault N., Roulin C., Roy M., Herbette A., Agrario C., Alberti C., Josserand V., Coll J.-L., Sastre-Garau X., Cosset J.-M., Larue L., Sun J.-S., Dutreix M. (2009) Small-molecule drugs mimicking DNA damage: A new strategy for sensitizing tumors to radiotherapy. *Clinical Cancer Research* 15, 1308-1316.

Ray A., Norden B. (2000) Peptide nucleic acid (PNA): its medical and biotechnical applications and promise for the future, *FASEB Journal* 14, 1041-1060.

Regulus P., Duroux B., Bayle P.-A., Favier, A., Cadet J., Ravanat J.-L. (2007) Oxidation of the sugar moiety of DNA by ionizing radiation or bleomycin could induce the formation of a cluster DNA lesion. *Proceedings of the National Academy of Sciences* 104, 14032–14037.

Richardson N.A., Gu J., Wang S., Xie Y., Schaefer H.F. III. (2004) DNA Nucleosides and Their Radical Anions: Molecular Structures and Electron Affinities. *Journal of the American Chemical Society*, 126, 4404–4411.

Romanelli A., Pedone C., Saviano M., Bianchi N., Borgatti M., Mischiati C., Gambari R. (2001) Molecular interactions between nuclear factor κB (NF-κB) transcription factors and a PNA-DNA chimera mimicking NF-κB binding sites. *European Journal of Biochemistry* 268, 6066-6075.

Sawada S., Okada S. (1972) Effects of BUdR-labelling on radiation-induced DNA breakage and subsequent rejoining in cultured mammalian cells. *International Journal of Radiation Biology* 21, 599-602.

Sczepanski J.T., Jacobs A.C., Greenberg M.M. (2008) Self-Promoted DNA Interstrand Cross-Link Formation by an Abasic Site. *Journal of the American Chemical Society*, 130, 9646–9647.

Sczepanski J.T., Jacobs A.C., Majumdar A., Greenberg M.M. (2009a) Scope and Mechanism of Interstrand Cross-Link Formation by the C4'-Oxidized Abasic Site. *Journal of the American Chemical Society*, 131, 11132–11139.

Sczepanski J., Jacobs A.C., Van Houten B., Greenberg M.M. (2009b) Double-Strand Break Formation during Nucleotide Excision Repair of a DNA Interstrand Cross-Link. *Biochemistry* 48, 7565–7567.

Sherer C., Cramer C.J. (2004) Structural and dynamic variations in DNA hexamers containing T-T and F-F single and tandem internal mispairs. *Theoretical Chemistry Accounts* 111, 311-327.

Smerdon M.J., Lieberman, M.W. (1978) Nucleosome rearrangement in human chromatin during UV-induced DNA-repair synthesis. *Proceedings of the National Academy of Sciences U.S.A.* 75, 4238-4241.

Špačková N., Berger I., Šponer J. (2000) Nanosecond Molecular Dynamics of Zipper-like DNA Duplex Structures Containing Sheared G·A Mismatch Pairs. *Journal of the American Chemical Society* 122, 7564–7572.

Stokes S.T., Li X., Grubisic A., Ko Y.J., Bowen K.H. (2007) Intrinsic electrophilic properties of nucleosides: Photoelectron spectroscopy of their parent anions. *Journal of Chemical Physics* 127, 084321.

Takata M., Sasaki M.S., Sonoda E., Morrison C., Hashimoto M., Utsumi H., Yamaguchi-Iwai Y., Shinohara A., Takeda S. (1998) Homologous recombination and non-homologous end-joining pathways of DNA double-strand break repair have overlapping roles in the maintenance of chromosomal integrity in vertebrate cells. *EMBO Journal* 17, 5497-5508.

Thoma F. (2005) Repair of UV lesions in nucleosomes - intrinsic properties and remodeling. *DNA Repair* 4, 855-869.

Van Attikum H., Gasser, S.M. (2005) The histone code at DNA breaks: A guide to repair? *Nature Reviews Molecular Cell Biology*. 6, 757-765.

Wang C.-R., Nguyen J., Lu Q.-B. (2009) Bond Breaks of Nucleotides by Dissociative Electron Transfer of Nonequilibrium Prehydrated Electrons: A New Molecular Mechanism for Reductive DNA Damage. *Journal of the American Chemical Society* 131, 11320-11322.

Wang C.-R., Lu Q.-B. (2010) Molecular Mechanism of the DNA Sequence Selectivity of 5-Halo-2'-Deoxyuridines as Potential Radiosensitizers. *Journal of the American Chemical Society* 132, 14710–14713.

Wang W. (2007) Emergence of a DNA-damage response network consisting of Fanconi anaemia and BRCA proteins. *Nature Reviews Genetics* 8, 735-748.

Weng X., Ren L., Weng L., Huang J., Zhu S., Zhou X., Weng L. (2007) Synthesis and Biological Studies of Inducible DNA Cross-Linking Agents. *Angewandte Chemie* 119, 8166–8169.

Yoshioka Y., Kitagawa Y., Takano Y., Yamaguchi K., Nakamura T., Saito I.J. (1999) Experimental and Theoretical Studies on the Selectivity of GGG Triplets toward One-Electron Oxidation in B-Form DNA. *American Chemical Society* 121, 8712-8719.

Zeng Y., Wang Y. (2006) Sequence-dependent formation of intrastrand crosslink products from the UVB irradiation of duplex DNA containing a 5-bromo-20-deoxyuridine or 5-bromo-20-deoxycytidine. *Nucleic Acids Research* 34, 6521–6529.

Zeng Y., Wang Y. (2007) UVB-induced formation of intrastrand cross-link products of DNA in MCF-7 cells treated with 5-bromo-20-deoxyuridine. *Biochemistry* 46, 8189–8195.

Zimbrick J.D., Ward J.F., Myers L.S. Jr. (1969a) Studies on the chemical basis of cellular radiosensitization by 5-bromouracil substitution in DNA. I. Pulse- and steady-state radiolysis of 5-bromouracil and thymine", *International Journal of Radiation Biology* 16, 505-523.

Zimbrick J.D., Ward J.F., Myers L.S. Jr. (1969b) Studies on the chemical basis of cellular radiosensitization by 5-bromouracil substitution in DNA. II. Pulse- and steady-state radiolysis of bromouracil-substituted and unsubstituted DNA, *International Journal of Radiation Biology* 16, 524-534.

# 19

# The Influence of Individual Genome Sensitivity in DNA Damage Repair Assessment in Chronic Professional Exposure to Low Doses of Ionizing Radiation

Mirta Milić[1], Ružica Rozgaj[1], Vilena Kašuba[1], Ana Marija Jazbec[2], Patrizia Hrelia[3] and Sabrina Angelini[3]
[1]*Institute for Medical Research and Occupational Health, Mutagenesis Unit, Zagreb*
[2]*Faculty of Forestry, University of Zagreb, Zagreb,*
[3]*Department of Pharmacology, University of Bologna, Bologna,*
[1,2]*Croatia*
[3]*Italy*

## 1. Introduction

During their working and living activities, humans are constantly exposed to different environmental genotoxic agents. Biological consequences of the exposure are accumulation of different mutations and DNA damage that can lead to disruption of genetic material. Numerous endogenous genotoxic agents can also cause DNA damage. Loss of normal cell function can cause cell death or can result in different health disorders, including teratogenic and cancerogenic effects (Jeggo & Lavin, 2009). There is an increasing concern about mutagenic and cancerogenic effects of genotoxic agents and their influence on individuals who are exposed to them by accident, or by living/working lifestyle (Au, 1991; Carrano & Natarajan, 1988; Kassie et al., 2000).
Exposure to ionising radiation, as a well known genotoxic agents (Balasem & Ali, 1991; Erexon et al., 1991; Fenech et al., 1990; He et al., 2000; Jeggo & Lavin, 2009), can leed to different DNA damage, such as oxidative damage, base and sugar modification in DNA, apurinic/apirimidinic places, single/double strand chromosomal breaks, adduct creation, inter/intra DNA cross linking and other types of damage (Hall & Giaccia, 2006). Numerous studies deal with ionising radiation exposure of individuals who are chronically professionally exposed to low doses (Andreassi, 2009; Au, 1991; Carrano & Natarajan, 1988; Kassie et al., 2000). The results showed the increase in chromosomal damage during chronically low dose exposure (Barquinero et al., 1993; Boutcher, 1985; Cardoso et al., 2001; Jha, 1991; Nowak & Jankowski, 1991), but without confirmed relationship between the received dose and the intensity of DNA damage (Bolus, 2001; Coates et al., 2004; Morgan, 2003; Mothersill et al., 2000, 2001; Seymour & Mothersill, 2000). The influence of chronically low dose exposure has been considered mutagenic and cancerogenic (Fachini et al., 2009). Although it is possible to estimate the influence of absorbed dose and the effect on the

exposed individuals, consequences of continuous low dose exposure are still a great topic of researches.

The medical stuff represents the best investigated group of professionals exposed to low levels of ionising radiation (UNSCEAR, 2000). During their work, all the employees wear dosimeters (film, TLD or electronic ones) that are analysed on monthly bases. In addition, they are under regular medical control.

Duration and the intensity of exposure to low doses of ionising radiation have significantly decreased over the last decades. The results of analysed dosimeters showed that the received doses are significantly below the regulatory threshold of 20 mSv per year, sometimes even under the dosimeters detection abilities (Kubelka et al., 2011).

Persons employed in emergency medical units and nuclear medicine workers are exposed to higher doses and show higher DNA damage than workers in diagnostic radiology departments (Sari-Minodier et al., 2007).

Andreassi et al. (2009) reported higher amount of DNA damage among interventional cardiologists when compared to clinical cardiologists. Epidemiological researches have shown the connection between the amounts of accumulated doses and the risk of tumour developing (Berrington et al., 2001; Maitre et al., 2003; Wang et al., 2002; Yoshinaga et al., 1999). Cardisi et al. (2005) reported the relationship between exposure to low doses of ionising radiation and cancer in study that involved 400 000 nuclear industry workers.

Today's general opinion is that initial event in radiation carcinogenesis is un/ missrepaired double strand break of DNA molecule, which is a major lesion that leads to developing of chromosomal abnormalities and genetic mutations (Little, 2000).

Accidental or therapeutical acute exposure to ionising radiation can cause different cytogenetic damage, including higher amount of micronuclei (small amount of chromatin in the shape of small nuclei in cytoplasm that was not divided into two new nuclei after first cell division) and chromosomal aberrations (single /double strand breaks of chromosome, inter/intra chromosomal exchange, dicentrics, acentrics, etc.). Recently, different biomarkers are used for monitoring of people occupationally exposed to chronical low doses of ionising radiation. The use of combined biomarkers can offer better assessment and health care of those individuals. With them a phenomenon of adaptive response has been observed. This response can be seen after the first adapting dose of ionising radiation is received (mostly under 10 cGy). After exposure to higher, so called challenging dose, above 100 cGy, those individuals show lower amount of DNA damage when compared to those who did not receive the first, adapting dose. There is also evidence that the amount of dose received can influence the adaptive response (Gourabi & Mozdarani, 1998). A great variability in DNA damage response to ionising radiation exposure of cell lines *in vitro* and individuals *in vivo* have been reported (Bosi & Olivieri, 1989; Shadley & Wiencke, 1989). Adaptive response has been shown also in persons after clinical, environmental or working exposure (Barquinero et al., 1993, 1995, 1996; Monsieurs et al., 2000; Padovani et al., 1995; Szumiel, 1998; Tedeschi et al., 1995, 1996). Individual differences in DNA repair genes can also influence on this response (Milić, 2010).

Molecular mechanisms of adaptive response are still not clear. It has been considered that it depends on the synthesis and/or protein expression, especially those involved in DNA repair mechanism (Boothman et al., 1989; Ikushima, 1989, 1996; Robson et al., 1999; Wolf et al., 1989, 1996; Youngblom et al., 1989). Early induction response (Okayasu et al., 2000;

Stecca & Gerber, 1998), changes in gene expression, gene transcription regulation are also related with adaptive response. Mutations in genes involved in DNA repair can cause DNA missrepair, chromosome endings fusion, fusion of unprotected telomere ends and double strand breaks after exposure to ionising radiation (Bailey et al., 2004; Bailey & Goodwin, 2004; Sasaki et al., 2002).

The accuracy of any risk assessment, especially low dose exposures, depends on both the resolution of the method, and the baseline data obtained in well-selected controls. Alkaline comet assay (single-cell gel electrophoresis, SCGE) is an easy-to-use, quick and very sensitive method for detecting primary DNA strand breaks, that is, direct DNA damage within single cells (Tice et al., 1990; Collins, 2004) and can be applied to proliferating and non proliferating cells (Kassie et al., 2000) to determine DNA damage as a result of endogenous factors, lifestyle (Hoffman & Speit, 2005), and occupational or environmental exposure (Valverde et al., 1999).

After relaxation, DNA can be seen as a comet during electrophoresis due to strand breaks (Singh, 2000). The advantages of this technique are sensitivity, reproducibility, easy to use, low expences. It is a rapid method and the amount of sample necessary for the analysis is very small. Comet assay enables analysis of any sort of cells, whether it is plant, animal or human origin, no matter are those single cells from the cell culture or from the tissue. Due to the short-time performance of this technique (it is possible to have results after few hours), it has become well accepted in investigation of different genotoxic agents both *in vitro* and *in vivo* conditions (Betti et al., 1994; Kassie et al., 2000; Kruszewski et al., 1998; McKelvey-Martin et al., 1993; Wojewodzka et al., 1998).

In this method, single cells are embedded into so called agarosis sandwich. Cytoplasm and membranic cell structures are lysed with high concentrated EDTA solution (ethylenediaminetetraacetic acid) and detergents, causing total cell DNA to be free. There are two comet assay protocols, whether alkaline or neutral denaturation is used.

Neutral version enables detection of double stranded DNA breaks (Olive et al., 1990). Under alkaline conditions, single stranded breaks, alkaline labile sites (AP, parts of DNA that can break easily in alkaline solutions), DNA-DNA and DNA protein crosslinking can be detected. Alkaline labile sites are apurinic and apirimidinic DNA bases that can break easily when exposed to alkaline conditions (Singh et al., 1988). After alkaline/neutral denaturation, the cells undergo electrophoresis. Concerning the high molecular weight of the entire DNA molecule, DNA can not pass through the agarose pores towards the anode. Only the small, damaged fragments can pass through. During electrophoresis, the velocity of those fragments that are caused by single or double chromosome breaks depends on their molecular weight. The smaller they are, the faster they get (Plappert et al., 1995). After electrophoresis, the slides are stained with fluorescent dye (usually ethidium bromide). Epifluorescent microscope is used for single cells analysing. Undamaged cells have round shape, while damaged one are similar to the shape of the comet. The mostly used parameters of comet assay are the tail length (TL), percentage of DNA in tail (TI) and the tail moment (TM). Tail length (usually expressed in micrometers) is measured from the centre of the comet head till the end of the comet tail (that is the distance of the fragments from the major DNA that have travelled through the gel during electrophoresis). It is proportional with DNA damage and with length of the fragments (Singh et al., 1988; Tice et al., 1990). TI is measured with computer programme for comet assay analysis. The amount of the damage is estimated based on the ratio of DNA percentage in head and in tail of a comet. Some researchers prefer tail moment as the most reliable marker of DNA damage, because it combines measurements of tail length and percentage of DNA in tail (Ashby et al., 1995; Hellman et al., 1995; 1997; Mc Kelvey-Martin et al., 1998). Collins (2004) emphasizes the advantage of TI considering that the percentage of the tail DNA reflects the real DNA damage. Comet assay can also detect apoptotic and necrotic cells. Apoptotic cells show small comet head, and most of DNA is spread in tail in the shape of a cloud (Fairbairn et al., 1995; Olive, 1999). Comet assay is also a valuable technique to study the kinetics of primary DNA damage. It enables to estimate the DNA damage level immediately after the exposure, even when the exposure included very small dose in very short exposure period (Tice et al., 1990; Plappert et al., 1995). Fast repair can represent a problem in DNA damage evaluation in populations occupationally exposed to low doses of ionising radiation and therefore the development of sensitive methods is necessary for those experiments. Most of the primary DNA damage is repaired 30 minutes after the exposure to ionising radiation (Frankenberg-Schwager, 1989), and 2 hours after the exposure to dose of 2 Gy, most of the damaged DNA is totally repaired (Plappert et al., 1997).

Polymorphism by definition is expression of different phenotypes in the same species due to the change/s in genotype. They usually include loss (deletion) of small or bigger part of DNA molecule, insertion of specific number of nucleotides or repetition of di-, three-, or oligonucleotides in variant number. The number or repeating differs among individuals.

Variations in human genome are usually caused by variations in DNA sequence, that is based on the change of only one nucleotide (one from the four nucleotides; A-adenine, T-thymine, C-cytosine or G-guanosine is replaced by the other) usually known as SNP polymorphism (*single nucleotide polymorphism*). Among almost 15 million of SNPs in human genome, 50.000 to 100. 000 of them can change the function or gene expression.

The connection of the change in only one nucleotide (that happens once in every 1000nucleotides in human genome) with the complex aetiology of malignant diseases is poorly investigated (Bonassi et al., 2005). More than 7 millions of well known SNPs in human genome appear with the allelic frequency higher than 5% of the entire population (Hinds et al., 2005). More than 70% of SNPs in human population have the frequency less than 5 % and those SNPs are called rare SNPs (Shastry, 2009). The results of new experiments have shown the connection between gene polymorphisms and risk association with disease developing (Norpa, 2004), especially in polymorphisms of DNA repair genes and folic acid metabolism. Polymorphisms can lead to different gene expression (decreased or increased) and through this process can influence on cell repair mechanisms (Hung et al., 2005; Parl, 2005; Weiss et al., 2005; Kotsopoulos et al., 2007). Variations in DNA repair capacity have been also observed among healthy individuals (Setlow, 1983).

Among 130 genes involved in DNA repair mechanisms, 80 of them are carriers of more than 400 SNPs (Mohrenweiser et al., 2003). DNA damage and repair correlate with the radiation sensitivity and are important in radiation protection and radiotherapy (Ross et al., 2000). Due to individual variations, some persons have higher sensitivity when compared with general population (Berwick, 2000). It has been estimated that 10 -15 percent of healthy people have phenotype that shows decreased possibility for successful DNA damage repair (Mohrenweiser & Jones, 1998; Hu et al., 2002a). Higher risk of mutations, genome instability and malignant tumours have been observed among persons with decreased DNA repair capacity (Berwick & Vineis, 2000; Chen et al., 2002; Collins & Harrington, 2002; Divine et al., 2001; Hou et al., 2002; Kumar et al., 2003; Sturgis et al., 1999; Winsey et al., 2000).

The connection between ionising radiation and SNPs in gene involved in DNA repair has been described by several authors (Aka et al., 2004; Hu et al., 2001; Lunn et al., 2000; Touil et al., 2002). There is an increased interest for exploring of SNPs of genes that are part of biological response to ionising radiation and connecting them with clinical sensibility. Those SNPs could be used for an estimation of exposure to ionising radiation (Andreassen, 2005).

Determination of high risk population on the basis of genetic polymorphism could help in tumour prevention. The influence of polymorphisms can be crucial in the exposure to low doses of ionising radiation (Boffetta et al., 1999).

## 2. Materials and methods

This study included 126 subjects, 70 medical workers occupationally exposed to low doses of ionising radiation (gastroenterologists, cardiologists, anaesthesiologists, surgeons, radiologists, radiology technicians, nurses) of both gender (45 females, 25 men; mean age was 40 years, from 20-60 years old) and 56 individuals in control group who were not exposed to neither ionising radiation nor to chemical mutagens (14 women and men; mean age 40 years, from 23 to 60 years old) (Table 1).

| | Control group | Exposed group |
|---|---|---|
| Subjects (No.)<br>F/M | 56<br>14/42 | 70<br>45/25 |
| Age±SD<br>(Min-Max) | 40.53±10.92<br>(23-60) | 40.27±10.8<br>(20-60) |
| Smoking, Y/N | 16/40 | 31/39 |
| Alcohol, Y/N | 35/21 | 21/49 |
| Years of exposure±SD<br>(Min-Max) | - | 12.22±8.65<br>(1-38) |

Table 1. Characteristics of the control and exposed group considering the gender, age, years of exposure, smoking status and alcohol consumption.

The examinees were informed of the study scope and experimental details, have filled a standardised questionnaire designed to obtain relevant information on the current health status, medical history, and lifestyle, and gave their written consent, submitted and approved by the local Ethics Committee. The questionnaire included data on the exposure to possible confounding factors: smoking, alcohol consumption, use of medicines, contraceptives, severe infections, or viral diseases over the past six months, vitamin intake, recent vaccinations, presence of known inherited genetic disorders and chronic diseases, family history of cancer, exposure to diagnostic X-rays. Subjects with history of previous radio- or chemotherapy were not included. Exposed group was under regular film dosimetry and the dose received did not exceed 20mSv/year (data not shown).

Two millilitres of venous blood was stored in heparinised vacutainers for comet assay and assessment of DNA repair kinetics and stored at +4°C before further procedure. Detailed protocol is described before (Milić et al., 2010). Five millilitres of venous blood was stored in vacutainers with EDTA (ethylenediaminetetraacetic acid) at -20°C until further DNA isolation (Milić et al., 2010). Blood samples were irradiated with 60Co (Alcyon, CGR-MeV, France). The doses used were 2 and 4 Gy, with the same distance from the source (80 cm). Irradiation field was 15 x 15 $cm^2$. After irradiation, samples were kept at + 4°C to prevent the repair of the damage. Details are also described before (Milić et al., 2010).

### 2.1 Comet assay

Alkaline version of comet assay (Singh et al., 1988) with small modifications was used. Detailed procedure is described elsewhere (Milić, 2010; Milić et al., 2010). The slides were marked and stored at +4°C till the beginning of the irradiation. Control samples were put into cold lysis solution immediately after preparation and left there for 24 hours at +4°C (Milić, 2010). Irradiated blood gel samples were incubated at 37°C in serum free RPMI 1640 medium. Zero samples were immediately immersed into lysis solution. DNA repair kinetics was measured at 0, 15, 30, 60 and 120 minutes after exposure, and additional 24 hours for samples irradiated with the dose of 4 Gy. Specific measure points were based on the results of other researches (Singh et al., 1988; Price, 1993; Tice, 1995). The 2 Gy dose was a standard daily dose in radiotherapy, while the 4 Gy dose was chosen as a ˝challenging˝ dose for the exposed group. After the repair, slides were vertically placed into cold lysis solution at 4°C, overnight. Protein denaturation and DNA unwinding were done at 4°C in denaturation buffer (1 mM Na2EDTA and 300 mM NaOH) (pH 13.0) for 20 minutes. Horizontal electrophoresis in fresh cold denaturation buffer was done at 300 mA and 25 V for 20 minutes. The slides were washed in neutralisation buffer (0.4 M Tris-HCl, pH 7.5) three times. Slides were stained with 50 µL of ethidium bromide solution (20 $\mu g mL^{-1}$, Sigma) (per slide), covered with cover slip and kept in container, in the dark conditions at 4°C.

The procedure was done under dimmed light, in order to avoid additional DNA damage caused by the exposure to the normal light. Each slide was examined using a 250x magnification fluorescence microscope (Zeiss, Germany) equipped with an excitation filter of 515-560 nm and a barrier filter of 590 nm. A total of 200 comets per sample and per interval were scored (100 from each of two replicate slides). Comets were randomly captured at a constant depth of the gel, avoiding the edges of the gel, occasional dead cells and superimposed comets. Using a black and white camera, the microscope image was transferred to a computer-based image analysis system (Comet Assay II, Perceptive Instruments Ltd., U.K.). To avoid the variability, one well-trained scorer scored all comets. Three parameters of DNA damage were analysed: tail length (TL, presented in micrometres), tail DNA (TI, %) and tail moment (TM).

### 2.2 DNA isolation

Genomic DNA was isolated from peripheral lymphocytes according to modified protocol by Daly et al. (1996) or according to protocol for genomic DNA lymphocyte isolation from QUIAGEN (mini KIT). DNA was purified with two times centrifugation at 4°C, 500 µL of 70 percent ethanol added every time. The pellet was dried overnight at room temperature and diluted in 100 μL of TE buffer (10mM Tris-HCl, pH 7.4; 1 mM EDTA, pH 8.0). Purity and concentration of DNA was specified by spectrophotometric method (NanoDrop ND- 1000 spectrophotometer, NanoDrop Technologies, Thermo Scientific, Wilmington, USA). Samples were diluted till concentration of 10 ng $\mu L^{-1}$ and kept at -20 °C till amplification. Specific polymorphisms were determined: in BER- (base excision repair) APE1- (apurinic/apirimidinic endonuclease, Asp148Glu), hOGG1 (human 8-oxoguanine DNA glycosylase, Ser326Cys), XRCC1 (X-ray repair cross-complementing protein-group 1, Arg194Trp); in NER- (nucleotide excision repair) XPD (Xeroderma pigmentosum-group D, Lys751Gln; DSBR- (double-strand-break repair) XRCC3 (X-ray repair cross-complementing protein-group 3, Thr241Met), PARP1 (poly (ADP-ribose) polymerase 1, Val762Ala); in DRR- (direct reversal repair) MGMT (O6-methylguanine-DNA methyltransferase, Leu84Phe) Genotyping was performed by either Real Time PCR (polymerase chain reaction) with Taqman assay, or after electrophoresis and fluorescence visualisation, DNA samples were cut with restriction enzymes.

### 2.3 Polymerase chain reaction-RFLP

In a total volume of 10 ml, 10 ng of genomic DNA was amplified for each sample. Compounds for the reaction mixture are given in Table 2.

PCR reaction was completed in six steps: (I) incubation at 94 °C (2 min) for Taq DNA polymerase activation; (II) incubation at 94 °C (30 s) for denaturation of double stranded DNA; (III) incubation at specific temperature that depended on the specific gene (30 s), for hybridisation of primers (Table 3); (IV) incubation at 72 °C (30 s) for DNA synthesis. Steps No.2 to No. 4 were repeated for 34 times. After that there were steps: (V) incubation at 72 °C (5 min) and (VI) incubation at 10 °C.

| Reaction mixture | Stock solution | Final concentration for PCR reaction |
|---|---|---|
| (DMSO) | (1x) | (for XRCC3-0.05x) |
| re$H_2O$ | 1x | 0.64x (for XRCC3-0.59x) |
| 10X BUFFER | 10x | 1.00 x |
| $MgCl_2$ | 50 mM | 2.00 mM |
| dNTP | 1.25 mM | 0.11 mM |
| Primer F | 20 μM | 0.30 μM |
| Primer R | 20 μM | 0.30 μM |
| DNA polymerase (Platinum Taq, Invitrogen) | 5 U $\mu l^{-1}$ | 0,03 U $\mu l^{-1}$ |

Table 2. Compounds for PCR-RFLP reaction (10 μl of reaction mixture (9 μl of Master Mix and 1 μl of DNA sample).

| GENE | rs | PCR method | primers | °C | Restriction enzyme |
|---|---|---|---|---|---|
| XPD ex 23 or ERCC2 | rs13181 [Aag > Cag; Lys751Gln] | RFLP (Angelini et al., 2005) | F CCC CTC TCC CTT TCC TCT GTT<br>R GCT GCC TTC TCC TGC GAT TA | 61 | PstI (37 °C, overnight)<br>CTGCA*G<br>G*ACGTC<br>HOwt-29,244bp; HE-29,63,181,244bp; HOSNP-29,63,181bp |
| XPD10 | rs1799793 [Gac > Aag; Asp312Asn] | Real Time TaqMan assay C_3145050_10 | none | none | none |
| XRCC1 ex10 | rs861539 [aCg > aTg; Trp194Arg] | RFLP (Angelini et al., 2005)<br>RT TaqMan assay C_622564_10 | F GCC CCT CAG ATC ACA CCT AAC<br>R CAT TGC CCA GCA CAG GAT AA | 61 | MspI (37 °C, overnight)<br>C*CGG<br>GGC*C<br>WT-161, 53 bp; HE-241, 161, 53 bp; SNP-214 bp |
| XRCC3 ex7 | rs861539 [aCg > aTg; Thr241Met] | RFLP (Angelini et al., 2005) | F GCT CGC CTG GTG GTC ATC<br>R CTT CCG CAT CCT GGC TAA AAA | 60 | Hin1 II/NIa III (37 °C, overnight) |
| hOGG1, ex4 | rs1052133 [tCc > tGc; Ser326cys] | RFLP (Godderis et al., 2006)<br>RT TaqMan assay C_3095552_1 | F CCCAACCCCAGTGGATTCTCATTGC<br>R GGTGCCCCATCTAGCCTTGCGGCCCTT | 60 | SatI/ Fnu4HI (37 °C, overnight)<br>GC*NGC<br>CGN*CG<br>HOwt-214,20pb; HE-214,165,49,20pb; HOSNP-165,49,20pb |
| PARP1 | - | RT TaqMan assay | Real time | none | none |
| APE1 | rs1130409 [gaT > gaG; Asp148Glu] | RFLP (Hu et al., 2002)<br>RT TaqMan assay C_8921503_10 | F CTGTTTCATTTCTATAGGCTA<br>R AGGAACTTGCGAAAGGCTTC | 57 | BfaI (37 °C, overnight)<br>(Asp/Asp 164bp, Asp/Glu 164,144,20bp; Glu/Glu-144,20bp) |
| MGMT C/T | rs12917, Leu84Phe | RT TaqMan assay | Real time | none | none |

Table 3. Gene, forward and reverse primers, method used for determination of polymorphism, hybridisation temperature, restriction enzymes and the DNA fragments.

After PCR reaction, DNA products were cut with specific restriction enzymes (Fermentas, Vilnius, Litva) that have cut DNA samples on specific places and have given different DNA fragments in order to recognize which samples were homozygote wild type, heterozygote and polymorphic homozygotes. Treatment with restriction enzymes was performed at 37 °C in a period of 3 hours or overnight (due to the specification of specific restriction enzyme used in the reaction). Enzymes, time intervals of cutting, the temperature for those enzymes and the resulting DNA fragments after the cutting are given in Table 3. After electrophoresis that lasted 30 minutes at 200 V, PCR products were analysed on 10%-polyacrilamid gel (Bio-Rad, Hercules, USA).

Genotype results were regularly confirmed by random repetition of the samples.

PCR products were also amplified with Real-Time PCR (Real-Time PCR ABI Prism 7300 thermocycler, Applied Biosystems, Foster City, USA) with TaqMan allelic discrimination assay (Applera, Foster City, USA). Allelic determination was done by their software. Compounds for the Real-Time PCR mixture is shown in Table 4. Forty cycluses were performed for division between VIC and FAM fluorescence stain. The intensity of those stains is selecting the samples into three categories (Angelini et al., 2005).

| Ingredients | Volume/µl |
|---|---|
| TaqMan Master Mix | 6.5 |
| re$H_2O$ | 5.33 |
| Specific primers for every gene | 0.65 |
| DNA sample | 0.5 |

Table 4. Compounds for Real Time PCR reaction. Steps in Real Time PCR-a were: (I) 95 °C (10 min); (II) 92 °C (15 s); and (III) 60 °C (10 min).

## 3. Results

DNA repair kinetics after the exposure to gamma radiation of 2 and 4 Gy was measured on a group of 126 subjects, 70 medical workers and 56 controls (Figure 1).

The groups differed in average age, gender, smoking status and alcohol consumption. The mean values for both groups did not significantly differ, although inter-individual differences were notable. In control group higher level of DNA damage compared to exposed group was observed, but without statistical difference. The repair dynamic was the same in both groups.

After genotyping, heterozygotes and polymorphic homozygotes were grouped together to evaluate polymorphic allele appearance. Number of individuals carrying particular gene is given in Table 5. Frequency of genotyping did not differ from expected Hardy-Weinberg equilibrium.

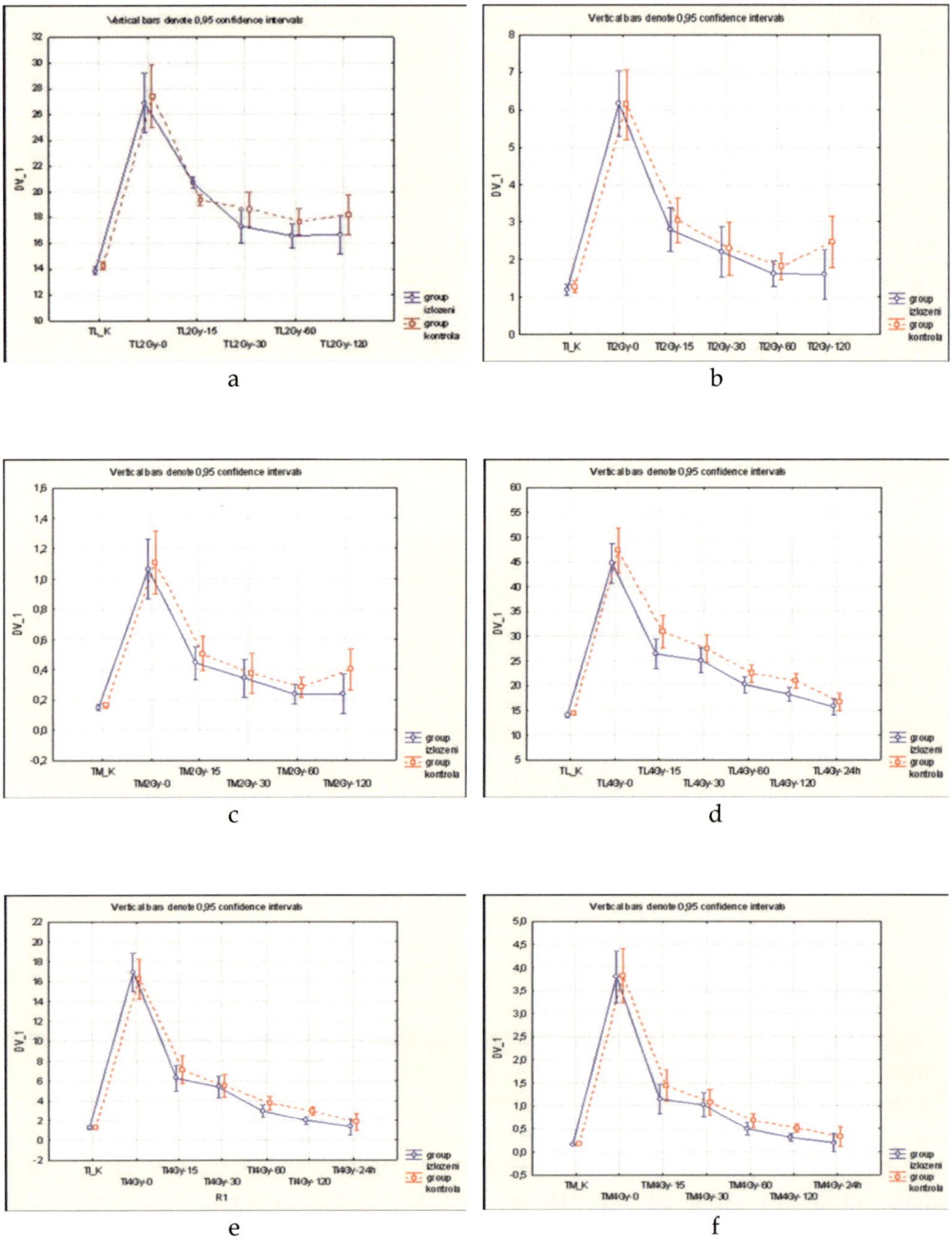


Fig. 1. Graphical results of DNA repair. Red colour - control group; blue - exposed group. a- TL after 2 Gy irradiation, b-TI after 2 Gy, c-TM after 2 Gy, d- TL after 4 Gy irradiation, e- TI after 4 Gy, f- TM after 4 Gy.

| Gene | Group (WT/HE/SNP) | Control (WT/HE/SNP) | Exposed (WT/HE/SNP) |
|---|---|---|---|
| XPD 23 | 42/58/26 | 15/33/8 | 27/25/18 |
| XPD 10 | 43/63/20 | 17/33/6 | 26/30/14 |
| XRCC1 | 47/67/12 | 22/25/9 | 25/42/3 |
| PARP1 | 83/37/6 | 33/18/5 | 50/19/1 |
| HOGG1 | 78/43/5 | 42/14/0 | 36/29/5 |
| APE1 | 43/57/26 | 19/27/10 | 24/30/16 |
| MGMT C/T | 87/34/5 | 39/16/1 | 48/18/4 |
| XRCC3 | 45/61/20 | 23/26/7 | 22/35/13 |

Table 5. Number of individuals in three genotyping groups for all genes (WT-homozygote wild type, HE-heterozygote, SNP-polymorphic homozygote).

| Variable | st | $\chi^2$ | p |
|---|---|---|---|
| XRCC1 | 1 | 0.1697 | 0.6804 |
| **hOGG1** | 1 | 7.3298 | **0.0068** |
| APE2 | 1 | 0.0018 | 0.9665 |
| XPD21 | 1 | 0.6372 | 0.4247 |
| PARP2 | 1 | 2.1624 | 0.1414 |
| MGMT C/T | 1 | 0.0167 | 0.8971 |
| XRCC3 | 1 | 1.6433 | 0.1999 |
| smoking | 1 | 1.7174 | 0.19 |
| **sex** | 1 | 13.2499 | **0.0003** |

Table 6. Results of $\chi 2$-test in the exposed and control group compared to genotype frequency, smoking and gender.

The differences between exposed and control group were analysed by $\chi 2$-test. Significant difference was found for hOGG1 gene and for gender (Table 6). Observed difference between smokers and non smokers was insignificant.

Multivariate regression analysis was used to estimate the influence of smoking, gender, age, years of exposure and genotypes on comet assay parameters immediately after and 120 minutes after exposure to 2 Gy and after 24 hours for the dose of 4 Gy.

Immediately after irradiation with the 2 Gy dose, exposed group had significantly lower amount of DNA damage than control group. Individuals with polymorphic variants of XRCC3 gene had higher TL than their homozygotes. Polymorphic variants of hOGG1 gene had higher TI than homozygotes. Polymorphic variants of hOGG1 gene had significantly higher TM than their homozygotes.

Tail length values significantly differed between the two groups both immediately after and also 120 minutes after irradiation with 2 Gy. Polymorphic variants of APE1 and XPD10 genes had higher TI and TM compared to homozygotes 120 min after irradiation with 2 Gy, and polymorphic variants of MGMT C/T and XRCC3 genes had significantly lower TI and TM than homozygotes (Table 7).

| Variable | PE | SE | Parc $R^2$ | F | p |
|---|---|---|---|---|---|
| **Log TL-2 Gy-0'** | | | | | |
| Group | -0.10669 | 0.04189 | 0.0468 | 6.49 | 0.0124 |
| XRCC3 | 0.09351 | 0.04390 | 0.0312 | 4.54 | 0.0357 |
| MTR | 0.07742 | 0.04335 | 0.0291 | 3.19 | 0.0772 |
| **Log TI-2 Gy-0'** | | | | | |
| hOGG1 | 0.14426 | 0.07300 | 0.0509 | 3.91 | 0.0376 |
| **Log TM-2 Gy-0'** | | | | | |
| TS | 0.16398 | 0.10332 | 0.1157 | 2.52 | 0.0243 |
| hOGG1 | 0.16083 | 0.09018 | 0.0776 | 3.18 | 0.0223 |
| **Log TL-2 Gy-120'** | | | | | |
| Group | 0.00069854 | 0.00019567 | 0.0914 | 12.74 | 0.0006 |
| XPD 10 | 0.00037667 | 0.00020220 | 0.0274 | 3.47 | 0.0655 |
| XRCC3 | 0.00031641 | 0.00020077 | 0.0220 | 2.48 | 0.1183 |
| **TI-2 Gy-120'** | | | | | |
| Group | 0.16440 | 0.04433 | 0.0004 | 13.75 | 0.1012 |
| APE1 | 0.08068 | 0.04704 | 0.0896 | 2.94 | 0.0217 |
| XPD10 | 0.09252 | 0.04627 | 0.0484 | 4.0 | 0.0239 |
| MGMT C/T | -0.07375 | 0.04608 | 0.1128 | 2.56 | 0.0217 |
| XRCC3 | -0.09915 | 0.04763 | 0.0401 | 4.33 | 0.0262 |
| **TM-2 Gy-120'** | | | | | |
| Group | 0.48944 | 0.12713 | 0.0002 | 14.82 | 0.1075 |
| APE1 | 0.23214 | 0.13490 | 0.0885 | 2.96 | 0.0217 |
| XPD10 | 0.26994 | 0.13268 | 0.0447 | 4.14 | 0.0247 |
| MGMT C/T | -0.20599 | 0.13216 | 0.1224 | 2.43 | 0.0204 |
| XRRC3 | -0.29847 | 0.13659 | 0.0313 | 4.77 | 0.0289 |

Table 7. Results of *stepwise* procedure in multivariate regression analysis for three comet assay parameters as a depended variable in the entire population immediately after radiation with 2 Gy dose and 120 minutes after irradiation (only the statistically significant results are shown in the Table).

Immediately after 4 Gy irradiation, multivariate regression analysis showed influence of smoking on TL. Polymorphic variants of SHMT1 genes had lower TL than their homozygotes. Gender had significant influence on TI. Polymorphic variants of SHMT1 and PARP1 genes had lower TI and TM when compared to their homozygotes.

Polymorphic variants of APE1 gene showed positive correlation with TL 24 hours after radiation with 4 Gy. Polymorphic variants of MGMT C/T gene had lower TL than homozygotes.

With the increase of age, significant increase in TI was measured 24 hours after exposure to 4 Gy. Polymorphic variants of PARP1 gene had lower values of TI than homozygotes. Age has shown positive correlation with TM. Lower values for TM were observed among polymorphic variants of PARP1 gene when compared to homozygotes (Table 8).

| Variable | PE | SE | Parc $R^2$ | F | p |
|---|---|---|---|---|---|
| **TL-4 Gy-0'** | | | | | |
| Smoking | 4.10520 | 2.19325 | 3.50 | 0.0642 | 0.0267 |
| SHMT1 | -3.74806 | 2.11391 | 3.14 | 0.0793 | 0.0297 |
| **TI-4 Gy-0'** | | | | | |
| Gender | 1.37561 | 0.94228 | 2.13 | 0.1475 | 0.0199 |
| SHMT1 | -1.65022 | 0.95455 | 2.99 | 0.0870 | 0.0294 |
| PARP1 | -1.63931 | 1.02226 | 2.57 | 0.1120 | 0.0257 |
| **TM-4 Gy-0'** | | | | | |
| SHMT1 | -0.14041 | 0.07716 | 3.31 | 0.0718 | 0.0304 |
| PARP1 | -0.13713 | 0.08267 | 2.75 | 0.1003 | 0.0260 |
| **TL-4 Gy-24h** | | | | | |
| Gender | 0.00036220 | 0.00017016 | 4.53 | 0.0361 | 0.0468 |
| MTR | 0.00047723 | 0.00017978 | 7.05 | 0.0094 | 0.0499 |
| APE1 | 0.00036597 | 0.00018268 | 4.01 | 0.0483 | 0.0329 |
| MGMT C/T | -0.00034719 | 0.00017942 | 3.74 | 0.0562 | 0.0359 |
| **TI-4 Gy-24h** | | | | | |
| Gender | 0.11087 | 0.04594 | 5.82 | 0.0180 | 0.0390 |
| Age | 0.00387 | 0.00203 | 3.63 | 0.0601 | 0.0376 |
| TS | -0.07933 | 0.05406 | 2.15 | 0.1461 | 0.0741 |
| MTHFR4 | 0.09859 | 0.04499 | 4.80 | 0.0313 | 0.0372 |
| PARP1 | -0.10466 | 0.04861 | 4.64 | 0.0342 | 0.0267 |
| **TM-4 Gy-24h** | | | | | |
| Gender | 2.03821 | 0.60467 | 11.36 | 0.0011 | 0.0869 |
| Age | 0.05384 | 0.02783 | 3.74 | 0.0565 | 0.0349 |
| MTHFR4 | 1.59011 | 0.62442 | 6.48 | 0.0127 | 0.0635 |
| MTR | 0.97502 | 0.62696 | 2.42 | 0.1238 | 0.0224 |
| PARP1 | -1.21130 | 0.67510 | 3.22 | 0.0765 | 0.0313 |

Table 8. Results of *stepwise* procedure in multivariate regression analysis for three comet assay parameters as a depended variable in the entire population immediately after radiation with 4 Gy dose and 24 hours after irradiation (only the statistically significant results are shown in the Table).

### 3.1 Discussion

Development of new methods in genotoxicology, especially on molecular level, has greatly improved the knowledge and understanding of processes that follow after the organism was exposed to ionising radiation. In the same time, better radiation protection, that includes more sophisticated handling of radiation sources, better education of personnel who are operating on those sources, precise dosimetry and the use of protection equipment have reduced health risk in specific population occupationally exposed to ionising radiation. Recent investigations in the field of radiation protection have focused on individual differences in radiosensitivity. It has been shown that DNA repair capability is regulated with different mechanisms that include great number of genes involved directly or indirectly in the repair process.

DNA damage kinetics of primary damage can give us first information about the level of the damage. Estimation of damage after exposure to low doses of ionising radiation is possible in a very short time period (Olive et al., 1990, 1995; Tice et al., 1990). Most of the DNA breaks can be repaired during 30 minutes from the exposure to ionising radiation (Frankenberg-Schwager, 1989), and two hours from the exposure, almost all the damage is repaired (Plappert et al., 1997). Since the repair is so quick, estimation of DNA damage represents a major problem in studies of occupationally exposed professionals and demands developing of sensitive methods for detecting the level of DNA damage after exposure to low doses of ionising radiation.

In this study the influence of gene polymorphisms on DNA repair after exposure to 2 and 4 Gy of gamma radiation was investigated. The analysis of comet assay parameters did not give consistent results. Immediately after the irradiation with the dose of 2 Gy, values for tail intensity, which is recently considered the most reliable parameter for DNA damage estimation (Collins, 2004), were higher than the values of other authors for the same dose (Cornetta et al., 2006). The exposed and control group also had significantly higher TL and TM for all observed time intervals when compared to the control values before irradiation in both groups. On the other hand, TI significantly decreased after 30 minutes from the exposure. After 60 minutes from the exposure, the values did not significantly differ from the control values before irradiation in both control and exposed group. Those results were different that the ones found by Cornetta et al. (2006) during DNA repair assessment after the exposure to the dose of 2 Gy. They have shown that even after 60 minutes from the exposure, TI were still significantly higher than before radiation. The differences in significance in TL and TI in our research showed different sensitivity of those two parameters. Tail length values implicate the existence of small DNA fragments that have created comet tail shape during electrophoresis and showed the length of travelling of small fragments from the nucleus. On the other hand, TI show the amount of damaged DNA in comet tail. Damaged DNA can be seen as small DNA fragments or relaxed DNA loops from the comet head created during electrophoresis. Tail moment shows the ratio of DNA in comet tail. Our results have shown that most of the DNA damage has been repaired during 30 minutes from the exposure to 2 Gy. The amount of the unrepaired damage did not significantly differ from the amount of the damage in samples that were not irradiated, but were also investigated in DNA repair process. The results showed that TI was better marker of DNA damage than TL. Those findings are in agreement with results of Kumaravel & Jha (2006), who have also estimated the reliability of comet assay parameter after the exposure of peripheral blood samples to gamma irradiation with the doses of 0, 1, 2, 4 and 8 Gy. Besides the fact that TI and TM showed greater reliability for DNA damage estimation, they have also showed strong correlation with the received dose of irradiation.

After 4 Gy irradiation, the values for all three parameters in both control and exposed groups were higher than after irradiation with 2 Gy. Tail length values in irradiated samples were significantly higher than non-irradiated samples for the time periods of 0, 15, 30, 60 and 120 minutes, but not after 24 hours for both exposed and control group.

Values for TI and TM in irradiated samples were significantly different from the values of non-irradiated samples for time period of 0, 15, 30 and 60 minutes, suggesting that most of DNA damage has been repaired during that period, although the values measured 120 minutes and 24 hours after the exposure did not reach the values before the exposure in exposed and control group. The results indicate the existence of small amount of DNA damage that is still present even after 24 hours from the exposure, independently of the dose level. The results could be explained by the difference in the repair of single stranded and double stranded DNA breaks. Single stranded DNA breaks are usually formed after the exposure to gamma or X-ray (90 %), while only small part of damage is created by double stranded breaks (10 %) (Cornetta et al., 2006). The repair of double stranded breaks after the exposure to ionising radiation usually lasts 12 or 16 hours (Vodicka et al., 2004), that is considerably longer than the repair of single stranded breaks. The amount of unrepaired damage in this experiment did not statistically differ from the control values before irradiation for both control and the exposed group. The difference between exposed and nonirradiated samples was higher for 2 Gy dose. The existence of small amount of unrepaired damage shows the importance of assessment of exposure to ionising radiation, especially to low doses and suggesting possible accumulation of primary, unrepaired damage that can lead to permanent damage and genome instability.

When the unrepaired amount of damage was compared, the results are implicating the existence of adaptive response in professionally exposed individuals to low doses of ionising radiation. Adaptive response in human lymphocytes has been described by other authors (Olivieri & Bosi, 1990; Sankaranarayanan et al., 1989; Shadley &Wolff, 1987; Wiencke et al., 1986; Wolff et al., 1990; Wolff, 1992, 1996). Aka et al. (2004) reported the existence of residual damage in tail intensity 60 and 120 minutes after the exposure to dose of 2 Gy. In their experiment, tail intensity values were also higher in the control group than the exposed one.

According to our results, despite the difference in the amount of damage, kinetics of repair after the exposure to both doses was similar to the one for the nonirradiated group. Unexpectedly, the difference between control and exposed group was significantly higher after 2 Gy than after 4 Gy exposure. These results were not in agreement with Wojcik et al. (1996) who claimed that kinetics of repair was faster in the exposed group. Aka et al. (2004) used comet assay for DNA repair assessment in human lymphocytes of male nuclear power plant workers and also for the control group (N=31). After the exposure, there was not significantly different repair kinetics between exposed and control group. Our results were comparable, indicating that healthy persons use the same repair mechanism, no matter if they are professionally exposed to ionising radiation or not. High standard deviation, also seen in the results of other author (DeMeo et al., 1991; Maluf et al., 2001; Maluf, 2004; Tice, 1995), implicated on the influence of interindividual differences. Since the comet assay measures primary DNA damage after the exposure, those results can be a marker of different gene activity. Besides the gene activity, the DNA repair can be influenced by the smoking status, gender, age and years of occupational exposure.

Smoking can also cause DNA damage when heavy and non heavy smokers were compared (Maluf et al., 2001; Maluf, 2004). Marcon et al. (2003) showed that heavy smokers can repair DNA damage after the exposure to 2 Gy faster than non smokers or non- heavy smokers. Olivieri et al. (1984) and Shadley (1994) suggested the existence of adaptive response that protects lymphocytes from oxidative damage. Smokers also showed lower levels of oxidised pyrimidinic bases in lymphocytes when compared to non-smokers (Berasati et al., 2001). Touil et al. (2002) showed that chemicals from the smoke can create covalent bonds between DNA and proteins, that can result with lower migration of DNA during electrophoresis, showing false results, that is lower damage. Cebulska et al. (2007) showed negative influence of smoking on the efficiency of DNA repair in lymphocytes. On the other hand, Rzeszowska-Wolny et al. (2005) did not find significant correlation between smoking and DNA damage and DNA repair after the irradiation of human lymphocytes with the dose of 2 Gy. Our results also did not show the influence of smoking on DNA repair of primary damage, except for the tail length after the exposure to 4 Gy dose. The results are similar to Aka et al. (2004) on nuclear power plant workers.

It is still not clear whether the basal damage differ due to gender. Dusinska et al. (2004a) did not find the difference in creation of strand breaks, nor in the amount of DNA damage sensitive to action of specific enzymes such as endonuclease III, or FPG enzyme or alkali labile sites, although male had lower DNA damage after the treatment with hydrogen peroxide (Dusinska et al., 2004a, b). Bajpayee et al. (2002) showed that healthy men have more basal damage in lymphocytes than women. Our results showed that difference was only seen after the 4 Gy dose, where women had higher values for DNA damage in all three parameters observed in comet assay immediately after and 24 hours after the irradiation. There was not similar number of male and female, and that could also influence the results. Trzeciak et al. (2008) showed that there are differences in the amount of damage and the repair rate after the exposure of whole blood sample to 6.3 Gy dose. But most of the experiments did not show the gender influence on DNA repair capacity (Muller et al., 2001, 2002; Rajaee-Behbahani et al., 2001; Marcon et al., 2003).

Age influence was not seen in this experiment. That is in agreement with other authors (Betti et al., 1994; Frenzili et al., 1997). Rzeszowska-Wolny et al. (2005) did not show the influence of sex on DNA damage level and DNA repair by the comet assay after the exposure to 2 Gy dose. Maluf et al. (2001) showed positive correlation of age and DNA repair in the exposed group. Singh et al. (1988) described positive correlation between the age and DNA damage in non-smokers.

Although former results showed the existence of radio adaptive response, our results did not confirm the relationship between primary DNA damage and adaptive response. Few authors have also shown lower DNA damage levels after the repeated exposure to ionising radiation (Sankaranarayanan et al., 1989; Wang et al., 1991; Ikushima, 1992; Domingues et al., 1993).

APE1 gene is involved in BER repair. Polymorphism in exon 5 is connected with hypersensitivity during the exposure to ionising radiation (Au et al., 2006). Results are in agreement with Au et al. (2006). There was positive correlation of polymorphic variants and DNA damage level 120 minutes after the exposure to 2 Gy.

Polymorphic variants of hOGG1 gene showed positive correlation with TI and TM measured immediately after the exposure to the dose of 2 Gy. The results are in agreement with Aka et al. (2004) who showed the connection between polymorphic variants of hOGG1 Ser326Cys with lower capability of repair of oxidative DNA damage in the exposed, but not in the control group measured 60 and 120 minutes after the exposure to 2 Gy. After 120 minutes from the exposure, 71 % of individuals with high level of DNA damage had polymorphic variant of hOGG1 gene. Cornetta et al. (2006) did not show the influence of hOGG1 polymorphism on DNA damage.

Goode et al. (2002)) showed the connection between polymorphic variants of hOGG1 with higher risk of lung, head and neck cancer. hOGG1 and XRCC1 are involved in the same repair pathway, while hOGG1 cuts oxidised base, XRCC1 together with ligase closes the break. Aka et al. (2004) and Matullo (2003) have described their connection. On the other hand, Cornetta et al. (2006), did not show significant difference between XRCC1, hOGG1 and XPC polymorphisms and DNA damage level measured 30 minutes from the exposure to 2 Gy dose. Yamane et al. (2004) showed that homozygotes differ for 2 fold factor in cutting of 8-oxodeoxiguanosine when compared to heterozygote.

XRCC1 polymorphism did not show the influence on DNA damage and repair, but polymorphic variants had lower levels of DNA damage for all three parameters measured. The results are not in agreement to those of Cornetta et al. (2006). Tail intensity values after the exposure to 2 Gy dose, immediatelly after, 30 minutes and 60 minutes after, homozygotes and polymorphic variants showed significant differences.

The two most common SNP polymorphisms in XPD gene are in exons 10 and 23. The results of studies of those polymorphisms are inconsistent. Naccarati et al. (2006) observed fewer number of single strand breaks in polymorphic homozygotes compared to heterozygotes and wild type of homozygotes. Similar results state Vodicka et al. (2004), analyzing chromosome aberrations frequency. Polymorphic XPD23 gene variants did not influence primary DNA damage, while polymorphic XPD10 gene variants showed positive correlation in all three comet assay parameters 120 min after exposure to 2 Gy of gamma radiation.

Polymorphic variants of XRCC3 in the exposed group had highest values for DNA damage. There was also positive correlation of polymorphic variants with TL immediately after the exposure to 2 Gy and negative correlation with TI and TL 120 minutes from the exposure to 2 Gy dose. Aka et al. (2004) did not find the correlation with primary damage, probably because this gene is involved in double strand breaks repair. PARP1 is important for integrity of chromosome ends and is involved in maintaining the integrity of BER and NHEJ repair. Our results showed negative correlation between polymorphic variants and TI values measured immediately after the exposure to 4 Gy and with TM values measured 24 hours after the exposure to 4 Gy.

MGMT C/T variants have higher risk of glioma (Liu et al., 2009), but there are no investigations that are connecting it with ionising radiation. In our study polymorphic variants have shown negative correlation with DNA damage level measured 120 minutes after the exposure to 2 Gy.

## 4. Conclusion

The results indicate that in addition to individual gene polymorphisms, the influence of combinations of polymorphic genes to DNA damage and repair should be tested.

## 5. Acknowledgment

This study was partly supported by the Ministry of Science, Education and Sports of the Republic of Croatia (grant number 0022-0222148-2137).

## 6. References

Aka, P.; Mateuca, R.; Buchet, J.P.; Thierens, H. & Kirsch-Volders, M. (2004) Are genetic polymorphisms in OGG1, XRCC1 and XRCC3 genes predictive for the DNA strand break repair phenotype and genotoxicity in workers xx)posed to low dose ionising radiations? *Mutat Res* 556: 169-181.

Andreassen, C.N. (2005) Can risk of radiotherapy-induced normal tissue complications be predicted from genetic profiles? *Acta Oncologica* 44: 801-815.

Andreassi, M.G.; Foffa, I.; Manfredi, S.; Botto, N.; Cioppa, A. & Picano, E. (2009) Genetic polymorphisms in XRCC1, OGG1, APE1 and XRCC3 DNA repair genes, ionizing radiation exposure and chromosomal DNA damage in interventional cardiologists. *Mutat Res* 666(1-2): 57-63.

Angelini, S.; Kumar, R.; Carbone, F.; Maffei, F.; Forti, G.C.; Violante, F.S.; Lodi, V.; Curti, S.; Hemminki, K. & Hrelia, P. (2005) Micronuclei in humans induced by exposure to low level of ionizing radiation: influence of polymorphims in DNA repair genes. *Mutat Res* 570: 105-117.

Ashby, J.; Tinwell, H.; Lefevre, P.A. & Browne, M.A. (1995) The single cell gel electrophoresis assay for induced DNA damage (comet assay): measurement of tail length and moment. *Mutagenesis* 10(2): 85-90.

Au, W.W. (1991) Monitoring human populations for effects of radiation and chemical exposures using cytogenetic techniques. *Occup Med* 4:597-611.

Au WW (2006) Heritable susceptibility factors for te development of cancer. *J Radiat Res* 47B: 13-17

Bailey, S. & Goodwin, E. (2004) DNA and telomeres: beginnings and endings. *Cytogenet Genome Res* 104: 109-115.

Bailey, S.; Cornforth, M.; Ullrich, R. & Goodwin, E. (2004) Dysfunctional mammalian telomeres join with DNA double-strand breaks. *DNA Repair* 3: 349-357.

Bajpayee, M.; Dhawan, A.; Parmar, D.; Pandey, A.K.; Mathur, N. & Seth, P.K. (2002) Gender-related differences in basal DNA damage inlymphocytes of a healthy Indian population using the alkaline Comet assay. *Mutat Res* 520: 83-91.

Balasem, A,N. & Ali, A.S.K. (1991) Establishment of dose–response relationships between doses of Cs137 gamma-rays and frequencies of micronuclei in human peripheral blood lymphocytes. *Mutat Res* 259:133–138.

Barquinero, J.F.; Barrios, L.; Caballin, M.R.; Miro, R.; Ribas, M.; Subias, A. & Egozcue, J. (1993) Cytogenetic analysis of lymphocytes from hospital workers occupationally exposed to low levels of ionizing radiation. *Mutat Res* 286: 275–279.

Barquinero, J.F.; Barrios, L.; Caballin, M.R.; Miro, R.; Ribas, M.; Subias, A. & Egozcue, J. (1995) Occupational exposure to radiation induces an adaptive response in human lymphocytes. *Int J Radiat Biol* 67 (2): 187-191.

Barquinero, J.F.; Barrios, L.; Caballin, M.R.; Miro, R.; Ribas, M.; Subias, A. & Egozcue, J. (1996) Decreased sensitivity to the cytogenetic effects of bleomycin in individuals occupationally exposed to ionizing radiation. *Mutat Res* 354:81-86.

Berasati Nia, A.; Van Schooten: F.J.; Schilderman, P.A.E.L.; De Kok, T.M.C.M.; Haenen, G.R.; Van Herwijnen, M.H.M.; Van Agen, E.; Pachen, D. & Kleinjans, J.C.S. (2001) A multi-biomarker approach to study the effects of smoking on oxidative DNA damage and repair and antioxidative defence mechanisms. *Carcinogenesis* 21: 395–401.

Berrington, A.; Darby, S.C.; Weiss, H.A. & Doll, R. (2001) 100 years of observation on British radiologists: mortality from cancer and other causes 1897–1997. *Br J Radiol* 34 74: 507–519.

Berwick, M. & Vineis, P. (2000) Markers of DNA repair and susceptibility to cancer in humans: An epidemiological review. *J Natl Cancer Inst* 91: 874-897.

Berwick, M. (2000) Gene-environment interaction in melanoma. *Forum Geneva* 10: 191- 200.

Betti, C.; Davini, T.; Gianessi, L.; Loprieno, N. & Barale, R. (1994) Microgel electrophoresis assay (comet test) and SCE analysis in human lymphocytes from 100 normal subjects. *Mutat Res* 307: 323-333.

Boffetta, P.; Caporaso, N.; Cuzick, J.; Lang, M.; Vineis, P.; Malats, N. & D'Errico, A. (1999) Metabolic polymorphisms and susceptibility to cancer. IARC Publications, 44 Lyon, France.

Bolus, N.E. (2001) Basic review of radiation biology and terminology. *J Nucl Med Technol* 46 29(2): 67-73. Review.

Bonassi, S.; Ugolini, D.; Kirsch-Volders, M.; Stromberg, U.; Vermeulen, R. & Tucker, J.D. (2005) Human population studies with cytogenetic biomarkers: review of the literature and future prospectives. *Environ Mol Mutagen* 45: 258–270.

Boothman, D.A.; Bouvard, I. & Hughes, E.N. (1989) Identification and characterisation of X-ray-induced proteins in human cells. *Cancer Res* 49 (11): 2871-2878.

Bosi, A. & Olivieri, G. (1989) Variability of the adaptive response to ionizing radiations in humans. *Mutat Res* 211(1): 13-17.

Boutcher, S. & Haas, T. (1985) External radiation doses to nuclear medicine technologists from procedures using 99mTc radiopharmaceuticals. *Can J Radiogr Radiother Nucl Med* 16: 161–165.

Cardisi, E.; Vrijheid, M.; Blettner, M.; Gilbert, E.; Hakama, M.; Hill, C.; Howe, G.; Kaldor, D.; Muirhead, C.R.; Schubauer-Berigan, M.; Yoshimura, T.; Bermann, F.; Cowper, G.; Fix, J.; Hacker, C.; Heinmiller, B.; Marshall, M.; Thierry-Chef, I.; Utterback, D.; Ahn, ,Y.O.; Amoros, E.; Ashmore, P.; Auvinen, A.; Bae, J.M.; Bernar Solano, J.; Biau, A.; Combalot, E.; Deboodt, P.; Diez Sacristan, A.; Eklof, M.; Engels, H.; Engholm, G.; Gulis, G.; Habib, R.; Holan, K;, Hyvonen, H.; Kerekes, A.; Kurtinaitis, J.; Malker, H.; Martuzzi, M.; Mastauskas, A.; Monnet, A.; Moser, M.; Pearce, M.S.; Richardson, D.B.; Rodriguez-Artalejo, F.; Rogel, A.; Tardy, H.; Telle-Lamberton, M.; Turai, I.; Usel, M. & Veress, K. (2005) Risk of cancer after low doses of ionising radiation: retrospective cohort study in 15 countries. *Br Med J* 331: 77–80.

Cardoso, R. S.; Takahashi-Hyodo, S.; Peitl Jr, P.; Ghilardi-Neto, T. & Sakamoto-Hojo, E.T. (2001) Evaluation of chromosomal aberrations, micronuclei, and sister chromatid exchanges in hospital workers chronically exposed to ionizing radiation. *Teratog Carcinog Mutagen* 21: 431–439.

Carrano, A.V. & Natarajan, A.T. (1988) Considerations for population monitoring using cytogenetic techniques. ICPEMC publication 14. *Mutat Res* 204: 379–406.

Cebulska-Wasilewska, A.; Pawłyk, I.; Panek, A.; Wiechec,´ A.; Kalina, I.; Popov, T.; Georgieva, T. & Farmer, P.B. (2007) Exposure to environmental polycyclic aromatic hydrocarbons: influences on cellularsusceptibility to DNA damage (sampling Kosice and Sofia). *Mutat Res* 620: 145–154.

Chen, S.; Tang, D.; Xue, K.; Xu, L.; Ma, G.; Hsu, Y. & Cho, S.S. (2002) DNA repair gene XRCC1 and XPD polymorphisms and risk of lung cancer in a Chinese population. *Carcinogenesis* 23: 1321-1325.

Coates, P.J.; Lorimore, S.A. & Wright, E.G. (2004) Damaging and protective cell signalling in the untargeted effects of ionizing radiation. *Mutat Res* 568: 5-20.

Collins, A. & Harrington, V. (2002) Repair of oxidative DNA damage: assessing its contribution to cancer prevention. *Mutagenesis* 17: 489-493.

Collins, A.R. (2004) The Comet Assay for DNA damage and repair: Principles, applications and limitations. *Mol Biotechnol* 26: 249-261.

Cornetta, T.; Festa, F.; Testa, A. & Cozzi, R. (2006) DNA damage repair and genetic polimorphisms: assessment of indivisual sensitivity and repair capacity. *Int J Radiation Oncology Biol Phys* 66 (2): 537-545.

Daly, A.K.; Steen, V.M.; Fairbrother, K.S. & Idle, J.R. (1996) CYP2D6 multiallelism. *Meth Enzymol* 272: 199–210.

DeMeo, M.; Laget, M.; Castegnaro, M. & Dumenil, G. (1991) Genotoxic activity of potassium permanganate in acidic solutions. *Mutat Res* 260: 295-306.

Divine, K.K.; Gilliland, F.D.; Crowell, R.E.; Stidley, C.A.; Bocklage, T.J.; Cook, D.L. & Belinsky, S.A. (2001) The XRCC1 399 glutamine allele is a risk factor for adenocarcinoma of the lung. *Mutat Res* 461: 273-278.

Domingues, I; Panneerselvam, N.; Escalza, P.; Natarajan, A.T. & Cortes, F. (1993) Adaptive response to radiation damage in human lymphocytes conditioned with hydrogen peroxide as measured by the cytokinesis-block micronucleus technique. *Mutat Res* 301: 135–141.

Dusinska, M.; Collins, A.; Kazimirova, A.; Barancokova, M.; Harrington, V.; Volkovova, K.; Staruchova, M.; Horska, A.; Wsolova, L.; Kocan, A.; Petrik, J.; Machata, M.; Ratcliffe, B. & Kyrtopoulos, S. (2004a) Genotoxic effects of asbestos in humans. *Mutat Res* 553: 91–102.

Dusinska, M.; Kazimirova, A.; Barancokova, M.; Horska, A.; Burghardtova, K.; Volkovova, K.; Staruchova, M.; Wsolova, L. & Collins, A.R. (2004b) Does occupational exposure to mineral fibres cause DNA or chromosome damage? *Mutat Res* 553: 103–110.

Erexon, G.L.; Kligerman, A.D.; Bryant, M.F.; Sontag, M.R. & Halperin, E.C. (1991) Induction of micronuclei by X-radiation in human, mouse and rat peripheral blood lymphocytes. *Mutat Res* 253: 193–198.

Fachini, A.L.; Mello, S.S.; Sandrin-Garcia, P.; Junta, C.M.; Ghilardi-Netto, T.; Donadi, E.A.; Da Silva, G.A.; Elza, P. & Sakamoto-Hojo, T. (2009) Gene expression profiles in radiation workers occupationally exposed to ionizing radiation. *J Radiat Res* 50: 61–71.

Fairbairn, D.W.; Olive, P.L.; O´Neill, K.L. (1995) The comet assay: a comprehensive review. *Mutat Res* 339: 37-59.

Fenech, M.; Denham, J.; Francis, W. & Morley, A.A. (1990) Micronuclei in cytokinesis blocked lymphocytes of cancer patients following fractionated partial-body radiotherapy. *Int J Radiat Biol* 57: 373–383.

Frankenberg-Schwager, M. (1989) Review of repair kinetics for DNA damage induced in eukaryotic ce,lls in vitro by ionizing radiation. *Radiother Oncol* 14: 307-320.

Frenzili, G.; Betti, C.; Davini, T.; Desideri, M.; Fornai, E.; Gianessi, L.; Maggiorelli, F.; Paoletti, P. & Barale, R. (1997) Evaluation of DNA damage in leukocytes of ex smokers by single cell gel electrophoresis. *Mutat Res* 375: 117-123.

Goode E.L-; Ulrich C.M. & Potter J.D. (2002) Polymorphisms in DNA repair genes and associations with cancer risk. *Cancer Epidemiol Biomarkers Prev* 11: 1513–1530.

Gourabi, H. & Mozdarani, H. (1998) A cytokinesis-blocked micronucleus study of the radioadaptive response of lymphocytes of individuals occupationally exposed to chronic doses of radiation. *Mutagenesis* 13(5): 475-480.

Hall, E.J. & Giaccia, A.J. (2006) Radiobiology for the Radiologist. 6th edn. Lippincott Williams & Wilkins, Philadelphia

He, J.L.; Chen, W.L.; Jin, L.F. & Jin, H.Y. (2000) Comparative evaluation of the in vitro micronucleus test and comet assay for the detection of genotoxic effects of X-ray radiation. *Mutat Res* 469:223–231.

Hellman, B.; Vaghef, H. & Bostrom, B. (1995) The concepts of tail moment and tail inertia in the single cell gel electrophoresis assay. *Mutat Res* 336: 123-131.

Hellman, B.; Vaghef, H.; Friis, L. & Edling, C. (1997) Alkaline single cell gel electrophoresis of DNA fragments in biomonitoring for genotoxicity: an introductiory study on healthy human volunteers. *International Archives of Occupational and Environmental Health* 69: 185-192.

Hinds, D.A.; Stuve, L.L.; Nilsen, G.B.; Halperin, E.; Eskin, E.; Ballinger, D.G.; Frazer, K.A. & Cox, D.R. (2005) Whole genome patterns of common DNA variation in three human populations. *Science* 307: 1072-1079.

Hoffmann H. & Speit G. (2005) Assessment of DNA damage in peripheral blood of heavy smokers with the comet assay and the micronucleus test. *Mutat Res* 581:105-14.

Hou, S.M.; Falt, S.; Angelini, S.; Yang, K.; Nyberg, F.; Lambert, B. & Hemminki, K. (2002) The XPD variant alleles are associated with increased aromatic DNA adduct level and lung cancer risk. *Carcinogenesis* 23: 599-603.

Hu, J.J.; Smith, T.R.; Miller, M.S.; Mohrenweiser, H.W.; Golden, A. & Case, L.D. (2001) Amino acid substitution variants of APE1 and XRCC1 genes associated with ionizing radiation sensitivity. *Carcinogenesis* 22: 917–922.

Hu, J.J.; Mohrenweiser, H.W.; Bell, D.A.; Leadon, S.A. & Miller, M.S. (2002a) Symposium overview: genetic polymorphisms in DNA repair and cancer risk. *Toxicol Appl Pharmacol* 185: 64–73.

Hu, J.J.; Smith, T.R.; Miller, M.S.; Lohman, K. & Case, L.D. (2002b) Genetic regulation of ionizing radiation sensitivity and breast cancer risk. *Environ Mol Mutagen* 39: 208-215.

Hu, Z.; Ma, H.; Chen, F.; Wei, Q. & Shen, H. (2005) XRCC1 polymorphisms and cancer risk: a meta-analysis of 38 case-control studies. *Cancer Epidemiol Biomarkers Prevent* 14:1810–1818.

Hung, R.J.; Hall, J.; Brennan, P. & Boffetta, P. (2005) Genetic polymorphisms in the base excision repair pathway and cancer risk: a HuGE review. *Am J Epidemiol* 162(10): 21 925-942.

Ikushima, T. (1989) Radio-Adaptive Response: Characterization of a cytogenetic repair induced by low-level ionizing radiation in cultured Chinese hamster cells. *Mutat Res* 227 (4): 241-246.

Ikushima, T. (1992) Radio-adaptive response: involvement of induction of specific gene expression by low doses of ionizing radiation. In: Sugahara T, Sagan L, Aoyama T(ed.) Low Dose Irradiation and Biological Defence Mechanisms. Elsevier Science Publishers BV, Amsterdam, 255–263.

Ikushima, T.; Aritomi, H. & Morisita, J. (1996) Radioadaptive Response: Efficient repair of radiation-induced DNA damage in adapted cells. *Mutat Res* 358(2):193-198.

Jeggo, P. & Lavin, M.F. (2009) Cellular radiosensitivity: how much better do we understand it? *Int J Radiat Biol* 85:1061-1081.

Jha, A.N. & Sharma, T. (1991) Enhanced frequency of chromosome aberrations in workers occupationally exposed to diagnostic X-rays. *Mutat Res* 260: 343–348.

Kassie, F.; Parzefall, W. & Knasmuller, S. (2000) Single cell gel electrophoresis assay: new technique for human biomonitoring studies. *Mutat Res* 463: 13–31.

Kotsopoulos, J.; Chen, Z.; Vallis, K.A.; Poll, A.; Ainsworth, P. & Narod, S.A. (2007) DNA repair capacity as a possible biomarker of breast cancer risk in female BRCA1 mutation carriers. *Br J Cancer* 96:118–125.

Kruszewski, M.; Wojewodzka, M.; Iwanenko, T.; Collins, A.R. & Szumiel, I. (1998) Application of the comet assay for monitoring DNA damage in workers exposed to chronic low-dose irradiation: II. Base damage. *Mutat Res* 416: 37–57.

Kubelka, D.; Sviličić, N.; Kralik, I.; Belamarić, N.; Faj, D.; Novosel, N.; Vukić, V. & Tečić Z. (2011) .Analiza učinkovitosti i usklanenosti s EU propisima zakonodavstva kojim se regulira radiološka i nuklearna sigurnost [Analysis of efficacy and conformity with the EU acquis communautaire of the radiation protection and nuclear safety legislative; *in Croatian*]. In: Krajcar Bronić I, Kopjar N, Milić M, 1 Branica G, editors. Proceedings of the 8th Symposium of the Croatian Radiation Protection Association; 13-15 Apr 2011; Krk, Croatia. Zagreb: Denona; p. 31-37.

Kumar, R.; Hoglund, L.; Zhao, Ch.; Forsti, A.; Snellman, E. & Hemminki, K. (2003) Single nucleotide polymorphisms in the XPG gene: determination of role in DNA repair and breast cancer risk. *Int J Cancer* 103: 671-675.

Kumaravel, T.S. & Jha, A.N. (2006) Reliable Comet assay measurements for detecting DNA damage induced by ionising radiation and chemicals. *Mutat Res* 605: 7-16.

Little, J.B. (2000) Radiation carcinogenesis. *Carcinogenesis* 21: 397–404.

Liu, Y.; Scheurer, M.E.; El-Zein, R.; Cao, Y.; Do, K.A.; Gilbert, M.; Aldape, K.D.; Wei, Q.; Etzel, C. & Bondy, M.L. (2009) Association and interactions between DNA repair gene polymorphisms and adult glioma. *Cancer Epidemiol Biomarkers Prev* 18(1): 204-214

Lunn, R.M.; Helzlsouer, K.J.; Parshad, R.; Umbach, M.D.; Harris, E.L.; Sanford, K.K. & Bell D.A. (2000) XPD polymorphisms: effects on DNA repair proficiency. *Carcinogenesis* 21: 551–555.

Maitre, A.; Colonna, M.; Gressin, C.; Menegoz, F. & de Gaudemaris, R. (2003) Increased incidence of haematological cancer among physicians in a University Hospital. *Int Arch Occup Environ Health* 76: 24–28.

Maluf, S. & Erdtmann, B. (2001a) Genomic instability in Down syndrome and Fanconi anemia assessed by micronucleus analysis and single-cell gel electrophoresis. *Cancer Genet Cytogenet* 124: 71–75.

Maluf, S.W.; Passos, D.F.; Bacelar, A.; Speit, G. & Erdtmann, B. (2001b) Assessment of DNA damage in lymphocytes of workers exposed to X-radiation using the micronucleus test and the comet assay. *Environ Mol Mutagen* 38: 311–315

Maluf, S.W. (2004) Monitoring DNA damage following radiation exposure using cytokinesis-block micronucleus method and alkaline single-cell gel electrophoresis. *Clinica Chimica Acta* 347: 15-24.

Marcon, F.; Andreoli, C.; Rossi, S.; Verdina, A.; Galati, R. & Crebelli, R. (2003) Assessment of individual sensitivity to ionizing radiation and DNA repair efficiency in a healthy population. *Mutation Research* 541: 1–8.

Matullo, G.; Peluso, M.; Polidoro, S.; Guarrera, S.; Munnia, A.; Krogh, V.; Masala, G.; Berrino, F.; Panico, S.; Tumino, R.; Vineis, P. & Palli, D. (2003) Combination of DNA repair gene single nucleotidepolymorphisms and increased levels of DNA adducts in a population-based study. *Cancer Epidemiol. Biomarkers Prev* 12: 674–677

McKelvey-Martin, V.J.; Green, M.H.L.; Schmezer, P.; Pool-Zobel, B.L.; De Me´o, M.P. & Collins, A. (1993) The single cell gel electrophoresis assay (comet assay): a European review. *Mutat Res* 288: 47–63.

McKelvey-Martin, V.J.; Ho, E.T.S.; McKeown, S.R.; Johnston, S.R.; McCarthy, P.J.; Rajab, N.F. & Downes, C.S. (1998) Emerging applications of the single cell gel electrophoresis (Comet) assay. I. Management of invasive transitionalcell human bladder carcinoma. II. Fluorescent in situ hybridization Comets for the identification of damaged and repaired DNA sequences in individual cells. *Mutagenesis* 13: 1–8.

Milić, M.; Rozgaj, R.; Kašuba, V.; Kubelka, D.; Angelini, S. & Hrelia, P. (2010) DNA repair genes and radiation sensitivity. *Arh Hig Rada Toksikol* 61 Supplement: 107-121.

Milić, M. (2010) Važnost individualne osjetljivosti za procjenu rizika od oštećenja genoma pri kroničnoj profesionalnoj izloženosti niskim dozama ionizirajućeg zračenja [The significance of individual genome sensitivity in risk assessment of chronic professional exposure to low doses of ionizing radiation; in Croatian]. [PhD thesis]. Zagreb: Faculty of Science, University of Zagreb.

Mohrenweiser, H.W. & Jones, I.M. (1998) Variation in DNA repair is 1 a factor in cancer susceptibility: a paradigm for the promises and perils of individual and population risk estimation? *Mutat Res* 400: 15–24.

Mohrenweiser, H.W.; Wilson, D.M. & Jones, I.M. (2003) Challenges and complexities in estimating both the functional impact and the disease risk associated with the extensive genetic variation in human DNA repair genes. *Mutat Res* 526: 93–125.

Monsieurs, M.A.; Thierens, H.M.; Vral, A.M.; Van De Wiele, C.; De Ridder, L.I. & Dierckx, R.A. (2000) Adaptive response in patients treated with 131I. *J Nucl Med* 41 (1): 17-22.

Morgan, W.F. (2003) Non-targeted and delayed effects of exposure to ionizing radiation: i. radiation-induced genomic instability and bystander effects *in vitro*. *Radiat Res* 159: 567-580.

Mothersill, C.; Kadhim, M.A.; O' Reilly, S.; Paphworth, D.; Mardsen, S.J.; Seaymoure, C.B. & Wright, E.G. (2000) Dose- and time-response relationships for lethal mutations and chromosomal instability induced by ionizing radiation in an immortalized human keratinocyte cell line. *Int Radiat Biol* 76 (6): 799-806.

Mothersill, C.; Rea, D.; Wright, E.G.; Lorimore, S.A.; Murphy, D.; Seymour, C.B. & O'Malley, K. (2001) Individual variation in the production of a bystander signal following irradiation of primary cultures of normal human urothelium. *Carcinogenesis* 22 (9): 1465-1471.

Muller, W.U.; Bauch, T.; Stuben, G.; Sack, H. & Streffer, C. (2001) Radiation sensitivity of lymphocytes from healthy individuals and cancer patients as measured by the comet assay. *Radiat Environ Biophys* 40: 83–89.

Muller, W.U.; Bauch, T.; Streffer, C. & von Mallek, D. (2002) Does radiotherapy affect the outcome of the comet assay? *Br J Radiol* 75: 608–614.

Naccarati, A.; Soucek, P.; Stetina, R.; Haufroid, V.; Kumar, R.; Vodickova, L.; Trtkova, K.; Dusinska, M.; Hemminki, K. & Vodicka, P. (2006) Genetic polymorphisms and possible gene-gene interactions in metabolic andDNA repair genes: Effects on DNA damage. *Mutat Res* 593: 22–31

Norppa, H. (2004) Cytogenetic biomarkers and genetic polymorphisms. *Toxicol Lett* 149: 309–334.

Nowak, B. & Jankowski, J. (1991) Occupational exposure in operational radiology. *Pol J Occup Med Environ Health* 4: 169–174.

Okayasu, R.; Suetomi, K.; Yu, Y.; Silver, A.; Bedford, J.; Cox, R. & Ullrich, R. (2000) A deficiency in DNA repair and DNA-PKcs expression in the radiosensitive BALB/c mouse. *Cancer Res.* 60: 4342-4345.

Olive, P.L.; Banath, J.P. & Durand, R.E. (1990) Heterogeneity in radiation-induced DNA damage and repair in tumor and normal cells using the "comet" assay. *Radiation Research* 122: 86-94.

Olive, P.L. (1999) DNA damage and repair in individual cells: aplications of the comet assay in radiobiology. *International Journal of Radiation Biology* 75(4): 395-405.

Olivieri, G.; Bodycote, J. & Wolff, S. (1984) Adaptive response of human lymphocytes to low concentrations of radioactive thymidine. *Science* 223: 594–597.

Olivieri, G. & Bosi, A. (1990) Possible causes of variability of the adaptive response in human lymphocytes. In: Obe G, Natarajan A T(ed.) Chromosomal Aberrations, Basic and Applied Aspects. Springer-Verlag, Berlin, 130–140.

Padovani, L.; Appolloni, M.; Anzidei, P.; Tedeschi, B.; Caporossi, D.; Vernole, P. & Mauro, F. (1995) Do human lymphocytes exposed to the fallout of the Chernobyl accident exhibit an adaptive response? I. Challenge with Ionizing Radiation. *Mutat Res* 332 (1-2): 33-38.

Parl, F.F. (2005) Glutathione S-transferase genotypes and cancer 1 risk. *Cancer Lett* 221:123–129.

Plappert, U.; Raddatz, K.; Roth, S. & Fliedner, T.M. (1995) DNA damage detection in man after radiation exposure-the comet assay- its possible application for human monitoring. *Stem Cells* 13(1): 215-222.

Plappert, U.G.; Stocker, B.; Fender, H. & Fliedner, T.M. (1997) Changes in the repair capacity of blood cells as a biomarker for chronic low-dose exposure to ionizing radiation. *Environ Mol Mutagen* 30(2): 153-160.

Price, A. (1993) The repair of ionising radiation- induced damage to DNA. *Cancer Biology* 4: 61-71.

Rajaee-Behbahani, N.; Schmezer, P.; Risch, A.; Rittgen, W; Kayser, K.W.; Dienemann, H.; Schulz, V.; Drings, P., Thiel, S. & Bartsch, H. (2001) Altered DNA repair capacity and bleomycin sensitivity as risk markers for non-small cell lung cancer. *Int J Cancer* 95: 86–91.

Robson, T., Joiner, M.C.; Wilson, G.D.; McCullough, W.; Price, M.E.; Logan, I.; Jones, H.; McKeown, S.R. & Hirst, D.G. (1999) A novel human stress response-related gene with a potential role in induced radioresistance. *Radiat Res* 152 (5): 451-461.

Roos, W.P.; Binder, A. & Bohm, L. (2000) Determination of the initial DNA damage and residual DNA damage remaining after 12 hours of repair in eleven cell lines at low doses of irradiation. *Int J Radiat Biol* 76: 1493-1500.

Rzeszowska-Wolny, J.; Polanska, J.; Pietrowska, M.; Palyvoda, O.; Jaworska, J.; Butkiewicz, D. & Hancock, R. (2005) Influence of polymorphisms in DNA repair genes XPD, XRCC1 and MGMT on DNA damage induced by gamma radiation and its repair in lymphocytes *in vitro*. *Radiat Res* 164: 132–140.

Sankaranarayanan, K.; Duyn, A.; Loos, M.J. & Natarajan, A.T. (1989) Adaptive response of human lymphocytes to low-level radiation from radioisotopes or X-rays. *Mutat Res* 211: 7–12.

Sari-Minodier, I.; Orsiere, T.; Auquier, P.; Martin, F. & Botta, A. (2007) Cytogenetic monitoring by use of the micronucleus assay among hospital workers exposed to low doses of ionizing radiation. *Mutat Res* 629(2): 111-121.

Sasaki, M.S.; Ejima, Y.; Tachibana, A.; Yamada, T.; Ishizaki, K.; Shimizu, T. & Nomura, T. (2002) DNA damage response pathway in radioadaptive response. *Mutat Res* 33 504: 101-118.

Setlow, R.B. (1983) Variations in DNA repair among humans. In: Harris CC, Autrup HN (ed.) Human Carcinogenesis. New York: Academic Press: 231-254.

Seymour, C.B. & Mothersill, C. (2000) Relative contribution of bystander and targeted cell killing to the low-dose region of the radiation dose-response curve. *Radiat Res* 153: 508-511.

Shadley, J.D. & Wiencke, J.K. (1989) Induction of the adaptive response by x-rays is dependent on radiation intensity. *Int J Radiat Biol* 56: 107-118.

Shadley, J.D. (1994) Chromosomal adaptive response in human lymphocytes. *Radiat Res* 138: S9–S12.

Shadley, J.D. & Wolff, S. (1987) Very low doses of X-rays can cause human lymphocytes to become less susceptible to ionizing radiation. *Mutagenesis* 2: 95–96.

Shastry, B.S. (2009) SNPs: impact on gene function and phenotype. *Methods Mol Biol* 578: 3-22.

Singh, N.P.; McCoy, M.T.; Tice, R.R. & Schneider, L.L. (1988) A simple technique for quantitation of low levels of DNA damage in individual cells. *Exp Cell Res* 175:184-191.

Singh, N.P. (2000) Microgels for estimation of DNA strand breaks, DNA protein crosslinks and apoptosis. *Mutat Res* 455: 111-127.

Stecca, C. & Gerber, G.B. (1998) adaptive response to dna-damaging agents: a review of potential mechanisms. *Biochem Pharmacol* 55 (7): 941-951.

Sturgis, E.M.; Castillo, E.J.; Li, L.; Zheng, R.; Eicher, S.A.; Clayman, G.L.; Strom, S.S.; Spitz, M.R. & Wei, Q. (1999) Polymorphisms of DNA repair gene XRCC1 in squamous cell carcinoma of the head and neck. *Carcinogenesis* 20: 2125-2129.

Szumiel, I. (1998) Monitoring and signaling of radiation-induced damage in mammalian cells. *Radiat Res* 150: 92-101.

Tedeschi, B.; Caporossi, D.; Vernole, P.; Padovani, L.; Appolloni, M.; Anzidei, P. & Mauro, F. (1995) Do Human lymphocytes exposed to the fallout of the Chernobyl accident exhibit an adaptive response? II. Challenge with bleomycin. *Mutat Res* 332 (1-2): 299-300.

Tedeschi, B.; Caporossi, D.; Vernole, P.; Padovani, L. & Mauro, F. (1996) Do human lymphocytes exposed to the fallout of the chernobyl accident exhibit an adaptive response? III. Challenge with bleomycin in lymphocytes from children hit by the initial acute dose of ionizing radiation. *Mutat Res* 354 (1): 77-80.

Tice, R.R.;Andrews, P.W.; Hirai, O. & Singh, N.P. (1990) The single cell gel (SCG) assay: an electrophoretic technique for the detection of DN damage in individual cells. In: Witmer, C.M., Snyder, R.R., Hollow, D.J., Kalf, G.F., Kocsis, J.J., Sipes, J.G. (ed.) Biological reactive intermediates, IV Molecular and cellular effects and their impact on human health. New York, Plenum Press, 157-164.

Tice, R.R. (1995) The single cell gel/comet assay: a microgel electrophoretic technique for the detection of DNA damage and repair in individual cells. In: Phillis DH, Venitt S (ed.) *Environmental Mutagenesis*. Bioscientific, Oxford, 315-339.

Touil, N.; Aka, P.V.; Buchet, J.P.; Thierens, H. & Kirsch-Volders, M. (2002) Assessment of genotoxic effects related to chronic low level exposureto ionizing radiation using biomarkers for DNA damage and repair. *Mutagenesis* 17: 223–232.

Trzeciak, A.R.; Barnes, J.; Ejiogu, N.; Foster, K.; Brant, L.J.; Zonderman, A.B. & Evans, M.K. (2008) Age, sex, and race influence single-strand break repair capacity in a human population. *Free Radic Biol Med* 45:1631-1641.

United Nations Scientific Committee on the Effects of Atomic Radiation, Sources and effects of ionizing radiation UNSCEAR 2000 report, vol. 1, http://www.unscear.org. UNSCEAR (United Nations Scientific Committee on theEffects of Atomic Radiation), 2000. Sources and effects of ionizing radiation. Report to the General Assembly.

Valverde, M.; Ostrosky-Wegman, P.; Rojas, E.; Fortoul, T.; Meneses, F.; Ramírez, M.; Díaz-Barriga, F. & Cebrian, M. The application of single cell gel electrophoresis or Comet assay to human monitoring studies. *Salud Publica Mex.* 1999;41 Suppl 2:S109-13.

Vodicka, P.; Kumar, R.; Stetina, R.; Sanyal, S.; Soucek, P.; Haufroid, V.; Dusinska, M.; Kuricova, M.; Zamecnikova, M., Musak, L.; Buchancova, J.; Norppa, H.; Hirvonen, A.; Vodickova, L.; Naccarati, A.; Matousu, Z. & Hemminki, K. (2004) Genetic polymorphismsin DNA repair genes and possible links with DNA repair rates, chromosomal aberrations and single-strand breaks in DNA. *Carcinogenesis* 25: 757-763.

Wang, J.X.; Zhang, L.A.; Li, B.X.; Zhao, Y.C.; Wang, Z.Q.; Zhang, J.Y. & Aoyama, T. (2002) Cancer incidence and risk estimation among medical X-ray workers in China, 1950-1995, *Health Phys* 82: 455–466.

Wang, Z.Q.; Saigusa, S. & Sasaki, M.S. (1991) Adaptive response to chromosome damage in cultured human lymphocytes primed with low doses of X-rays. *Mutat Res* 246: 179-186.

Weiss, J.M.; Goode, E.L.; Ladiges, W.C. & Ulrich, C.M. (2005) Polymorphic variation in hOGG1 and risk of cancer: a review of the functional and epidemiologic literature. *Mol Carcinog* 42: 127–141.

Wiencke, J.K.; Afzal, V; Olivieri, G. & Wolff, S. (1986) Evidence that the (3h) thymidine induced adaptive response of human lymphocytes to subsequent doses of x-rays involves the induction of a chromosomal repair mechanism. *Mutagenesis* 1(5): 375-380.

Winsey, S.L.; Haldar, N.A.; Marsh, H.P.; Bunce, M.; Marshall, S.E.; Harris, A.L.; Wojnarowska, F. & Welsh, K.I. (2000) A variant within theDNA repair gene XRCC3 is associated with the development of melanoma skin cancer. *Cancer Res* 60: 5612-5616.

Wojcik, A.; Sauer, K.; Zolzer, F.; Bauch, T. & Muller, W.U. (1996) Analyses of DNA damage recovery processes in the adaptive response to ionising radiation in human lymphocytes. *Mutagenesis* 11: 291–297.

Wojewodzka, M.; Kruszewski, M.; Iwanenko, T.; Collins, A.R. & Szumiel, I. (1998) Application of the comet assay for monitoring DNA damage inworkers exposed to chronic low-dose irradiation: I. Strand breakage. *Mutat Res* 416:21–35.

Wolff, S.; Wiencke, J.K. & Afzal, V. (1989) Biological Bases of Risk Assessment. In: Baverstock KF and Stather JW (ed.) Low Dose Radiation. Taylor and Francis, London, 439-445.

Wolff, S.; Oliviery, G. & Afzal, V. (1990) Adaptation of human lymphocytes to radiation or chemical mutagens: differences in cytogenetic repair. In: Obe G., Natarajan, A.T. (ed.) Chromosomal Aberrations, Basic and Applied Aspects. Springer-Verlag, Berlin, 140–149.

Wolff, S. (1992) Low-dose exposures and the induction of adaptation. In: Sugahara, T., Sagan, L.A., Aoyama, T. (ed.) Low Dose Irradiation and Biological Defence Mechanisms. Elsevier Science Publishers BV, Amsterdam, 21–28.

Wolff, S. (1996) Aspects of the adaptive response to very low doses of radiation and other agents. *Mutat Res* 358: 135–142.

Yamane, A.; Kohno, T.; Ito, K.; Sunaga, N.; Aoki, K.; Yoshimura, K.; Murakami, H.; Nojima, Y. & Yokota, J. (2004) Differential ability of polymorphic OGG1 proteins to suppress mutagenesis induced by 8-hydroxyguanine in human cell in vivo. *Carcinogenesis* 25: 1689-1694

Yoshinaga, S.; Aoyama, T.; Yoshimoto, Y. & Sugahara, T. (1999) Cancer mortality among radiological technologists in Japan: updated analysis of follow-up data from 1969 to 1993. *J Epidemiol* 9: 61–72.

Youngblom, J.H.; Wiencke, J.K. & Wolff, S. (1989) Inhibition of the adaptive response of human lymphocytes to very low doses of ionizing radiation by the protein synthesis inhibitor cycloheximide. *Mutat Res* 227(4):257-261.

20

# Application of Host Cell Reactivation in Evaluating the Effects of Anticancer Drugs and Environmental Toxicants on Cellular DNA Repair Activity in Head and Neck Cancer

Yi-Shan Tsai[1], Jau-Ling Huang[2] and Chang-Shen Lin[3]
*[1]Center of Excellence for Environmental Medicine, Kaohsiung Medical University, Kaohsiung*
*[2]Department of Bioscience Technology, Chang Jung Christian University, Tainan*
*[3]Graduate Institute of Medicine, Kaohsiung Medical University, Kaohsiung*
*Taiwan*

## 1. Introduction

DNA repair pathways are targets of numerous anticancer drugs including natural and chemical compounds, which direct cancer cells toward apoptosis. However, different types of cancer cells consist of various alterations in DNA repair genes that make cancer cells become drug-resistant and lead to treatment failure and disease recurrence. On the contrary, cancer cells may also possess defects in certain DNA repair pathway that make them are susceptible to certain compounds, which inhibit another DNA repair pathway inside the cancer cells. As a result, these compounds selectively kill the cancer cells and are less harmful to the normal ones. Understanding the effects of anticancer drugs on DNA repair as well as the DNA repair activity of cancer cells themselves are important for improvement of anticancer treatment. Similarly, this information is helpful for elucidation of the carcinogenicity of environmental toxicants. This chapter introduces the crosstalk between anticancer drugs, environmental toxicants and DNA repair pathways in head and neck cancer. In addition, the application of an easy, fast and measurable *in vivo* functional assay for nucleotide excision repair (NER) and DNA repair via homologous recombination (HR) and non-homologous end-joining (NHEJ) pathways is shown to examine the cellular DNA repair activity responding to anticancer drugs or environmental toxicants. By which the functional roles of DNA repair genes in response to anticancer treatments and genotoxic substances could be evolved in head and neck cancer cells.

## 2. Roles of DNA repair genes/pathways in cancer development and treatment

DNA repair genes play a pivotal role in the maintenance of genome integrity. Defects or dysregulation of DNA repair genes can result in genomic instability (GIN), which is a common feature of cancer cells (Hanahan & Weinberg, 2000). To prevent this, human cells evolve several

DNA repair pathways that may interplay each other to repair various types of DNA damages. These DNA repair mechanisms include pathways of base excision repair (BER), nucleotide excision repair (NER), mismatch repair (MMR), double strand break (DSB) repair through homologous recombination (HR) or non-homologous end-joining (NHEJ) and direct repair of DNA lesions such as $O^6$-methylguanine by $O^6$-methylguanine-DNA methyltransferase (Sancar et al., 2004). Collectively, there are hundreds of DNA repair genes involved in various DNA repair pathways that include processes of sense and recognition of DNA lesions, amplification and transmission of the damage signal, recruitment of repair proteins to the damage sites, and execution of DNA repair (Sancar et al., 2004; Wood et al., 2005).

### 2.1 DNA repair genes/signaling in HR and NER pathways

Upon DNA damaged, histone H2AX, a histone H2A variant, is quickly phosphorylated (denoted as γ-H2AX) in an ataxia telangiectasia mutated (*ATM*)-dependent manner (Uziel et al., 2003). The phosphorylated H2AX serves as an important marker for DNA damages. Some genes are also involved in the recognition of DNA damages. They are members of MRN complex (*Mre11A, RAD50, NBN*) for DSB and damage-specific DNA binding protein 1 and 2 (*DDB1* and *DDB2*), Xeroderma pigmentosum (XP) complementation group C (*XPC*) for UV-induced damages and bulky DNA adducts, which are produced by DNA-damaging chemotherapeutic drugs and can be repaired through NER pathway. In addition to H2AX, ATM also phosphorylates p53, BRCA1, CHEK1/2 and results in activation of various DNA repair pathways as well as induction of cell cycle arrest (Sancar et al., 2004). Generally, the genes involved in HR repair include *BRCA1, BRCA2*, members of *RAD51* and Fanconi anemia (FA) families, as well as the Bloom syndrome, RecQ helicase-like (*BLM*) and Werner syndrome, RecQ helicase-like (*WRN*). The genes in NER pathway consists of XP complementation group A to G (*XPA* to *XPG*), XP complementation group variant (*XPV*), excision repair cross-complementing rodent repair deficiency, complementation group 1 (*ERCC1*), replication protein A (*RPA*), and so on (Sancar et al., 2004; Wood et al., 2005).

*ATM* is the key gene for initiating DNA repair signaling. Its downstream targets, both *TP53* and *BRCA1* are capable of regulating multiple DNA repair pathways (Deng, 2006; Helton & Chen, 2007). *BRCA1* encodes a multifunctional protein that maintains genome integrity through regulating gene transcription, cell cycle checkpoints, DNA repair (Deng, 2006; Yoshida & Miki, 2004), and centrosome duplication (Deng, 2002; Xu et al., 1999). In addition to the role in HR, BRCA1 is involved in NER through transactivating the expression of *DDB2* and *XPC* (Hartman & Ford, 2002; Takimoto et al., 2002), both of them can also be transactivated by p53 (Adimoolam & Ford, 2002; Hwang et al., 1999). Thus, both *BRCA1* and *TP53* can regulate NER pathway. RAD51 is the human homolog of bacteria *recA* and forms a complex with BRCA1 and BRCA2. This interaction is important for proper regulation of RAD51 activity inside a cell. Loss of the binding between RAD51 and BRCA complex may be a key event leading to GIN and tumorigenesis (Martin et al., 2007). RAD51 contributes the key step of HR by mediating homologous pairing and strand exchange between two homologous DNA (Richardson, 2005). It has been shown that *RAD51* overexpression is correlated with GIN and that p53 can transcriptionally inhibits *RAD51* expression (Arias-Lopez et al., 2006; Richardson et al., 2004).

### 2.2 DNA repair activity is important for preventing cancer development

Activation of DNA repair genes has been shown as a critical anticancer barrier in early human tumorigenesis. By examining various stages from precancerous lesions to late-stage tumor tissues, DNA repair genes, including *ATM, CHEK1/2,* and *TP53,* are found predominantly to be highly activated in the precancerous stage of bladder, colon and lung epithelia when DNA damages are emerging inside these cells (Bartkova et al., 2005; Gorgoulis et al., 2005; Venkitaraman, 2005). Further, DNA repair genes also play a key role in the oncogene-induced senescence and prevent cell transformation (Bartkova et al., 2006; Braig et al., 2005; Di Micco et al., 2006). In other word, cells that are unable to activate DNA repair genes in the early-stage of tumorigenesis are susceptible for malignant transformation. These data demonstrated in somatic cancers strongly indicate that defects or inactivations of DNA repair genes/pathways are prerequisite for tumor development. Besides, several cancer predisposition syndromes are linked to hereditary mutations or deletions of DNA repair genes, such as *ATM* in ataxia telangiectasia, *BRCA1* and *BRCA2* in familial breast and ovarian cancers, *XPC* and *DDB2* in Xeroderma pigmentosum. Hence, people with, either inherited or sporadic, inactivated DNA repair genes/pathways are prone to cancer development. In this chapter, we will use head and neck cancer as an example to illustrate the important role of DNA repair genes/pathways in the development and treatment of this malignancy, and demonstrate the application of a functional DNA repair assay, host cell reactivation (HCR), in cancer research.

### 2.3 DNA repair activity is a critical determinant for efficacy of anticancer treatment using chemotherapy or radiotherapy

The cell-killing mechanisms of radiotherapy and most regimens of chemotherapy are dependent on the induction of severe DNA damages, which result in apoptosis of cancer cells. Therefore, the DNA repair activity of cancer cells can play an important role in modulating patient's response to these anticancer treatments. For example, the platinum-based anticancer chemical, cisplatin is one of the most popular DNA-damaging chemotherapeutic drugs used in clinical management. It causes DNA adducts by interstrand crosslinking, which is repaired by a combination of NER and HR (Helleday et al., 2008; Miyagawa, 2008). Mutations of NER genes, such as *XPF* or *ERCC1,* may increase the sensitivity of cells toward cisplatin (Martin et al., 2008; Saldivar et al., 2007). In contrast, elevated expression of NER genes usually confers resistance to chemotherapy using DNA-damaging regimens. The expression level of *BRCA1,* which plays a primary role in HR and may has a regulatory role in NER (Hartman & Ford, 2002; Takimoto et al., 2002), is also correlated with chemotherapy efficacy. It has been shown that cells with reduced or inactivated *BRCA1* are more sensitive to cisplatin but, in contrast, are resistant to taxanes, the microtubule-interfering drugs (Husain et al., 1998; Lafarge et al., 2001; Mullan et al., 2001). Overexpression of *RAD51,* a member of BRCA/FA complex involved in HR, is also correlated with cisplatin resistance (Bhattacharyya et al., 2000). For *ATM,* an *in vitro* study showed that partial loss of distal 11q (*ATM* locus) was associated with decreased IR sensitivity in head and neck cancer cell lines (Parikh et al., 2007). Therefore, understanding the status of DNA repair genes/activity is thought to be important for the selection of appropriate chemotherapeutic regimens and may have a great impact on the clinical treatment as well as the patient's outcome.

## 3. Head and neck cancer

Head and neck squamous cell carcinoma (HNSCC) is the most popular head and neck cancer and is the sixth most common cancer in the world. They include malignancies originated from the epithelia of larynx, pharynx, oral and nasal cavities.

### 3.1 Some HNSCC risk factors are able to inhibit DNA repair

Epidemiological evidences have demonstrated that alcohol drinking, betel quid (BQ) chewing (especially in South Asia and South-West Pacific area including Taiwan), cigarette smoking, and infection of human papillomavirus are risk factors for HNSCC development (Haddad & Shin, 2008; IARC, 2004). The carcinogenicity of betel nut has been approved by the International Agency for Research on Cancer (IARC), a WHO organization, in 2004 (IARC, 2004), although the molecular mechanism underlying its carcinogenicity is not fully elucidated. In this regard, we have explored the possible effect of arecoline, a major alkaloid in betel nut, on DNA repair activity using HCR. We found that arecoline could inhibit the repair of UV-induced DNA damages, at least partly, through inactivating p53's expression and transactivation activity (Tsai et al., 2008). Besides, we also showed that arecoline could affect mitotic spindles and deregulated mitotic checkpoint, another key guardian of genome integrity (Wang et al., 2010). These results provide molecular explanation for BQ-associated carcinogenicity that has been shown previously by an increase of mitosis errors and micronucleus (MN) in mammalian cells (Lin, 2010). Micronucleus is a typical sign of GIN and is derived from either DNA strand breaks (clastogenic effect) or whole chromosome lagging during mitosis (aneugenic effect) (Norppa & Falck, 2003).

Epidemiological studies also show that the probability of HNSCC development is synergistically increased by simultaneous exposure of BQ, cigarette, and alcohols (Ko et al., 1995; Lee et al., 2005). Regarding the carcinogenic role of cigarette on the aspect of DNA repair, we also found that benzo(a)pyrene (BaP), an important carcinogen in cigarette (IARC, 2010), exhibited negative effects on DNA repair (Lin et al., 2011 manuscript in preparation). The mechanistic study regarding the synergistic effect of arecoline and BaP on regulating DNA repair, especially via p53- and aryl hydrocarbon receptor-dependent pathway, is worthy to be investigated further.

### 3.2 Alterations of DNA repair genes/activity in HNSCC and the relationship with HNSCC development, treatment, as well as patient's outcome

GIN is a hallmark of most human malignancies including HNSCC that elevated microsatellite instability, aneuploidy and various genomic alterations have been found by genome-wide analyses (Bockmuhl et al., 1996; Brieger et al., 2003; Friedlander, 2001; Partridge et al., 1999; Sparano et al., 2006), suggesting that GIN may be involved in the development of HNSCC. Some studies also show that DNA repair activity is reduced in the peripheral blood cells of HNSCC patients when compared with normal individuals (Cheng et al., 1998; Paz-Elizur et al., 2006), implying that altered DNA repair genes and/or activity may play a critical role in the development of HNSCC.

Studies using comparative genomic hybridization (CGH) have shown that gene copy numbers at chromosome 11q22-23 (*ATM* locus) are frequently lost in HNSCC (Bockmuhl et al., 1996; Brieger et al., 2003; van den Broek et al., 2007). Lazar et al. also showed loss of heterozygosity (LOH) at 11q23 in 25% (13/52) of primary HNSCC (Lazar et al., 1998). In addition, we have reported that *ATM* mRNA is down-regulated in 81.3% (65/80) of laryngeal and pharyngeal cancers, and further show that lower *ATM* expression (tumor/normal < 0.3) was an independent risk factor for patient's survival (Lee et al., 2011). This is the first study showing that *ATM* expression is a valuable prognostic marker for HNSCC. One study also shows an absent or reduced ATM protein expression in 31.25% (10/32) of oral cancer (He et al., 2008). These results suggest that alteration of *ATM*, either in gene sequence or in expression level may be associated with HNSCC.

Previous investigations showed that LOH of chromosome 17q (*BRCA1* locus) were found in 35% to 56% of laryngeal cancer (Kiaris et al., 1995; Rizos et al., 1998). In contrast, studies using CGH found an overrepresentation of 17q in 9% to 47% of HNSCC (Bockmuhl et al., 1996; Brieger et al., 2003), and one array-CGH reported the gain of 17q21 in 33% (7/21) of oral cancer (Sparano et al., 2006). These controversial results by genome-wide analyses may be due to the physically close localization of *ERBB2* (HER-2/neu) oncogene and the results need to be clarified by specifically looking at the *BRCA1* gene locus. Regarding the expression of *BRCA1* in HNSCC, one study showed that BRCA1 immunostaining positivity was lost in 34% (26/77) of tongue cancers, which might be correlated with early-stage tumor progression (Vora et al., 2003).

The results of genome-wide studies also suggest that genetic alterations at *RAD51* (15q15.1) and *XPC* (3p25) loci may be present in HNSCC (Bockmuhl et al., 1996; Brieger et al., 2003; Partridge et al., 1999; Sparano et al., 2006; van den Broek et al., 2007). Altered RAD51 protein expression has been reported by one pilot study with twelve head and neck cancer patients (Connell et al., 2006). The patients with high RAD51 protein levels in their pre-treatment tumor biopsies demonstrate poorer cancer-specific survival rates than those with lower RAD51 levels (33.3% vs. 88.9% at 2 years; $P = 0.025$). These results suggest that RAD51 expression may influence the outcome of with head and neck cancer patients who receive chemotherapy and radiotherapy (Connell et al., 2006). Other reports regarding altered expression of DNA repair genes in HNSCC include Ku80 (Chang et al., 2006), NBN and ERCC1 (Hsu et al., 2010; Yang et al., 2006). It has been shown that ERCC1 expression is associated with cisplatin resistance (Handra-Luca et al., 2007; Hsu et al., 2010) and NBN is correlated with outcome of advanced HNSCC patients (Yang et al., 2006). Inactivation of the BRCA/FA pathway via promoter methylation has also been described in HNSCC, and may be related to tobacco and alcohol exposure and survival of these patients (Marsit et al., 2004).

### 3.3 Treatment of HNSCC

Since HNSCC and its treatment can affect important physiological functions, such as speaking, breathing, and swallowing, it is important for choosing the appropriate treatment that not only cures but also benefits to the preservation of organs, physiological functions, and quality of life. The standard treatment for resectable HNSCC is surgical resection with or without postoperative concurrent chemotherapy (cisplatin plus 5-fluorouracil) and radiotherapy (CCRT). Around two-thirds of HNSCC are in advanced stage at time of diagnosis (Specenier & Vermorken, 2009). The majority of these patients with advanced stage tumors finally relapse locoregionally or at distant sites. These patients are usually qualified for palliative treatment only. Recent advances in using cetuximab (anti-EGFR) to prolong patient's survival time in locally advanced HNSCC is a big, but still not a fully satisfied progress (Vermorken et al., 2008). The use of docetaxel (a spindle poison and mitotic catastrophe inducer) can enhance the efficacy of chemotherapy using cisplatin/fluorouracil and improve slightly the overall survival rates of HNSCC patients (Hitt et al., 2005; Posner et al., 2007; Vermorken et al., 2007). These results suggest that a combination regimen exploiting different cell-killing mechanisms may be superior to monotherapy. However, an ideal combination regimen with lower adverse and side effects for efficient treatment of HNSCC is still under looking for.

### 3.4 Understanding the status of DNA repair genes in HNSCC is important for design of an effective therapeutic strategy for this malignancy

Since DNA repair genes/activity play a key role in cancer development and treatment, understanding their expression and genomic/functional alterations may facilitate the identification of new predictive or prognostic markers and new therapeutic targets for treatment of HNSCC. For example, recent studies using the strategy of synthetic lethal interaction (SLI) to improve efficacy of cancer treatment have become an attractive strategy (Helleday et al., 2008). Cancer cells that can survive from innumerable genetic alterations are largely dependent on the activities of multiple DNA repair pathways. However, cancer cells may also be defective in certain DNA repair pathway that is inherent or arises during tumorigenesis. Therefore, inhibition of one DNA repair pathway may increase selectively killing of cancer cells that already have another defective DNA repair pathway. For examples, some clinical trials have shown the efficient killing of *BRCA1*- or *BRCA2*-defective cancer cells (with defective HR repair) by using *PARP1* inhibitors, which block BER pathway (Annunziata & O'Shaughnessy, 2010; Bryant et al., 2005; Farmer et al., 2005; Underhill et al., 2010). Notably, such kind of treatment is less toxic than conventional radiotherapy and chemotherapy. This may benefit to organ preservation of HNSCC patients if one can identify SLI targets (DNA repair genes are good candidates) and develop corresponding regimens for treatment. For this reason, some clinical trials are ongoing to examine the efficacy of anticancer treatments by modulating DNA repair activities that are involved in different DNA repair pathways (Bolderson et al., 2009; Helleday, 2010; Helleday et al., 2008).

## 4. Host cell reactivation (HCR) assay

As mentioned above, DNA repair activity plays a critical role in maintaining genome integrity. Regardless the alterations of DNA repair genes at the levels of gene expression or DNA sequence, measurement of DNA repair activity can reflect the overall biological effects that are as consequences of these molecular changes and/or anticancer drug responses. Here we describe an easy and fast functional assay (HCR) to evaluate cellular DNA repair activity *in vivo*. This method uses a plasmid that can produce luciferase in mammalian cells as a reporter. We choose luciferase as a reporter since its characteristics of high sensitivity and wide dynamic linear range for quantification. Of course, other commonly used reporters, such as chloramphenicol acetyltransferase (CAT), secreted alkaline phosphatase (SEAP) or green fluorescent protein (GFP) can also be used.

The reporter is damaged *in vitro* first and is transfected into host cells. If the damaged reporter plasmid can be repaired in the host cells, the luciferase will be re-expressed. Otherwise, the luciferase activity will be much lower than that transfected with undamaged control plasmid. By this way, one can determine the DNA repair capacity by simply measuring luciferase activity. The reporter plasmid can be damaged using various methods such as UV, chemicals or restriction enzymes and serve as substrates for different DNA repair pathways. In this chapter, we will demonstrate the use of HCR in evaluating DNA repair capacities via NER, HR and NHEJ pathways.

### 4.1 HCR for NER

NER is responsible for the repair of bulky DNA lesions induced by UV and a lot of anticancer drugs. Here we use UV as a method to damage a luciferase reporter plasmid. Other chemicals (such as cisplatin) that cause bulky DNA adducts can also be used.

#### 4.1.1 Materials

1. The reporter plasmid: pCMV-Luc (Liu et al., 2004). The firefly luciferase is driven by the cytomegalovirus (CMV) immediate early (IE) gene promoter.

2. The internal control plasmid used for calibrating transfection efficiency: pRL-CMV (Promega, Cat. No. E2261). The *Renilla* luciferase is driven by the CMV IE promoter.
3. Transfection reagents: Lipofectamine™ 2000 (Invitrogen, Cat. No. 11668) and Opti-MEM® I reduced serum medium (Invitrogen, Cat. No. 31985).
4. The Dual-Glo™ Luciferase assay system (Promega, Cat. No. E2940) for analyzing firefly and *Renilla* luciferase activities.

#### 4.1.2 Substrate preparation for NER

1. Amplify the pCMV-Luc and pRL-CMV plasmids in *E. coli* (Fig. 1A).
2. Harvest bacteria by centrifugation at 13,000 rpm for 15 minutes, discard the supernatant completely and purify plasmids using the Plasmid Midi Kit (Geneaid, Cat. No. PI025).
3. Determine plasmid DNA concentration and purity by measuring the absorbance at 260 nm and 280 nm with a UV spectrophotometer.
4. Prepare UV-damaged luciferase reporter plasmid (pCMV-Luc) with a UV-crosslinker (CL-1000, UVP). The plasmids are placed within inner side of an opened eppendorf lid (Fig. 1B) or 35 mm petri dish without lid. The UV dose for irradiation is dependent on cell types because of differential intrinsic DNA repair capacities of various cells. We use 1000 $J/m^2$ for 293 (human embryonic kidney), Beas-2B (human bronchial epithelium), H1299 (human lung cancer), HEp-2 (human laryngeal cancer), SAS, Ca9-22, (human oral cancer) and 500 $J/m^2$ for KB (human oral cancer) cells. It is important to keep above parameters (the same plasmid amount in a fixed volume for UV irradiation) consistently in each experiment, or prepare an enough quantity of UV-dameged plasmids that can be stored in aliquots at -80°C once for all experiments.

#### 4.1.3 Transfection

1. The HEp-2 cells ($6\times10^4$) are seeded in 24-well plates 24 h prior to transfection (the appropriate cell numbers for seeding are dependent on cell types).
2. Prepare DNA-Lipofectamine™ 2000 (Invitrogen) complexes for each sample as follows:
   a. Add 0.5 μg of UV-damaged or undamaged (serve as a control) pCMV-Luc together with 0.05 μg of internal control plasmid (pRL-CMV, Promega) in 50 μl of Opti-MEM (Invitrogen) medium, mix gently.
   b. Mix 1 μl Lipofectamine™ 2000 gently in 50 μl of Opti-MEM medium and incubate for 5 minutes at room temperature.
   c. Combine the diluted DNA with the diluted Lipofectamine™ 2000 (total volume is 100 μl). Mix gently and incubate for 20 min at room temperature to allow the formation of DNA-Lipofectamine™ 2000 complexes.
3. Add the 100 μl of DNA-Lipofectamine™ 2000 complexes to each well and incubate at 37°C in a $CO_2$ incubator for 6 h. Then the cells can be treated with toxicants (such as arecoline) or anticancer drugs for another 24 h. Note: cells can be treated with toxicants or anticancer drugs prior to transfection that is dependent on experimental design.

#### 4.1.4 Dual-luciferase assay

1. After 24 h post-transfection, cells are harvested in 100 μl (adjustable) lysis buffer (0.1 M HEPES, pH 7.8, 1% Triton X-100, 1 mM $CaCl_2$ and 1 mM $MgCl_2$) with cell scrapers.
2. The cell lysates are transferred to eppendorf tubes and centrifuged at 13,000 rpm at 20°C for one minute.

3. The supernatants (50 µl, adjustable) are transferred into a 96-well plate and 20 µl of Dual-Glo™ Luciferase Reagent (Promega) are added to each well.
4. Ten minutes later, the firefly luminescence is measured by a microplate luminometer (Centro LB 960, Berthold, Bad Wildbad, Germany).
5. Add 20 µl of Dual-Glo™ Stop & Glo® Reagent (Promega) to each well and wait for 10 minutes, then the *Renilla* luminescence is read.
6. The transfection efficiency-adjusted firefly luciferase activity is obtained by dividing the *Renilla* luciferase activity.

#### 4.1.5 Representation of NER activity by HCR assay

Since the pCMV-Luc is damaged by UV, the DNA repair activity (responsible to UV) can be represented as the *Renilla*–calibrated firefly luciferase activity derived from UV-damaged pCMV-Luc verse to those from undamaged pCMV-Luc. By this way, one can compare the effects of various environmental toxicants on cellular DNA repair capacity. For example, an inhibitory effect of arecoline on the repair of UV-damaged pCMV-Luc can be found by using HCR assay (Fig. 1C).

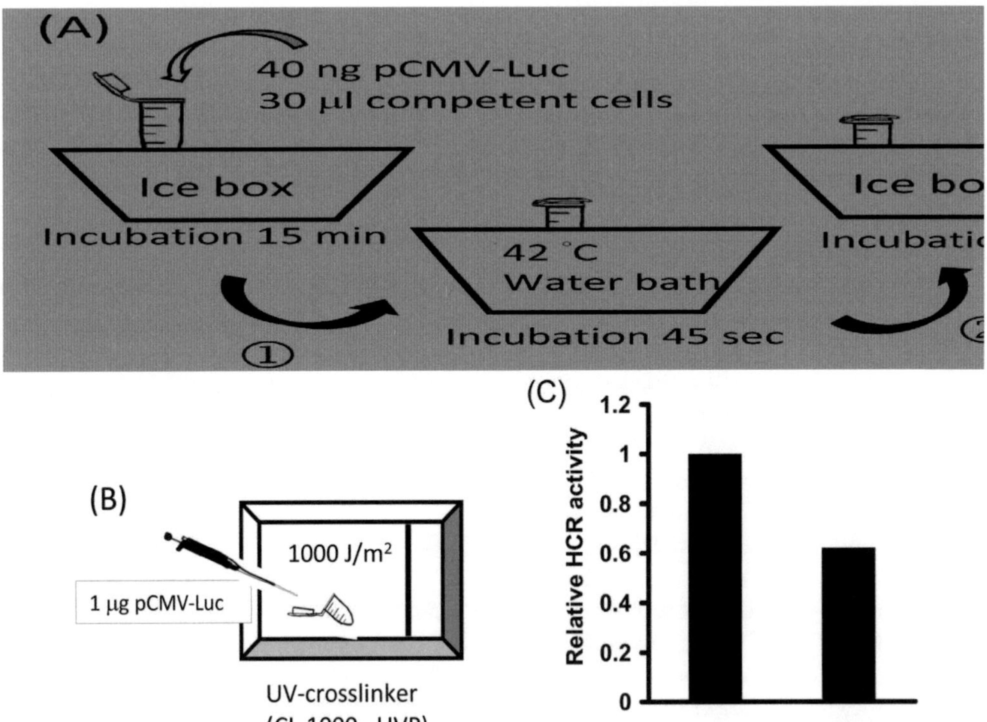


Fig. 1. Schematic illustration of host cell reactivation (HCR) assay for examination of nucleotide excision repair.
(A) The reporter plasmid pCMV-Luc is prepared in *E. coli*.
(B) The pCMV-Luc is damaged by 1000 J/m² of UV light.
(C) Comparison of the effects of arecoline (ARE, 0.3 mM) and its vehicle (distilled water) on the repair of UV-damaged pCMV-Luc in HEp-2 cells.

### 4.2 HCR for HR repair

HR is a reliable mechanism to accurately repair DNA double strand breaks. Here we use PCR to generate two overlapping DNA fragments that contain i) CMV IE promoter and 5'-part of *Renilla* luciferase gene, ii) 3'-part of *Renilla* luciferase gene and poly-A tail sequence from pRL-CMV (Fig. 2A) and serve as substrates for HR (Fig. 2B). The two overlapping DNA fragments can also be produced by restriction enzyme digestion and gel elution.

#### 4.2.1 Materials

1. Plasmids: pRL-CMV (Promega, Cat. No. E2261) and pCMV-Luc (Liu et al., 2004).
2. PCR primers: RL_1: 5'-AGA TCT TCA ATA TTG GCC ATT AGC; RL_2: 5'-TTC TTA TTT ATG GCG ACA TGT TGT; RL_3: 5'-ACG AGG CCA TGA TAA TGT TGG ACG; RL_4: 5'-CTT ATC GAT TTT ACC ACA TTT GTA.
3. DNA Polymerase: *Ex Taq*™ Polymerase (Takara, Cat No. RR001A).
4. Gel-M™ Gel Extraction System (Viogene, Cat No. EG1002).

#### 4.2.2 Substrate preparation for HR repair

1. Set up PCR reaction as below:

| Reaction mixtures | HR_13 (μl) | HR_24 (μl) |
|---|---|---|
| 10×PCR buffer | 5 | 5 |
| dNTP (2.5 mM) | 4 | 4 |
| RL_1 primer (10 μM) | 2 | - |
| RL_3 primer (10 μM) | 2 | - |
| RL_2 primer (10 μM) | - | 2 |
| RL_4 primer (10 μM) | - | 2 |
| ExTaq polymerase (5u/μl) | 0.25 | 0.25 |
| Template (40 ng/μl) | 1 | 1 |
| DNA/RNAase free- $H_2O$ | 35.75 | 35.75 |
| Total volume (μl) | 50 | 50 |

2. Incubate the PCR reaction mixtures at 94°C for 2 min, then run for 30 cycles of amplification (94°C, 45 sec; 55°C, 1 min; 72°C, 1 min) and additional extension step at 72°C for 5 min.
3. Purify the PCR products of HR13 fragments (1730 bp, containing CMV IE promoter and 5'-part of *Renilla* luciferase gene) and HR24 fregments (1023 bp, containing 3'-part of *Renilla* luciferase gene and poly-A tail) from 0.8% agarose gels (Fig. 2C) using the Gel-M™ Gel Extraction System kit (Viogene).
4. Determine DNA concentration and purity by measuring the absorbance at 260 nm and 280 nm with a UV spectrophotometer. Dilute the HR13-PCR products to 17 ng/μl and HR24-PCR products to 10 ng/μl with distilled $H_2O$ to make the molar ratio of HR13:HR24 = 1:1, by which the same volume of the two DNA fragments can be used for transfection. Store the purified DNA in aliquots at -20°C.

Alternative: the two DNA fragments used for HR can also be generated by using a combination of restriction endonucleases *Bgl*II/*Nhe*I and *Pst*I/*Bam*HI for pRL-CMV (Progema). The use of former restriction enzymes will produce a DNA fragment containing

CMV IE promoter and 5′-part of *Renilla* luciferase gene, the later ones result in 3′-part of *Renilla* luciferase gene and the poly-A signal. These two DNA fragments contain a 222-bp overlapping region for recombination (Fig. 2D).

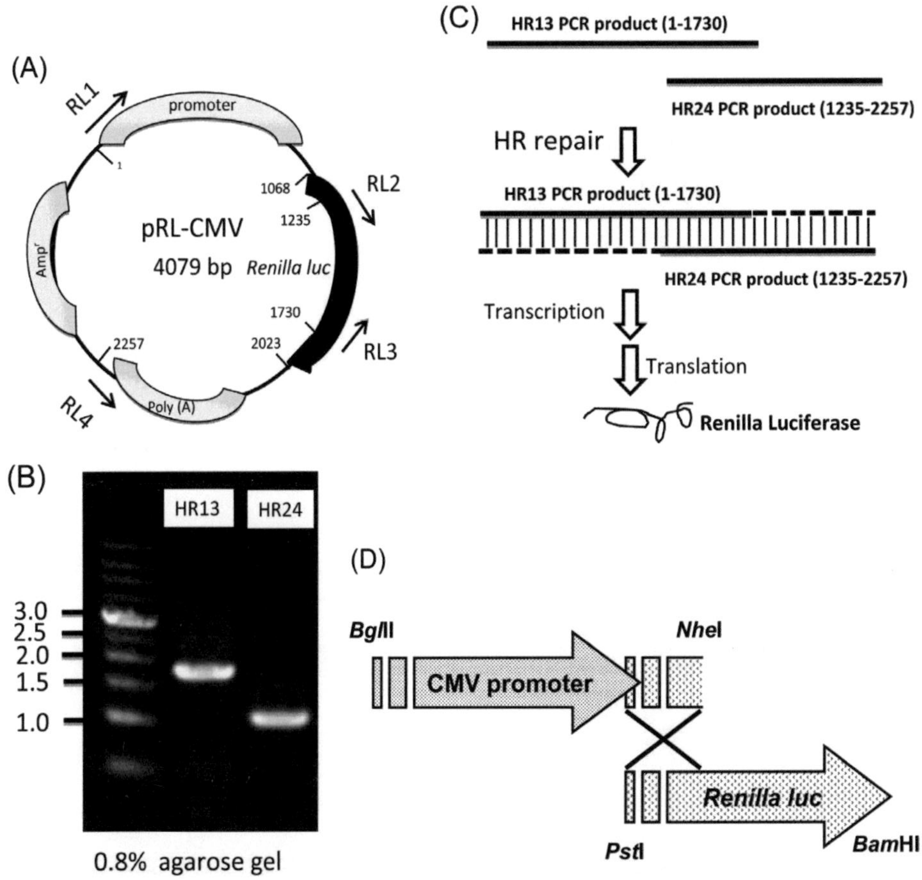


Fig. 2. Schematic representation of substrate preparation for HCR assay of homologous recombination (HR) repair.
(A) Location of PCR primers on the pRL-CMV reporter plasmid.
(B) Agarose gel electrophoresis of the PCR products, which serve as HR substrates.
(C) Homologous recombination of the two PCR fragments results in expression of luciferase.
(D) An alternative way to produce DNA fragments for HR by using restriction enzymes.

#### 4.2.3 Transfection, dual-luciferase assay and representation of HR repair activity

1. The HEp-2 cells ($6 \times 10^4$) are seeded in 24-well plates 24 h prior to transfection (the appropriate cell numbers for seeding are dependent on cell types).
2. Prepare DNA-Lipofectamine™ 2000 (Invitrogen) complexes for each sample as follows:
   a. Add 4 µl each of HR13 and HR24 DNA fragments together with 0.25 µg of internal control plasmid (pCMV-Luc) in 50 µl of Opti-MEM (Invitrogen) medium, mix gently.
   b. Mix 1 µl Lipofectamine™ 2000 gently in 50 µl of Opti-MEM medium and incubate for 5 minutes at room temperature.

c. Combine the diluted DNA with the diluted Lipofectamine™ 2000 (total volume is 100 µl). Mix gently and incubate for 20 min at room temperature to allow the formation of DNA-Lipofectamine™ 2000 complexes.

3. Add the 100 µl of DNA-Lipofectamine™ 2000 complexes to each well and incubate at 37°C in a $CO_2$ incubator for 6 h. Then the cells can be treated with toxicants (such as areca nut extracts, ANE) or anticancer drugs for another 24 h. Note: cells can be treated with toxicants or anticancer drugs prior to transfection that is dependent on experimental design.
4. Perform dual-luciferase assay as section 4.1.4.
5. Determine the HR activity by comparing the firefly luciferase-calibrated *Renilla* luciferase activities between the environmental toxicants- or anticancer drugs-treated cells and vehicle-treated control cells. For examples, the treatment of anticancer drug camptothecin (CPT, a topoisomerase I inhibitor) can potentiate HR repair activity but the areca nut extracts (ANE) repress HR repair in HEp-2 cells (Fig. 3).

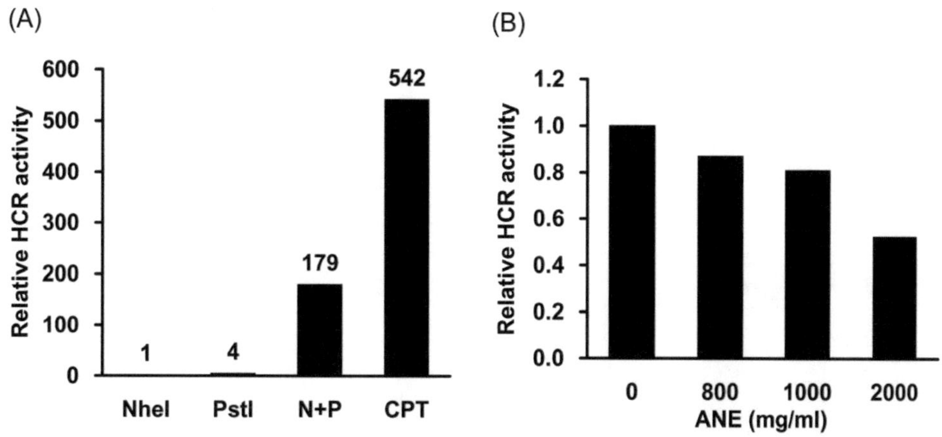


Fig. 3. The use of HCR assays in evaluating the effects of camptothecin and areca nut extracts on homologous recombination repair.
(A) Using the method illustrated in Fig. 2D, the *Renilla* luciferase activity (reflecting the HCR activity in Y-axis) can only be detected in the presence of both two DNA fragments (N+P, lane 3) but not in cells transfected with only one fragment (NheI or PstI, lanes 1 and 2). Treatment of camptothecin (CPT) stimulates HR repair efficiency in the cells (lane 4).
(B) Dose-dependent repression of HR repair activity by areca nut extracts (ANE).

### 4.3 HCR for NHEJ repair

NHEJ is another DNA repair mechanism responsible to DSB. Unlike HR repair using sister-chromatids as templates, NHEJ directly joins the broken DNA ends by trimming a few nucleotides on the ends. Therefore, it is thought as an error-prone repair system. In this regard, we prepare two kinds of reporter DNA substrates that are suitable for analyzing the precise and overall NHEJ repair activities, respectively.

For overall NHEJ repair, pRL-CMV is linearized with *Hin*dIII that cuts the flanking sequence between CMV promoter and the Renilla luciferase coding sequence. The luciferase will express after re-ligation regardless the loss of some nucleotides. For examining precise

NHEJ, *Afl* III that digests the coding region of *Renilla* luciferase gene is used and the luciferase can only be expressed after exact repair (Fig. 4A). The linearized reporter DNA fragments are purified, transfected into host cells and examined for luciferase activity as described above. Below is an example of evaluating the effect of areca nut extracts on precise and overall NHEJ repair (Fig. 4B).

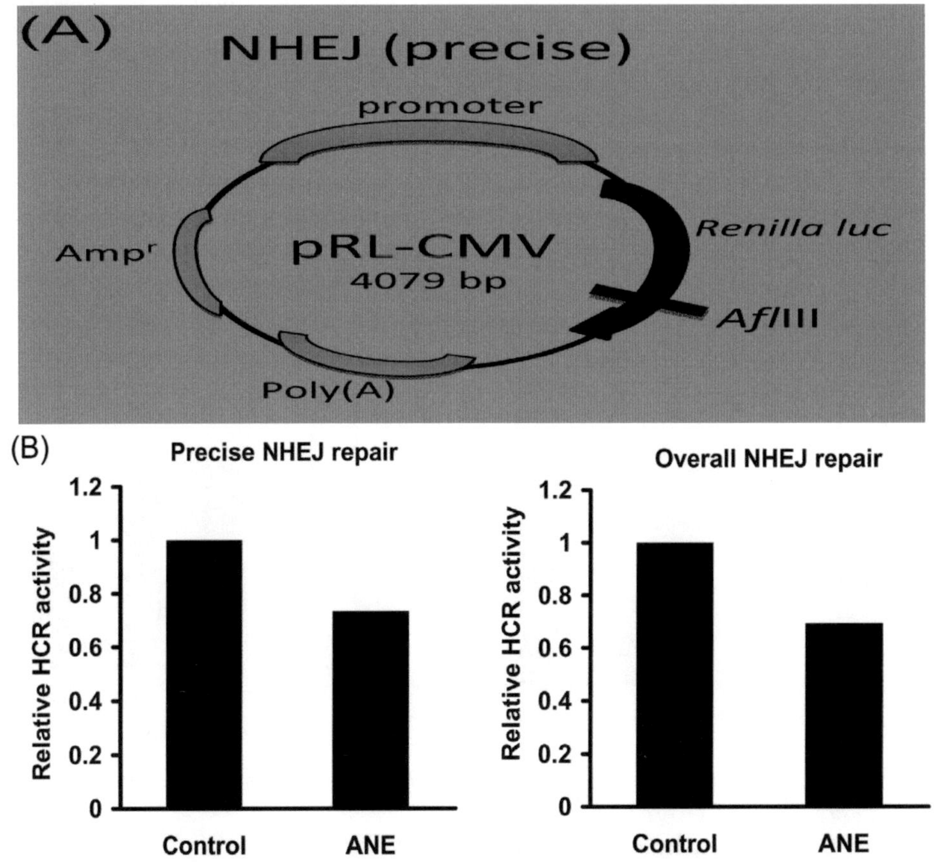


Fig. 4. HCR assay for non-homologous end-joining (NHEJ) repair.
(A) The *Afl* III-digested pRL-CMV is used as a substrate for analyzing precise NHEJ repair activity because of the need of exact joining of the *Renilla* luciferase coding sequence. For overall NHEJ, *Hind* III that cuts the flanking sequence between CMV promoter and the *Renilla* luciferase gene is used. The expression of luciferase is not affected by loss of a few nucleotides in this region during the end-joining process.
(B) The effect of areca nut extracts (ANE, 800 mg/ml for 24 h) on precise (left panel) and overall (right panel) NHEJ repair.

## 5. Conclusion

DNA repair genes play a pivotal role in the maintenance of genome integrity. Alterations of various DNA repair genes, either in gene sequence/structure or in gene expression, are frequently found in most of human malignancies. Since DNA repair activity is able to modulate cellular response to DNA-damaging anticancer drugs, alterations of DNA repair genes may be involved in the development of resistance to chemotherapy and radiotherapy. In addition, DNA repair activity plays an important role in preventing the mutagenicity and cytotoxicity induced by numerous environmental carcinogens and toxicants. Cells with reduced DNA repair activity may thus be prone to pathological transformation. Therefore, examining the DNA repair activity of a cell can help us to understand the probability of cellular tumorigenicity associated with exposure of environmental carcinogens and is able to assess the responses of various regimens of anticancer treatment. HCR assay is an easy and fast functional assay that can be applied to investigate several DNA repair pathways and is one of the most useful methods for evaluating cellular DNA repair activity *in vivo*.

## 6. Acknowledgment

The authors thank the financial support (grant No. NSC97-2311-B-037-002-MY3 to C.S.L. and NSC99-2314-B-309-004-MY2 to J.L.H.) from the National Science Council, Taiwan.

## 7. References

Adimoolam, S. & Ford, J.M. (2002) p53 and DNA damage-inducible expression of the xeroderma pigmentosum group C gene. *Proc Natl Acad Sci U S A*, Vol. 99, No.20, pp. 12985-12990.

Annunziata, C.M. & O'Shaughnessy, J. (2010) Poly (adp-ribose) polymerase as a novel therapeutic target in cancer. *Clin Cancer Res*, Vol. 16, No.18, pp. 4517-4526.

Arias-Lopez, C., Lazaro-Trueba, I., Kerr, P., Lord, C.J., Dexter, T., Iravani, M., Ashworth, A. & Silva, A. (2006) p53 modulates homologous recombination by transcriptional regulation of the RAD51 gene. *EMBO Rep*, Vol. 7, No.2, pp. 219-224.

Bartkova, J., Horejsi, Z., Koed, K., Kramer, A., Tort, F., Zieger, K., Guldberg, P., Sehested, M., Nesland, J.M., Lukas, C., Orntoft, T., Lukas, J. & Bartek, J. (2005) DNA damage response as a candidate anti-cancer barrier in early human tumorigenesis. *Nature*, Vol. 434, No.7035, pp. 864-870.

Bartkova, J., Rezaei, N., Liontos, M., Karakaidos, P., Kletsas, D., Issaeva, N., Vassiliou, L.V., Kolettas, E., Niforou, K., Zoumpourlis, V.C., Takaoka, M., Nakagawa, H., Tort, F., Fugger, K., Johansson, F., Sehested, M., Andersen, C.L., Dyrskjot, L., Orntoft, T., Lukas, J., Kittas, C., Helleday, T., Halazonetis, T.D., Bartek, J. & Gorgoulis, V.G. (2006) Oncogene-induced senescence is part of the tumorigenesis barrier imposed by DNA damage checkpoints. *Nature*, Vol. 444, No.7119, pp. 633-637.

Bhattacharyya, A., Ear, U.S., Koller, B.H., Weichselbaum, R.R. & Bishop, D.K. (2000) The breast cancer susceptibility gene BRCA1 is required for subnuclear assembly of Rad51 and survival following treatment with the DNA cross-linking agent cisplatin. *J Biol Chem*, Vol. 275, No.31, pp. 23899-23903.

Bockmuhl, U., Schwendel, A., Dietel, M. & Petersen, I. (1996) Distinct patterns of chromosomal alterations in high- and low-grade head and neck squamous cell carcinomas. *Cancer Res*, Vol. 56, No.23, pp. 5325-5329.

Bolderson, E., Richard, D.J., Zhou, B.B. & Khanna, K.K. (2009) Recent advances in cancer therapy targeting proteins involved in DNA double-strand break repair. *Clin Cancer Res*, Vol. 15, No.20, pp. 6314-6320.

Braig, M., Lee, S., Loddenkemper, C., Rudolph, C., Peters, A.H., Schlegelberger, B., Stein, H., Dorken, B., Jenuwein, T. & Schmitt, C.A. (2005) Oncogene-induced senescence as an initial barrier in lymphoma development. *Nature*, Vol. 436, No.7051, pp. 660-665.

Brieger, J., Jacob, R., Riazimand, H.S., Essig, E., Heinrich, U.R., Bittinger, F. & Mann, W.J. (2003) Chromosomal aberrations in premalignant and malignant squamous epithelium. *Cancer Genet Cytogenet*, Vol. 144, No.2, pp. 148-155.

Bryant, H.E., Schultz, N., Thomas, H.D., Parker, K.M., Flower, D., Lopez, E., Kyle, S., Meuth, M., Curtin, N.J. & Helleday, T. (2005) Specific killing of BRCA2-deficient tumours with inhibitors of poly(ADP-ribose) polymerase. *Nature*, Vol. 434, No.7035, pp. 913-917.

Chang, H.W., Kim, S.Y., Yi, S.L., Son, S.H., Song do, Y., Moon, S.Y., Kim, J.H., Choi, E.K., Ahn, S.D., Shin, S.S., Lee, K.K. & Lee, S.W. (2006) Expression of Ku80 correlates with sensitivities to radiation in cancer cell lines of the head and neck. *Oral Oncol*, Vol. 42, No.10, pp. 979-986.

Cheng, L., Eicher, S.A., Guo, Z., Hong, W.K., Spitz, M.R. & Wei, Q. (1998) Reduced DNA repair capacity in head and neck cancer patients. *Cancer Epidemiol Biomarkers Prev*, Vol. 7, No.6, pp. 465-468.

Connell, P.P., Jayathilaka, K., Haraf, D.J., Weichselbaum, R.R., Vokes, E.E. & Lingen, M.W. (2006) Pilot study examining tumor expression of RAD51 and clinical outcomes in human head cancers. *Int J Oncol*, Vol. 28, No.5, pp. 1113-1119.

Deng, C.X. (2002) Roles of BRCA1 in centrosome duplication. *Oncogene*, Vol. 21, No.40, pp. 6222-6227.

Deng, C.X. (2006) BRCA1: cell cycle checkpoint, genetic instability, DNA damage response and cancer evolution. *Nucleic Acids Res*, Vol. 34, No.5, pp. 1416-1426.

Di Micco, R., Fumagalli, M., Cicalese, A., Piccinin, S., Gasparini, P., Luise, C., Schurra, C., Garre, M., Nuciforo, P.G., Bensimon, A., Maestro, R., Pelicci, P.G. & d'Adda di Fagagna, F. (2006) Oncogene-induced senescence is a DNA damage response triggered by DNA hyper-replication. *Nature*, Vol. 444, No.7119, pp. 638-642.

Farmer, H., McCabe, N., Lord, C.J., Tutt, A.N., Johnson, D.A., Richardson, T.B., Santarosa, M., Dillon, K.J., Hickson, I., Knights, C., Martin, N.M., Jackson, S.P., Smith, G.C. & Ashworth, A. (2005) Targeting the DNA repair defect in BRCA mutant cells as a therapeutic strategy. *Nature*, Vol. 434, No.7035, pp. 917-921.

Friedlander, P.L. (2001) Genomic instability in head and neck cancer patients. *Head Neck*, Vol. 23, No.8, pp. 683-691.

Gorgoulis, V.G., Vassiliou, L.V., Karakaidos, P., Zacharatos, P., Kotsinas, A., Liloglou, T., Venere, M., Ditullio, R.A., Jr., Kastrinakis, N.G., Levy, B., Kletsas, D., Yoneta, A., Herlyn, M., Kittas, C. & Halazonetis, T.D. (2005) Activation of the DNA damage checkpoint and genomic instability in human precancerous lesions. *Nature*, Vol. 434, No.7035, pp. 907-913.

Haddad, R.I. & Shin, D.M. (2008) Recent advances in head and neck cancer. *N Engl J Med*, Vol. 359, No.11, pp. 1143-1154.

Hanahan, D. & Weinberg, R.A. (2000) The hallmarks of cancer. *Cell*, Vol. 100, No.1, pp. 57-70.

Handra-Luca, A., Hernandez, J., Mountzios, G., Taranchon, E., Lacau-St-Guily, J., Soria, J.C. & Fouret, P. (2007) Excision repair cross complementation group 1 immunohistochemical expression predicts objective response and cancer-specific survival in patients treated by Cisplatin-based induction chemotherapy for locally advanced head and neck squamous cell carcinoma. *Clin Cancer Res*, Vol. 13, No.13, pp. 3855-3859.

Hartman, A.R. & Ford, J.M. (2002) BRCA1 induces DNA damage recognition factors and enhances nucleotide excision repair. *Nat Genet*, Vol. 32, No.1, pp. 180-184.

He, Y., Chen, Q. & Li, B. (2008) ATM in oral carcinogenesis: association with clinicopathological features. *J Cancer Res Clin Oncol*, Vol. 134, No.9, pp. 1013-1020.

Helleday, T. (2010) Homologous recombination in cancer development, treatment and development of drug resistance. *Carcinogenesis*, Vol. 31, No.6, pp. 955-960.

Helleday, T., Petermann, E., Lundin, C., Hodgson, B. & Sharma, R.A. (2008) DNA repair pathways as targets for cancer therapy. *Nat Rev Cancer*, Vol. 8, No.3, pp. 193-204.

Helton, E.S. & Chen, X. (2007) p53 modulation of the DNA damage response. *J Cell Biochem*, Vol. 100, No.4, pp. 883-896.

Hitt, R., Lopez-Pousa, A., Martinez-Trufero, J., Escrig, V., Carles, J., Rizo, A., Isla, D., Vega, M.E., Marti, J.L., Lobo, F., Pastor, P., Valenti, V., Belon, J., Sanchez, M.A., Chaib, C., Pallares, C., Anton, A., Cervantes, A., Paz-Ares, L. & Cortes-Funes, H. (2005) Phase III study comparing cisplatin plus fluorouracil to paclitaxel, cisplatin, and fluorouracil induction chemotherapy followed by chemoradiotherapy in locally advanced head and neck cancer. *J Clin Oncol*, Vol. 23, No.34, pp. 8636-8645.

Hsu, D.S., Lan, H.Y., Huang, C.H., Tai, S.K., Chang, S.Y., Tsai, T.L., Chang, C.C., Tzeng, C.H., Wu, K.J., Kao, J.Y. & Yang, M.H. (2010) Regulation of excision repair cross-complementation group 1 by Snail contributes to cisplatin resistance in head and neck cancer. *Clin Cancer Res*, Vol. 16, No.18, pp. 4561-4571.

Husain, A., He, G., Venkatraman, E.S. & Spriggs, D.R. (1998) BRCA1 up-regulation is associated with repair-mediated resistance to cis-diamminedichloroplatinum(II). *Cancer Res*, Vol. 58, No.6, pp. 1120-1123.

Hwang, B.J., Ford, J.M., Hanawalt, P.C. & Chu, G. (1999) Expression of the p48 xeroderma pigmentosum gene is p53-dependent and is involved in global genomic repair. *Proc Natl Acad Sci U S A*, Vol. 96, No.2, pp. 424-428.

IARC. (2004) Betel-quid and areca-nut chewing and some areca-nut-derived nitrosamines. *IARC Monographs on the Evaluation of Carcinogenic Risks to Humans*, Vol. 85, The International Agency for Research on cancer, World Health Organization, Lyon, France.

IARC. (2010) Some non-heterocyclic polycyclic aromatic hydrocarbons and some related exposures. *IARC Monographs on the Evaluation of Carcinogenic Risks to Humans*, Vol. 92, The International Agency for Research on cancer, World Health Organization, Lyon, France.

Kiaris, H., Spanakis, N., Ergazaki, M., Sourvinos, G. & Spandidos, D.A. (1995) Loss of heterozygosity at 9p and 17q in human laryngeal tumors. *Cancer Lett*, Vol. 97, No.1, pp. 129-134.

Ko, Y.C., Huang, Y.L., Lee, C.H., Chen, M.J., Lin, L.M. & Tsai, C.C. (1995) Betel quid chewing, cigarette smoking and alcohol consumption related to oral cancer in Taiwan. *J Oral Pathol Med*, Vol. 24, No.10, pp. 450-453.

Lafarge, S., Sylvain, V., Ferrara, M. & Bignon, Y.J. (2001) Inhibition of BRCA1 leads to increased chemoresistance to microtubule-interfering agents, an effect that involves the JNK pathway. *Oncogene*, Vol. 20, No.45, pp. 6597-6606.

Lazar, A.D., Winter, M.R., Nogueira, C.P., Larson, P.S., Finnemore, E.M., Dolan, R.W., Fuleihan, N., Chakravarti, A., Zietman, A. & Rosenberg, C.L. (1998) Loss of heterozygosity at 11q23 in squamous cell carcinoma of the head and neck is associated with recurrent disease. *Clin Cancer Res*, Vol. 4, No.11, pp. 2787-2793.

Lee, K.W., Kuo, W.R., Tsai, S.M., Wu, D.C., Wang, W.M., Fang, F.M., Chiang, F.Y., Ho, K.Y., Wang, L.F., Tai, C.F., Kao, E.L., Chou, S.H., Lee, C.H., Chai, C.Y. & Ko, Y.C. (2005) Different impact from betel quid, alcohol and cigarette: risk factors for pharyngeal and laryngeal cancer. *Int J Cancer*, Vol. 117, No.5, pp. 831-836.

Lee, K.W., Tsai, Y.S., Chiang, F.Y., Huang, J.L., Ho, K.Y., Yang, Y.H., Kuo, W.R., Chen, M.K. & Lin, C.S. (2011) Lower ataxia telangiectasia mutated (ATM) mRNA expression is correlated with poor outcome of laryngeal and pharyngeal cancer patients. *Ann Oncol*, Vol. 22, No.5, pp. 1088-1093.

Lin, C.S. (2010) Carcinogenicity of arecoline, an alkaloid of betel nut. In: *SciTopics* , Date of access: 20 August 2010, Available from: http://www.scitopics.com/Carcinogenicity_of_arecoline_an_alkaloid_of_betel_nut.html

Liu, M.T., Chen, Y.R., Chen, S.C., Hu, C.Y., Lin, C.S., Chang, Y.T., Wang, W.B. & Chen, J.Y. (2004) Epstein-Barr virus latent membrane protein 1 induces micronucleus formation, represses DNA repair and enhances sensitivity to DNA-damaging agents in human epithelial cells. *Oncogene*, Vol. 23, No.14, pp. 2531-2539.

Marsit, C.J., Liu, M., Nelson, H.H., Posner, M., Suzuki, M. & Kelsey, K.T. (2004) Inactivation of the Fanconi anemia/BRCA pathway in lung and oral cancers: implications for treatment and survival. *Oncogene*, Vol. 23, No.4, pp. 1000-1004.

Martin, L.P., Hamilton, T.C. & Schilder, R.J. (2008) Platinum resistance: the role of DNA repair pathways. *Clin Cancer Res*, Vol. 14, No.5, pp. 1291-1295.

Martin, R.W., Orelli, B.J., Yamazoe, M., Minn, A.J., Takeda, S. & Bishop, D.K. (2007) RAD51 up-regulation bypasses BRCA1 function and is a common feature of BRCA1-deficient breast tumors. *Cancer Res*, Vol. 67, No.20, pp. 9658-9665.

Miyagawa, K. (2008) Clinical relevance of the homologous recombination machinery in cancer therapy. *Cancer Sci*, Vol. 99, No.2, pp. 187-194.

Mullan, P.B., Quinn, J.E., Gilmore, P.M., McWilliams, S., Andrews, H., Gervin, C., McCabe, N., McKenna, S., White, P., Song, Y.H., Maheswaran, S., Liu, E., Haber, D.A., Johnston, P.G. & Harkin, D.P. (2001) BRCA1 and GADD45 mediated G2/M cell cycle arrest in response to antimicrotubule agents. *Oncogene*, Vol. 20, No.43, pp. 6123-6131.

Norppa, H. & Falck, G.C. (2003) What do human micronuclei contain? *Mutagenesis*, Vol. 18, No.3, pp. 221-233.

Parikh, R.A., White, J.S., Huang, X., Schoppy, D.W., Baysal, B.E., Baskaran, R., Bakkenist, C.J., Saunders, W.S., Hsu, L.C., Romkes, M. & Gollin, S.M. (2007) Loss of distal 11q is associated with DNA repair deficiency and reduced sensitivity to ionizing radiation in head and neck squamous cell carcinoma. *Genes Chromosomes Cancer*, Vol. 46, No.8, pp. 761-775.

Partridge, M., Emilion, G., Pateromichelakis, S., A'Hern, R., Lee, G., Phillips, E. & Langdon, J. (1999) The prognostic significance of allelic imbalance at key chromosomal loci in oral cancer. *Br J Cancer*, Vol. 79, No.11-12, pp. 1821-1827.

Paz-Elizur, T., Ben-Yosef, R., Elinger, D., Vexler, A., Krupsky, M., Berrebi, A., Shani, A., Schechtman, E., Freedman, L. & Livneh, Z. (2006) Reduced repair of the oxidative 8-oxoguanine DNA damage and risk of head and neck cancer. *Cancer Res*, Vol. 66, No.24, pp. 11683-11689.

Posner, M.R., Hershock, D.M., Blajman, C.R., Mickiewicz, E., Winquist, E., Gorbounova, V., Tjulandin, S., Shin, D.M., Cullen, K., Ervin, T.J., Murphy, B.A., Raez, L.E., Cohen, R.B., Spaulding, M., Tishler, R.B., Roth, B., Viroglio Rdel, C., Venkatesan, V., Romanov, I., Agarwala, S., Harter, K.W., Dugan, M., Cmelak, A., Markoe, A.M., Read, P.W., Steinbrenner, L., Colevas, A.D., Norris, C.M., Jr. & Haddad, R.I. (2007) Cisplatin and fluorouracil alone or with docetaxel in head and neck cancer. *N Engl J Med*, Vol. 357, No.17, pp. 1705-1715.

Richardson, C. (2005) RAD51, genomic stability, and tumorigenesis. *Cancer Lett*, Vol. 218, No.2, pp. 127-139.

Richardson, C., Stark, J.M., Ommundsen, M. & Jasin, M. (2004) Rad51 overexpression promotes alternative double-strand break repair pathways and genome instability. *Oncogene*, Vol. 23, No.2, pp. 546-553.

Rizos, E., Sourvinos, G. & Spandidos, D.A. (1998) Loss of heterozygosity at 8p, 9p and 17q in laryngeal cytological specimens. *Oral Oncol*, Vol. 34, No.6, pp. 519-523.

Saldivar, J.S., Wu, X., Follen, M. & Gershenson, D. (2007) Nucleotide excision repair pathway review I: implications in ovarian cancer and platinum sensitivity. *Gynecol Oncol*, Vol. 107, No.1 Suppl 1, pp. S56-71.

Sancar, A., Lindsey-Boltz, L.A., Unsal-Kacmaz, K. & Linn, S. (2004) Molecular mechanisms of mammalian DNA repair and the DNA damage checkpoints. *Annu Rev Biochem*, Vol. 73, No., pp. 39-85.

Sparano, A., Quesnelle, K.M., Kumar, M.S., Wang, Y., Sylvester, A.J., Feldman, M., Sewell, D.A., Weinstein, G.S. & Brose, M.S. (2006) Genome-wide profiling of oral squamous cell carcinoma by array-based comparative genomic hybridization. *Laryngoscope*, Vol. 116, No.5, pp. 735-741.

Specenier, P.M. & Vermorken, J.B. (2009) Current concepts for the management of head and neck cancer: chemotherapy. *Oral Oncol*, Vol. 45, No.4-5, pp. 409-415.

Takimoto, R., MacLachlan, T.K., Dicker, D.T., Niitsu, Y., Mori, T. & el-Deiry, W.S. (2002) BRCA1 transcriptionally regulates damaged DNA binding protein (DDB2) in the DNA repair response following UV-irradiation. *Cancer Biol Ther*, Vol. 1, No.2, pp. 177-186.

Tsai, Y.S., Lee, K.W., Huang, J.L., Liu, Y.S., Juo, S.H., Kuo, W.R., Chang, J.G., Lin, C.S. & Jong, Y.J. (2008) Arecoline, a major alkaloid of areca nut, inhibits p53, represses DNA repair, and triggers DNA damage response in human epithelial cells. *Toxicology*, Vol. 249, No.2-3, pp. 230-237.

Underhill, C., Toulmonde, M. & Bonnefoi, H. (2011) A review of PARP inhibitors: from bench to bedside. *Ann Oncol*, Vol. 22, No. 2, pp. 268-279.

Uziel, T., Lerenthal, Y., Moyal, L., Andegeko, Y., Mittelman, L. & Shiloh, Y. (2003) Requirement of the MRN complex for ATM activation by DNA damage. *Embo J*, Vol. 22, No.20, pp. 5612-5621.

van den Broek, G.B., Wreesmann, V.B., van den Brekel, M.W., Rasch, C.R., Balm, A.J. & Rao, P.H. (2007) Genetic abnormalities associated with chemoradiation resistance of head and neck squamous cell carcinoma. *Clin Cancer Res*, Vol. 13, No.15 Pt 1, pp. 4386-4391.

Venkitaraman, A.R. (2005) Medicine: aborting the birth of cancer. *Nature*, Vol. 434, No.7035, pp. 829-830.

Vermorken, J.B., Mesia, R., Rivera, F., Remenar, E., Kawecki, A., Rottey, S., Erfan, J., Zabolotnyy, D., Kienzer, H.R., Cupissol, D., Peyrade, F., Benasso, M., Vynnychenko, I., De Raucourt, D., Bokemeyer, C., Schueler, A., Amellal, N. & Hitt, R. (2008) Platinum-based chemotherapy plus cetuximab in head and neck cancer. *N Engl J Med*, Vol. 359, No.11, pp. 1116-1127.

Vermorken, J.B., Remenar, E., van Herpen, C., Gorlia, T., Mesia, R., Degardin, M., Stewart, J.S., Jelic, S., Betka, J., Preiss, J.H., van den Weyngaert, D., Awada, A., Cupissol, D., Kienzer, H.R., Rey, A., Desaunois, I., Bernier, J. & Lefebvre, J.L. (2007) Cisplatin, fluorouracil, and docetaxel in unresectable head and neck cancer. *N Engl J Med*, Vol. 357, No.17, pp. 1695-1704.

Vora, H.H., Shah, N.G., Patel, D.D., Trivedi, T.I. & Choksi, T.J. (2003) BRCA1 expression in leukoplakia and carcinoma of the tongue. *J Surg Oncol*, Vol. 83, No.4, pp. 232-240.

Wang, Y.C., Tsai, Y.S., Huang, J.L., Lee, K.W., Kuo, C.C., Wang, C.S., Huang, A.M., Chang, J.Y., Jong, Y.J. & Lin, C.S. (2010) Arecoline arrests cells at prometaphase by deregulating mitotic spindle assembly and spindle assembly checkpoint: implication for carcinogenesis. *Oral Oncol*, Vol. 46, No.4, pp. 255-262.

Wood, R.D., Mitchell, M. & Lindahl, T. (2005) Human DNA repair genes, 2005. *Mutat Res*, Vol. 577, No.1-2, pp. 275-283.

Xu, X., Weaver, Z., Linke, S.P., Li, C., Gotay, J., Wang, X.W., Harris, C.C., Ried, T. & Deng, C.X. (1999) Centrosome amplification and a defective G2-M cell cycle checkpoint induce genetic instability in BRCA1 exon 11 isoform-deficient cells. *Mol Cell*, Vol. 3, No.3, pp. 389-395.

Yang, M.H., Chiang, W.C., Chou, T.Y., Chang, S.Y., Chen, P.M., Teng, S.C. & Wu, K.J. (2006) Increased NBS1 expression is a marker of aggressive head and neck cancer and overexpression of NBS1 contributes to transformation. *Clin Cancer Res*, Vol. 12, No.2, pp. 507-515.

Yoshida, K. & Miki, Y. (2004) Role of BRCA1 and BRCA2 as regulators of DNA repair, transcription, and cell cycle in response to DNA damage. *Cancer Sci*, Vol. 95, No.11, pp. 866-871.

21

# Role of Radioprotectors in the Inhibition of DNA Damage and Modulation of DNA Repair After Exposure to Gamma-Radiation

Dharmendra Kumar Maurya and Thomas Paul Asir Devasagayam
*Radiation Biology and Health Sciences Division,*
*Bhabha Atomic Research Centre, Mumbai,*
*India*

## 1. Introduction

Radiation has been considered an enigma to the general public and the use of radiation for therapeutic and other uses has always been associated with some skepticism. Presently, ionizing radiation is being used in a large number of therapeutic, industrial and other applications apart from for the generation of nuclear power, developing new varieties of high-yielding crops and enhancing storage period of food materials. Radiation treatment is an important therapeutic option for a number of malignancies, but its use is frequently limited due to adverse effects on normal tissues because it generates reactive oxygen species (ROS) such as hydroxyl radical ($^{\cdot}OH$), superoxide radicals ($O_2^{-\cdot}$), singlet oxygen and peroxyl radicals ($ROO^{\cdot}$) in irradiated tissue that induce several pathophysiological changes in the body. The goal of most cancer treatments is to maximize the antineoplastic effect while minimizing harmful side effects for the patient.

Due to the increased use of ionizing radiation in various aspects of human life, there is a need to develop an effective and non-toxic radioprotector. Radioprotectors are compounds that are designed to reduce the damage in normal tissues caused by radiation. These compounds are often antioxidants and must be present before or at the time of radiation for their effectiveness. Other agents, termed mitigators, may be used to minimize toxicity even after radiation has been delivered. Many natural and synthetic chemicals have been investigated in the recent past for their efficacy to protect against radiation-induced damage in biological systems (Maurya et al. 2006). Though a large number of compounds have been shown to be promising as radioprotectors in laboratory studies, few could pass the transition from bench to bedside. In fact, no radioprotective agent is now available, either alone or in combination to meet all the requisites of an ideal radioprotector. Amifostine is the only one that is currently in use having good radioprotection, even though there are reports about contraindications in some cases. Different radioprotectors offer protection to cellular molecules by different mechanisms (Maurya et al. 2006). Some of these compounds protect the target molecules because of their antioxidant mechanism by neutralizing the free radical, some enhances the cellular DNA repair (Maurya et al. 2005a; Maurya et al. 2005b), some modified the signaling pathways, some modulate the immune system and some contribute to a combination of all above mentioned mechanisms.

Radiation-induced DNA double-strand breaks are believed to be important lesions and the key trigger leading to a series of cellular consequences related to cell killing, gene mutation, induction of chromosome aberrations and carcinogenesis. There are two major cellular intrinsic factors deciding the extent of DNA damage in the irradiated cells, i.e. the activity of antioxidant systems and the capacity of DNA repair. There are two distinct but complementary mechanisms for DNA DSB repair namely; non-homologous end joining (NHEJ) and homologous recombination (HR) involving various repair proteins to execute the repair process. When discussing about a single or a group of radioprotectors, one has to keep in mind that radioprotective effect is an ability of radioprotectors to inhibit indirect effect and to repair direct and indirect damages occurred in the cells after radiation exposure. Discussions of all the molecular steps are out of the chapter's scope. In this chapter we are going to discuss a series of consequences happening after irradiation, types of damages induced, possible role of radioprotectors in preventing DNA damage and modulating DNA repair. At the end the future prospects for radioprotectors in mitigation of radiation damage will be discussed.

## 2. Consequences of radiation exposure on cells/ tissues and possible role of radioprotectors

Exposure of living cells/ tissues to ionizing radiation causes damages by transfer of energy to atoms and molecules in the cellular structure. Ionizing radiation causes either excitation or ionization or both to atoms and molecules. These excitations and ionizations can lead to following events inside the cells/ tissues;

i. Generation of free radicals
ii. Breakage of chemical bonds
iii. Formation of new chemical bonds and cross-linkage between macromolecules.
iv. Damage to biomolecules (e.g. DNA, RNA, lipids, proteins) which regulate vital cell processes

To understand the mechanism of action of radioprotectors, an in-depth knowledge of fundamental radiobiological events happening during and shortly after irradiation in tissues and cells is essential. Scheme 1 depicts the series of events happening in cells/ tissues following radiation exposure. Radiation causes damage to cells/ tissues by both direct and indirect actions. During direct action, the radiation is directly causing irreparable damage to critical targets within the cell, such as DNA, RNA, proteins and lipids. In indirect action, radiation interacts with other molecules of the cell that are not critical targets but are close enough to pass on this damage, typically in the form of free radicals. Indirect action of ionizing radiation is due to free radicals, generated during radiolysis. Because body is composed of >80% water, indirect effect is important due to the radiolytic products, mainly the hydroxyl free radical, which is an effective oxidant capable of breaking chemical bonds, initiating lipid peroxidation, in the nano- to microsecond timeframe. After radiation exposures following changes are observed in DNA at the molecular level namely single- or double-strand breaks (DSB), base damage, and DNA-DNA or DNA-protein cross-links (Maurya et al. 2006). If different damages following radiation exposure not repaired, they affect the cell structure and function. After DNA damage has occurred, a number of processes occur in the damaged cell, tissue, or organism, including activation of DNA repair, activation of signal transduction, expression of radiation response genes and stimulation of proliferation etc. These pathways can be important for cell or tissue recovery after radiation exposure but may also play a role in the development of toxicity.

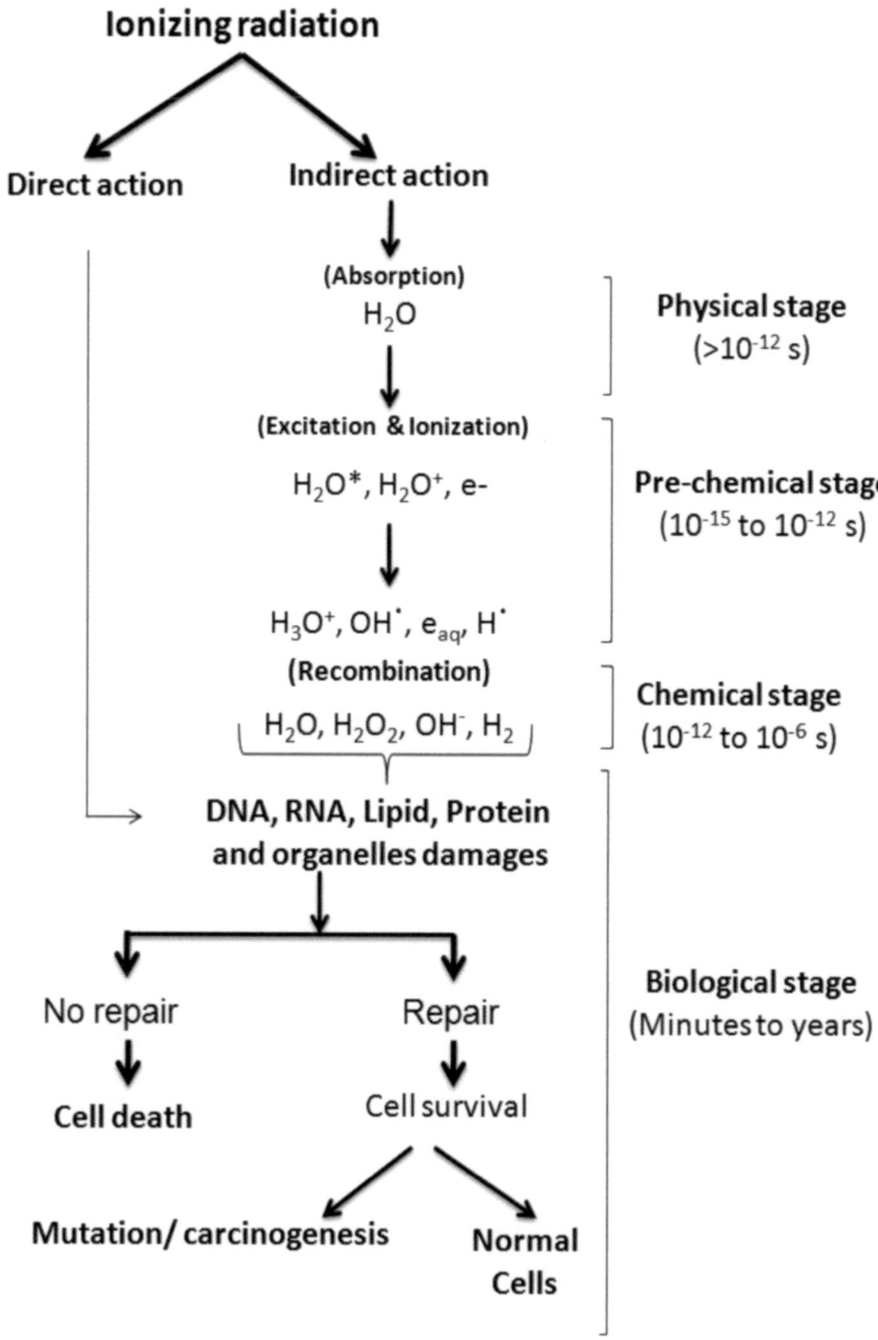


Fig. 1. Chain of the cellular event occurring in the cell/ tissue after ionizing radiation exposure.

## 3. Types of damages induced after radiation exposure

Ionizing radiation can produce different types of damage to DNA, RNA, proteins and other biomolecules. DNA is the major target of radiation induced damage where as membrane is an alternative target. Because the portion of water in living matter is quite high, radiolytic product of the water, mainly hydroxyl radical is responsible for most damages to biomolecules. Hydroxyl radical causes damages to biomolecules by abstracting an H-atom from the biomolecules (from the sugar moiety of the DNA or from the peptide chain of a protein) or by addition of the double bonds of aromatic moieties (DNA bases or aromatic moieties of protein side chain) (Spothem-Maurizot et al. 2008).

Ionizing radiation causes the formation of strand breaks in cellular DNA, as well as other types of lesions in the chromatin of cells(Roots et al. 1985). The amount of DNA damage induced is determined by type of radiation as well as the presence of other molecular components in close proximity to DNA, in particular the presence of proteins because it is well known that most molecular interactions between proteins and DNA occur via amino acids. It is estimated each gray (Gy) of radiation leads to about 100,000 ionizations within a cell, damage to over 1,000 bases, about 1,000 SSBs and about 20 – 40 DSBs. Despite this, 1 Gy kills only 30% of mammalian cells due to the effectiveness of DNA repair - particularly for non-DSB lesions (Spothem-Maurizot et al. 2008).

Lipid peroxidation has been found as the main damage to membrane lipids and lipoproteins. Ionizing radiation induced lipid oxidative modifications of poly unsaturated fatty acids (PUFAs) appears as a dynamic process initiated by hydroxyl free radicals generated by water radiolysis, amplified by a propagating-chain mechanism involving alkyl and peroxyl free radicals, and leading not only to hydroperoxides but also to a lot of other lipidic oxidized end-products, lipid hydroperoxides and conjugated dienes which are early products of lipid peroxidation (Spothem-Maurizot et al. 2008).

During ionizing radiation induced damage to protein, the type of reactions and consequences are quite similar to those of DNA; abstraction of H atoms and binding to aromatic rings, leading to backbone breakage and modification of side chains. All these event leads to peptide chain fragmentation and modification of amino acid side chain (e.g.Trp/formylkynurenine, Tyr/bityrosine,Cys/disulfide) (Spotheim-Maurizot and Davidkova 2011).

## 4. Classification of radioprotective agents

Radioprotective agent can be defined as "any agent that protects against radiation-induced damage, whether administered before, during, or after irradiation". They have been classified into three categories; *i. Prophylactic agents, ii. Mitigators,* and *iii. Therapeutic agents* (Stone et al. 2004). Prophylactic agents are administered before radiation exposure to prevent damage. 'Mitigators' designates agents that are administered during or after radiation exposure with the aim of preventing or reducing the action of radiation on tissues before the appearance of symptoms. These agents include decorporation and chelating agents that mitigate injury from internal radionuclide exposure. They also include blocking agents that mitigate the uptake of radionuclides by specific organs; for example, potassium iodide (KI) protects the thyroid from radioiodine. Therapeutic agents are administered after radiation exposure to treat or facilitate recovery from various aspects of the acute radiation syndrome (ARS) and delayed effects of radiation exposure(Weiss and Landauer 2009). The putative mechanism of radioprotection by plant and herbal radioprotectors may be mediated through several mechanisms, since they are complex mixtures of many chemicals (Jagetia 2007) but this may or may not be true with the pure compounds. Table 1 is a list of some radioprotective agents with their possible radioprotective properties.

| Radioprotectors/ mitigators and therapeutics | Protective property | Ref. |
|---|---|---|
| Amifostine (WR-2721) | This is the most effective thiol protector still today. Administration of WR-2721 intramuscularly (IM) at 300 mg/kg in mice 15 min before radiation, a DRF of 2.7 was obtained with protection observed when injected up to 2 h before irradiation. | (Kuna 1983) |
| Manganese (III) tetrakis (N-methyl-2-pyridyl)porphyrin | Administration for 14 days at a daily dosage of 5 mg/kg provided protection against oxidative damage and lethality in mice exposed to total body irradiation (TBI). | (Lee and Park 2004) |
| Melatonin | Oral administration of 20 mg/ mouse (approximately 800 mg/kg) of melatonin 30 min before irradiation significantly protected intestinal crypt cells. It inhibits chromosomal aberrations and micronuclei formation in lymphocytes. When melatonin treated mice were irradiated at an $LD_{50/30}$ dose (8.15 Gy), survival increased to 85% in the group injected with 250 mg/kg melatonin administered 1 h before irradiation. In a model of acute lung injury in rats, administration of 100 mg/kg melatonin before radiation exposure resulted in decreased inflammation but promoted fibrosis. | (Monobe et al. 2005); (Vijayalaxmi et al. 1999); (Vijayalaxmi et al. 1996); (Serin et al. 2007) |
| ACE inhibitors | They prevent the development of radiation-induced late effects including damage to the kidney and lung. When the ACE inhibitor perindopril was administered to mice for two days before and two days after a lethal dose of gamma-radiation, a significant increase in survival was observed ACE inhibition accelerated hematopoietic recovery and increased the number of hematopoietic stem cells. Protection was mediated by inhibition of the angiotensin II pathway through the AT1 receptor because similar effects were obtained with an AT1 receptor antagonist. | (Charrier et al. 2004; Moulder and Cohen 2007) |
| CDK4/6 inhibitors | Entry into the cell cycle is mediated by cyclin-dependent kinase 4/6 (CDK4/6) activation, followed by CDK2 activation. Johnson et al. have explored the role of cyclin-dependent kinase inhibitors (CDKIs) in the control of the transition from G1 to S phase in ionizing radiation-induced cell toxicity. They confirmed that inhibitors specific for CDK4/6, specifically PD0332991 and 2BrIC, caused reversible G1 arrest (pharmacological quiescence) exclusively in Rb-positive and not Rb-deficient human cells. They also reported that in mice, oral administration of PD0332991 resulted in reversible inhibition of proliferation of different populations of bone marrow cells. Same group also found that PD0332991 markedly enhanced the survival of mice, when applied as late as 20 h after total body irradiation, thus, it acted as a radiomitigator. | (Johnson et al. 2010) |
| Growth factors such as Palifermin, | They are FDA approved growth factors. Palifermin specifically decrease the incidence and duration of severe oral mucositis in | (Spielberger et al. 2004) |

| Radioprotectors/ mitigators and therapeutics | Protective property | Ref. |
|---|---|---|
| Filgrastim | patients with hematologic cancers undergoing high-dose chemotherapy, with or without irradiation, followed by bone marrow transplantation. | |
| Chelators such as diethylenetriamene pentaacetate (DTPA) | DTPA is a FDA-approved agents and includes the calcium and zinc salts, used for the chelation of the transuranic radionuclides plutonium, americium, and curium; Prussian blue for decorporation of $^{137}Cs$; and KI to block uptake of radioactive iodine by the thyroid. | |
| Selenium compounds such as Selenomethionine (SeM) and Sodium selenite | SeM is a naturally occurring derivative of selenium, found in soya, grains, legumes, and selenium-enriched yeast (Whanger 2002). When administered i.p., SeM (4 mg/kg Se) significantly increased the survival of mice irradiated at 10-Gy $^{60}Co$ at a low dose rate (0.2 Gy/min). | (Damron et al. 2004; Diamond et al. 1996) |
| Orientin and vicenin from *Ocimum sanctum* | DRF for 30-days survival in mice treated 30 min before irradiation with low doses (50 mg/kg) i.p. were 1.30 for orientin and 1.37 for vicenin. The same low doses of orientin or vicenin provided efficient protection against bone marrow damage, as measured by chromosomal aberrations and stem cell survival using the exogenous colony-forming unit spleen (CFU-S) assay. | (Nayak and Devi 2005; Uma Devi et al. 2000) |
| Genistein | A DRF of 1.16 was obtained at a genistein dose (200 mg/kg SC) that did not result in any adverse pathology or behavioural toxicity. | (Landauer et al. 2003) |

Table 1. A list of well known radioprotectors, mitigators and therapeutics.

## 5. Role of radioprotectors in inhibition of DNA damages and enhancement of DNA repair after radiation exposure

In order to restore the cellular function DNA repair is our important parameter that can be modified by radioprotective compounds to improve the radioprotection. Most of the cellular alterations induced by ionizing radiation is indirect and is mediated by the generation of free radicals and related reactive species, mainly derived from oxygen. Hence natural compounds with antioxidant activity have potential as good radioprotectors. Though a large variety of compounds have shown promise as radioprotector in laboratory studies, most of them failed even before reaching the preclinical stage due to toxicity and side effects.

Protection of cellular molecules including DNA from radiation can be achieved by various mechanisms. Protection to cellular DNA can be achieved by reducing the quantity of damage (by radical scavenging and chemical repair) followed by enhancement of biochemical repair of DNA to improved protection and recovery. Thus DNA repair is one of the important parameters that can be modified to attain improved protection. Many natural and related compounds are shown to be effective radioprotectors. They protect cellular molecules including DNA by various mechanisms. These include their antioxidant capacity and induction of repair mechanisms. Our studies have identified many compounds with radioprotective ability using *in vitro, ex vivo* and *in vivo* model systems. The systems used are rat liver and brain sub-cellular organelles, plasmid DNA, human lymphocytes, mammalian cells in culture and mouse. Different parameters also have been used to estimate damage and protection. Our studies have identified caffeine, chlorophyllin, flavonoid troxerutin, ferulic acid present in cereals, the food flavoring agent vanillin and tocopherol-mono-glucoside among others as effective radioprotectors. Details of some of these molecules are given below.

### 5.1 Alpha tocopherol monoglucoside (TMG)

TMG, a water-soluble derivative of Vitamin E, has been reported to be a good radioprotector with low toxicity (Kapoor et al. 2002; Nair et al. 2004; Rajagopalan et al. 2002). It has been reported that an oral administration of 2 g/kg body weight of TMG, five minutes prior to radiation exposure, resulted in early recovery of the radiation-induced weight loss (Nair et al. 2003). Embryonic death, resulting from exposure to 2 Gy radiation in pregnant mice, was reduced by 75% with a single intra peritoneal injection of TMG (0.6 g/kg body weight) prior to the radiation exposure. However, the administration of TMG after the radiation exposure did not have any effect on the embryonic mortality (Nair et al. 2003). A single intra peritoneal injection of TMG (0.6 g/kg) to mice, after whole body irradiation, elevated the $LD_{50\,(30)}$ from 6 to 6.72 Gy (Nair et al. 2003). Radiation induced formation of micronucleated polychromatic and normochromatic erythrocytes in mouse bone marrow cells was inhibited by a single injection of TMG (0.6 g/kg body weight) i.p. after the radiation exposure with a dose reduction factor of 0.5 (Satyamitra et al. 2001). Our in vitro studies, either with humans or mice, peripheral blood leucocytes showed that the presence of TMG (0.5 mM) in post-irradiation incubation medium did not enhance the repair of DNA strand breaks(Salvi et al. 2007). TMG is also effective in preventing radiation-induced bone marrow death in mice and enhance hematopoietic recovery (Ueno et al. 2009), (Cherdyntseva et al. 2005).

### 5.2 Baicalein

Baicalein (scheme 2A), has been reported to possess lipid peroxidation inhibitory activity. Our results indicate that baicalein is a potent radioprotector at micromolar (5-50) levels. The protective effect, at 5 μM, was 80% against formation of thiobarbituric acid reactive substances (TBARS) and 50% against lipid hydroperoxide. The protective ability against protein carbonyl formation was 50% and protein hydroperoxide formation 85% at the same concentration. Similar protective effects were also observed against damage to glutathione peroxidase and superoxide dismutase. A concentration dependent effect also was seen with most of the parameters examined. Single-strand break formation induced by radiation also was accentuated with baicalein. It also inhibited the DNA binding caused by radiation. (Tilak and Devasagayam 2003). Recently it was found that baicalein has a radioprotective effect against NF-κB-mediated inflammatory response through MAPKs and the Akt pathway (Lee et al. 2011).

### 5.3 Caffeine

Caffeine is a bitter, white crystalline xanthine alkaloid that is a psychoactive stimulant present in coffee and cola-based soft drinks. In humans, caffeine acts as a central nervous system (CNS) stimulant, temporarily warding off drowsiness and restoring alertness. We have shown that caffeine protected against DNA strand breaks in plasmid pBR322, a system devoid of repair and replication machinery (Kumar et al. 2001). This protective effect was related to the demonstrated antioxidant properties of caffeine in vitro, including scavenging of primary and secondary ROS (Devasagayam et al. 1996). Pretreatment with caffeine at doses of 5 or 15 mg/kg, administered either i.p. or in drinking water, reduced radiation-induced frequency of chromosomal aberrations. Farooqi and Kesavan, had shown that administration immediately after radiation exposure also significantly reduced chromosome aberrations (Farooqi and Kesavan 1992). In our other study, George et al showed that when caffeine (80 mg/kg) was administered i.p. 1 h before irradiation it increases the survival of the mice (George et al. 1999). Radioprotection in mice at the same dose of caffeine may be related to modulation of radiation-induced apoptotic genes, for example, the depression of bax mRNA (Kim et al. 2003). This same high dose of caffeine protected against local radiation (35 Gy) skin reactions of mice. However, caffeine injection into a mouse fibrosarcoma did not affect the tumor response to irradiation (Hebbar et al. 2002).

### 5.4 Chlorophyllin

Chlorophyllin (CHL) (scheme 2B), is a water-soluble mixture of sodium-copper salts of green plant pigment, chlorophyll. CHL is widely marketed for a variety of dietary and medicinal uses. Recently, it has also been shown to occur naturally in a constituent of traditional Chinese medicine (Chiu et al. 2003). It has chemopreventive, antimutagenic and anticarcinogenic properties (Egner et al. 2001; Guo et al. 1995). Our lab has explored it radioprotective property in various model systems. It exhibited protection against radiation and chemical induced cytogenetic damage (Kumar et al. 1999)). CHL inhibited lipid peroxidation induced by 2,2'-azobis(2-propionimidinedihydrochloride) (AAPH) in lymphocytes in vitro. It also partially prevented radiation-induced suppression of mitogenic stimulation of lymphocytes in vitro (Kumar et al. 2004).

### 5.5 Ferulic acid

Ferulic acid (FA) (Scheme 2C) is a monophenolic phenylpropanoid occurring in plant materials such as rice, green tea and coffee beans. It is well known antioxidant and has ability to scavenge the free radicals. As for toxicity of this compound, no *in vivo* data is available, but *in vitro* cytotoxicity in rat hepatocytes showed an $LD_{50}$ of 25 mM (Maurya et al. 2005b). We have explored the effect of ferulic acid on gamma-radiation-induced relaxation of plasmid pBR322 DNA and induction of DNA strand breaks in peripheral blood leukocytes and bone marrow cells of mice exposed to whole body gamma-radiation. Presence of 0.5 mM ferulic acid significantly inhibited the disappearance of supercoiled (ccc) plasmid pBR322 with a dose modifying factor (DMF) of 2.0. Intraperitoneal administration of different amounts (50, 75 and 100 mg/kg body weight) of FA 1 h prior to 4Gy gamma-radiation exposure showed dose-dependent decrease in the yield of DNA strands breaks in murine peripheral blood leukocytes and bone marrow cells as evidenced from comet assay. The dose-dependent protection was more pronounced in bone marrow cells than in the blood leukocytes. It was observed that there was a time-dependent disappearance of radiation induced strand breaks in blood leukocytes (as evidenced from comet parameters) following whole body radiation exposure commensurate with DNA repair (Maurya et al. 2005b). Administration of 50 mg/kg body weight of FA after whole body irradiation of mice resulted disappearance of DNA strand breaks at a faster rate compared to irradiated controls, suggesting enhanced DNA repair in FA treated animals. When normal and tumor cells were treated with FA and the DNA damage measured after radiation exposure it was found that FA is having preferential protection to normal cells compared to tumor cells both under *ex vivo* and *in vivo* conditions (Maurya and Nair 2006). Recently, Ma et al have suggested that the radioprotective efficacy by FA may be a result of early recovery of hematopoietic cells due to enhanced production of G-CSF and erythropoietin (Ma et al. 2011a). They have also reported that FA had a radioprotective effect through the ERK pathway to inhibit apoptosis and oxidation (Ma et al. 2011b).

### 5.6 Troxerutin

Troxerutin (Scheme 2D), a derivative of the natural flavonoid rutin extracted from *Sophora japonica* (Japanese pogoda tree) has been commonly used in the treatment of Chronic Venous Insufficiency (CVI) disease (Lefebvre and Lacombe 1991). In clinical trials, troxerutin has been given in doses up to 7 g per day orally for up to 6 months with no contraindications (Glacet-Bernard et al. 1994). It has been reported that during radiotherapy of head and neck cancer, administration of a mixture of troxerutin and coumarin offered protection to salivary glands and mucosa. We have shown that troxerutin inhibited lipid peroxidation in membrane of sub-cellular organelles as well as normal tissues of tumor-bearing mice exposed to gamma-radiation. Further, it was found that administration of troxerutin resulted in differential protection of DNA in blood leucocytes and bone marrow cells and not in cells of tumor in whole body irradiated tumor-bearing mice. Troxerutin protected the human peripheral blood leucocytes from radiation-induced DNA strand breaks in a concentration dependent manner under *ex vivo* condition of irradiation (2Gy)

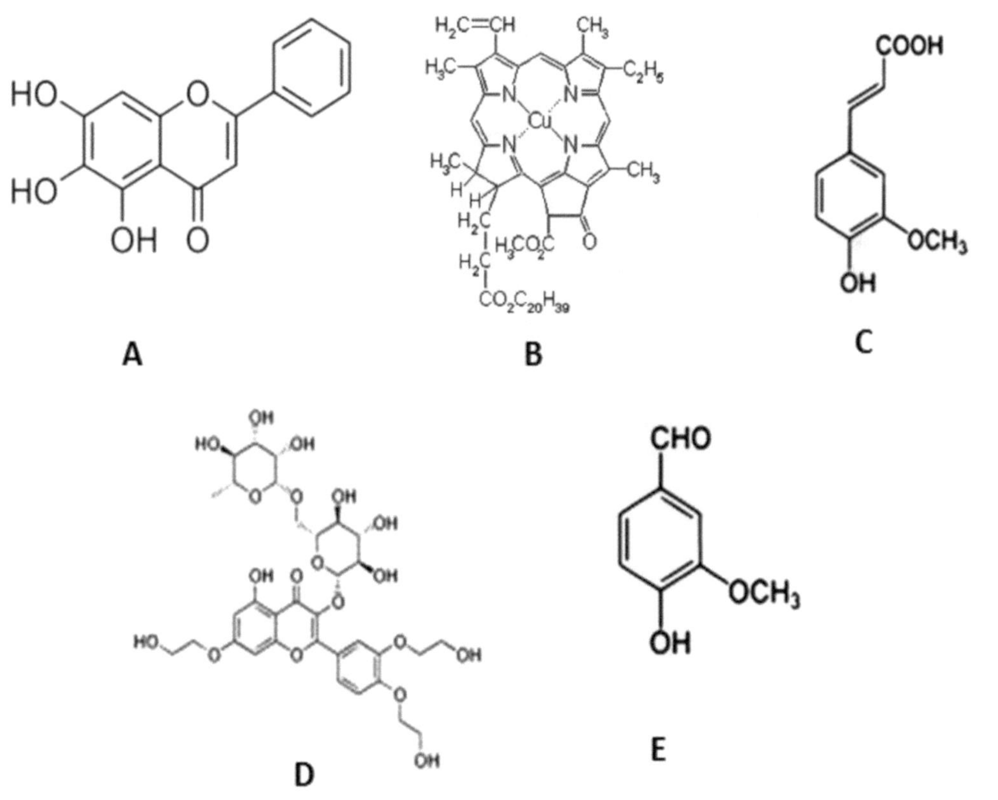


Fig. 2. A. Baicalein, B. Chlorophyllin, C. Ferulic acid, D. Troxerutin, E. Vanillin.

(Maurya et al. 2004). Intraperitoneal administration of troxerutin (175 mg/kg body weight) to mice before and after whole body radiation exposure inhibited micronuclei formation in blood reticulocytes significantly. The administration of different doses (75, 125 and 175 mg/kg body weight) of troxerutin 1 h prior to 4 Gy gamma-radiation exposure showed dose-dependent decrease in the yield of DNA strand breaks in murine blood leucocytes and bone marrow cells. The dose-dependent protection was more pronounced in bone marrow cells than in blood leucocytes. Administration of 175 mg/kg body weight of the drug (i.p.) 1 h prior or immediately after whole body irradiation of mice showed that the decrease in strand breaks depended on the post-irradiation interval at which the analysis was done. Measurement of DNA repair potential of the troxerutin shows that it enhances the DNA repair (Maurya et al. 2005a). So the observed time-dependent decrease in the DNA strand breaks could be attributed to enhanced DNA repair in troxerutin administered animals.

### 5.7 Vanillin

Vanillin (4-hydroxy-3-methoxybenzaldehyde), scheme 2E, is a compound used as a flavoring agent and as a dietary component. It is the major component of natural vanilla, which is one of the most widely used and important flavoring materials throughout the world. The source of vanilla is the bean, or pod, of the tropical Vanilla orchid (principally *Vanilla planifolia* Andrews, syn. *V. fragrans* (Salisb. Ames)). Vanillin is an antioxidant capable of protecting membrane against lipid peroxidation and DNA against strand breaks induced by reactive oxygen species like singlet oxygen. Vanillin and its analogs were strongly anti-mutagenic or anti-genotoxic in most studies. Vanillin also suppresses the chromosomal aberrations induced by X-rays in V79 cells *in vitro* (Keshava et al. 1998) and in mice *in vivo* (Sasaki et al. 1990). Imanishi et al. have shown anti-mutagenic effect of vanillin against UV and X-rays in Chinese hamster V79 cells (Imanishi et al. 1990). We have explored the effect of vanillin on radiation-induced DNA damage in plasmid pBR322 (*in vitro*), human peripheral blood leucocytes and mouse splenic lymphocytes (*ex vivo*) and in mouse (*in vivo*), besides the possible mechanisms involved in terms of scavenging radiation related free radicals by pulse radiolysis. Our finding shows that presence of 0.5mM vanillin has a dose-modifying factor (DMF) of 6.75 for 50% inactivation of ccc form. Exposure of human peripheral blood leucocytes (*ex vivo*) to radiation causes strand breaks in the cellular DNA, as assessed by comet assay. When leucocytes were exposed to 2 Gy of -radiation there was an increase in parameters of comet assay such as %DNA in tail, tail length, 'tail moment' and 'Olive tail moment'. The presence of 0.5 mM vanillin during irradiation significantly reduced these parameters. Damage to DNA in mouse peripheral blood leucocytes after whole-body exposure of mice (*in vivo*) to radiation was studied at 1 and 2 h post-irradiation. There was recovery of DNA damage in terms of the above-mentioned parameters at 2h post-irradiation. This was more than that observed at 1 h (Maurya et al. 2007). The recovery was more in vanillin treated mice. Hence our studies showed that vanillin offers protection to DNA against radiation-induced damage possibly imparting a role other than modulation of DNA repair (Maurya et al. 2007).

## 6. Future prospects for radioprotectors in mitigation of radiation damage

Research in the development of radioprotectors worldwide has focused on screening a variety of chemical and biological compounds (Maurya et al. 2006; Nair et al. 2001; Weiss and Landauer 2009). Various natural or synthetic compounds having either antioxidant or cytoprotective or immunomodulatory property or their combination have been evaluated extensively for their radioprotective potentials in both in vitro and in vivo models (Maurya et al. 2006; Weiss and Landauer 2009). So far no synthetic radioprotective molecule is available that is perfectly safe and effective. Herbal origin radioprotectors have a hope to overcome the toxicity issues seen with the synthetic compounds. There are many reports on the pre-irradiation radioprotectors, using synthetic or natural compounds. There are hardly a few post-irradiation radioprotectors. Such radioprotectors based on induction of DNA repair and related mechanisms will have great potential in reducing accidental exposure such as those that occur due to natural calamities like earthquakes and tsunami as in the case of Fukushima daiichi nuclear reactors. To overcome this kind of situation, there is a need to locate more effective post-irradiation effective radioprotector that can enhance the DNA repair. Since the DNA is the critical target for ionizing radiation, future, studies should focus on compounds that have potential to enhance the process of DNA repair which is essential after radiation exposure. These also can be used in other cases of exposure such as that of radiotherapy for cancer.

## 7. References

Charrier, S., Michaud, A., Badaoui, S., Giroux, S., Ezan E, Sainteny, F., Corvol, P., & Vainchenker, W. (2004). Inhibition of angiotensin I-converting enzyme induces radioprotection by preserving murine hematopoietic short-term reconstituting cells. *Blood* Vol.104, No.4, pp. 978-985

Cherdyntseva, N., Shishkina, A., Butorin, I., Murase, H., Gervas, P., & Kagiya, T.V. (2005). Effect of tocopherol-monoglucoside (TMG), a water-soluble glycosylated derivate of vitamin E, on hematopoietic recovery in irradiated mice. *Journal of Radiation Research,* Vol.46, No.1 pp.37-41

Chiu LC, Kong CK, and Ooi VE. (2003). Antiproliferative effect of chlorophyllin derived from a traditional Chinese medicine Bombyx mori excreta on human breast cancer MCF-7 cells. *International Journal of Oncology,* Vol. 23, No.3, pp.729-735

Damron, T.A., Spadaro, J.A., Horton, J.A., Margulies, B.S., Strauss, J.A., & Farnum, C.E. (2004). Novel radioprotectant drugs for sparing radiation-induced damage to the physis. *International Journal of Radiation Biology,* Vol. 80, No. 3, pp.217-228

Devasagayam, T.P., Kamat, J.P., Mohan, H., & Kesavan, P.C. (1996). Caffeine as an antioxidant: inhibition of lipid peroxidation induced by reactive oxygen species. *Biochim Biophys Acta, Vol.* 1282, No 1, pp.63-70

Diamond, A.M., Dale, P., Murray, J.L., & Grdina, D.J. (1996). The inhibition of radiation-induced mutagenesis by the combined effects of selenium and the aminothiol WR-1065. *Mutation Research,* Vol. 356, No.2, pp.147-154

Egner, P.A., Wang, J.B., Zhu, Y.R., Zhang, B.C., Wu, Y., Zhang, QN., Qian, G.S., Kuang, S.Y., Gange, S.J, Jacobson, L.P., et al. (2001). Chlorophyllin intervention reduces aflatoxin-DNA adducts in individuals at high risk for liver cancer. *Proceeding In National Academy of Science,* U S A, Vol. 98, No.25, pp.14601-14606

Farooqi, Z., & Kesavan, P.C. (1992). Radioprotection by caffeine pre- and post-treatment in the bone marrow chromosomes of mice given whole-body gamma-irradiation. *Mutation Research,* Vol. 269, No.2, pp.225-230

George, K.C., Hebbar, S.A., Kale, S.P., & Kesavan, P.C. (1999). Caffeine protects mice against whole-body lethal dose of gamma-irradiation. *Journal of Radiological Protection,* Vol.19, No.2, pp.171-176

Glacet-Bernard, A., Coscas, G., Chabanel, A., Zourdani, A., Lelong, F., & Samama, M.M. (1994). A randomized, double-masked study on the treatment of retinal vein occlusion with troxerutin. *Americal Journal of Ophthalmology,* Vol. 118, No.4, pp.421-429

Guo, D., Horio, D.T., Grove, J.S., & Dashwood, R.H. (1995). Inhibition by chlorophyllin of 2-amino-3-methylimidazo-[4,5-f]quinoline-induced tumorigenesis in the male F344 rat. *Cancer Letters,* Vol. 95, No.1-2, pp.161-165

Hebbar, S.A., Mitra, A.K., George, K.C., & Verma, N.C. (2002). Caffeine ameliorates radiation-induced skin reactions in mice but does not influence tumour radiation response. *Journal of Radiological Protection,* Vol. 22, No.1, pp.63-69

Imanishi, H., Sasaki, Y.F., Matsumoto, K., Watanabe ,M., Ohta, T., Shirasu, Y., & Tutikawa, K. (1990). Suppression of 6-TG-resistant mutations in V79 cells and recessive spot formations in mice by vanillin. *Mutation Research,* Vol. 243, No.2, pp.151-158

Jagetia, G.C. (2007). Radioprotective Potential of Plants and Herbs against the Effects of Ionizing Radiation. *Journal of Clinical Biochemistry and Nutrition,* Vol. 40, No.2, pp.74-81

Johnson, S. M., Torrice, C. D., Bell, J. F., Monahan, K. B., Jiang, Q., Wang, Y., Ramsey, M. R., Jin, J., Wong, K., Su, L., Zhou, D., & Sharpless, N. E. (2010). Mitigation of hematologic radiation toxicity in mice through pharmacological quiescence induced by CDK4/6 inhibition. *The Journal of Clinical Investigation,* Vol 120, No. 7, pp.2528–2536.

Kapoor, S., Mukherjee, T., Kagiya, T.V., & Nair, C.K. (2002). Redox reactions of tocopherol monoglucoside in aqueous solutions: a pulse radiolysis study. *Journal of Radiation Research (Tokyo),* Vol. 43, No.1, pp.99-106

Keshava, C., Keshava, N., Ong, T.M., & Nath, J. (1998). Protective effect of vanillin on radiation-induced micronuclei and chromosomal aberrations in V79 cells. Mutation Research, Vol. 397, No.2, pp.149-159

Kim, J.K., Kim, J.H., & Yoon, Y.D. (2003). Evaluation of caffeine as a radioprotector in whole-body irradiated male mice. *In Vivo,* Vol.17, No.2, pp.197-200

Kumar, S.S., Chaubey, R.C., Devasagayam, T.P.A., Priyadarsini, K.I., & Chauhan, P.S. (1999). Inhibition of radiation-induced DNA damage in plasmid pBR322 by chlorophyllin and possible mechanism(s) of action. *Mutation Research,* Vol. 425, No.1, pp.71-79

Kumar, S.S., Devasagayam, T.P.A., Jayashree, B., & Kesavan, P.C. (2001). Mechanism of protection against radiation-induced DNA damage in plasmid pBR322 by caffeine. *International Journal of Radiation Biology,* Vol. 77, No.5, pp.617-623

Kumar, S.S., Shankar, B., & Sainis, K.B. (2004). Effect of chlorophyllin against oxidative stress in splenic lymphocytes in vitro and in vivo. *Biochim Biophys Acta,* Vol.1672, No.2, pp.100-111

Kuna, P. (1983). Duration and degree of radioprotection of WR-2721 in mice following its intraperitoneal, intramuscular and subcutaneous administration. *Radiobiological Radiotherapy (Berl),* Vol.24, No.3, pp.357-364

Landauer, M.R., Srinivasan, V., & Seed, T.M.. (2003). Genistein treatment protects mice from ionizing radiation injury. *Journal of Applied Toxicology,* Vo. 23, No.6, pp.379-385

Lee, E.K., Kim, J.M., Choi, J., Jung, K.J., Kim, D.H., Chung, S.W., Ha, Y.M., Yu, B.P., & Chung, H.Y. (2011). Modulation of NF-kappaB and FOXOs by baicalein attenuates the radiation-induced inflammatory process in mouse kidney. *Free Radicical Research,* Vol. 45, No.5, pp.507-517

Lee, J.H., & Park, J.W. (2004). A manganese porphyrin complex is a novel radiation protector. *Free Radical Biology in Medicine,* Vol. 37, No.2, pp.272-283

Lefebvre, G., & Lacombe, C. (1991). Venous insufficiency in the pregnant woman. Rheological correction by troxerutin. *Rev Fr Gynecol Obstet*, Vol.86(2 Pt 2), pp.206-208

Ma, Z.C., Hong, Q., Wang, Y.G., Tan, H.L., Xiao, C.R., Liang, Q.D., Lu, B.B., & Gao, Y. (2011a). Effects of ferulic acid on hematopoietic cell recovery in whole-body gamma irradiated mice. *International Journal of Radiation Biology*. (doi:10.3109/09553002.2011.548438)

Ma, Z.C., Hong, Q., Wang, Y.G., Tan, H.L., Xiao, C.R., Liang, Q.D., Wang, D.G., & Gao, Y. (2011b). Ferulic acid protects lymphocytes from radiation-predisposed oxidative stress through extracellular regulated kinase. *International Journal of Radiation Biology*, Vol.87, No.2, pp.130-140

Maurya, D.K., Adhikari, S., Nair, C.K.K., & Devasagayam T.P.A. (2007). DNA protective properties of vanillin against gamma-radiation under different conditions: possible mechanisms. *Mutation Research*, Vol. 634, No.1-2, pp.69-80

Maurya, D.K., Balakrishnan, S., Salvi, V.P., & Nair, C.K.K. (2005a). Protection of cellular DNA from gamma-radiation-induced damages and enhancement in DNA repair by troxerutin. *Molecular and Cellular Biochemistry*, Vol. 280, No.1-2, pp.57-68

Maurya, D.K., Devasagayam, T.P.A., & Nair, C.K.K. (2006). Some novel approaches for radioprotection and the beneficial effect of natural products. Indian Journal of Experimental Biology, Vol. 44, No.2, pp.93-114

Maurya, D.K., & Nair, C.K.K. (2006). Preferential radioprotection to DNA of normal tissues by ferulic acid under ex vivo and in vivo conditions in tumor bearing mice. *Molecular and Cellular Biochemistry*, Vol. 285, No.1-2, pp.181-190

Maurya, D.K., Salvi, V.P., & Nair, C.K.K. (2004). Radioprotection of normal tissues in tumor-bearing mice by troxerutin. *Journal of Radiation Research* (Tokyo), Vol. 45, No.2, pp.221-228

Maurya, D.K., Salvi, V.P., & Nair, C.K. K.(2005b). Radiation protection of DNA by ferulic acid under in vitro and in vivo conditions. *Molecular and Cellular Biochemistry*, Vol. 280, No.1-2, pp.209-217

Monobe, M., Hino, M., Sumi, M., Uzawa, A., Hirayama, R., Ando, K., & Kojima, S. (2005). Protective effects of melatonin on gamma-ray induced intestinal damage. *International Journal of Radiation Biology*, Vo. 81, No.11, pp.855-860

Moulder, J.E., & Cohen, E.P. (2007). Future strategies for mitigation and treatment of chronic radiation-induced normal tissue injury. *Seminal in Radiation Oncology*, Vol. 17, No.2, pp.141-148

Nair, C.K.K., Parida, D.K., & Nomura, T. (2001). Radioprotectors in radiotherapy. Journal of Radiatin Research (Tokyo), Vol. 42, No.1, pp.21-37

Nair, C.K.K., Salvi, V., Kagiya, T.V., & Rajagopalan, R. (2004). Relevance of radioprotectors in radiotherapy: studies with tocopherol monoglucoside. *Journal of Environmental Pathology, Toxicology and Oncology*, Vol 23, No.2, pp.153-160

Nair, C.K.K., Devi, P.U., Shimanskaya, R., Kunugita, N., Murase, H., Gu, Y-H., & Kagiya, T.V. (2003). Water soluble vitamin E (TMG) as a radioprotector. *Indian Journal of Experimental Biology*, Vol.41, pp.1365-1371

Nayak, V., & Devi, P.U.( 2005). Protection of mouse bone marrow against radiation-induced chromosome damage and stem cell death by the ocimum flavonoids orientin and vicenin. *Radiation Research*, Vol. 163, No.2, pp.165-171

Rajagopalan, R., Wani, K., Huilgol, N.G., Kagiya, T.V., & Nair, C.K.K. (2002). Inhibition of gamma-radiation induced DNA damage in plasmid pBR322 by TMG, a water-soluble derivative of vitamin E. *Journal of Radiation Research* (Tokyo), Vol. 43, No.2, pp.153-159

Roots, R., Kraft, G., & Gosschalk, E. (1985). The formation of radiation-induced DNA breaks: the ratio of double-strand breaks to single-strand breaks. International Journal of Radiation Oncology Biology and Physics, Vol. 11, No.2, pp.259-265

Salvi, V.P., Maurya, D.K., Kagiya, T.V., & Nair, C.K.K. (2007). Enhancement in repair of radiation-induced DNA strand breaks in vivo by tocopherol monoglucoside. *International Journal of Low Radiation*, Vol.4, No.1, pp.43-52

Sasaki, Y.F., Ohta, T., Imanishi, H., Watanabe, M., Matsumoto, K., Kato, T., & Shirasu, Y. (1990). Suppressing effects of vanillin, cinnamaldehyde, and anisaldehyde on chromosome aberrations induced by X-rays in mice. *Mutation Research*, Vol. 243, No.4, pp.299-302

Satyamitra, M., Devi ,P.U., Murase, H, & Kagiya, V.T. (2001). In vivo radioprotection by alpha-TMG: preliminary studies. *Mutation Research*, Vol. 479, No.1-2, pp.53-61

Serin, M., Gulbas, H., Gursces, I., Erkal, H.S., & Yucel, N. (2007). The histopathological evaluation of the effectiveness of melatonin as a protectant against acute lung injury induced by radiation therapy in a rat model. *International Journal of Radiation Biology*, Vol. 83, No.3, pp.187-193

Spielberger, R., Stiff, P., Bensinger, W., Gentile, T., Weisdorf, D., Kewalramani, T., Shea, T., Yanovich, S., Hansen, K., Noga, S., et al. (2004). Palifermin for oral mucositis after intensive therapy for hematologic cancers. *New England Journal of Medicine*, Vol. 351, No.25, pp.2590-2598

Spotheim-Maurizot, M., & Davidkova, M. (2011). Radiation damage to DNA in DNA-protein complexes. Journal of Physics: Conference Series 261 (2011) (doi:10.1088/1742-6596/261/1/012010)

Spothem-Maurizot, M., Mostafavi, M., Douki, T., & Belloni, J., editors. (2008). Radiation Chemistry: from basics to applications in material and life science: EDP Science.

Stone, H.B., Moulder, J.E., Coleman, C.N., Ang, K.K., Anscher, M.S., Barcellos-Hoff, M.H., Dynan, W.S., Fike, J.R., Grdina, D.J., Greenberger, J.S., et al. (2004). Models for evaluating agents intended for the prophylaxis, mitigation and treatment of radiation injuries. Report of an NCI Workshop, December 3-4, 2003. *Radiation Research*,Vol. 162, No.6, pp.711-728

Tilak, J.C., & Devasagayam, T.P.A. (2003). Radioprotective property of baicalein. *BARC Newsletter*, Vol. 249, pp.98–104

Ueno, M., Inano. H., Onoda, M., Murase, H., Ikota, N., Kagiya, T.V., & Anzai, K. (2009). Modification of mortality and tumorigenesis by tocopherol-mono-glucoside (TMG) administered after X irradiation in mice and rats. *Radiation Research*, Vol. 172, No.4, pp.519-524

Devi, P.U., Ganasoundari, A., Vrinda, B., Srinivasan, K.K., & Unnikrishnan, M.K. (2000). Radiation protection by the ocimum flavonoids orientin and vicenin: mechanisms of action. *Radiation Research*, Vol 154, No.4, pp.455-460

Vijayalaxmi, Meltz, M.L., Reiter, R.J., Herman, T.S., & Kumar, K.S. (1999). Melatonin and protection from whole-body irradiation: survival studies in mice. Mutation Research, Vol. 425, No.1, pp.21-27

Vijayalaxmi, Reiter, R.J., Herman, T.S., & Meltz, M.L. (1996). Melatonin and radioprotection from genetic damage: in vivo/in vitro studies with human volunteers. *Mutation Research*, Vol. 371, No.3-4, pp.221-228

Weiss, J.F., & Landauer, M.R. (2009). History and development of radiation-protective agents. International Journal of Radiation Biology, Vo. 85, No.7, pp.539-573

# 22

# DNA-Binding Radioprotectors

Pavel Lobachevsky[1], Alesia Ivashkevich[1],
Olga A. Martin[1,2] and Roger F. Martin[1]
[1]*Laboratory of Molecular Radiation Biology,*
*Peter MacCallum Cancer Centre*
[2]*Laboratory of Molecular Pharmacology,*
*Center for Cancer Research, National Cancer Institute*
[1]*Australia*
[2]*USA*

## 1. Introduction

For decades the world of radioprotectors has been dominated by the aminothiols, in particular WR1065 and its prodrug amifostine. These drugs emerged from an extensive programme of synthesis and evaluation under the auspices of the Walter Reed Army Institute of Research starting in the early 1950s (Sweeny, 1979). As discussed in detail in section 4 below, structure-activity studies on a series of aminothiols in John Ward's lab at the University of San Diego established a relationship between net charge and radioprotective activity. Positive charge conferred a DNA binding capability, by ionic interaction, and improved radioprotective activity. This was consistent with the fact that an important aspect of the mechanism of radioprotection by WR1065 is its radical scavenging activity. Given the limited range of diffusion of hydroxyl radicals generated from ionisation of water molecules, it makes sense that the radical scavengers will be most effective when located in the close vicinity of DNA. This basic rationale prompted the synthesis and evaluation of an aminothiol tethered to a DNA intercalating agent (Laayoun et al., 1994), but there is no evidence in the literature of a systematic follow-up.

Also, the new DNA binding radioprotector methylproamine emerged not from a rational design premise, but rather, from the serendipitous discovery of radioprotective activity of a minor groove binder Hoechst 33342 synthesized by the Hoechst company as part of a program aimed at developing antihelminthics. From that starting point, a modest lead optimisation program guided by a mechanistic hypothesis showed that radioprotective activity was enhanced by the introduction of more electron-rich substituents into the phenyl ring of the molecule.

Thus, this article links two groups of radioprotectors with the common feature of DNA-binding, albeit with quite different affinities. The dissociation constant for the WR1065-DNA interaction is in the mM range (Smoluk et al., 1986), whereas that for methylproamine is a few hundred nM (Martin et al., 2004). Accordingly, the relative radioprotective potency of WR1065 and methylproamine differs by more than 2-orders of magnitude. In contrast to this focus, other publications review a much wider range of radioprotectors (Hosseinimehr, 2007; Weiss & Landauer, 2009; Citrin, 2010).

## 2. DNA damage and biological response to radiation

Both the hazards and potential beneficial uses of ionizing radiation (IR) were realised soon after the discovery of X-rays by Wilhelm Conrad Roentgen in 1895. Studies of Hiroshima and Nagasaki survivors, reconstructed dosimetry, and unfortunate accidents at nuclear plants documented a pattern of events following a whole-body IR exposure, confirmed by extensive animal experiments. Exposure to high doses of IR (100-150 Gy) leads to death within a few hours which results from neurological and cardiovascular breakdown. At intermediate dose levels (5-12 Gy), death occurs within a few days and is associated with gastrointestinal syndrome. At lower doses (2.5-5 Gy) death occurs within several weeks due to haematopoietic syndrome (Hall, 1973). All these effects are attributable to killing of critical cells, and the question of how IR kills cells has stimulated much research. A key milestone was the identification of DNA as the critical molecular target. This research was prompted by both the potential uses of IR, for example in cancer therapy, and by concerns about effects of IR on health. Potentially damaging exposure may come from diagnostic radiology such as computed tomography as well as from cosmic rays, the sun and radioactive nuclides in the ground (e.g. radon), during high altitude journeys, or in space. Such concerns about occupational and environmental radiation exposure have prompted much scientific and legislative activity, the latter leading to the establishment of the International Commission on Radiological Protection.

It is a commonly recognised concept that two distinct mechanisms are responsible for induction of DNA damage by IR; one involves direct ionisation of atoms in the DNA molecule and usually is referred to as the direct effect, and another that results from DNA attack by free radicals generated as a result of the radiolysis of surrounding water molecules and is referred to as the indirect effect (Hall, 1973; Hall et al., 1988). The major contributor to the indirect effect is the hydroxyl radical (HO•) as evidenced by studies using compounds that scavenge hydroxyl radicals (Roots & Okada, 1972). The direct DNA damage is considered to include the damage that is produced by hydroxyl radicals generated in water molecules intimately associated with DNA water layer since these radicals cannot be scavenged (Ward, 1994a). It is estimated that two-thirds of DNA damage is caused indirectly by scavengeable radicals (Roots & Okada, 1972).

IR induces a wide variety of mainly isolated DNA lesions, including strand breaks (single strand breaks – SSB) and damage that involves DNA bases (modified bases and abasic sites). Isolated DNA lesions are normally easily repaired by cells (Ward, 1994a; Sutherland et al., 2000), without serious biological consequences. It is believed that cytotoxic and mutagenic effects of IR originate from so called clustered DNA damage when two or more lesions occur close to each other in both DNA strands (Goodhead, 1994; Ward, 1994a; Goodhead & Nikjoo, 1997; Nikjoo et al., 1997; Nikjoo et al., 1998; Sutherland et al., 2000). This type of DNA damage was initially termed locally multiply damaged sites (LMDS) (Ward, 1994a), but more recently the term LDMS has been largely replaced by the synonym oxidative clustered DNA lesions (OCDL) (Sutherland et al., 2000; Georgakilas, 2008). Formation of strand breaks in opposite DNA strands results in a double strand break (DSB), that represents a particular case of OCDL (Purkayastha et al., 2007). Assuming that base damage (BD) occurs more frequently than SSB (Ward, 1994b; Ward, 1994a), it is expected that the majority of OCDL are not frank DSB but contain two BD or BD and SSB in opposite strands (Goodhead & Nikjoo, 1997). While isolated DNA lesions are generally repaired efficiently, OCDL are more difficult to resolve (Ward, 1981; Harrison et al., 1999; Georgakilas et al.,

2002; Georgakilas, 2008). An attempt to process by the base excision repair (BER) a modified base that constitute an OCDL with a SSB in opposite strand may result in formation of a DSB, which also can be formed when an unprocessed OCDL interferes with either DNA replication and transcription (Bonner et al., 2008; Sedelnikova et al., 2010). Although DNA DSB can be repaired in cells by non-homologous end joining (NHEJ) and homologous recombination (HR) (Matsumoto et al., 1994; Memisoglu & Samson, 2000; Wilson et al., 2003; Cadet et al., 2010; Hinz, 2010; Lieber, 2010; Mladenov & Iliakis, 2011), DSB are among the most toxic IR-induced DNA lesions. If not properly repaired, both accumulated DSB and OCDL lead to cytotoxicity, genome instability and carcinogenesis (Jeggo & Lobrich, 2007; McKinnon & Caldecott, 2007).

It is established that a substantial level of oxidative DNA lesions may be present in normal cells and tissues, usually a few isolated oxidative DNA lesions per Mbp (Nakamura & Swenberg, 1999; De Bont & van Larebeke, 2004). These lesions are believed to be generated by free radicals that originate from endogenous reactive oxygen species (ROS) (Riley, 1994; Mikkelsen & Wardman, 2003). Two of the biologically important endogenous ROS are superoxide anion radical $O_2^{-}\bullet$ and hydrogen peroxide $H_2O_2$. Endogenous superoxide is produced in cells mainly as a result of mitochondrial respiration (Mikkelsen & Wardman, 2003), and then is efficiently converted to hydrogen peroxide by cellular superoxide dismutase (SOD). Although the superoxide and hydrogen peroxide are relatively long lived species and are able to diffuse in cells over considerable distance (Riley, 1994), these endogenous species are produced in cytoplasm and also they are not able to damage DNA directly. The genotoxic effect of the endogenous ROS is mainly mediated by their ability to give rise to hydroxyl radicals from hydrogen peroxide by a redox reaction with traces of reduced transitional metal ions, mainly ferrous via Fenton chemistry (Mikkelsen & Wardman, 2003). Since ROS represent potential risk for cells, an antioxidant defense system has been developed in cells to maintain a steady state level of ROS.

Exogenous cytotoxic agents can lead to the increase above the steady state in the ROS level thus creating an oxidative stress that can result in induction of additional oxidative DNA damage (Sedelnikova et al., 2010). Exposure to IR is also known to cause the oxidative stress however, interestingly, the level of ROS generated directly from radiolysis of water at biologically relevant doses is much less that the level of the endogenous ROS. This follows from the estimation that for example a 100 Gy radiation dose would be required to double the endogenous level of one of the major types of DNA base damage 7,8-dihydro-8-oxoguanine (8-oxoG) (Ward, 1994b). There is also experimental evidence that the transient increase in the cellular ROS level following irradiation is dependent on mitochondria respiration, however it is dose independent in the range of biologically relevant doses (1 - 10 Gy) with the fraction of cells exhibiting the increased ROS level being dose dependent (Leach et al., 2001). These observations underline the minimal impact of isolated DNA lesions and the critical role of clustered lesions for cyto- and genotoxic consequences of IR. The major difference between endogenous ROS and those generated by IR is that while the spatial distribution of hydroxyl radicals produced from endogenous ROS is random, IR is also able to generate clusters of hydroxyl radicals within a nanometre scale resulting in the multiple radical attack on DNA within small volume from a single track of a charged particle (Goodhead, 1994; Goodhead & Nikjoo, 1997; Nikjoo et al., 1997; Nikjoo et al., 1998). As a result, the relative frequency of OCDL is much higher for damage induced by IR as compared to endogenous oxidative DNA damage for which OCDL are very rare. The frequency of endogenous OCDL is estimated to be a few per Gbp in normal tissues (Bennett et al., 2005), and can probably be formed as a result of two isolated oxidative lesions occurring close to each other spatially and temporally. The radiation induced OCDL can also be more complex since consisting of more than two individual lesions in a cluster (Ward, 1994a; Bennett et al., 2005).

Recently, the dogma that cells subjected to IR are killed solely through direct energy deposition within a cell, with the effect being proportional to dose, has been reconsidered in view of the discovery of the radiation-induced bystander effect (RIBE). The neighbours of irradiated cells respond as if they themselves have been irradiated. The RIBE is now a well-established consequence of exposure to IR and is manifested as increased genomic abnormalities and loss of viability in unirradiated ("bystander") cells associated with the targeted cells. Affected bystander cells exhibit increased levels of micronuclei, apoptosis, mutations, altered DNA damage and repair, and senescence arrest (Sokolov et al., 2005; Sedelnikova et al., 2007; Prise & O'Sullivan, 2009). DSB appear in the DNA of bystander cells, invoking the existence of some kind of biological "danger signal" that is sent from irradiated to bystander cell. Possible mediators of the RIBE include various inflammation-related cytokines and ROS including nitric oxide that have been found at elevated levels in medium conditioned by irradiated cells (Dickey et al., 2009; Prise & O'Sullivan, 2009; Hei et al., 2010; Ivanov et al., 2010).

## 3. Radiation therapy of tumours and the role of radioprotectors

The detrimental consequences of IR for cells and tissues can be harnessed in cancer radiation therapy. Radiation therapy exploits the cytotoxic effect of IR on cancer cells (Lawrence et al., 2008) and represents one of the three major treatment modalities for cancer, along with surgery and cytotoxic chemotherapy. Radiotherapy is used in approximately half of all patients diagnosed with cancer at some stage of their illness. Technological advances in the physical targeting of radiation to the tumour are extensively exploited, reflecting the simple idea that the most efficient radioprotection strategy is to exclude normal tissues from irradiated volume. These include such techniques as conformal radiotherapy, intensity modulated therapy, image guided radiotherapy etc (Brizel, 2005). Although still in the pre-clinical stage of development, microbeam radiotherapy (MRT), in which the X-ray beam is split into an array of planar parallel microbeams, shows much greater therapeutic index than conventional radiotherapy. Studies of synchrotron MRT in animal models indicated that tumours can be ablated by MRT at radiation levels that spare normal tissues (Dilmanian et al., 2002; Dilmanian et al., 2003; Crosbie et al., 2010). Nevertheless, whether used alone or in combination with other treatment modalities, the dose of radiation that can be safely delivered is limited by radiation induced injury to the normal tissues in the irradiated volume. This gives rise to the concept of "treatment to tolerance" i.e. the administration of the maximally tolerated dose (MTD) imposed by the normal tissues which is often less than required to effect a high probability of tumour eradication. Clearly, any strategy that selectively increases the MTD improves the chances of tumour cure, and one of such strategies is the selective pharmacologic modification of the normal tissue response with radiation modifiers/protectors. These agents alter the response of normal tissues to irradiation when present in tissues prior or after exposure to IR (Citrin, 2010). This approach can also be viewed as an attractive countermeasure for possible nuclear/radiological terrorism and radiation accidents, but without the important constraint to avoid protection of the tumour that is imperative in the use of radioprotectors in radiation oncology.

The US National Cancer Institute Workshop have developed recommendations for the terminology and classification of the agents used to ameliorate the biological consequences of the exposure to IR (Stone, 2003). The classification implies that there are different mechanisms of action of these agents, and therefore they may be efficient when administered appropriately with regard to the time of the exposure to IR. Accordingly, there are three groups of such agents. Prophylactic agents/protectors are administered before exposure to IR and mainly act by chemically preventing the initial radiochemical damage; mitigators are given during or soon after exposure to IR to prevent development of tissue damage; and treatment agents are administered after exposure to IR to reduce symptoms developed as a result of this exposure.

Apart from normal tissue damage, another major concern associated with cancer radiotherapy is the potential for emergence of secondary radiation-induced cancers, affecting more than 1% of patients (Hall, 2006). Such an outcome can arise in two ways, the first being the induction of mutagenic DNA damage in nearby normal tissues. The second is associated with a phenomenon similar to RIBE in *in vitro* settings that has been reported by cancer radiotherapists more than 50 years ago and termed the abscopal effect (Mole, 1953; Kaminski et al., 2005). It is defined as a change in an organ or tissue distant from the irradiated region. Since these non-targeted effects include malignant transformation (Hall & Hei, 2003; Mancuso et al., 2008), the abscopal effect represents a serious risk factor in radiotherapy.

Therefore, efforts to reduce radiation toxicity in normal tissues and/or in a whole organism are of significant clinical importance and an area of active research. The development of radioprotectors can be regarded as an important strategy to achieve these objectives.

## 4. Aminothiols as radioprotectors

Of the thousands of compounds synthesised and tested at the Walter Reed Army Institute of Research in the 1960's search for radioprotectors, aminothiols emerged as the most promising compounds. The persistent motif associated with radioprotective activity of aminothiols is a thiol separated from an aliphatic amino group by a two carbon chain (Brown et al., 1982). The simplest example is cysteamine (chemical formula $H_2N$-$CH_2$-$CH_2$-SH). One of the most studied aminothiols is the radioprotector WR1065 (2-[aminopropyl)amino]ethanethiol, Figure 1), which is the active thiol metabolite of amifostine (WR2721).

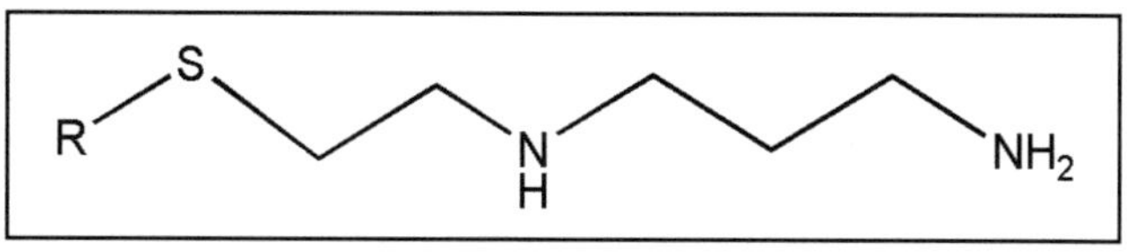


Fig. 1. Structure of WR1065 (R = H) and its prodrug amifostine (R = $H_2PO_3$).

WR1065 protects cultured cells against radiation induced clonogenic death. A dose modification factor (DMF) of 1.9 is achieved for V79 cells pre-incubated 30 min with 4mM of WR1065 before irradiation (Grdina et al., 1985). DMF is defined as the ratio of radiation doses producing the same degree of radiation effect, in the presence and absence of the radiomodifier. In the context of radioprotection, and particularly for *in vivo* endpoints, DRF, dose reduction factor is often used. It has been shown using neutral elution technique that

the number of radiation induced DNA DSB in V79 cells is reduced by 4 mM WR1065 with a DMF of 1.8 (Sigdestad et al., 1987). WR1065 also protects against the mutagenic effect of radiation as demonstrated for the hypoxanthine-guanine phosphoribosyl transferase locus in V79 cells (Grdina et al., 1985). Radioprotection by WR1065 and WR2721 *in vivo* has been demonstrated using the Withers assay that is based on histological staining and counting of the repopulating crypt clonogens in mouse jejunum (Withers & Elkind, 1969; Withers & Elkind, 1970). A DMF of 1.8 - 2.0 has been reported for this assay (Murray et al., 1988a), however much smaller DMF values of 1.1 - 1.3 have been obtained for the DNA SSB induction end point in the same system. Reduction of the radiation induced phosphorylated histone H2AX (γH2AX) level by WR1065 has been observed in human endothelial cells in accordance with increasing clonogenic survival (Kataoka et al., 2007). The phosphorylation of the histone H2AX occurs in response to IR exposure in the regions of chromatin adjacent to the sites of radiation induced DNA DSB (Rogakou et al., 1998; Rogakou et al., 1999; Sedelnikova et al., 2003) and is considered as a marker for DNA DSB (Sedelnikova et al., 2002; Sedelnikova et al., 2003).
Amongst the different mechanisms that have been suggested for radioprotection by WR1065 and other aminothiols, the most likely are the scavenging of hydroxyl radicals, the chemical repair of DNA radicals and the depletion of oxygen (Purdie et al., 1983; Smoluk et al., 1988a). It has been demonstrated that the radioprotective ability of aminothiols is dependent on their positive charge (Aguilera et al., 1992; Zheng et al., 1992). This observation is attributed to the phenomenon of the counterion condensation that results in high local concentration of cationic aminothiols near DNA (Smoluk et al., 1988b). At neutral pH, the WR1065 molecule has a positive charge of +2 and therefore protects better than cysteamine with a charge of +1. Experiments with plasmid DNA demonstrated however, that radioprotection by aminothiols cannot be accounted solely by scavenging of hydroxyl radicals (Zheng et al., 1992). This follows from the fact that WR1065 protects DNA much better than cystamine (a disulfide form of cysteamine, chemical formula $H_2N\text{-}(CH_2)_2\text{-}S\text{-}S\text{-}(CH_2)_2\text{-}NH_2$) which has the same positive charge and higher hydroxyl radical scavenging capacity (Zheng et al., 1992). Investigators comparing radioprotective effects of aminothiols on DNA damage endpoints, with clonogenic survival (Murray et al., 1988b; Aguilera et al., 1992) or repopulating crypt clonogens in the *in vivo* mouse jejunum model (Murray et al., 1988a), also conclude that the radioprotective mechanism is more complex than just scavenging of hydroxyl radicals. Studies aimed at investigating the role of chemical repair of DNA in radioprotection of V79 cells suggest that this becomes the dominant mechanism for aminothiols with increasing positive charge (Aguilera et al., 1992). The oxygen depletion hypothesis emerged from the studies of radioprotection in mouse skin by WR2721 under different oxygen tension that demonstrated decrease in radioprotection from a DMF of 1.95 in air, down to 1.1 and less, at 5% oxygen and less (Denekamp et al., 1982). This hypothesis has been further supported by the finding of the rapid oxygen consumption in cell culture medium following addition of WR1065 and WR2721 (Purdie et al., 1983). Cell culture studies with V79 cells have also indicated the decrease in radioprotection by WR1065 under hypoxia (DMF of 1.4) as compared to oxic conditions (DMF of 1.9) (Grdina et al., 1989).
With regard to clinical application, attention has focussed on WR2721 (amifostine, Ethyol), which is a phosphorylated form of the WR1065 (Figure 1). Amifostine has FDA approval for use as a radioprotector for a subgroup of patients undergoing radiation therapy. Following administration, amifostine is dephosphorylated by alkaline phosphatase to convert it to WR1065, which actually affords protection against IR. Amifostine has undergone extensive

testing as a potential adjuvant to radiotherapy and chemotherapy. The drug has been shown conclusively to have protective activity against both radiation and cisplatin induced toxicity without demonstrable protection of tumours (Wasserman, 1994). One randomised trial of amifostine in patients with inoperable, unresectable, or recurrent rectal cancers (Liu et al., 1992), showed a significant reduction in morbidity in the treated group. Despite these results, and those of subsequent clinical studies, including differing routes of administration, the drug has not found wide clinical acceptance in radiation oncology, because of its toxicity especially hypotension and severe malaise, and the requirement that it be administered systemically (with monitoring of blood pressure) before each radiation treatment. The topical application of WR2721 to rat colon (France et al., 1986) conferred substantial protection, namely a DMF of 1.8. Subsequent clinical trials, the most recent in 2008, employing amifostine doses up to 2 g in a 30 ml enema, did report some clinical benefit, especially for the higher of two doses (Simone et al., 2008). These results underline the low potency of this agent.

## 5. Radioprotection by methylproamine

### 5.1 Methylproamine as a DNA binding antioxidant

Methylproamine is a radioprotector, which belongs to a family of DNA minor groove binders featuring a common bi-benzimidazole structure (Figure 2). Two commercially available bi-benzimidazoles Hoechst 33258 and Hoechst 33342 are widely used as fluorescent DNA binding dyes.

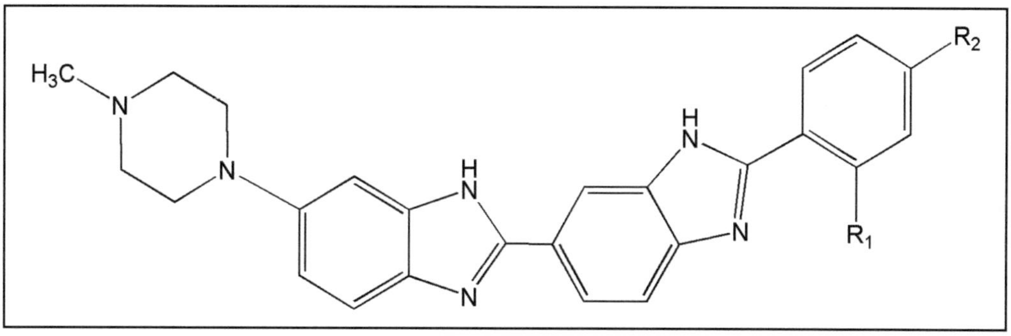


Fig. 2. Chemical structure of bibenzimidazoles. $R_1$ = H and $R_2$ = $OCH_2CH_3$ (Hoechst 33342); $R_1$ = $CH_3$ and $R_2$ = $N(CH_3)_2$ (methylproamine); $R_1$ = H and $R_2$ = $N(CH_3)_2$ (proamine).

Some protective activity against IR was initially discovered for Hoechst 33342 in cultured cells (Smith & Anderson, 1984; Young & Hill, 1989) and followed by reports of radioprotection of isolated DNA (Denison et al., 1992; Martin & Denison, 1992) and *in vivo* radioprotection of mouse lung (Martin et al., 1996) and brain (Lyubimova et al., 2001). New analogues of Hoechst 33342 were designed to improve the radioprotective activity, resulting in synthesis of more efficient compounds proamine (Figure 2) (Martin et al., 1996) and methylproamine (Figure 2) (Martin et al., 2004). Incubation of V79 Chinese Hamster cells in 30 μM of methylproamine before and during γ-irradiation increases clonogenic survival with a DMF of 2.1 (Martin et al., 2004). *In vivo* radioprotection by methylproamine has been demonstrated in mouse jejunum using the Withers assay with a DMF of 1.2 - 1.3.
Methylproamine, like other DNA binding bi-benzimidazoles, has a binding preference for AT-rich sequences, the consensus binding site being 3-4 consecutive AT base pairs as

established by footprinting (Harshman & Dervan, 1985) and affinity cleavage (Martin & Holmes, 1983; Martin et al., 1990; Murray & Martin, 1994) studies, and confirmed by X-ray crystallography studies (Martin et al., 2004).

### 5.2 Electron transport is involved in radioprotection by methylproamine

In the 70's and 80's considerable effort was devoted to the development of hypoxic cell radiosensitisers and it was well established that these agents were electron-affinic. From this dogma, that withdrawing electron density from DNA confers radiosensitivity, it can be inferred that increasing electron density in DNA would have radioprotective effect. It was this simple idea that guided the modification of Hoechst 33342 by the substitution of electron rich groups, and this improved radioprotective activity. Pulse radiolysis studies of methylproamine/DNA complexes provided further information on the movement of an electron from DNA-bound radioprotector to oxidising lesions on DNA (Martin & Anderson, 1998). In these studies, the spectral changes associated with oxidation of the DNA ligand were followed by time resolved spectrophotometry. Moreover, by studying the effect of the drug loading of DNA on the rate of oxidation of the ligand, the range of electron movement from the bound ligand to oxidising lesion could be estimated. The results indicated that for methylproamine, the maximum range was several base pairs (Martin & Anderson, 1998).

The phenomenon of electron donation as the basis for radioprotection also emerged from the studies of tyrosine containing peptides which have been modelled of naturally occurring nuclear proteins involved in the endogenous radioprotection (Tsoi et al., 2010).

From consideration of studies of the chemical mechanism of radioprotection by thiols, the alternative mechanisms of H-atom donation and electron donation have been discussed. The close relationship between these two mechanisms of reduction is also invoked in the combination of electron and proton transfer in a concerted mechanism. Indeed this mechanism is well established in radiation chemistry of DNA (Kumar & Sevilla, 2010). These considerations have lead to the hypothesis that radioprotection by methylproamine involves repair of transient radiation induced species on DNA by electron donation from the DNA bound ligand. An alternative mechanistic concept would invoke the DNA bound ligand as the sink for "holes" produced in irradiated DNA. It is well established that radical cations produced on DNA by powerful oxidants move to the most easily oxidisable base pair, namely GC. The presence of DNA-bound methylproamine would constitute an alternative destination for the hole, thus reducing the yield of oxidised bases. A redox potential of 0.84 - 0.9 volt has been reported for Hoechst 33342 (Adhikary et al., 2000) so it is reasonable to assume that the redox potential for methylproamine is similar and therefore consistent with the hole trapping hypothesis.

### 5.3 DNA bound methylproamine is responsible for radioprotection of cells

The results of pulse radiolysis studies of methylproamine-DNA complexes indicated that intramolecular electron transfer from the ligand to radiation induced oxidising species on DNA is involved in the oxidation of methylproamine, and this process can be implicated in radioprotective activity of methylproamine (Martin & Anderson, 1998). Radioprotection *in vivo* however occurs in a different environment than reduction of oxidising species on DNA in pulse radiolysis experiments, and other processes may contribute to radioprotection *in vivo* such as for example scavenging of hydroxyl radicals by free methylproamine. To clarify the role of DNA bound methylproamine in radioprotection we have undertaken extensive studies of radioprotection using clonogenic survival of human cultured keratinocytes as an endpoint (Lobachevsky et al., 2011). The dose response curves of clonogenic survival have been established for FEP-1811 keratinocytes pre-incubated with various concentrations of methylproamine from 0.5 to 10 μM for 30 min before irradiation with $^{137}Cs$ γ-rays. The DMF calculated for each survival curve has increased from 1.01 at 0.5 μM to 1.97 at 10 μM of methylproamine.

In parallel experiments the uptake of methylproamine in cells and nuclei has been measured by extracting the drug from nuclear and cellular pellets and measurement by liquid chromatography. It was found that while the cellular uptake increased as a linear function of methylproamine concentration (up to 4 fmole/cell at 10 μM of methylproamine), the nuclear uptake indicated the presence of the major saturated and minor linear components. The saturated component reflects in our opinion accumulation of DNA bound methylproamine and saturation of high affinity binding sites at high concentrations. The saturation level has been estimated to be 0.173 fmole per nucleus and corresponds to approximately 1 ligand per 58 bp. This value is similar to the size of the binding site calculated from *in vitro* DNA binding studies with methylproamine and analogues (Loontiens et al., 1990; Martin et al., 2004). The fraction of DNA bound methylproamine is not less than 98% as estimated assuming nucleus radius of 5 μm (DNA concentration 26 mM bp), binding dissociation constant $K_d$ = 100 nM and methylproamine concentration 450 μM (total nuclear uptake 0.234 fmole at 10 μM in medium). This result in combination with the presence of the saturated component indicates that the majority of the nuclear methylproamine is in the DNA bound form. The presence of the linear component of the nuclear uptake may result from the heterogeneity in the affinity of binding sites so that "weaker" sites are occupied at increasing methylproamine concentrations.

Values of DMF obtained at various concentrations of methylproamine have been analysed in conjunction with results of cellular and nuclear uptake studies (Lobachevsky et al., 2011). Correlation has been studied between DMF values and each of the cellular uptake, nuclear uptake and saturated and linear components of nuclear uptake. The best correlation have been achieved for the total nuclear uptake of methylproamine ($R^2$ = 0.97) and the least correlation for the cellular uptake ($R^2$ = 0.87). These results, along with the finding that the majority of the nuclear methylproamine is present in DNA bound form, support the hypothesis that it is the DNA associated drug that is responsible for radioprotection of cells.

### 5.4 Methylproamine reduces radiation induced DNA damage in cells

In addition to radioprotection at the clonogenic survival endpoint, the effect of methylproamine on the induction by radiation of γH2AX foci has been studied (Sprung et al., 2010; Lobachevsky et al., 2011). γH2AX can be detected microscopically using immunofluorescence technique as a distinct focus that is associated with a DNA DSB (Sedelnikova et al., 2002; Sedelnikova et al., 2003). The dose response curves of γH2AX focus number per cell were established following irradiation of FEP-1811 keratinocytes pre-incubated with 20 μM of methylproamine for the time intervals of 1, 5 and 15 min before irradiation with $^{137}Cs$ γ-rays (Lobachevsky et al., 2011). The results have demonstrated the reduction by methylproamine of the number of radiation induced γH2AX foci. The extent of this reduction is consistent with pre-incubation interval as indicated by DMF values of 1.4, 1.9 and 3.5 for 1, 5 and 15 min respectively. The efficient reduction of the number of radiation induced γH2AX foci by pre-incubation with methylproamine has been also demonstrated with three lymphoblast cell lines derived from the blood of the radiotherapy patients with different DNA repair capacity (Sprung et al., 2005; Sprung et al., 2008). In these experiments (Sprung et al., 2010), cells have been irradiated with $^{137}Cs$ γ-rays following 15 min pre-incubation with 20 μM methylproamine. Radioprotection has been observed in all three cell lines including those obtained from a radiosensitive patient and with a defective DNA ligase IV that is critical for DNA DSB repair pathway. This finding demonstrates the ability of methylproamine to reduce the amount of radiation induced DNA damage.

To further investigate the effect of methylproamine on the radiation induced DNA damage in cells, the pulsed field gel electrophoresis (PFGE) assay has been exploited (Sprung et al., 2010). For this assay, lymphoblast cells have been irradiated with γ-ray doses of 20, 40 and 80 Gy in the presence or without 20 μM methylproamine. DNA was extracted from the cells, analysed on PFGE and the fraction of lower molecular weight DNA released from the wells has been quantified (Sprung et al., 2010). The results demonstrate substantial decrease of the low molecular weight fraction in all irradiated samples pre-treated with methylproamine as compared to the irradiated only samples thus indicating prevention by methylproamine of DNA fragmentation due to radiation induced DSB.

### 5.5 Methylproamine protects against breaks and base damage in plasmid DNA

A series of observations such as the role of DNA bound methylproamine in the radioprotection of cells, the requirement for methylproamine to be present in cells at the time of irradiation and demonstration that electron transport is involved in radioprotection support the hypothesis that the chemical reduction of transient radiation induced oxidative species on DNA by donation of an electron from methylproamine constitutes the main mechanism of radioprotection. This hypothesis however, in conjunction with the observation that methylproamine prevents formation of radiation induced DSB in cells, as demonstrated by pulsed field gel electrophoresis studies and the reduction of the yield of γH2AX foci, prompts the question of what are those oxidative DNA species that are reduced by methylproamine and how the chemical reduction can repair or prevent the formation of a DNA DSB. A further insight into the mechanisms of radioprotection can be obtained from investigation of DNA damage of isolated DNA using a plasmid model.

Plasmid DNA is a convenient tool to assay DNA strand breakage. It exploits conformational changes of the supercoiled plasmid to the relaxed open circle form following induction of a SSB and to the linear form following induction of a DSB (Freifelder & Trumbo, 1969; Cowan et al., 1987; Lobachevsky et al., 2004). Three plasmid forms can be separated using agarose gel electrophoresis and numbers of SSB and DSB calculated from fractions of the linear and relaxed forms (Cowan et al., 1987). Combination of the plasmid DNA breakage assay and treatment of DNA with base excision repair enzymes (endonucleases) that recognise various DNA base lesions and convert them to strand breaks allows quantitation of radiation induced base lesions (Milligan et al., 2000a). One of such enzymes is the endonuclease formamidopyrimidine-DNA N-glycosylase (FPG) from Escherichia coli (O'Connor & Laval, 1989). FPG recognises oxidised purines, in particular 8-oxoG (Chetsanga & Lindahl, 1979; Milligan et al., 2002) and possesses both glycosylase and endonuclease activity to excise the modified base and then produce a nick at this abasic site (O'Connor & Laval, 1989), thus converting the base damage to a SSB.

Early experiments with plasmid DNA model have demonstrated ability of methylproamine analogues Hoechst 33342 and Hoechst 33258 to protect DNA from radiation induced SSB (Denison et al., 1992; Martin & Denison, 1992) with a linear increase in the DMF from approximately 2 to more than 10 with the ligand concentration changing from 5 to 50 μM (Martin & Denison, 1992). Two modes of protection have been suggested: the site-specific and global protection. The site-specific protection occurs at the site of the ligand binding on DNA and has been suggested to involve direct block of the radical attack by the ligand occupying DNA minor groove and/or electron or H-atom transfer from the ligand to DNA. However, since only limited DNA regions (less than 20%) can by occupied by bound ligand, the site-specific protection can not account completely for the observed extent in the SSB reduction (up to DMF of 10). Therefore the idea of global protection has been suggested that implies radioprotection between ligand binding sites. Given that the linear relationship between the extent of radioprotection and the ligand concentration has been observed, the most likely mechanism of global protection detected in these experiments is the scavenging of hydroxyl radicals by free ligand in solution. This suggestion is supported by the much smaller extent of radioprotection by 25 μM of Hoechst 33258 in the presence of 100 mM mannitol that efficiently scavenges hydroxyl radicals: a DMF of 1.4 as compared to 9.6 for 25 μM of Hoechst 33258 in phosphate buffer (Martin & Denison, 1992), and the fact that majority of the ligand binding sites (94-100%) are occupied within the range of the studied concentrations of Hoechst 33258 (5 - 50 μM) indicating that the radioprotection by DNA bound ligand wouldn't change significantly at this condition.

Although the site-specific protection by methylproamine analogues partially prevents formation of SSB, and the global protection by DNA bound ligand in cells can also potentially reduce the yield of SSB, it is unlikely that these mechanisms of radioprotection by methylproamine will affect the yield of DSB as to account for the observed radioprotection at the clonogenic survival and γH2AX induction endpoints with DMF of 2 and more. A more likely mechanism is the chemical reduction by DNA bound methylproamine of the initial oxidative DNA lesion that results in base damage constituting a part of OCDL. Such OCDL represent a difficult challenge for the cellular DNA repair machinery and potentially can result in enzymatic DNA DSB. However, following reduction by methylproamine of the radical precursor of the lesion that otherwise would constitute a part of an OCDL, the formation of this OCDL can be prevented, thus preventing potential formation of an enzymatic DSB. The ability of methylproamine to reduce oxidative base lesions has also been demonstrated using plasmid DNA model.

In our experiments pBR322 plasmid DNA has been irradiated with $^{137}Cs$ γ-rays in the PTP buffer (Figure 3) containing thiocyanate ions, as described by (Milligan et al., 2000b; Milligan et al., 2001). In this buffer, the thiocyanate ion ($SCN^-$) is the main scavenger of radiation induced hydroxyl radicals ($HO^\bullet$) that otherwise would be responsible for the induction of the majority of DNA breakage.

Interaction of $SCN^-$ with $HO^\bullet$ results in formation of highly reactive radical species $SCN^\bullet$ and/or $(SCN)_2^{\bullet-}$ that are the major mediators of the radiation induced DNA damage in this buffer. In contrast to $HO^\bullet$ radicals that are efficient in induction of DNA breaks, $SCN^\bullet/(SCN)_2^{\bullet-}$ radicals produce oxidative lesions of DNA bases. Guanine is considered as the most frequently damaged site oxidation of which results in formation of guanyl radical that eventually is converted mainly to 8-oxoG. Compared to $HO^\bullet$ radicals, with a reduction potential (E) of 2.3 V, $SCN^\bullet/(SCN)_2^{\bullet-}$ are more moderate oxidants (E = 1.62/1.32 V), but nevertheless powerful enough to oxidise guanines in DNA (E = 1.29 V). Thus irradiation in PTP buffer results in selective damage; primarily oxidation of guanine.

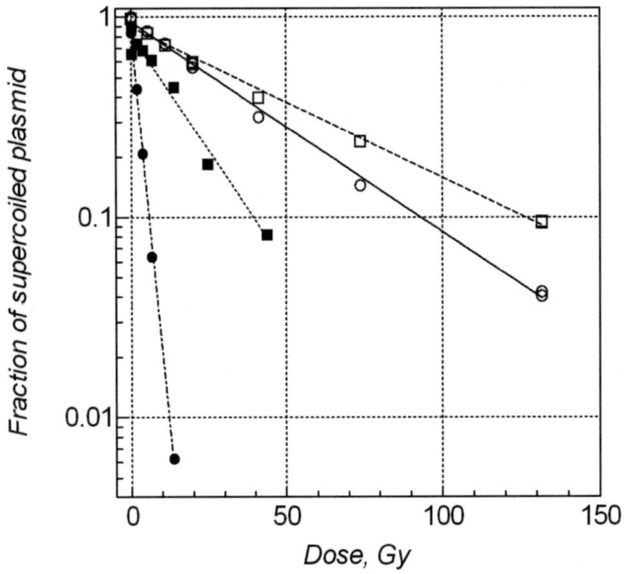


Fig. 3. Loss of supercoiled plasmid with increasing radiation dose. A solution of 7.5 μg/mL of pBR322 (11.4 μM bp) in a buffer containing 5 mM sodium phosphate, pH 7.0, 1 mM sodium thiocyanate and 110 mM sodium perchlorate (PTP buffer) has been irradiated with $^{137}Cs$ γ-rays without (circles) or with 5 μM of methylproamine (squares). Irradiated samples were analysed by agarose gel electrophoresis to assay frank SSB (open symbols) or after treatment with FPG to assay total frank SSB and enzymatic SSB (base damage) (closed symbols).

The yield of FPG sensitive lesions (FPG enzymatic SSB) in pBR322 following irradiation in the thiocyanate buffer is more than 10-fold higher than the yield of frank SSB (Figure 3, Table 1).

| | Yield of SSB and BD $10^{-2}$ per plasmid per Gy | | DMF | |
|---|---|---|---|---|
| Buffer | Frank SSB | BD (enzymatic SSB) | Frank SSB | BD (enzymatic SSB) |
| PTP | 2.45 ± 0.05 | 31.8 ± 1.2 | | |
| PTP+1.25 μM methylproamine | 1.76 ± 0.03 | 3.16 ± 0.29 | 1.39 | 10.1 |
| PTP+2.5 μM methylproamine | 1.67 ± 0.01 | 2.45 ± 0.13 | 1.47 | 13.0 |
| PTP+5 μM methylproamine | 1.52 ± 0.01 | 2.08 ± 0.09 | 1.61 | 15.3 |

Table 1. Effect of methylproamine on the yield of frank and enzymatic SSB in irradiated pBR322 plasmid DNA.

Methylproamine at concentration as low as 1.25 μM protects plasmid DNA against enzymatic SSB with a DMF of 10 while against frank SSB with a moderate DMF of 1.4 (Table 1), thus demonstrating much higher extent of protection against base damage than against frank SSB. A possible candidate lesion for repair by methylproamine is a guanyl radical cation that results, if not repaired, in formation of 8-oxoG, a modified base that is recognised and converted to SSB by FPG. The most critical question with regard to mechanisms of such efficient protection against base damage is whether radioprotection is mediated by DNA bound or free methylproamine and is achieved via the reduction by methylproamine of oxidative lesions on DNA or scavenging $SCN^{\bullet}/(SCN)_2^{\bullet -}$ radicals in solutions that cause DNA lesions.

The results presented in Table 1 for radioprotection at 1.25 and 5 μM of methylproamine indicate a moderate decrease in the yield of base damage from $3.16\text{x}10^{-2}$ to $2.08\text{x}10^{-2}$ (34%) that resulted from 4-fold increase in methylproamine concentration. While addition of 1.25 μM methylproamine to PTP buffer prevents formation of 90% of base damage, second addition of 1.25 μM (from 1.25 to 2.5 μM) prevents formation of only 22% of the remaining base damage. It is important to note that the change in the fraction of pBR322 DNA binding sites occupied by methylproamine is minimal (estimated from 85 to 97% as methylproamine concentration changes from 1.25 to 2.5 μM). The results therefore are consistent with the hypothesis that the radioprotection against base damage is mainly mediated by DNA bound methylproamine. In general, these results demonstrate the ability of methylproamine to protect against radiation induced base damage and therefore support the hypothesis that reduction of the oxidative DNA lesions by methylproamine accounts for radioprotection of cells.

## 6. Cytotoxicity of DNA binding ligands

The strong high affinity binding of bibenzimidazoles in the minor groove of DNA is a factor that determines the high radioprotective potency of methylproamine: substantial radioprotection of clonogenic survival is achieved at concentrations as low as a few μM in cell culture medium (a DMF 1.6 at 2 μM) (Lobachevsky et al., 2011), and at even lower concentrations for base damage in the plasmid model (a DMF of 10 at 1.25 μM) (Table 1). On the other hand, it is logical to expect that the tightly DNA associated bisbenzimidazole molecule will interfere with normal DNA metabolic processes such as replication, transcription, repair etc and such an interaction may result in adverse cytotoxic and mutagenic effects. While no effect of methylproamine on the clonogenic survival of human keratinocytes has been detected following 60 min incubation with 10 μM of the drug, at 20 μM of methylproamine the clonogenic survival has been reduced to 80% (Lobachevsky et al., 2011). Mechanisms of this cytotoxicity have not been fully investigated. The cytotoxicity of Hoechst 33342 has prompted consideration and further development of bibenzimidazoles as potential antitumour agents (Baraldi et al., 2004). Inhibition of DNA synthesis has been demonstrated in V79 cells exposed to 5 and 10 μM of Hoechst 33342. This inhibition results in substantial changes in the progression of cells through cell cycle as manifested by appearance of increased S-phase population and $S/G_2$ block (Durand & Olive, 1982). One of the potential mechanisms of the Hoechst 33342 cytotoxicity is its interaction with topoisomerase I. Inhibition of the topoisomerase I activity by Hoechst 33342 and 33258 has been demonstrated using both the relaxation and cleavage assays (Chen et al., 1993). The inhibition activity of the Hoechst ligands in the relaxation assay might indicate their interaction with the binding of topoisomerase I with DNA. In the cleavage assay, a DNA SSB is induced that is attributed to the trapping by Hoechst ligands of topoisomerase I cleavable complexes (Chen et al., 1993; Bailly, 2000).

## 7. Conclusion

Given the central role of DNA as radiobiological target, the design of radioprotectors which bind to DNA is an obvious strategy, however neither of the DNA binding radioprotectors discussed in this paper arose from such a deliberate design plan. WR1065 and amifostine emerged from an empirical drug development program, and the association between radioprotective efficacy and DNA binding only became evident in retrospect. In the case of methylproamine, derived from a minor groove DNA binding ligand developed for an entirely different purpose, and found to have a serendipitous radioprotective activity, incorporation electron-rich substituents has improved radioprotective activity compared to Hoechst 33342. No doubt this rational thread might be followed more explicitly in the design of future radioprotectors, but it remains to be seen whether it is possible to design DNA-binding radioprotectors that are devoid of any toxicity derived from the DNA-binding property.

## 8. Acknowledgement

This work was supported by licensing agreement between Sirtex Medical Inc and Peter MacCallum Cancer Centre and by the Intramural Research Program of the National Cancer Institute, National Institutes of Health.

## 9. References

Adhikary, A., Bothe, E., Jain, V. & Von Sonntag, C. (2000). Pulse radiolysis of the DNA-binding bisbenzimidazole derivatives Hoechst 33258 and 33342 in aqueous solutions. *Int J Radiat Biol*, Vol. 76, No. 9, pp. 1157-1166.

Aguilera, J. A., Newton, G. L., Fahey, R. C. & Ward, J. F. (1992). Thiol uptake by Chinese hamster V79 cells and aerobic radioprotection as a function of the net charge on the thiol. *Radiat Res*, Vol. 130, No. 2, pp. 194-204.

Bailly, C. (2000). Topoisomerase I poisons and suppressors as anticancer drugs. *Curr Med Chem*, Vol. 7, No. 1, pp. 39-58.

Baraldi, P. G., Bovero, A., Fruttarolo, F., Preti, D., Tabrizi, M. A., Pavani, M. G. & Romagnoli, R. (2004). DNA minor groove binders as potential antitumor and antimicrobial agents. *Med Res Rev*, Vol. 24, No. 4, pp. 475-528.

Bennett, P. V., Cuomo, N. L., Paul, S., Tafrov, S. T. & Sutherland, B. M. (2005). Endogenous DNA damage clusters in human skin, 3-D model, and cultured skin cells. *Free Radic Biol Med*, Vol. 39, No. 6, pp. 832-839.

Bonner, W. M., Redon, C. E., Dickey, J. S., Nakamura, A. J., Sedelnikova, O. A., Solier, S. & Pommier, Y. (2008). GammaH2AX and cancer. *Nat Rev Cancer*, Vol. 8, No. 12, pp. 957-967.

Brizel, D. M. (2005). *Strategies for protecting normal tissues in the treatment of head and neck cancer*. Totowa, NJ, Humana Press.

Brown, D. Q., Pittock, J. W., 3rd & Rubinstein, J. S. (1982). Early results of the screening program for radioprotectors. *Int J Radiat Oncol Biol Phys*, Vol. 8, No. 3-4, pp. 565-570.

Cadet, J., Douki, T. & Ravanat, J. L. (2010). Oxidatively generated base damage to cellular DNA. *Free Radic Biol Med*, Vol. 49, No. 1, pp. 9-21.

Chen, A. Y., Yu, C., Bodley, A., Peng, L. F. & Liu, L. F. (1993). A new mammalian DNA topoisomerase I poison Hoechst 33342: cytotoxicity and drug resistance in human cell cultures. *Cancer Res*, Vol. 53, No. 6, pp. 1332-1337.

Chetsanga, C. J. & Lindahl, T. (1979). Release of 7-methylguanine residues whose imidazole rings have been opened from damaged DNA by a DNA glycosylase from Escherichia coli. *Nucleic Acids Res*, Vol. 6, No. 11, pp. 3673-3684.

Citrin, D., Cotrim, A.P., Hyodo, F., Baum, B.J., Krishna, M.C., Mitchell, J.B. (2010). Radioprotectors and Mitigators of Radiation-Induced Normal Tissue Injury. *The Oncologist*, Vol. 15, No., pp. 360-371.

Cowan, R., Collis, C. M. & Grigg, G. W. (1987). Breakage of double-stranded DNA due to single-stranded nicking. *J Theor Biol*, Vol. 127, No. 2, pp. 229-245.

Crosbie, J. C., Anderson, R. L., Rothkamm, K., Restall, C. M., Cann, L., Ruwanpura, S., Meachem, S., Yagi, N., Svalbe, I., Lewis, R. A., Williams, B. R. & Rogers, P. A. (2010). Tumor cell response to synchrotron microbeam radiation therapy differs markedly from cells in normal tissues. *Int J Radiat Oncol Biol Phys*, Vol. 77, No. 3, pp. 886-894.

De Bont, R. & van Larebeke, N. (2004). Endogenous DNA damage in humans: a review of quantitative data. *Mutagenesis*, Vol. 19, No. 3, pp. 169-185.

Denekamp, J., Michael, B. D., Rojas, A. & Stewart, F. A. (1982). Radioprotection of mouse skin by WR-2721: the critical influence of oxygen tension. *Int J Radiat Oncol Biol Phys*, Vol. 8, No. 3-4, pp. 531-534.

Denison, L., Haigh, A., D'Cunha, G. & Martin, R. F. (1992). DNA ligands as radioprotectors: molecular studies with Hoechst 33342 and Hoechst 33258. *International Journal of Radiation Biology*, Vol. 61, No., pp. 69-81.

Dickey, J. S., Baird, B. J., Redon, C. E., Sokolov, M. V., Sedelnikova, O. A. & Bonner, W. M. (2009). Intercellular communication of cellular stress monitored by gamma-H2AX induction. *Carcinogenesis*, Vol. 30, No. 10, pp. 1686-1695.

Dilmanian, F. A., Button, T. M., Le Duc, G., Zhong, N., Pena, L. A., Smith, J. A., Martinez, S. R., Bacarian, T., Tammam, J., Ren, B., Farmer, P. M., Kalef-Ezra, J., Micca, P. L., Nawrocky, M. M., Niederer, J. A., Recksiek, F. P., Fuchs, A. & Rosen, E. M. (2002). Response of rat intracranial 9L gliosarcoma to microbeam radiation therapy. *Neuro Oncol*, Vol. 4, No. 1, pp. 26-38.

Dilmanian, F. A., Morris, G. M., Zhong, N., Bacarian, T., Hainfeld, J. F., Kalef-Ezra, J., Brewington, L. J., Tammam, J. & Rosen, E. M. (2003). Murine EMT-6 carcinoma: high therapeutic efficacy of microbeam radiation therapy. *Radiat Res*, Vol. 159, No. 5, pp. 632-641.

Durand, R. E. & Olive, P. L. (1982). Cytotoxicity, Mutagenicity and DNA damage by Hoechst 33342. *J Histochem Cytochem*, Vol. 30, No. 2, pp. 111-116.

France, H. G., Jr., Jirtle, R. L. & Mansbach, C. M., 2nd (1986). Intracolonic WR 2721 protection of the rat colon from acute radiation injury. *Gastroenterology*, Vol. 91, No. 3, pp. 644-650.

Freifelder, D. & Trumbo, B. (1969). Matching of single-strand breaks to form double-strand breaks in DNA. *Biopolymers*, Vol. 7, No., pp. 681-693.

Georgakilas, A. G. (2008). Processing of DNA damage clusters in human cells: current status of knowledge. *Mol Biosyst*, Vol. 4, No. 1, pp. 30-35.

Georgakilas, A. G., Bennett, P. V. & Sutherland, B. M. (2002). High efficiency detection of bi-stranded abasic clusters in gamma-irradiated DNA by putrescine. *Nucleic Acids Res*, Vol. 30, No. 13, pp. 2800-2808.

Goodhead, D. T. (1994). Initial events in the cellular effects of ionizing radiations: clustered damage in DNA. *Int J Radiat Biol*, Vol. 65, No. 1, pp. 7-17.

Goodhead, D. T. & Nikjoo, H. (1997). Clustered damage in DNA: estimates from track structure simulations. *Radiation Research*, Vol. 148, No. 5, pp. 485-486.

Grdina, D. J., Nagy, B., Hill, C. K. & Sigdestad, C. P. (1989). Protection against radiation-induced mutagenesis in V79 cells by 2-[(aminopropyl)amino] ethanethiol under conditions of acute hypoxia. *Radiat Res*, Vol. 117, No. 2, pp. 251-258.

Grdina, D. J., Nagy, B., Hill, C. K., Wells, R. L. & Peraino, C. (1985). The radioprotector WR1065 reduces radiation-induced mutations at the hypoxanthine-guanine phosphoribosyl transferase locus in V79 cells. *Carcinogenesis*, Vol. 6, No. 6, pp. 929-931.

Hall, E. J. (1973). *Radiobiology for the radiologist*. Hagerstown, MD, New York, Evanston, San Francisco, and London, Harper & Raw.

Hall, E. J. (2006). Intensity-modulated radiation therapy, protons, and the risk of second cancers. *Int J Radiat Oncol Biol Phys*, Vol. 65, No. 1, pp. 1-7.

Hall, E. J., Astor, M., Bedford, J., Borek, C., Curtis, S. B., Fry, M., Geard, C., Hei, T., Mitchell, J., Oleinick, N. & et al. (1988). Basic radiobiology. *Am J Clin Oncol*, Vol. 11, No. 3, pp. 220-252.

Hall, E. J. & Hei, T. K. (2003). Genomic instability and bystander effects induced by high-LET radiation. *Oncogene*, Vol. 22, No. 45, pp. 7034-7042.

Harrison, L., Hatahet, Z. & Wallace, S. S. (1999). In vitro repair of synthetic ionizing radiation-induced multiply damaged DNA sites. *J Mol Biol*, Vol. 290, No. 3, pp. 667-684.

Harshman, K. D. & Dervan, P. B. (1985). Molecular recognition of B-DNA by Hoechst 33258. *Nucleic Acids Research*, Vol. 13, No. 13, pp. 4825-4835.

Hei, T. K., Zhou, H., Chai, Y., Ponnaiya, B. & Ivanov, V. N. (2010). Radiation Induced Non-targeted Response: Mechanism and Potential Clinical Implications. *Curr Mol Pharmacol*, Vol., No., pp.

Hinz, J. M. (2010). Role of homologous recombination in DNA interstrand crosslink repair. *Environ Mol Mutagen*, Vol. 51, No. 6, pp. 582-603.

Hosseinimehr, S. J. (2007). Trends in the development of radioprotective agents. *Drug Discov Today*, Vol. 12, No. 19-20, pp. 794-805.

Ivanov, V. N., Zhou, H., Ghandhi, S. A., Karasic, T. B., Yaghoubian, B., Amundson, S. A. & Hei, T. K. (2010). Radiation-induced bystander signaling pathways in human fibroblasts: a role for interleukin-33 in the signal transmission. *Cell Signal*, Vol. 22, No. 7, pp. 1076-1087.

Jeggo, P. A. & Lobrich, M. (2007). DNA double-strand breaks: their cellular and clinical impact? *Oncogene*, Vol. 26, No. 56, pp. 7717-7719.

Kaminski, J. M., Shinohara, E., Summers, J. B., Niermann, K. J., Morimoto, A. & Brousal, J. (2005). The controversial abscopal effect. *Cancer Treat Rev*, Vol. 31, No. 3, pp. 159-172.

Kataoka, Y., Murley, J. S., Baker, K. L. & Grdina, D. J. (2007). Relationship between phosphorylated histone H2AX formation and cell survival in human microvascular endothelial cells (HMEC) as a function of ionizing radiation exposure in the presence or absence of thiol-containing drugs. *Radiat Res*, Vol. 168, No. 1, pp. 106-114.

Kumar, A. & Sevilla, M. D. (2010). Proton-coupled electron transfer in DNA on formation of radiation-produced ion radicals. *Chem Rev*, Vol. 110, No. 12, pp. 7002-7023.

Laayoun, A., Coulombeau, C., Constant, J. F., Berger, M., Cadet, J. & Lhomme, J. (1994). Aminothiols linked to quinoline and acridine chromophores efficiently decrease 7,8-dihydro-8-oxo-2'-deoxyguanosine formation in gamma-irradiated DNA. *Int J Radiat Biol*, Vol. 66, No. 3, pp. 259-266.

Lawrence, T. S., Ten Haken, R. K. & Giaccia, A. (2008). Principles of Radiation Oncology. *Cancer: Principles and Practice of Oncology*. D. V. Jr., T. S. Lawrence and S. A. Rosenberg. Philadelphia, Lippincott Williams and Wilkins.

Leach, J. K., Van Tuyle, G., Lin, P. S., Schmidt-Ullrich, R. & Mikkelsen, R. B. (2001). Ionizing radiation-induced, mitochondria-dependent generation of reactive oxygen/nitrogen. *Cancer Res*, Vol. 61, No. 10, pp. 3894-3901.

Lieber, M. R. (2010). The mechanism of double-strand DNA break repair by the nonhomologous DNA end-joining pathway. *Annu Rev Biochem*, Vol. 79, No., pp. 181-211.

Liu, T., Liu, Y., He, S., Zhang, Z. & Kligerman, M. M. (1992). Use of radiation with or without WR-2721 in advanced rectal cancer. *Cancer*, Vol. 69, No. 11, pp. 2820-2825.

Lobachevsky, P. N., Karagiannis, T. C. & Martin, R. F. (2004). Plasmid DNA breakage by decay of DNA-associated Auger electron emitters: approaches to analysis of experimental data. *Radiat Res*, Vol. 162, No. 1, pp. 84-95.

Lobachevsky, P. N., Vasireddy, R. S., Broadhurst, S., Sprung, C. N., Karagiannis, T. C., Smith, A. J., Radford, I. R., McKay, M. J. & Martin, R. F. (2011). Protection by methylproamine of irradiated human keratinocytes correlates with reduction of DNA damage. *Int J Radiat Biol*, Vol. 87, No. 3, pp. 274-283.

Loontiens, F. G., Regenfuss, P., Zechel, A., Dumortier, L. & Clegg, R. M. (1990). Binding Characteristics of Hoechst 33258 with Calf Thymus DNA, Poly[d(A-T)], and d(CCGGAATTCCGG): Multiple Stoichiometries and Determination of Tight Binding with a Wide Spectrum of Site Affinities. *Biochemistry*, Vol. 29, No. 38, pp. 9029-9039.

Lyubimova, N. V., Coultas, P. G., Yuen, K. & Martin, R. F. (2001). In vivo radioprotection of mouse brain endothelial cells by Hoechst 33342. *Br J Radiol*, Vol. 74, No. 877, pp. 77-82.

Mancuso, M., Pasquali, E., Leonardi, S., Tanori, M., Rebessi, S., Di Majo, V., Pazzaglia, S., Toni, M. P., Pimpinella, M., Covelli, V. & Saran, A. (2008). Oncogenic bystander radiation effects in Patched heterozygous mouse cerebellum. *Proc Natl Acad Sci U S A*, Vol. 105, No. 34, pp. 12445-12450.

Martin, R. F. & Anderson, R. F. (1998). Pulse radiolysis studies indicate that electron transfer is involved in radioprotection by Hoechst 33342 and methylproamine. *International Journal of Radiation Oncology Biology Physics*, Vol. 42, No. 4, pp. 827-831.

Martin, R. F., Broadhurst, S., D'Abrew, S., Budd, R., Sephton, R., Reum, M. & Kelly, D. P. (1996). Radioprotection by DNA ligands. *British Journal of Cancer Supplement*, Vol. 27, No., pp. S99-101.

Martin, R. F., Broadhurst, S., Reum, M. E., Squire, C. J., Clark, G. R., Lobachevsky, P. N., White, J. M., Clark, C., Sy, D., Spotheim-Maurizot, M. & Kelly, D. P. (2004). In vitro studies with methylproamine: a potent new radioprotector. *Cancer Research*, Vol. 64, No. 3, pp. 1067-1070.

Martin, R. F. & Denison, L. (1992). DNA ligands as radiomodifiers: studies with minor-groove binding bibenzimidazoles. *International Journal of Radiation Oncology Biology Physics*, Vol. 23, No. 3, pp. 579-584.

Martin, R. F. & Holmes, N. (1983). Use of an 125I-labelled DNA ligand to probe DNA structure. *Nature*, Vol. 302, No. 5907, pp. 452-454.

Martin, R. F., Murray, V., D'Cunha, G., Pardee, M., Kampouris, E., Haigh, A., Kelly, D. P. & Hodgson, G. S. (1990). Radiation sensitization by an iodine-labelled DNA ligand. *International Journal of Radiation Biology*, Vol. 57, No. 5, pp. 939-946.

Matsumoto, Y., Kim, K. & Bogenhagen, D. F. (1994). Proliferating cell nuclear antigen-dependent abasic site repair in Xenopus laevis oocytes: an alternative pathway of base excision DNA repair. *Mol Cell Biol*, Vol. 14, No. 9, pp. 6187-6197.

McKinnon, P. J. & Caldecott, K. W. (2007). DNA strand break repair and human genetic disease. *Annu Rev Genomics Hum Genet*, Vol. 8, No., pp. 37-55.

Memisoglu, A. & Samson, L. (2000). Base excision repair in yeast and mammals. *Mutat Res*, Vol. 451, No. 1-2, pp. 39-51.

Mikkelsen, R. B. & Wardman, P. (2003). Biological chemistry of reactive oxygen and nitrogen and radiation-induced signal transduction mechanisms. *Oncogene*, Vol. 22, No. 37, pp. 5734-5754.

Milligan, J. R., Aguilera, J. A., Mares, E. J., Paglinawan, R. A. & Ward, J. F. (2001). Reaction of guanyl radicals in plasmid DNA with biological reductants: chemical repair of DNA damage produced by the direct effect of ionizing radiation. *Int J Radiat Biol*, Vol. 77, No. 11, pp. 1095-1108.

Milligan, J. R., Aguilera, J. A., Nguyen, T. T., Paglinawan, R. A. & Ward, J. F. (2000a). DNA strand-break yields after post-irradiation incubation with base excision repair endonucleases implicate hydroxyl radical pairs in double-strand break formation. *Int J Radiat Biol*, Vol. 76, No. 11, pp. 1475-1483.

Milligan, J. R., Aguilera, J. A., Paglinawan, R. A., Nguyen, K. J. & Ward, J. F. (2002). Modification of ionizing radiation clustered damage: estimate of the migration distance of holes through DNA via guanyl radicals under physiological conditions. *Int J Radiat Biol*, Vol. 78, No. 8, pp. 733-741.

Milligan, J. R., Aguilera, J. A., Paglinawan, R. A. & Ward, J. F. (2000b). Mechanism of DNA damage by thiocyanate radicals. *Int J Radiat Biol*, Vol. 76, No. 10, pp. 1305-1314.

Mladenov, E. & Iliakis, G. (2011). Induction and repair of DNA double strand breaks: The increasing spectrum of non-homologous end joining pathways. *Mutat Res*, Vol., No., pp.

Mole, R. H. (1953). Whole body irradiation; radiobiology or medicine? *Br J Radiol*, Vol. 26, No. 305, pp. 234-241.

Murray, D., Milas, L. & Meyn, R. E. (1988a). Radioprotection of mouse jejunum by WR-2721 and WR-1065: effects on DNA strand-break induction and rejoining. *Radiat Res*, Vol. 114, No. 2, pp. 268-280.

Murray, D., VanAnkeren, S. C., Milas, L. & Meyn, R. E. (1988b). Radioprotective action of WR-1065 on radiation-induced DNA strand breaks in cultured Chinese hamster ovary cells. *Radiat Res*, Vol. 113, No. 1, pp. 155-170.

Murray, V. & Martin, R. F. (1994). Ultraviolet light-induced cleavage of DNA in the presence of iodoHoechst 33258: the sequence specificity of the reaction. *Nucleic Acids Research*, Vol. 22, No. 3, pp. 506-513.

Nakamura, J. & Swenberg, J. A. (1999). Endogenous apurinic/apyrimidinic sites in genomic DNA of mammalian tissues. *Cancer Res*, Vol. 59, No. 11, pp. 2522-2526.

Nikjoo, H., O'Neill, P., Goodhead, D. T. & Terrissol, M. (1997). Computational modelling of low-energy electron-induced DNA damage by early physical and chemical events. *Int J Radiat Biol*, Vol. 71, No. 5, pp. 467-483.

Nikjoo, H., Uehara, S., Wilson, W. E., Hoshi, M. & Goodhead, D. T. (1998). Track structure in radiation biology: theory and applications. *Int J Radiat Biol*, Vol. 73, No. 4, pp. 355-364.

O'Connor, T. R. & Laval, J. (1989). Physical association of the 2,6-diamino-4-hydroxy-5N-formamidopyrimidine-DNA glycosylase of Escherichia coli and an activity nicking DNA at apurinic/apyrimidinic sites. *Proc Natl Acad Sci U S A*, Vol. 86, No. 14, pp. 5222-5226.

Prise, K. M. & O'Sullivan, J. M. (2009). Radiation-induced bystander signalling in cancer therapy. *Nat Rev Cancer*, Vol. 9, No. 5, pp. 351-360.

Purdie, J. W., Inhaber, E. R., Schneider, H. & Labelle, J. L. (1983). Interaction of cultured mammalian cells with WR-2721 and its thiol, WR-1065: implications for mechanisms of radioprotection. *Int J Radiat Biol*, Vol. 43, No. 5, pp. 517-527.

Purkayastha, S., Milligan, J. R. & Bernhard, W. A. (2007). On the chemical yield of base lesions, strand breaks, and clustered damage generated in plasmid DNA by the direct effect of X rays. *Radiat Res*, Vol. 168, No. 3, pp. 357-366.

Riley, P. A. (1994). Free radicals in biology: oxidative stress and the effects of ionizing radiation. *Int J Radiat Biol*, Vol. 65, No. 1, pp. 27-33.

Rogakou, E. P., Boon, C., Redon, C. & Bonner, W. M. (1999). Megabase chromatin domains involved in DNA double-strand breaks in vivo. *Journal of Cell Biology*, Vol. 146, No. 5, pp. 905-916.

Rogakou, E. P., Pilch, D. R., Orr, A. H., Ivanova, V. S. & Bonner, W. M. (1998). DNA double-stranded breaks induce histone H2AX phosphorylation on serine 139. *Journal of Biological Chemistry*, Vol. 273, No. 10, pp. 5858-5868.

Roots, R. & Okada, S. (1972). Protection of DNA molecules of cultured mammalian cells from radiation-induced single-strand scissions by various alcohols and SH compounds. *Int J Radiat Biol Relat Stud Phys Chem Med*, Vol. 21, No. 4, pp. 329-342.

Sedelnikova, O. A., Nakamura, A., Kovalchuk, O., Koturbash, I., Mitchell, S. A., Marino, S. A., Brenner, D. J. & Bonner, W. M. (2007). DNA double-strand breaks form in bystander cells after microbeam irradiation of three-dimensional human tissue models. *Cancer Res*, Vol. 67, No. 9, pp. 4295-4302.

Sedelnikova, O. A., Pilch, D. R., Redon, C. & Bonner, W. M. (2003). Histone H2AX in DNA damage and repair. *Cancer Biology and Therapy*, Vol. 2, No. 3, pp. 233-235.

Sedelnikova, O. A., Redon, C. E., Dickey, J. S., Nakamura, A. J., Georgakilas, A. G. & Bonner, W. M. (2010). Role of oxidatively induced DNA lesions in human pathogenesis. *Mutat Res*, Vol. 704, No. 1-3, pp. 152-159.

Sedelnikova, O. A., Rogakou, E. P., Panyutin, I. G. & Bonner, W. M. (2002). Quantitative detection of (125)IdU-induced DNA double-strand breaks with gamma-H2AX antibody. *Radiation Research*, Vol. 158, No. 4, pp. 486-492.

Sigdestad, C. P., Treacy, S. H., Knapp, L. A. & Grdina, D. J. (1987). The effect of 2-[(aminopropyl)amino] ethanethiol (WR-1065) on radiation induced DNA double strand damage and repair in V79 cells. *Br J Cancer*, Vol. 55, No. 5, pp. 477-482.

Simone, N. L., Menard, C., Soule, B. P., Albert, P. S., Guion, P., Smith, S., Godette, D., Crouse, N. S., Sciuto, L. C., Cooley-Zgela, T., Camphausen, K., Coleman, C. N. & Singh, A. K. (2008). Intrarectal amifostine during external beam radiation therapy for prostate cancer produces significant improvements in Quality of Life measured by EPIC score. *Int J Radiat Oncol Biol Phys*, Vol. 70, No. 1, pp. 90-95.

Smith, P. J. & Anderson, C. O. (1984). Modification of the radiation sensitivity of human tumour cells by a bis-benzimidazole derivative. *International Journal of Radiation Biology and Related Studies in Physics, Chemistry and Medicine*, Vol. 46, No. 4, pp. 331-344.

Smoluk, G. D., Fahey, R. C., Calabro-Jones, P. M., Aguilera, J. A. & Ward, J. F. (1988a). Radioprotection of cells in culture by WR-2721 and derivatives: form of the drug responsible for protection. *Cancer Res*, Vol. 48, No. 13, pp. 3641-3647.

Smoluk, G. D., Fahey, R. C. & Ward, J. F. (1986). Equilibrium dialysis studies of the binding of radioprotector compounds to DNA. *Radiat Res*, Vol. 107, No. 2, pp. 194-204.

Smoluk, G. D., Fahey, R. C. & Ward, J. F. (1988b). Interaction of glutathione and other low-molecular-weight thiols with DNA: evidence for counterion condensation and coion depletion near DNA. *Radiat Res*, Vol. 114, No. 1, pp. 3-10.

Sokolov, M. V., Smilenov, L. B., Hall, E. J., Panyutin, I. G., Bonner, W. M. & Sedelnikova, O. A. (2005). Ionizing radiation induces DNA double-strand breaks in bystander primary human fibroblasts. *Oncogene*, Vol. 24, No. 49, pp. 7257-7265.

Sprung, C. N., Chao, M., Leong, T. & McKay, M. J. (2005). Chromosomal radiosensitivity in two cell lineages derived from clinically radiosensitive cancer patients. *Clin Cancer Res*, Vol. 11, No. 17, pp. 6352-6358.

Sprung, C. N., Davey, D. S., Withana, N. P., Distel, L. V. & McKay, M. J. (2008). Telomere length in lymphoblast cell lines derived from clinically radiosensitive cancer patients. *Cancer Biol Ther*, Vol. 7, No. 5, pp. 638-644.

Sprung, C. N., Vasireddy, R. S., Karagiannis, T. C., Loveridge, S. J., Martin, R. F. & McKay, M. J. (2010). Methylproamine protects against ionizing radiation by preventing DNA double-strand breaks. *Mutat Res*, Vol. 692, No. 1-2, pp. 49-52.

Stone, H. B., Moulder, J.E., Coleman, C.N., Ang, K.K., Anscher, M.S., Barcellos-Hoff, M.H., Dynan, W.S., Fie, J.R., Grdina, D.J., Greenberger, J.S., Hauer-Jensen, M., Hill, R.P., Kolesnick, R.N., Macvittie, T.J., Marks, C., McBride, W.H., Metting, N., Pellmar, T., Purucker, M., Robbins, M.E., Schiestl, R.H., Seed, T.M., Tomaszewski, J.E., Travis, E.L., Wallner, P.E., Wolpert, M., Zaharevitz, D. (2003). Models for evaluating agents intended for the prophylaxis, mitigatin and treatment of radiation injuries. *Radiation Research*, Vol. 162, No. 6, pp. 711-728.

Sutherland, B. M., Bennett, P. V., Sidorkina, O. & Laval, J. (2000). Clustered DNA damages induced in isolated DNA and in human cells by low doses of ionizing radiation. *Proc Natl Acad Sci U S A*, Vol. 97, No. 1, pp. 103-108.

Sweeny, T. R. (1979). *Survey of Compounds from the Antiradiation Drug Development Program of the U.S. Army Medical Research and Development Command.* Washington, DC, Walter Reed Institute of Research

Tsoi, M., Do, T. T., Tang, V. J., Aguilera, J. A. & Milligan, J. R. (2010). Reduction of electron deficient guanine radical species in plasmid DNA by tyrosine derivatives. *Org Biomol Chem*, Vol. 8, No. 11, pp. 2553-2559.

Ward, J. F. (1981). Some biochemical consequences of the spatial distribution of ionizing radiation-produced free radicals. *Radiat Res*, Vol. 86, No. 2, pp. 185-195.

Ward, J. F. (1994a). The complexity of DNA damage: relevance to biological consequences. *Int J Radiat Biol*, Vol. 66, No. 5, pp. 427-432.

Ward, J. F. (1994b). DNA damage as the cause of ionizing radiation-induced gene activation. *Radiat Res*, Vol. 138, No. 1 Suppl, pp. S85-88.

Wasserman, T. H. (1994). Radiotherapeutic studies with amifostine (Ethyol). *Semin Oncol*, Vol. 21, No. 5 Suppl 11, pp. 21-25.

Weiss, J. F. & Landauer, M. R. (2009). History and development of radiation-protective agents. *Int J Radiat Biol*, Vol. 85, No. 7, pp. 539-573.

Wilson, D. M., 3rd, Sofinowski, T. M. & McNeill, D. R. (2003). Repair mechanisms for oxidative DNA damage. *Front Biosci*, Vol. 8, No., pp. d963-981.

Withers, H. R. & Elkind, M. M. (1969). Radiosensitivity and fractionation response of crypt cells of mouse jejunum. *Radiat Res*, Vol. 38, No. 3, pp. 598-613.

Withers, H. R. & Elkind, M. M. (1970). Microcolony survival assay for cells of mouse intestinal mucosa exposed to radiation. *Int J Radiat Biol Relat Stud Phys Chem Med*, Vol. 17, No. 3, pp. 261-267.

Young, S. D. & Hill, R. P. (1989). Radiation sensitivity of tumour cells stained in vitro or in vivo with the bisbenzimide fluorochrome Hoechst 33342. *British Journal of Cancer*, Vol. 60, No. 5, pp. 715-721.

Zheng, S., Newton, G. L., Ward, J. F. & Fahey, R. C. (1992). Aerobic radioprotection of pBR322 by thiols: effect of thiol net charge upon scavenging of hydroxyl radicals and repair of DNA radicals. *Radiat Res*, Vol. 130, No. 2, pp. 183-193.

# 23

# DNA Damage Response and Repair: Insights into Strategies for Radiation Sensitization

Joshua D. Lawson[1], Kristopher T. Kahle[2], Kimberly Ng[3], Bob Carter[4], Santosh Kesari[5] and Clark C. Chen[3]
[1]*Department of Radiation Oncology, Moores Cancer Center, University of California, San Diego, La Jolla, CA*
[2]*Department of Neurosurgery, Massachusetts General Hospital and Harvard Medical School, Boston, MA*
[3]*Department of Radiation Oncology, Division of Genomic Stability and DNA Repair, Dana-Farber Cancer Institute, Boston, MA*
[4]*Center for Theoretical and Applied Neuro-Oncology, Moores Cancer Center, University of California, San Diego, La Jolla, CA*
[5]*Department of Neurosciences, Moores Cancer Center, University of California, San Diego, La Jolla, CA*
*USA*

## 1. Introduction

Glioblastoma is the most common form of primary brain tumors [1]. About 10,000 new patients each year in the US are diagnosed with GBM. Despite its comparatively low incidence of about 2-3 new cases per 100,000 people per year (for comparison, the incidence of colon cancer in the US is approximately 1 new case per 1,800 people per year), the total number of deaths per year attributable to glioblastoma rivals that of other major cancers. This disparity reflects the lethal nature of the disease. If untreated, patients with glioblastoma generally die within 3 months of their diagnosis [2]. Diffuse invasion into the surrounding normal cerebral parenchyma is a cardinal feature of glioblastoma, preventing surgical cure. In this context, it is not surprising that surgical resection alone does not significantly prolong patient survival [2]. When maximal surgical resection is combined with radiation and the chemotherapeutic agent, temozolomide, the median survival of patients improved to 14.6 months [3]. While this regimen achieves an approximate 10% five-year progression free survival [4], the majority of the afflicted patients succumb to the disease within a year of diagnosis. Effective therapeutic strategies are desperately needed.

Despite the abundance of strategies and agents that have been tested over the last half-century for the treatment of GBM, the single most efficacious modality and significant advance has been the use of post-resection radiation therapy. In 1966, the Montreal Neurology Institute published the first large case series that suggested a survival advantage in patients who received an average total post-resection IR dose of 5,000–6,000 cGy [5]. Over the next decade, other case series corroborated those data, suggesting an improvement in patient survival with post-resection IR [6-9]. Although interpretation of these case series is confounded by their retrospective, non-randomized nature, and wide variations in radiation dose regimen, an overall trend of improved patient survival was seen.

The efficacious nature of radiation therapy in glioblastoma was subsequently confirmed in three subsequent randomized control trials. *BTSG 66-01,* the first of the initial three clinical studies that randomized patients with newly-diagnosed malignant gliomas to with Whole-Brain RadioTherapy (WBRT) with or without mithramycin [10]. While mithramycin did not significantly impact survival, the survival of patients who received adjuvant WBRT were extended to about 5 months on average. *BTSG 69-01* randomized patients post-surgical resection to best supportive care or chemotherapy (BCNU), with or without WBRT. Overall patient *survival* was improved with radiation therapy (with or without BCNU) when compared to supportive care alone. The median survival for the surgery only patient was 14 weeks. The median survival for patients who underwent surgery followed by radiation therapy was 36 weeks ($p<0.05$). Similar results were seen in another randomized trial, *BTSG72-01.*

A meta-analysis of *66-01, 69-01,* and *72-01* [11]showed that patients who did not receive radiation or were treated with less than 4,500 cGy exhibited poor survival (median survival of 4.2 and 3.1 months, respectively). On the other hand, patients treated with 5,000, 5,500, and 6,000 cGy showed improved survival (median survival of 6.5, 8.4, and 9.8 months, respectively). Subsequent dose escalation beyond 6,000 cGy revealed increased neuro-toxicity without significant therapeutic gain [12]. These studies collectively established the dosimetry for modern glioblastoma therapy.

It is important to note that, as a single agent, the efficacy of radiation therapy as a glioblastoma therapeutic has yet been matched by any chemotherapy [12]. For this reason, radiation therapy remains a universal component in clinical trials with curative intent for treatment of newly diagnosed glioblastomas. Identification of agents that augment the efficacy of radiation therapy remains a promising strategy for glioblastoma therapy. In this context, we will review the molecular mechanism underlying cellular response to radiation.

## 2. DNA repair and damage response following ionizing radiation

While Ionizing Radiation (IR) has been shown to induce a plethora of cellular effects, it is widely held that its tumoricidal activity is largely related its effect on DNA [13]. IR induces multiple types of DNA lesions, including damages to the nucleobase, sugar, and phosphate back bone [13]. Ultimately, these lesions, if unrepaired, are converted into Double Stranded DNA Breaks (DSBs). DSBs are highly cytotoxic as the presence of a single DSB in a cell is sufficient to induce death [14-19]. Our understanding of DNA damage response and DSB repair has expanded exponentially in the past decade. To make this vast information more accessible to the reader, we will organize the information into the following sections: 1) general mechanism of DSB repair, 2) mechanism by which DNA damage response activates DSB repair, and 3) effect of DNA damage on cell cycle progression.

### 2.1 General mechanism of DSB repair

DSBs are repaired by two major mechanisms: Non-Homologous End Joining (NHEJ) or Homologous Recombination (HR) [20, 21]. The simplest way of repairing DSB is by re-ligation. This process is termed NHEJ since no significant DNA sequence homology at the broken ends is required. Instead, the NHEJ enzymatic machinery relies on limited processing of the DNA ends followed by annealing short stretches of complementary DNA sequences.

Because short stretches of complementary sequences occur at some regularity in the human genome, NHEJ is prone to the generation of mutations, deletions, as well as chromosomal rearrangements[22].

The second major DSB repair process is termed HR. HR initiates with extensive 5′ to 3′ end processing of the broken ends into large regions of single stranded tails. The resultant 3′ single stranded tail invades a homologous donor sequence. This strand invasion is mediated by enzyme(s) termed "recombinase" that coats the single stranded tail. Subsequent strand extension and Holliday junction resolution result in restoration of DNA continuity. The resolution is mediated by specific enzymes(s) termed "resolvase" [21]. Because the process cannot proceed without extensive sequence homology, HR tends to be less prone to mutagenesis relative to NHEJ. Because of the requirement for a homologous donor sequence, HR occurs only in the S/G2/M phases of the cell cycle while NHEJ occurs throughout the cell cycle. Both HR and NHEJ contribute to the repair of RT induced DSBs, suggesting that these pathways may be functionally compensatory [23-25]. Given the critical role of these two processes, it is not surprising they are subject to complex regulation.

In mammalian cells, both are carried out by multi-step processes facilitated by a large number of proteins. The mechanistic details of these processes remain an active area of investigation. Working models are described as follows.

For NHEJ, upon DNA damage response activation (see below), the Ku70/Ku 80 heterodimer is recruited to the break site. This protein complex forms a ring shaped structure to protect the broken DNA ends [26]. Additionally, the heterodimer serves as a platform for binding of the critical kinase, DNA-PK [27], and the XRCC4-Ligase IV-XLF4 complex [28]to the site of damage. DNA-PK performs two important functions: 1) it phosphorylates the Ligase IV complex to facilitate the joining of DNA ends; and 2) in cases where DNA end processing is required before rejoining, DNA-PK binds to and recruits the Artemis endonuclease to perform this function. While other proteins also participate in NHEJ [21], *in vitro* reconstitution of NHEJ with these seven proteins (Ku70, Ku80, DNA-PK, XRCC4-Ligase IV-XLF4 complex, and Artemis) suggest that they are essential for this process.

In comparison, the genetics of HR is more complex and far less well understood. Upon DNA damage response activation, it is thought that the BRCA1 and BRCA2 protein are recruited to the site of DNA damage. These two proteins were cloned by virtue of their inactivation in familial breast cancer cohorts (BReast CAncer genes 1 and 2) [29-31]. Both proteins encode large molecular weight proteins that mediate multiple cellular processes to suppress tumor formation. One of these critical functions involves HR. It's proposed that BRCA1 and 2 bind to aberrant DNA structures related to DSB ends [32, 33]. Through BRCA2, the mammalian recombinase, RAD51, is recruited to the site of damage [34]. RAD51 coats the DNA and facilitates the strand exchange reaction in homologous recombination [35-37]. After strand invasion, resolution of the Holliday intermediate is mediated by a protein complex consisting of XRCC3 and RAD51C (two homologues of RAD51) [21, 38].

The mechanism by which HR and NHEJ is activated in response to DNA damage is discussed below.

### 2.2 DNA damage response

The DNA Damage Response (DDR) refers to the signal transduction cascades that are triggered by DNA damages. These cascades coordinate DNA repair, cell cycle progression, and cell death mechanisms to facilitate the faithful transmission of genetic material after

DNA damage. The process initiates with the recognition of DNA damage by specialized "sensor" proteins. These sensor proteins, in turn, recruit and/or activate "transducer" proteins required for subsequent signaling to "effector" responses, such as cell cycle arrest, apoptosis, transcription, and DNA repair [39]. Defects in DNA damage response have been associated with genomic instability, sensitivity to genotoxic agents, and cancer predisposition [40].

Upon DNA damage, the strand discontinuities trigger complex changes in DNA topology secondary to histone acetylation and phosphorylation of chromatin proteins [41]. The unveiled strand break is recognized by the Mre11-Rad50-Nbs1 (MRN) complex. In addition to serving as an exo/endonuclease to process the DSBs into single stranded DNA tails [42], the MRN complex also recruits the Ataxia Telangiectasia Mutated (ATM) protein kinase to the site of the DSB [43, 44]. When recruited to DSBs, ATM - normally existing in an inactive dimeric form - dissociates and autophosphorylates on multiple residues that are thought to be important for activation of ATM's kinase activity [45]. The activated ATM phosphorylates the histone protein, H2AX, over a region of megabases surrounding a DSB [46, 47]. The phosphorylated H2AX (also known as γ-H2AX), in turn, recruits the Mediator of DNA Checkpoint (MDC1) protein [48, 49]. The MDC1 protein serves as a scaffold protein for docking of the E3 ubiquitin ligase complex, UBC13-RNF8 [50], which serves to poly-ubiquitinate H2AX. Completion of this poly-ubiquitination reaction requires a second ubiquitin ligase, RNF168 [51]. RNF168 is recruited to the site of DNA damage through its interaction with HERC2 and RNF8 [52]. The poly-ubiquitination reaction alters local chromatin structure as well as provides docking site for the ubiquitin binding protein, RAP80. RAP80, in turn, recruits the BRCA1/BRCA2/RAD51 repair complex by direct physical interaction[53]. This complex initiates DSB repair by HR as well as arrests cell cycle progression in a process known as DNA damage checkpoint activation (see ensuing section).

It is important to note that while the above damage response is described in a linear manner, parallel interactions occur at each step. For instance, MDC1, in addition to recruiting UBC13-RNF8, also interacts with ATM [48] and MRN [54] to stabilize the repair complex. The aggregate effect of these other complex interactions induces chromatin state changes surrounding the DSB and the localization of numerous proteins required for coordinating DNA repair and checkpoint regulation.

Similar to HR, the NHEJ process can be initiated by the MRN complex upon DDR activation. The Mre11 protein in the complex can directly interact with the Ku70 subunit [55]. Moreover, the RAD50 protein in the MRN complex encodes a high-affinity DNA binding domain and a second domain that facilitates homodimeric interactions that holds DNA ends in close proximity [56] to facilitate subsequent NHEJ.

Since the MRN complex may initiate either HR or NHEJ, a central question in the field of DNA repair involves the mechanism of this regulation. Inappropriate activation of HR in the G1 phase of the cell cycle could lead to cell death. Similarly, activation of NHEJ during the S/G2 phases of the cell cycle could increase the rate of mutagenesis. One of the key mediators of this regulatory process involves the protein CTBP Interacting Protein (CTIP). In a landmark study [57], CTIP was found to interact with the MRN complex to promote its exo/endonuclease activity and process DSBs into single stranded DNA ends. Importantly, this activity is regulated by cell cycle dependent phosphorylation events mediated by Cyclin-Dependent Kinases (CDKs). In the S/G2 phase of the cell cycle, CTIP is phosphorylated. Thus, the MRN complex processes DSBs into single stranded tails required for the initiation of HR. On the other hand, in the G1 phase of the cell cycle, CTIP remains unphosphorylated, and the MRN complex remains inactive as an exo/endo-nuclease. Without this processing, HR cannot be initiated. Thus, NHEJ becomes the predominant repair process.

### 2.3 Effect of DNA damage on cell cycle progression

In addition to the assembly of repair complexes as above described, DNA damage triggers signaling to proteins required for cell cycle progression, such as the CDK/cyclin complex. Generally speaking, DNA damage checkpoint regulation occurs at three distinct phases of the cell cycle: the G1-S transition, the intra-S-phase, and the G2-M transition. Most of what we understand of this transduction process involves protein phosphorylation cascades, though the importance of other types of reversible modifications, such as ubiquitination and sumoylation, are become increasingly apparent [58]. Here, we will review an illustrative example of signal transduction between DNA damage sensors and cell cycle regulation. Upon recognition of DSB, the MRN complex recruits and activates the critical ATM kinase. The ATM kinase, in turn, phosphorylates the tumor suppressor p53 and another kinase termed Chk2 (Checkpoint Kinase 2) [59]. ATM phosphorylation of Chk2 activates its kinase activity which, in turn, phosphorylates both p53 and MDM2. These phosphorylation events stabilize p53 by interrupting its association with its negative regulator, MDM2 [60]. Activated p53 then induces the transcription of its target genes, which include the critical regulator of the G1-S transition, p21 [61]. The binding of p21 to the CDK-cyclin complexes and prevents phosphorylation of the retinoblastoma protein (pRb). When in a hypophosphorylated state, pRb blocks cell proliferation by sequestering and altering the function of E2F transcription factors that control transcription of genes required for progression from G1 into S phase. Disruption of the pRb pathway - as occurs with mutant p53 or p21 - liberates E2Fs and allows cell proliferation, which renders cells insensitive to DNA damage-induced anti-growth signals that normally operate to inhibit passage through G1 phase of the cell cycle [62]. With regards to the G2-M checkpoint, ATM release inhibition of p53 additionally results in the transcriptional induction of 14-3-3σ in addition to p21. The 14-3-3σ protein sequesters the cyclinB-cdc2 kinase complex in the cytoplasm and prevents nuclear phosphorylation events required for G2/M progression [63]. Additionally, p21 binds to any residual cdc2 that enters the nucleus to prevent its activation. These and other ATM events prevent progression through the G2/M transition and afford time for DSB repair [64].

## 3. Strategies for sensitization

A prediction of the above presented model is that inhibition of any of the proteins required for DDR or DSB repair should lead to radiation sensitization. In general, this prediction has been confirmed [65]. However, therapeutic agents that directly inhibit these critical proteins are still years from reaching clinical trial. Encouragingly, several FDA-approved agents have recently been shown to modulate DNA damage response. This property may be explored as therapeutic strategy.

### 3.1 Molecular rationale for therapeutic window

Before considering the strategy of radiation sensitization, one must first consider the molecular rationale for therapeutic window. After all, if normal and tumor cells were equally sensitized by the agent, then no therapeutic efficacy is gained.

A large body has yielded data suggesting that oncogene activation creates a tumor state that increases the accumulation of DNA damage [66-69]. This damage, if unrepaired, can be converted into DSBs that eventually lead to cell death. To compensate for this increased DNA damage, the tumor cells require increased utilization of DNA repair processes [69]. In this context, the administration of radiation introduces additional DNA damage that further taxes the already over-utilized repair process. This situation, in turn, increases the likelihood of an unrepaired DSB causing cell death. The same effect can be achieved by inhibition of DSB repair. The following sections will review FDA-approved agents with such properties. It is important to note that these agents induce pleiotropic effects beyond DSB repair inhibition.

### 3.2 DNA damaging agents

Conventional chemotherapy involves DNA damaging agents that are often used in conjunction with radiation. In this context, these FDA-approved agents often sensitize the tumoricidal effects of radiation. The mechanism of this sensitization is thought to be related to the generation of DNA damages that sequester critical DNA repair proteins. For instance, lesions generated by cisplatin bind to and sequester the Ku70/80 heterodimer and thereby compromise the efficiency of NHEJ [70]. Further, most DNA damages induced by conventional chemotherapy are ultimately converted to DSBs [71]. These DSBs will titrate away the repair proteins available to repair the DSBs induced by subsequent radiation. These types of mechanisms likely account for the increased glioblastoma patient survival observed in the context of concurrent radiation/ temozolomide treatment relative to radiation treatment alone [3, 4].

### 3.3 Proteasome inhibitors

As a result of extreme aneuploidy, copy-number variation, and transcriptional alteration that are present in many cancer cells, there is increased stress on the chaperone pathways (such as heat shock proteins) to maintain folding of over-expressed proteins. When the capacity of these chaperone proteins becomes saturated, the unfolded proteins require degradation by the proteasome complex [72]. Thus, tumor cells exhibit increased dependency on proteasome function. Indeed, proteasome inhibition has been demonstrated to selectively ablate cancer cells both *in vitro* and *in vivo* [73]. The proteasome inhibitor bortezomib has attained FDA-approval as a treatment for multiple myeloma and mantle cell lymphoma.

Recent studies implicate proteasome function in DSB repair. The yeast Sem1 protein is a subunit of the 19S proteasome that is required for efficient HR [74]. The human Sem1 homologue, DSS1, physically interacts with the HR protein, BRCA2, and is required for its stability and function [75-77]. Using the DR-GFP assay to directly assess HR efficiency, Murakawa et al. demonstrated that HR efficiency is significantly reduced by proteasome inhibition [78]. As a whole, these studies suggest proteasome inhibition as a means to target HR in cancer therapy.

The mechanism by which proteasome inhibition modulates HR remains an area of investigation. One hypothesis frequently put forth is the following. The proteins destined for proteasome degradation are typically modified by attachment of multiple ubiquitin moieties [74]. Processing of the tagged protein releases the tagged ubiquitin to replete the intracellular pool. Proteasome inhibition, thus, leads to accumulation of ubiquitinated proteins. This accumulation, in turn, depletes the intracellular ubiquitin pool. Since free ubiquitins are required to activate HR, the repair process is compromised by proteasome inhibition.

### 3.4 Epidermal Growth Factor Receptor (EGFR) inhibitors

EGFR is frequently amplified or mutated in several cancer types, including Non-Small Cell Lung Cancer (NSCLC) and glioblastomas [79-81]. As aberrant EGFR signaling is required to sustain tumor survival and proliferation in some cancers, targeted inhibition has led to selective tumor ablation [79]. Clinical trial success has led to FDA-approval for treatment of NSCLC.

Several studies have demonstrated that EGFR inhibition sensitized tumor cells to radiation [65]. Insights into the mechanism underlying this sensitization have been provided by several recent studies. One series of studies demonstrate that a subset of EGFR travels to the nucleus where it binds to and enhances DNA-PK activity to enhance NHEJ [82, 83]}. Indeed, glioblastomas over-expressing an over-active form of EGFR (termed EGFRvIII) exhibit radiation resistance that can be abridged by treatment with DNA-PK inhibitors [84]. Another series of studies reveal that EGFR inhibition leads to retention of BRCA1 in the cytoplasm, thereby causing defective HR [85]. Finally, other downstream effectors of EGFR, including the Extracellular signal Regulated Kinase (ERK1/2) also modulates HR efficiency [86]. It is likely that the radiation sensitization effect of EGFR inhibition represents a culmination of these individual effects.

### 3.5 Other late stage clinical trial agents

There are several other agents that are in mid- to late- clinical trial testing that have also been shown to inhibit DNA damage response. For instance, Histone DeACetylase (HDAC) inhibitors have been shown to down regulate the transcript level of BRCA1 [87]. These agents have also been shown to disrupt the chromatin re-organization required for ATM activation [41]. As another example, Heat Shock Protein 90 (HSP90, the prototypical chaperone protein) inhibitor treatment inhibits ATM autophosphorylation upon DNA damage [88] and destabilizes the MRN complex [89, 90], thereby inhibiting HR. Finally, CDK1 inhibition causes the loss of a critical phosphorylation event on BRCA1 required for its HR function [91].

There are additional modulators of DDR and DNA repair not described here [65]. Indeed, the number of pharmacologic inhibitors that either directly or indirectly inhibit DSB repair is being uncovered at a rapid pace. Careful consideration should be given for combination with radiation therapy in clinical trial design.

## 4. Closing remarks

Radiotherapy is the most effective post-surgical treatment modality in the management of glioblastoma. Adjuvant radiotherapy alone provides a more than doubling of median survival. Incremental gains with additional medical therapy have proven elusive, with most agents showing moderate activity *in vitro* or with encouraging early clinical experience only to demonstrate a lack of benefit in larger trials. Attempts at treatment intensification with radiotherapy have been similarly disappointing. Molecular understanding of DNA damage response and repair, on the other hand, has now afforded novel therapeutic targets. These targets are particularly attractive in the context that oncogenes induce increased DNA damage accumulation and cause tumors to become hyper-dependent on DNA damage response pathways. Encouragingly, several FDA-approved agents modulate critical proteins in DNA damage response/repair, including conventional DNA damaging agents, proteasome inhibitors, and EGFR inhibitors. Clinical trials involving these and other agents modulating DNA damage response should be designed with this consideration.

## 5. References


[1] Louis DN. Molecular pathology of malignant gliomas. *Annu Rev Pathol.* 2006;1:97-117.

[2] Walker MD, Alexander E, Jr., Hunt WE, et al. Evaluation of BCNU and/or radiotherapy in the treatment of anaplastic gliomas. A cooperative clinical trial. *J Neurosurg.* Sep 1978;49(3):333-343.

[3] Stupp R, Mason WP, van den Bent MJ, et al. Radiotherapy plus concomitant and adjuvant temozolomide for glioblastoma. *N Engl J Med.* Mar 10 2005;352(10):987-996.

[4] Stupp R, Hegi ME, Mason WP, et al. Effects of radiotherapy with concomitant and adjuvant temozolomide versus radiotherapy alone on survival in glioblastoma in a randomised phase III study: 5-year analysis of the EORTC-NCIC trial.

[5] Uihlein A, Colby MY Jr, Layton DD. Comparisons of surgery and surgery plus irradiation in the treatment of supratentorial gliomas. *Acta Radiol Ther Phys Biol.* 1966;3:67-78.

[6] Stage WS, Stein JJ. Treatment of malignant astrocytomas. *Am J Roentgenol Radium Ther Nucl Med.* Jan 1974;120(1):7-18.

[7] Sheline GE. Radiation therapy of brain tumors. *Cancer.* Feb 1977;39(2 Suppl):873-881.

[8] Sheline G. Conventional radiation therapy of gliomas. *Recent Results in Cancer Research. Gliomas: Current Concepts in Biology, Diagnosis, and Therapy.* New York: Springer-Verlag; 1975:125-134.

[9] Kramer S. Radiation therapy in the management of malignant gliomas. *Cancer of the Central Nervous System: Seventh National Cancer Conference Proceedings.* Philadelphia: Lippincott Company; 1973:823-826.

[10] Walker MD, Alexander E, Jr., Hunt WE, et al. Evaluation of mithramycin in the treatment of anaplastic gliomas. *J Neurosurg.* Jun 1976;44(6):655-667.

[11] Walker MD, Strike TA, Sheline GE. An analysis of dose-effect relationship in the radiotherapy of malignant gliomas. *Int J Radiat Oncol Biol Phys.* Oct 1979;5(10):1725-1731.

[12] Chang JE, Khuntia D, Robins HI, Mehta MP. Radiotherapy and radiosensitizers in the treatment of glioblastoma multiforme. *Clin Adv Hematol Oncol.* Nov 2007;5(11):894-902, 907-815.

[13] Hall E, ed *Radiobiology for the radiologist.* 6th ed. Philadelphia, PA: Lippincott Williams and Wilkins; 2006.

[14] Bennett CB, Lewis AL, Baldwin KK, Resnick MA. Lethality induced by a single site-specific double-strand break in a dispensable yeast plasmid. *Proc Natl Acad Sci U S A.* Jun 15 1993;90(12):5613-5617.

[15] Bennett CB, Westmoreland TJ, Snipe JR, Resnick MA. A double-strand break within a yeast artificial chromosome (YAC) containing human DNA can result in YAC loss, deletion or cell lethality. *Mol Cell Biol.* Aug 1996;16(8):4414-4425.

[16] Dugle DL, Gillespie CJ, Chapman JD. DNA strand breaks, repair, and survival in x-irradiated mammalian cells. *Proc Natl Acad Sci U S A.* Mar 1976;73(3):809-812.

[17] Game JC, Mortimer RK. A genetic study of X-ray sensitive mutants in yeast. *Mutat Res.* 1974;24:281-292.

[18] Lee SE, Moore JK, Holmes A, Umezu K, Kolodner RD, Haber JE. Saccharomyces Ku70, mre11/rad50 and RPA proteins regulate adaptation to G2/M arrest after DNA damage. *Cell.* Aug 7 1998;94(3):399-409.

[19] Sandell LL, Zakian VA. Loss of a yeast telomere: arrest, recovery, and chromosome loss. *Cell.* Nov 19 1993;75(4):729-739.
[20] Hartlerode AJ, Scully R. Mechanisms of double-strand break repair in somatic mammalian cells. *Biochem J.* Oct 15 2009;423(2):157-168.
[21] Wyman C, Kanaar R. DNA double-strand break repair: all's well that ends well. *Annu Rev Genet.* 2006;40:363-383.
[22] Lieber MR, Ma Y, Pannicke U, Schwarz K. Mechanism and regulation of human non-homologous DNA end-joining. *Nat Rev Mol Cell Biol.* Sep 2003;4(9):712-720.
[23] Ristic D, Modesti M, Kanaar R, Wyman C. Rad52 and Ku bind to different DNA structures produced early in double-strand break repair. *Nucleic Acids Res.* Sep 15 2003;31(18):5229-5237.
[24] Schar P, Herrmann G, Daly G, Lindahl T. A newly identified DNA ligase of Saccharomyces cerevisiae involved in RAD52-independent repair of DNA double-strand breaks. *Genes Dev.* Aug 1 1997;11(15):1912-1924.
[25] Takata M, Sasaki MS, Sonoda E, et al. Homologous recombination and non-homologous end-joining pathways of DNA double-strand break repair have overlapping roles in the maintenance of chromosomal integrity in vertebrate cells. *EMBO J.* Sep 15 1998;17(18):5497-5508.
[26] Walker JR, Corpina RA, Goldberg J. Structure of the Ku heterodimer bound to DNA and its implications for double-strand break repair. *Nature.* Aug 9 2001;412(6847):607-614.
[27] Gottlieb TM, Jackson SP. The DNA-dependent protein kinase: requirement for DNA ends and association with Ku antigen. *Cell.* Jan 15 1993;72(1):131-142.
[28] Nick McElhinny SA, Snowden CM, McCarville J, Ramsden DA. Ku recruits the XRCC4-ligase IV complex to DNA ends. *Mol Cell Biol.* May 2000;20(9):2996-3003.
[29] Futreal PA, Liu Q, Shattuck-Eidens D, et al. BRCA1 mutations in primary breast and ovarian carcinomas. *Science.* Oct 7 1994;266(5182):120-122.
[30] Miki Y, Swensen J, Shattuck-Eidens D, et al. A strong candidate for the breast and ovarian cancer susceptibility gene BRCA1. *Science.* Oct 7 1994;266(5182):66-71.
[31] Wooster R, Bignell G, Lancaster J, et al. Identification of the breast cancer susceptibility gene BRCA2. *Nature.* Dec 21-28 1995;378(6559):789-792.
[32] Paull TT, Cortez D, Bowers B, Elledge SJ, Gellert M. Direct DNA binding by Brca1. *Proc Natl Acad Sci U S A.* May 22 2001;98(11):6086-6091.
[33] Yang H, Jeffrey PD, Miller J, et al. BRCA2 function in DNA binding and recombination from a BRCA2-DSS1-ssDNA structure. *Science.* Sep 13 2002;297(5588):1837-1848.
[34] Powell SN, Kachnic LA. Roles of BRCA1 and BRCA2 in homologous recombination, DNA replication fidelity and the cellular response to ionizing radiation. *Oncogene.* Sep 1 2003;22(37):5784-5791.
[35] Galkin VE, Esashi F, Yu X, Yang S, West SC, Egelman EH. BRCA2 BRC motifs bind RAD51-DNA filaments. *Proc Natl Acad Sci U S A.* Jun 14 2005;102(24):8537-8542.
[36] Shin DS, Chahwan C, Huffman JL, Tainer JA. Structure and function of the double-strand break repair machinery. *DNA Repair (Amst).* Aug-Sep 2004;3(8-9):863-873.
[37] Shivji MK, Venkitaraman AR. DNA recombination, chromosomal stability and carcinogenesis: insights into the role of BRCA2. *DNA Repair (Amst).* Aug-Sep 2004;3(8-9):835-843.

[38] Liu Y, Masson JY, Shah R, O'Regan P, West SC. RAD51C is required for Holliday junction processing in mammalian cells. *Science.* Jan 9 2004;303(5655):243-246.
[39] Harper JW, Elledge SJ. The DNA damage response: ten years after. *Mol Cell.* Dec 14 2007;28(5):739-745.
[40] Jackson SP, Bartek J. The DNA-damage response in human biology and disease. *Nature.* Oct 22 2009;461(7267):1071-1078.
[41] van Attikum H, Gasser SM. The histone code at DNA breaks: a guide to repair? *Nat Rev Mol Cell Biol.* Oct 2005;6(10):757-765.
[42] D'Amours D, Jackson SP. The Mre11 complex: at the crossroads of dna repair and checkpoint signalling. *Nat Rev Mol Cell Biol.* May 2002;3(5):317-327.
[43] Lee JH, Paull TT. ATM activation by DNA double-strand breaks through the Mre11-Rad50-Nbs1 complex. *Science.* Apr 22 2005;308(5721):551-554.
[44] Paull TT, Lee JH. The Mre11/Rad50/Nbs1 complex and its role as a DNA double-strand break sensor for ATM. *Cell Cycle.* Jun 2005;4(6):737-740.
[45] Bakkenist CJ, Kastan MB. DNA damage activates ATM through intermolecular autophosphorylation and dimer dissociation. *Nature.* Jan 30 2003;421(6922):499-506.
[46] Paull TT, Rogakou EP, Yamazaki V, Kirchgessner CU, Gellert M, Bonner WM. A critical role for histone H2AX in recruitment of repair factors to nuclear foci after DNA damage. *Curr Biol.* Jul 27-Aug 10 2000;10(15):886-895.
[47] Rogakou EP, Boon C, Redon C, Bonner WM. Megabase chromatin domains involved in DNA double-strand breaks in vivo. *J Cell Biol.* Sep 6 1999;146(5):905-916.
[48] Lou Z, Minter-Dykhouse K, Franco S, et al. MDC1 maintains genomic stability by participating in the amplification of ATM-dependent DNA damage signals. *Mol Cell.* Jan 20 2006;21(2):187-200.
[49] Stucki M, Clapperton JA, Mohammad D, Yaffe MB, Smerdon SJ, Jackson SP. MDC1 directly binds phosphorylated histone H2AX to regulate cellular responses to DNA double-strand breaks. *Cell.* Dec 29 2005;123(7):1213-1226.
[50] Huen MS, Grant R, Manke I, et al. RNF8 transduces the DNA-damage signal via histone ubiquitylation and checkpoint protein assembly. *Cell.* Nov 30 2007;131(5):901-914.
[51] Doil C, Mailand N, Bekker-Jensen S, et al. RNF168 binds and amplifies ubiquitin conjugates on damaged chromosomes to allow accumulation of repair proteins. *Cell.* Feb 6 2009;136(3):435-446.
[52] Bekker-Jensen S, Rendtlew Danielsen J, Fugger K, et al. HERC2 coordinates ubiquitin-dependent assembly of DNA repair factors on damaged chromosomes. *Nat Cell Biol.* Jan 2010;12(1):80-86; sup pp 81-12.
[53] Kim H, Chen J, Yu X. Ubiquitin-binding protein RAP80 mediates BRCA1-dependent DNA damage response. *Science.* May 25 2007;316(5828):1202-1205.
[54] Chapman JR, Jackson SP. Phospho-dependent interactions between NBS1 and MDC1 mediate chromatin retention of the MRN complex at sites of DNA damage. *EMBO Rep.* Aug 2008;9(8):795-801.
[55] Goedecke W, Eijpe M, Offenberg HH, van Aalderen M, Heyting C. Mre11 and Ku70 interact in somatic cells, but are differentially expressed in early meiosis. *Nat Genet.* Oct 1999;23(2):194-198.
[56] Dinkelmann M, Spehalski E, Stoneham T, et al. Multiple functions of MRN in end-joining pathways during isotype class switching. *Nat Struct Mol Biol.* Aug 2009;16(8):808-813.

[57] Sartori AA, Lukas C, Coates J, et al. Human CtIP promotes DNA end resection. *Nature.* Nov 22 2007;450(7169):509-514.
[58] Abraham RT. Cell cycle checkpoint signaling through the ATM and ATR kinases. *Genes Dev.* Sep 1 2001;15(17):2177-2196.
[59] Peters M, DeLuca C, Hirao A, et al. Chk2 regulates irradiation-induced, p53-mediated apoptosis in Drosophila. *Proc Natl Acad Sci U S A.* Aug 20 2002;99(17):11305-11310.
[60] Cheng Q, Chen J. Mechanism of p53 stabilization by ATM after DNA damage. *Cell Cycle.* Feb 1 2010;9(3):472-478.
[61] Waldman T, Kinzler KW, Vogelstein B. p21 is necessary for the p53-mediated G1 arrest in human cancer cells. *Cancer Res.* Nov 15 1995;55(22):5187-5190.
[62] Shapiro GI, Harper JW. Anticancer drug targets: cell cycle and checkpoint control. *J Clin Invest.* Dec 1999;104(12):1645-1653.
[63] Bunz F, Dutriaux A, Lengauer C, et al. Requirement for p53 and p21 to sustain G2 arrest after DNA damage. *Science.* Nov 20 1998;282(5393):1497-1501.
[64] Chan TA, Hermeking H, Lengauer C, Kinzler KW, Vogelstein B. 14-3-3Sigma is required to prevent mitotic catastrophe after DNA damage. *Nature.* Oct 7 1999;401(6753):616-620.
[65] Ljungman M. Targeting the DNA damage response in cancer. *Chem Rev.* Jul 2009;109(7):2929-2950.
[66] Denko NC, Giaccia AJ, Stringer JR, Stambrook PJ. The human Ha-ras oncogene induces genomic instability in murine fibroblasts within one cell cycle. *Proc Natl Acad Sci U S A.* May 24 1994;91(11):5124-5128.
[67] Lee AC, Fenster BE, Ito H, et al. Ras proteins induce senescence by altering the intracellular levels of reactive oxygen species. *J Biol Chem.* Mar 19 1999;274(12):7936-7940.
[68] Lo HW, Hsu SC, Ali-Seyed M, et al. Nuclear interaction of EGFR and STAT3 in the activation of the iNOS/NO pathway. *Cancer Cell.* Jun 2005;7(6):575-589.
[69] Nitta M, Kozono D, Kennedy R, et al. Targeting EGFR induced oxidative stress by PARP1 inhibition in glioblastoma therapy. *PLoS One.* 2010;5(5):e10767.
[70] Turchi JJ, Henkels KM, Zhou Y. Cisplatin-DNA adducts inhibit translocation of the Ku subunits of DNA-PK. *Nucleic Acids Res.* Dec 1 2000;28(23):4634-4641.
[71] Stojic L, Mojas N, Cejka P, et al. Mismatch repair-dependent G2 checkpoint induced by low doses of SN1 type methylating agents requires the ATR kinase. *Genes Dev.* Jun 1 2004;18(11):1331-1344.
[72] Luo J, Solimini NL, Elledge SJ. Principles of cancer therapy: oncogene and non-oncogene addiction. *Cell.* Mar 6 2009;136(5):823-837.
[73] Rajkumar SV, Richardson PG, Hideshima T, Anderson KC. Proteasome inhibition as a novel therapeutic target in human cancer. *J Clin Oncol.* Jan 20 2005;23(3):630-639.
[74] Krogan NJ, Lam MH, Fillingham J, et al. Proteasome involvement in the repair of DNA double-strand breaks. *Mol Cell.* Dec 22 2004;16(6):1027-1034.
[75] Gudmundsdottir K, Lord CJ, Witt E, Tutt AN, Ashworth A. DSS1 is required for RAD51 focus formation and genomic stability in mammalian cells. *EMBO Rep.* Oct 2004;5(10):989-993.
[76] Li J, Zou C, Bai Y, Wazer DE, Band V, Gao Q. DSS1 is required for the stability of BRCA2. *Oncogene.* Feb 23 2006;25(8):1186-1194.

[77] Marston NJ, Richards WJ, Hughes D, Bertwistle D, Marshall CJ, Ashworth A. Interaction between the product of the breast cancer susceptibility gene BRCA2 and DSS1, a protein functionally conserved from yeast to mammals. *Mol Cell Biol.* Jul 1999;19(7):4633-4642.

[78] Murakawa Y, Sonoda E, Barber LJ, et al. Inhibitors of the proteasome suppress homologous DNA recombination in mammalian cells. *Cancer Res.* Sep 15 2007;67(18):8536-8543.

[79] da Cunha Santos G, Shepherd FA, Tsao MS. EGFR mutations and lung cancer. *Annu Rev Pathol.* Feb 28 2011;6:49-69.

[80] Parsons DW, Jones S, Zhang X, et al. An integrated genomic analysis of human glioblastoma multiforme. *Science.* Sep 26 2008;321(5897):1807-1812.

[81] TCGA. Comprehensive genomic characterization defines human glioblastoma genes and core pathways. *Nature.* Oct 23 2008;455(7216):1061-1068.

[82] Dittmann K, Mayer C, Fehrenbacher B, et al. Radiation-induced epidermal growth factor receptor nuclear import is linked to activation of DNA-dependent protein kinase. *J Biol Chem.* Sep 2 2005;280(35):31182-31189.

[83] Liccardi G, Hartley JA, Hochhauser D. EGFR nuclear translocation modulates DNA repair following cisplatin and ionizing radiation treatment. *Cancer Res.* Feb 1 2011;71(3):1103-1114.

[84] Mukherjee B, McEllin B, Camacho CV, et al. EGFRvIII and DNA double-strand break repair: a molecular mechanism for radioresistance in glioblastoma. *Cancer Res.* May 15 2009;69(10):4252-4259.

[85] Li L, Wang H, Yang ES, Arteaga CL, Xia F. Erlotinib attenuates homologous recombinational repair of chromosomal breaks in human breast cancer cells. *Cancer Res.* Nov 15 2008;68(22):9141-9146.

[86] Golding SE, Rosenberg E, Neill S, Dent P, Povirk LF, Valerie K. Extracellular signal-related kinase positively regulates ataxia telangiectasia mutated, homologous recombination repair, and the DNA damage response. *Cancer Res.* Feb 1 2007;67(3):1046-1053.

[87] Burkitt K, Ljungman M. Phenylbutyrate interferes with the Fanconi anemia and BRCA pathway and sensitizes head and neck cancer cells to cisplatin. *Mol Cancer.* 2008;7:24.

[88] Koll TT, Feis SS, Wright MH, et al. HSP90 inhibitor, DMAG, synergizes with radiation of lung cancer cells by interfering with base excision and ATM-mediated DNA repair. *Mol Cancer Ther.* Jul 2008;7(7):1985-1992.

[89] Camphausen K, Tofilon PJ. Inhibition of Hsp90: a multitarget approach to radiosensitization. *Clin Cancer Res.* Aug 1 2007;13(15 Pt 1):4326-4330.

[90] Dote H, Burgan WE, Camphausen K, Tofilon PJ. Inhibition of hsp90 compromises the DNA damage response to radiation. *Cancer Res.* Sep 15 2006;66(18):9211-9220.

[91] Johnson N, Cai D, Kennedy RD, et al. Cdk1 participates in BRCA1-dependent S phase checkpoint control in response to DNA damage. Mol Cell. Aug 14 2009;35(3):327-339.

# 24

# The Botanical Extract Feverfew PFE Reduces DNA Damage and Induces DNA Repair Processes

Michael D. Southall, Simarna Kaur and Khalid Mahmood
*The Johnson & Johnson Skin Research Center, CPPW, a division of Johnson & Johnson Consumer Companies, Inc. Skillman, New Jersey, USA*

## 1. Introduction

Our skin is equipped with specialized cells and mechanisms that defend our bodies against pathogens, heat, and water loss. Today, our skin is exposed to increased environmental stress including solar ultraviolet radiation (which results in direct and indirect DNA damage) and atmospheric pollutants. Ozone depletion from the earth's atmosphere as well as expanding industrial processes has led to increased exposure to pollutants including pesticides and cigarette smoke. While UV radiation, and in particular its UV-B component (280-315 nm), has several health benefits (including production of vitamin $D_3$) (Reichrath, 2008) continuous exposure is the primary source of UV-induced DNA damage.

The sun produces UV radiation classified into three broad bands. The highest energy UV-C (100-280 nm) radiation is largely absorbed by the earth's atmosphere and thus does not affect humans. Meanwhile, the UV-B component is partially absorbed by the atmosphere and UV-A (315-400 nm) is primarily unabsorbed. While lower energy UV-A radiation penetrates beyond the epidermis, higher energy UV-B radiation primarily affects the outermost epidermal layer of skin.

Harm to the body's barrier can lead to DNA mutation or DNA replication inhibition in the skin and eyes (cataracts) and may lead to broader immunosuppression (Britt, 1995). The most serious skin cancer (malignant melanoma) occurs when excitation of a chromophore leads to either direct reaction of the excited molecule with DNA or in the production of a free radical which may also react with DNA. Since the body produces oxygen free radicals (ROS) as part of normal metabolism (during ATP production), it is able to combat oxidative stress through endogenous antioxidants.

The body's protective system, however, may become overwhelmed and compromised by environmental factors, age, or disease. Aging leads not only to increased total exposure but also to a decrease in production of endogenous antioxidants (enzymes and vitamins) and an increased risk of DNA damage. Oxidative stress can also lead to damage to other cellular components including lipids and proteins. A naturally-derived method to enhance protection against environmental factors that eventually overwhelm the body's defense mechanisms is discussed. Another major risk of UV radiation is oxidative damage to lipids (peroxidation) and proteins. Cell membranes, which are composed of lipids, are especially prone to the damaging effect of free radicals (Sen, et al., 2010). Prolonged oxidative stress to the lipid bilayer can lead to membrane rupture and apoptosis. Lipid peroxidation is, in fact, used as a marker of oxidative stress since the lipid membrane is easily attacked by free radicals.

Cellular DNA damage caused by UV radiation may be classified into two components. The first is that caused by an immediate photochemical reaction (direct) while the other is caused by the formation of ROS (indirect). Direct damage (through direct UV absorption) results primarily in the DNA product cyclobutane-pyrimidine dimer (CPD) (Farage, et al., 2010). On the other hand, indirect damage (through ROS formation) causes DNA mutation due to a replication error induced by modified guanine base (8-oxo-guanine). Direct UV absorption also leads to the formation of 8-oxo-guanine (8oGua) as well as the photoproduct pyrimidine (6-4) pyrimidinone although in proportionally lower amounts.

## 2. Free radicals & ROS

The negative effect of free radicals may be mitigated by antioxidants primarily through their radical-scavenging ability. These antioxidants stabilize radicals by donating electrons and thus preventing oxidation of DNA or other cellular components. While the body is equipped with its own defense system against reactive oxygen species (ROS) and other free radicals produced in the body, it also relies on external (exogenous) antioxidants including those contained in food. As environmental conditions lead to premature aging, a search for a suitable antioxidant product is vital.

Free radicals cause damage in the body because of their instability and high reactivity. ROS are of particular interest. During aerobic respiration, mitochondrial electron transport results in the formation of a ROS (superoxide) as a by-product. Solar UV radiation also leads to formation of ROS. Oxygen is particularly vulnerable to radical formation due to its electronic configuration with two valence shell unpaired electrons. Thus, there are several types of ROS including superoxide, hydrogen peroxide, nitric oxide, and hydroxyl radical. Free radicals of other atomic species specifically nitrogen are also formed within the body.

ROS can potentially react with other cellular entities including DNA which can lead to DNA modification and ultimately bodily harm. The guanine base in DNA is particularly susceptible to attack by ROS formed by solar UV radiation. Oxidation reactions which modify the guanine base may also lead to single-strand breaks in DNA (Held, 2010).

While the effects of oxidative stress on the body vary according to type and duration, cells often halt division (enter $G_0$ phase) and may even undergo apoptosis under severe stress. The general response to oxidative stress is cell cycle arrest through the expression of various inhibitor proteins (such as p21). Nevertheless, ROS also serve useful roles within the body including intracellular and intercellular communication (Held, 2010).

## 3. Antioxidants combat oxidative stress

While broad-spectrum sunscreens which absorb and reflect harmful solar radiation remain the most effective protection against immediate solar UV damage (which result in CPD formation), antioxidants are crucial in combating oxidative stress caused by ROS. Skin's antioxidant system consists of vitamins (vitamins C and E), enzymes (catalase and superoxide dismutase), glutathione, and coenzyme Q10 ($CoQ_{10}$). As these antioxidants perform their protective actions and are degraded by ROS, they are reactivated by other antioxidants. Because several types of ROS may be formed through environmental insult, several types of antioxidants are produced in the skin. Thus antioxidants come in various forms (vitamins, enzymes, etc.) and may be either lipophilic or hydrophilic to function in a variety of areas.

## 4. DNA repair mechanism in plants

In plants, UV radiation-induced DNA damage can lead to DNA replication inhibition. Although plants exhibit mechanisms by which they are able tolerate some DNA damage, DNA mutation can still lead to transcription and replication blocks. Since plants, like humans, are subjected to oxidative stress (including that induced by UV radiation), an investigation into the evolutionary response by plants to this stress may allow us to apply these findings in a clinical setting.

By their nature, plants are subjected to solar UV radiation indiscriminately. They must necessarily, then, possess inherent methods to prevent and repair DNA damage. While plants are better able to absorb the high energy UV radiation through various photon-absorbing structures, they are still at high risk for oxidative modification of DNA. DNA repair mechanisms in plants such as Arabidopsis thaliana have been investigated and serve as a foundation for the search of a botanical extract that can effectively combat UV-induced DNA damage.

Repair mechanisms increase the likelihood of the accurate transmission of genetic information from parent to daughter cell and thus the survival of the species. Although plants have developed methods to minimize the toxic effects of DNA damage including DNA translesion synthesis and recombination (Schmitz-Hoerner and Weissenbock, 2003), they also have active repair pathways. These pathways include photoreactivation (via photolyase), nucleotide excision repair, base excision repair, and mismatch repair (Kimura et al., 2004).

Plants and some other organisms are able to use light energy (UV and visible) to reverse DNA damage. The enzyme photolyase binds to CPDs and via photoreactivation removes UV-induced lesions. Additionally, excision repair pathways work by replacing damaged DNA with new nucleotides. Base excision repair (BER) employs various DNA glycosylases to remove modified DNA. On the other hand, nucleotide excision repair (NER) is essential in solar radiation protection and in repairing a wide range of DNA lesions. A complex array of proteins recognize, bind to, excise, and repair DNA irregularities in both excision repair pathways.

Humans share repair pathways with plants, particularly nucleotide excision repair (NER). NER is essential in removing major damage to DNA which interferes with the genetic code. Due to similarities in DNA damage and repair mechanisms in plants and humans, metabolites produced by plants may provide beneficial effects in humans.

## 5. Botanical extracts | Feverfew PFE as an antioxidant

Feverfew (*Tanacetum parthenium*) is a plant that has been used as a medicinal herb for centuries throughout Eastern Europe and more recently North America. Traditionally, it was used for its anti-inflammatory properties to treat migraine headaches, fever, and arthritis. Additionally, feverfew has shown to exhibit powerful antioxidant activity. Although feverfew leaves contain skin irritating compounds called parthenolides, purification processes are available to create feverfew parthenolide-free extract (Feverfew PFE) which does not produce skin irritation and is free of sensitization potential (Kurtz, et al., 2005).

### 5.1 Feverfew PFE reduces UV and external aggression induced reactive oxygen species formation

Reactive Oxygen Species are produced in skin following UV irradiation and is a major mediator of oxidative damage to the skin (Pathak and Stratton, 1968). Hydrogen Peroxide ($H_2O_2$) and peroxyl radicals are produced in skin following UVB irradiation (Stewart et al., 1996) and can induce oxidative damage to DNA and other cellular constituents. Singlet oxygen can be generated from the action of UVA and endogenous photosensitizers, such as porphyrins and flavins (Cadet et al., 1997), which can produce DNA damage. In addition external aggression such as cigarette smoke can induce oxidative stress in human tissues. Cigarette smoke not only contains peroxy radicals but also contains nitric oxide which can facilitate conversion of peroxy radicals into the more highly reactive alkoxy and hydroxy radicals. Exposure to cigarette smoke depletes the intracellular antioxidant thiol glutathione, decreases phagocytic cell chemotaxis, increases epithelial cell permeability and pro-inflammatory cytokine release, reduces epithelial cell repair processes and can result in cell death (Rahman and MacNee, 1999), (Rusznak et al., 2000).
Feverfew PFE has been shown to directly scavenging a wide range of free radicals, thereby reducing the oxidative damage to skin that can result from the presence of the free radicals. Feverfew PFE had the greatest scavenging activity against ferric radicals, followed by oxygen, hydroxyl, peroxynitrate radicals respectively (Martin et al., 2008). In comparison to the reference antioxidant, Ascorbic acid (Vitamin C), Feverfew PFE has a 5-fold greater scavenging activity for oxygen and hydroxyl radicals than Ascorbic acid, and 3-fold greater scavenging activity for ferric radicals than Ascorbic acid. Feverfew PFE was also 13-fold greater than Ascorbic acid in scavenging the superoxide anion.
Functionally Feverfew PFE was also shown to reduce UV-induced cellular damage in primary human keratinocytes. Exposing normal human keratinocytes to UV increases the production of hydrogen peroxide ($H_2O_2$). $H_2O_2$ production is represented as mean fluorescent units (MFU). The production of hydrogen peroxide occurs during exposure to UV, so that measurements of hydrogen peroxide immediately after UV exposure can detect significant increases in hydrogen peroxide. A dose of 4.2 $kJ/m^2$ (at 360nm) from a solar simulator increased intracellular hydrogen peroxide by 73%.
Preincubation with Feverfew PFE at concentrations from 3.1 to 100 µg/mL significantly attenuated hydrogen peroxide production in a dose-dependent manner (*$P<0.05$ compared with UV exposed vehicle treated control keratinocytes). At concentrations greater than 10 µg/mL the suppression of hydrogen peroxide production was less than in non-irradiated controls indicating that Feverfew PFE reduced the basal level of hydrogen peroxide present in keratinocytes due to metabolism (Tierney, et al., 2005). The activity of Feverfew PFE reducing oxidative stress in keratinocytes was not limited to UV exposure. Exposure to external aggressors such as cigarette smoke was found to increase free radical formation in keratinocytes which was inhibited by Feverfew PFE in a dose dependent manner at concentrations as low as 6 µg/mL. The reduction of oxidative stress in skin cells also helped to preserve the levels of endogenous cellular antioxidants. In cells exposed to cigarette smoke treatment with Feverfew PFE maintained the cellular thiol content at levels similar to

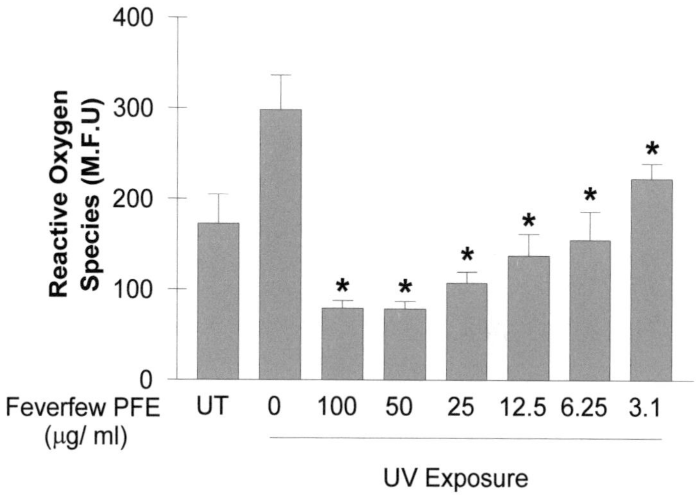


Fig. 1. Feverfew PFE inhibits Reactive Oxygen Species.

those in the no-smoke exposed control (Martin et al., 2008). Through free radicals scavenging activity and preserving endogenous antioxidant levels, Feverfew PFE may protect skin from oxidative stress that could result in DNA damage.

### 5.2 Feverfew PFE inhibits cellular inflammation

UV irradiation has been shown to induce the release of various inflammatory cytokines such as IL-1α, IL-6, TNF-α, that are involved in the pathophysiology of UV-induced inflammation (Aubin, 2003). Inflammation has been linked to epithelial skin tumors, and anti-inflammatory drugs are being studied for the prevention and treatment of non-melanoma skin cancers (Mueller, 2006).

Feverfew PFE can reduce the release of pro-inflammatory mediators through inhibition of enzymes involved in production and regulation of inflammation. Feverfew PFE directly inhibited the activity of 5-lipoxygenase (5-LOX), phosphodiesterase-3 (PDE3) and phosphodiesterase-4 (PDE4) with IC50 values 11.8 ± 4.8 μg/ ml, 35.2 ± 12.3 μg/ml and 20.8 ± 9.4 μg/ml respectively (Martin et al., 2008).

Feverfew PFE also reduced $PGE_2$ secretion from human skin equivalents and inhibited p38 MAP kinase activation in vitro (Martin et al., 2005). Feverfew PFE had no direct effect on COX-2, this indicates the mechanism of inhibiting $PGE_2$ formation may be upstream to COX-2. Human skin equivalents were pretreated with Feverfew PFE and then thoroughly washed prior to UV exposure. In the absence of treatment, UV irradiation induced inflammatory cytokine release. Pretreatment with Feverfew PFE significantly reduced UV-induced cytokine release by more than 60% over placebo treated control skin equivalents.

Topical application of Feverfew PFE was examined in an investigator blinded, placebo-controlled clinical study for their effect on UV-induced erythema. Subjects were exposed to UVB irradiation of 0.5 to 1.5 MED (Minimal Erythema Dose), followed by daily applications of Feverfew PFE. Chromameter, diffused reflectance spectroscopy measurements and independent dermatologist assessment concluded that Feverfew PFE significantly reduced the UV-induced erythema at 24 and 48 hrs after UV exposure (Tierney et al., 2005). This clinical study clearly demonstrates that Feverfew PFE can reduce the skin inflammation and damage resulting from UV exposure.

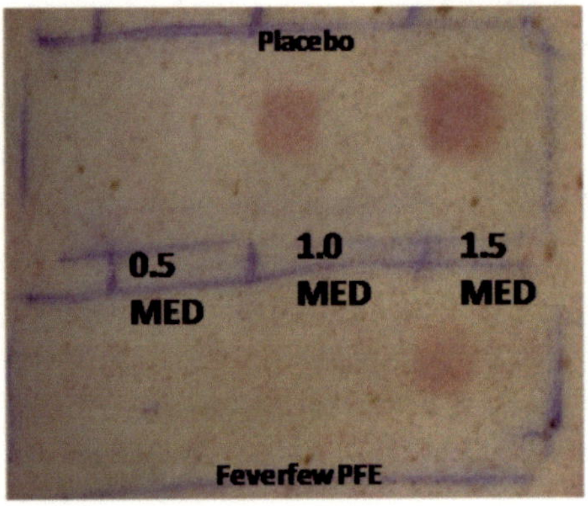


Fig. 2. Feverfew PFE mitigates UV-induced erythema.

### 5.3 Feverfew PFE reduces DNA damage

One of the major adverse effects of UV irradiation is damage to DNA. DNA damage by UVB irradiation results from photochemical reactions consequent to direct absorption of photons by DNA bases. The UV-induced DNA lesions that have been studied in most detail are the cyclobutane pyrimidine dimer (CPD) and the 6-4 pyrimidine-pyrimidone photoproduct (6-4PP) at adjacent pyrimidines (Nakajima et al., 2004). Nuclear DNA strand breaks are produced by incubation of keratinocytes with hydrogen peroxide (Armeni et al., 2001) and hydroxyl radicals, which are generated from hydrogen peroxide through $Fe^{2+}$-mediated Fenton-type reactions (Stewart et al., 1996).

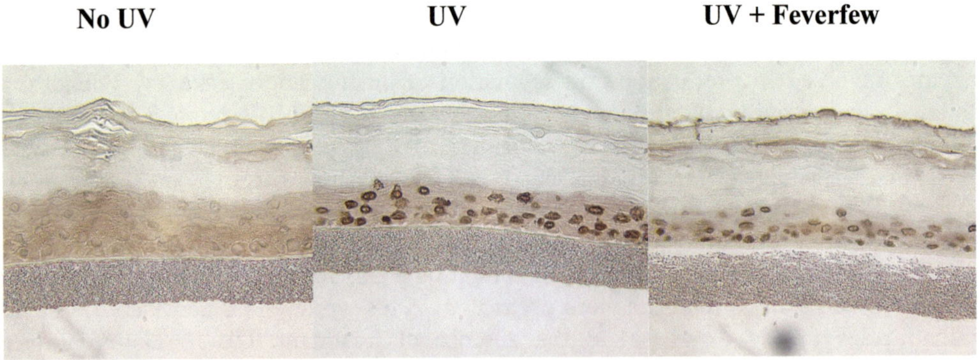


Fig. 3. Treatment with Feverfew PFE inhibits UV-induced T-T dimer formation.

UV light exposure induces a dose dependent increase in Thymine dimer immunostaining of human skin equivalent tissue. Exposure to 65 $kJ/m^2$ of UV produced a 10-fold increase in T-T dimer formation and 160 $kJ/m^2$ increased T-T dimers approximately 14-fold. Feverfew

PFE decreased UV induced TT dimer formation by nearly 50% compared to UV alone (Martin etal 2008). Thus the antioxidant properties of Feverfew PFE can block the cascade of events taking place between UV irradiation and DNA damage.
In addition to having direct effects on mitigating DNA damage, Feverfew PFE may also aid the DNA repair process via an indirect mechanism, such as induction of the Nrf2/ARE pathway and downstream activation of several genes involved in oxidative stress response.

## 6. The NRF2/ARE pathway and its effect on reducing oxidative damage and DNA damage

### 6.1 Antioxidant Response Element (ARE)

The antioxidant response element is a *cis*-acting enhancer sequence that mediates transcriptional activation of genes in cells exposed to oxidative stress. It was initially identified in the promoters of the cell detoxification enzymes, GSTA2 (glutathione S-transferase A2) and NQO1 (NADPH: quinone oxidoreductase 1) (Friling et al., 1990; Li and Jaiswal, 1992; Rushmore and Pickett, 1990). The ARE possesses structural and biological features that characterize its unique responsiveness to oxidative stress, and its consensus sequence was identified to be 5′-TGACnnnGC-3′ (Rushmore et al., 1991). In addition to being involved in inducible gene expression, the antioxidant response element is also responsible for the low-level basal expression of several genes, and is therefore crucial for maintaining cellular redox homeostasis under a variety of cell conditions. Proteins that are encoded by the ARE include enzymes associated with glutathione biosynthesis (Moinova and Mulcahy, 1998; Wild et al., 1998), redox proteins with active sulfhydryl moieties (Ishii et al., 2000; Kim et al., 2001), and drug-metabolizing enzymes (Favreau and Pickett, 1991; Rushmore and Pickett, 1990). Several of these proteins have an endogenous role in protecting the cells from oxidative damage, for example, enzymes such as GST, NQO1, and HO-1 (heme oxygenase-1) function to detoxify harmful by-products of oxidative stress. Other phase II enzymes induced by ARE activation include aldehyde dehydrogenase, glutathione peroxidase, glutathione transferases, superoxide dismutase, quinone reductase, epoxide hydrolase, UDP-glucuronosyl transferases, and gamma-glutamylcysteine synthetase, etc. The human 8-oxoguanine DNA glycosylase (OGG1) enzyme has also been shown to contain the binding sites for transcription factor Nrf2 in its promoter region (Dhenaut et al., 2000). Human OGG1 functions to remove 8-oxoG, a mutagenic base byproduct which occurs as a result of exposure to reactive oxygen, from damaged DNA and initiates base excision DNA repair.

### 6.2 Transcription factor Nrf2

Transcription factor Nrf2 (Nuclear factor E2-related factor 2) binds to and induces activation of the ARE. Nrf2 was first isolated by an expression cloning procedure using an oligonucleotide containing the NF-E2 DNA binding motif as a probe to screen for closely related proteins (Moi et al., 1994). Nrf2 belongs to the cap-and-collar family of basic region-leucine zipper transcription factors, and is an essential component of the ARE-mediated transcriptional machinery. It has been shown that Nrf2 mediates both the basal and inducible activity of the ARE, and the loss of Nrf2 results in a profound reduction in the enzyme activities of NQO1 and certain GST isoenzymes (Itoh et al., 1997). These observations also correlate well with the ubiquitous expression of Nrf2 at steady-state levels in various tissues and cell lines (Nguyen et al., 2004). As a result, the function of Nrf2 and its downstream target genes are vital for protection against cellular damage induced by oxidative stress or chemicals. Several studies have shown that Nrf2 knockout mice having decreased levels of phase II detoxification enzymes and antioxidant proteins are highly sensitive to cytotoxic electrophiles compared to their wild-type littermates (Lee and Johnson, 2004; Leung et al., 2003). The upregulation of protective detoxification and antioxidant genes by Nrf2/ARE pathway can synergistically increase the efficiency of our cellular defense system.

### 6.3 Activation of the Nrf2/ARE pathway by oxidative stress

The induction of several cytoprotective enzymes in response to reactive chemical entities or oxidative stress is regulated at the transcriptional level via activation of Nrf2. This transcriptional response is mediated by the ARE, and is activated in response to $H_2O_2$ (Purdom-Dickinson et al., 2007) and by chemical compounds with the capacity to either undergo redox cycling or be metabolically transformed to a reactive or electrophilic intermediate (Nguyen et al., 2003). Several electrophiles, including diethyl maleate, tert-butylhydroquinone, sulforaphane (Zhang et al., 1992) and curcumin (Balogun et al., 2003) have been shown to induce Nrf2-dependent transcriptional activation of downstream target genes. In addition, several phytochemicals, such as Sulforaphane obtained from cruciferous vegetables (Zhang et al., 1992), Resveratrol (Kode et al., 2008), and Celastrol from the medicinal plant Tripterygium wilfordii (Seo et al.) have also been shown to activate the antioxidant response element . Chemical compounds such as the isothiocyanates and diethyl maleate can directly react with sulfhydryl groups and do not require metabolism. They can mimic an oxidative insult by oxidizing cysteine residues and depleting reduced cellular glutathione (GSH). Elevated levels of reactive oxygen and other electrophilic species followed by a reduced antioxidant capacity can lead to the alteration of the cellular redox status and trigger the transcriptional response mediated by Nrf2/ARE (Nguyen et al., 2009).

### 6.4 Pathways/mechanism that regulate Nrf2/ARE

The major signaling pathways implicated in the modulation of ARE/Nrf2 activity include mitogen activated protein (MAP) kinases, phosphatidylinositol-3-kinase (PI3 kinase), and Protein kinase C (PKC). Activation of ERK signaling by sulforaphane and other agents was shown to be involved in ARE/Nrf2 induction (Yu et al., 1999), while p38 MAPK was found to negatively regulate ARE/Nrf2 in certain cell types (Keum et al., 2006; Yu et al., 2000a; Yu et al., 2000b). The PI3 kinase pathway has also been demonstrated to be a key component of ARE/Nrf2 regulation; induction of ARE-driven antioxidant genes by sulforaphane was abrogated by blocking PI3 kinase (Nakaso et al., 2003; Wang et al., 2008). Direct involvement of PKC in Nrf2 phosphorylation and ARE activation has also been established (Huang et al., 2000, 2002; Numazawa et al., 2003).

### 6.5 Activation of the Nrf2/ARE pathway by Feverfew PFE

Human epidermoid KB cells expressing the antioxidant response element promoter were treated with Feverfew PFE or with the well-known ARE-inducing agent Sulforaphane (Zhang et al., 1992) for a period of 24 hr. Treatment with Feverfew PFE led to 2-fold activation of the ARE promoter, which was at par with the induction mediated by Sulforaphane.

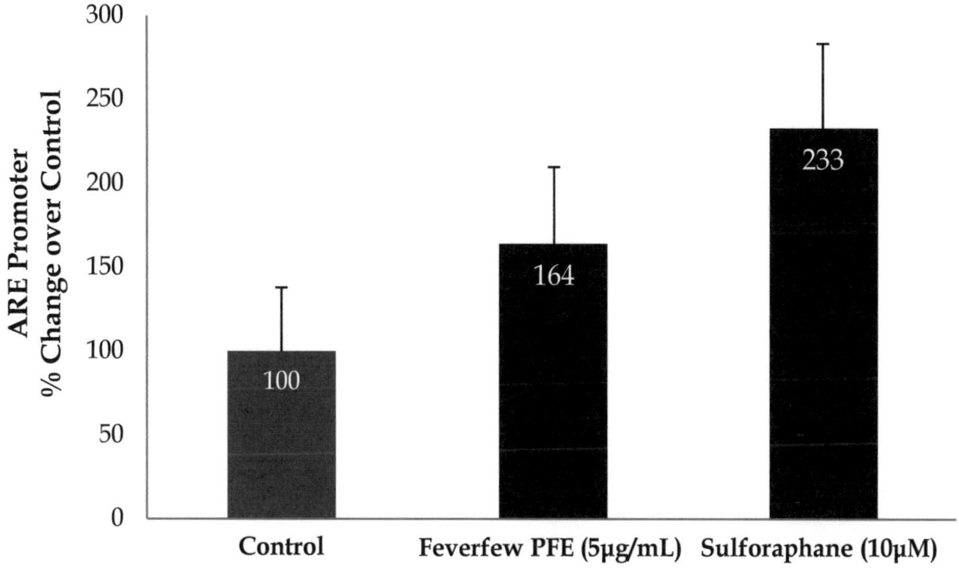


Fig. 4. Feverfew PFE induces activation of the ARE promoter.

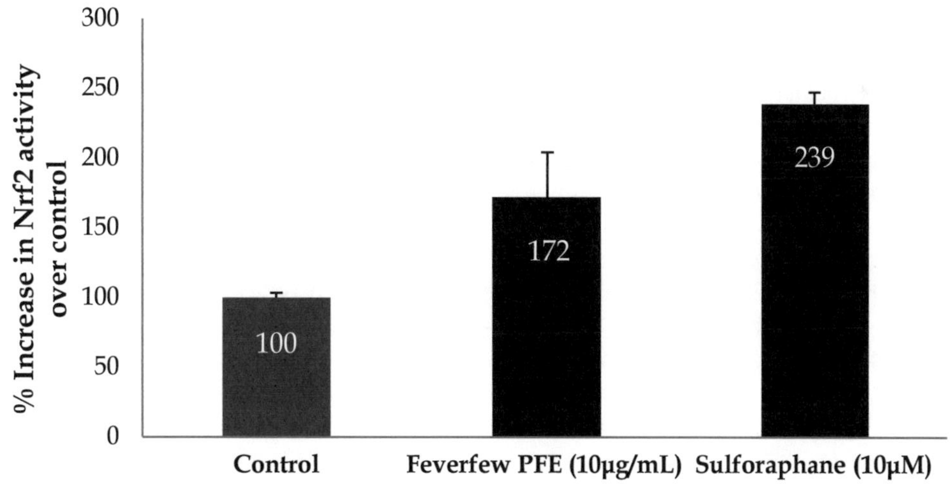


Fig. 5. Feverfew PFE activates the Nrf2 transcription factor.

In order to analyze the effects of Feverfew PFE on the transcription factor, Nrf2, a TransAM ELISA was utilized. Primary human keratinocytes were treated with Feverfew PFE or Sulforaphane for 24 hr, following which the nuclear and cytoplasmic cell lysate fractions were separated. Translocation of Nrf2 was analyzed in the nuclear fractions. Feverfew PFE enhanced the nuclear translocation of Nrf2 by more than 70%.

The downstream functional effects of Nrf2/ARE activation by Feverfew PFE were analyzed by using an Oxidative Stress and Antioxidant Defense PCR array. Human epidermal skin equivalents treated with Feverfew PFE for 24 hr were analyzed using the PCR array. Feverfew PFE led to more than 2-fold increase in the expression of several genes involved in antioxidant defense and oxidative stress. These genes included Lactoperoxidase, an antioxidant-related gene which functions as a natural antibacterial agent, Glutathione Peroxidase which functions to protect the organism from oxidative damage by reducing free hydrogen peroxide to water, inducible Nitric Oxide Synthase-2 involved in superoxide metabolism, and G protein-coupled receptor-156 which is implicated in oxidative stress response.

| Gene | Fold-increase in Feverfew PFE-treated sample over vehicle control |
|---|---|
| Lactoperoxidase | 2 |
| Glutathione Peroxidase | 2 |
| Inducible-Nitric Oxide synthase-2 (iNOS2) | 3 |
| G-protein coupled Receptor-156 (GPR156) | 3 |

Table 1. Fevefew PFE leads to induction of antioxidant defense genes.

## 7. Feverfew PFE increases expression of DNA repair enzymes

Skin is continously exposed to numerous aggressors that can cause oxidative DNA damage. The age-related accumulation of somatic damage is worsened by sun exposure, leading to an increased incidence of skin disorders and skin cancer. Chemical entities such as $O_2^{\cdot}$, $H_2O_2$, $OH^{\cdot}$ are also generated in cells as a result of several endogenous processes including normal cellular metabolism and mitochondrial respiration (Verjat et al., 2000). Some of these chemical species are highly reactive and can interact with DNA, lipids and proteins (Ames and Shigenaga, 1992) causing damage. Oxidative DNA damage can arise through the direct interaction of reactive species with genomic DNA, or via oxidation of DNA precursors in the nucleotide pool (Rai, 2010). One of the major DNA oxidation products formed as a result of such damage is 8-oxo-7,8-dihydro-2'-deoxyguanosine (8-oxo-dG). Mammalian cells have evolved several DNA-repair pathways to remove all the categories of DNA base lesions, relying in particular on DNA excision mechanisms. One of these, nucleotide excision repair, removes bulky adducts and is thus an essential mechanism for correcting UV-induced DNA damage (Sarasin, 1999). The base excision repair pathway corrects small base modifications such as oxidized and alkylated bases (Almeida and Sobol, 2007). The importance of repair mechanisms is demonstrated by the hazardous consequences of genetic defects in DNA repair (Friedberg, 2001).

Feverfew PFE increases the enzymatic activity of DNA repair enzymes in human epidermal keratinocytes. Feverfew PFE directly induced DNA repair via the nucleotide excision repair process resulting in the repair of CPD damage induced by UV exposure. Feverfew PFE also induced the repair of DNA caused by exposure to agents that produce oxidative damage in skin. The chemotherapeutic agent, Cisplatin, and the photodynamic agent, Psoralen both induce oxidative stress which can produce DNA damage (Martin et al., 2008). Feverfew PFE induced DNA repair activity in DNA damaged by Cisplatin or Psoralen. Thus Feverfew PFE can activate the endogenous nucleotide excision repair in human epidermal keratinocytes, which could repair DNA damaged by extrinsic or intrinsic ROS formation.

In addition to the direct effects of Feverfew PFE on DNA repair enzymes, activation of the ARE/Nrf2 pathway by Feverfew might also play a crucial role in preventing DNA damage and augmenting DNA repair. Daily exposure to UV, smoke, and other external aggressors leads to the generation of high levels of reactive oxygen species in the body. In order to avoid the deleterious effects of reactive oxidative species, cells have developed different defensive mechanisms including antioxidant molecules such as glutathione, alpha-tocopherol, vitamins A and C, and enzymes such as superoxide dismutase (SOD) and catalase (Ames et al., 1993; Verjat et al., 2000). When the cellular balance between antioxidants and pro-oxidants is upset, free radicals lead to the formation of lesions in the DNA causing damage, which in most cases is endogenously repaired in the cells by several repair mechanisms. The Nrf2/ARE pathway induces production of a battery of downstream genes that mitigate damage from reactive oxygen species, and aid DNA repair (Villeneuve et al., 2009). It has been shown that activation of Nrf2 generates a glutathione gradient to protect skin from the damaging effects of UVB (Saw et al., Schafer et al.), and reduces UVA-induced apoptosis in fibroblasts (Hirota et al., 2005). Thus, Feverfew PFE may help protect the skin from DNA damage incurred by UV and other environmental aggressors by boosting the cellular antioxidant defense machinery.

## 8. Summary and conclusions: The use of botanical extracts for protection from DNA damage and DNA repair

Skin is under continual assault from a variety of damaging environmental factors such as ultraviolet irradiation and atmospheric pollutants. As organisms age the cumulative damage exceeds the capacity of endogenous antioxidant defenses resulting in oxidative damage. Plants have adapted to chronic exposure to ultraviolet irradiation by producing phytochemicals which can mitigate reactive oxygen species and repair damaged DNA. Botanical extracts such as Feverfew PFE, containing naturally occurring antioxidants can replenish the depleted cutaneous stores and perhaps prevent oxidative stress. Feverfew has been shown to contain chlorogenic acid (Wu et al., 2007), which can activate the Nrf2-ARE pathway (Feng et al., 2005), increase DNA repair enzyme expression (Bernstein et al., 2007), and induce repair of DNA (Huang et al., 2008). Furthermore, chlorogenic acid might be one of several phytochemicals present in Feverfew that could protect from DNA damage and induce the DNA repair process. Through the ability to scavenge free radicals, preserve endogenous antioxidant levels, reduce DNA damage and induce repair of damaged DNA, Feverfew PFE may protect skin from numerous external aggressions encountered daily and reduce the damage to oxidatively challenged skin.

## 9. Acknowledgements

The authors would like to thank Katharine Martin, Neena Tierney, Peter Lyte, Dara Miller, Thierry Oddos, Karien Rodriguez and Dr. Balz Frei (Linus Pauling Institute, Oregon State University) for research and discussions on Feverfew PFE.

## 10. References


Almeida, K. H., Sobol, R. W., 2007. A unified view of base excision repair: lesion-dependent protein complexes regulated by post-translational modification. DNA Repair (Amst) 6, 695-711.

Ames, B. N., Shigenaga, M. K., 1992. Oxidants are a major contributor to aging. Ann N Y Acad Sci 663, 85-96.

Ames, B. N., Shigenaga, M. K., Hagen, T. M., 1993. Oxidants, antioxidants, and the degenerative diseases of aging. Proc Natl Acad Sci U S A 90, 7915-7922.

Armeni, T., Battino, M., Stronati, A., Pugnaloni, A., Tomassini, G., Rosi, G., Biagini, G., Principato, G., 2001. Total antioxidant capacity and nuclear DNA damage in keratinocytes after exposure to H2O2. Biol Chem 382, 1697-1705.

Aubin, F., 2003. Mechanisms involved in ultraviolet light-induced immunosuppression. Eur J Dermatol 13, 515-523.

Balogun, E., Hoque, M., Gong, P., Killeen, E., Green, C. J., Foresti, R., Alam, J., Motterlini, R., 2003. Curcumin activates the haem oxygenase-1 gene via regulation of Nrf2 and the antioxidant-responsive element. Biochem J 371, 887-895.

Bernstein, H., Crowley-Skillicorn, C., Bernstein, C., Payne, C., Dvorak, K., Garewal, H., 2007. Dietary Compounds that Enhance DNA Repair and their Relevance to Cancer and Aging, In: *New research on DNA repair,* Landseer, B. R., 99-113, Nova Science Publishers, Inc., 1-60021-385-5, New York.

Cadet, J., Berger, M., Douki, T., Morin, B., Raoul, S., Ravanat, J. L., Spinelli, S., 1997. Effects of UV and visible radiation on DNA-final base damage. Biol Chem 378, 1275-1286.

Dhenaut, A., Boiteux, S., Radicella, J. P., 2000. Characterization of the hOGG1 promoter and its expression during the cell cycle. Mutat Res 461, 109-118.

Favreau, L. V., Pickett, C. B., 1991. Transcriptional regulation of the rat NAD(P)H:quinone reductase gene. Identification of regulatory elements controlling basal level expression and inducible expression by planar aromatic compounds and phenolic antioxidants. J Biol Chem 266, 4556-4561.

Feng, R., Lu, Y., Bowman, L. L., Qian, Y., Castranova, V., Ding, M., 2005. Inhibition of activator protein-1, NF-kappaB, and MAPKs and induction of phase 2 detoxifying enzyme activity by chlorogenic acid. J Biol Chem 280, 27888-27895.

Friedberg, E. C., 2001. How nucleotide excision repair protects against cancer. Nat Rev Cancer 1, 22-33.

Friling, R. S., Bensimon, A., Tichauer, Y., Daniel, V., 1990. Xenobiotic-inducible expression of murine glutathione S-transferase Ya subunit gene is controlled by an electrophile-responsive element. Proc Natl Acad Sci U S A 87, 6258-6262.

Hirota, A., Kawachi, Y., Itoh, K., Nakamura, Y., Xu, X., Banno, T., Takahashi, T., Yamamoto, M., Otsuka, F., 2005. Ultraviolet A irradiation induces NF-E2-related factor 2 activation in dermal fibroblasts: protective role in UVA-induced apoptosis. J Invest Dermatol 124, 825-832.

Huang, H. C., Nguyen, T., Pickett, C. B., 2000. Regulation of the antioxidant response element by protein kinase C-mediated phosphorylation of NF-E2-related factor 2. Proc Natl Acad Sci U S A 97, 12475-12480.

Huang, H. C., Nguyen, T., Pickett, C. B., 2002. Phosphorylation of Nrf2 at Ser-40 by protein kinase C regulates antioxidant response element-mediated transcription. J Biol Chem 277, 42769-42774.

Huang, J., Li, T., Chen, Z., Liu, X., Liu, S., 2008. Rapid electrochemical detection of DNA damage and repair with epigallocatechin gallate, chlorogenic acid and ascorbic acid. Electrochemistry Communications 10, 1198-1200.

Ishii, T., Itoh, K., Takahashi, S., Sato, H., Yanagawa, T., Katoh, Y., Bannai, S., Yamamoto, M., 2000. Transcription factor Nrf2 coordinately regulates a group of oxidative stress-inducible genes in macrophages. J Biol Chem 275, 16023-16029.

Itoh, K., Chiba, T., Takahashi, S., Ishii, T., Igarashi, K., Katoh, Y., Oyake, T., Hayashi, N., Satoh, K., Hatayama, I., Yamamoto, M., Nabeshima, Y., 1997. An Nrf2/small Maf heterodimer mediates the induction of phase II detoxifying enzyme genes through antioxidant response elements. Biochem Biophys Res Commun 236, 313-322.

Keum, Y. S., Yu, S., Chang, P. P., Yuan, X., Kim, J. H., Xu, C., Han, J., Agarwal, A., Kong, A. N., 2006. Mechanism of action of sulforaphane: inhibition of p38 mitogen-activated protein kinase isoforms contributing to the induction of antioxidant response element-mediated heme oxygenase-1 in human hepatoma HepG2 cells. Cancer Res 66, 8804-8813.

Kim, Y. C., Masutani, H., Yamaguchi, Y., Itoh, K., Yamamoto, M., Yodoi, J., 2001. Hemin-induced activation of the thioredoxin gene by Nrf2. A differential regulation of the antioxidant responsive element by a switch of its binding factors. J Biol Chem 276, 18399-18406.

Kimura, S., Tahira, Y., Ishibashi, T., Mori, Y., Mori, T., Hashimoto, J., Sakaguchi, K., 2004. DNA repair in higher plants; photoreactivation is the major DNA repair pathway in non-proliferating cells while excision repair (nucleotide excision repair and base excision repair) is active in proliferating cells. Nucleic Acids Res 32, 2760-2767.

Kode, A., Rajendrasozhan, S., Caito, S., Yang, S. R., Megson, I. L., Rahman, I., 2008. Resveratrol induces glutathione synthesis by activation of Nrf2 and protects against cigarette smoke-mediated oxidative stress in human lung epithelial cells. Am J Physiol Lung Cell Mol Physiol 294, L478-488.

Lee, J. M., Johnson, J. A., 2004. An important role of Nrf2-ARE pathway in the cellular defense mechanism. J Biochem Mol Biol 37, 139-143.

Leung, L., Kwong, M., Hou, S., Lee, C., Chan, J. Y., 2003. Deficiency of the Nrf1 and Nrf2 transcription factors results in early embryonic lethality and severe oxidative stress. J Biol Chem 278, 48021-48029.

Li, Y., Jaiswal, A. K., 1992. Regulation of human NAD(P)H:quinone oxidoreductase gene. Role of AP1 binding site contained within human antioxidant response element. J Biol Chem 267, 15097-15104.

Martin, K., Sur, R., Liebel, F., Tierney, N., Lyte, P., Garay, M., Oddos, T., Anthonavage, M., Shapiro, S., Southall, M., 2008. Parthenolide-depleted Feverfew (Tanacetum parthenium) protects skin from UV irradiation and external aggression. Arch Dermatol Res 300, 69-80.

Moi, P., Chan, K., Asunis, I., Cao, A., Kan, Y. W., 1994. Isolation of NF-E2-related factor 2 (Nrf2), a NF-E2-like basic leucine zipper transcriptional activator that binds to the tandem NF-E2/AP1 repeat of the beta-globin locus control region. Proc Natl Acad Sci U S A 91, 9926-9930.

Moinova, H. R., Mulcahy, R. T., 1998. An electrophile responsive element (EpRE) regulates beta-naphthoflavone induction of the human gamma-glutamylcysteine synthetase regulatory subunit gene. Constitutive expression is mediated by an adjacent AP-1 site. J Biol Chem 273, 14683-14689.

Mueller, M. M., 2006. Inflammation in epithelial skin tumours: old stories and new ideas. Eur J Cancer 42, 735-744.

Nakajima, S., Lan, L., Kanno, S., Takao, M., Yamamoto, K., Eker, A. P., Yasui, A., 2004. UV light-induced DNA damage and tolerance for the survival of nucleotide excision repair-deficient human cells. J Biol Chem 279, 46674-46677.

Nakaso, K., Yano, H., Fukuhara, Y., Takeshima, T., Wada-Isoe, K., Nakashima, K., 2003. PI3K is a key molecule in the Nrf2-mediated regulation of antioxidative proteins by hemin in human neuroblastoma cells. FEBS Lett 546, 181-184.

Nguyen, T., Nioi, P., Pickett, C. B., 2009. The Nrf2-antioxidant response element signaling pathway and its activation by oxidative stress. J Biol Chem 284, 13291-13295.

Nguyen, T., Sherratt, P. J., Pickett, C. B., 2003. Regulatory mechanisms controlling gene expression mediated by the antioxidant response element. Annu Rev Pharmacol Toxicol 43, 233-260.

Nguyen, T., Yang, C. S., Pickett, C. B., 2004. The pathways and molecular mechanisms regulating Nrf2 activation in response to chemical stress. Free Radic Biol Med 37, 433-441.

Numazawa, S., Ishikawa, M., Yoshida, A., Tanaka, S., Yoshida, T., 2003. Atypical protein kinase C mediates activation of NF-E2-related factor 2 in response to oxidative stress. Am J Physiol Cell Physiol 285, C334-342.

Pathak, M. A., Stratton, K., 1968. Free radicals in human skin before and after exposure to light. Arch Biochem Biophys 123, 468-476.

Purdom-Dickinson, S. E., Sheveleva, E. V., Sun, H., Chen, Q. M., 2007. Translational control of nrf2 protein in activation of antioxidant response by oxidants. Mol Pharmacol 72, 1074-1081.

Rahman, I., MacNee, W., 1999. Lung glutathione and oxidative stress: implications in cigarette smoke-induced airway disease. Am J Physiol 277, L1067-1088.

Rai, P., Oxidation in the nucleotide pool, the DNA damage response and cellular senescence: Defective bricks build a defective house. Mutat Res 703, 71-81.

Rushmore, T. H., Morton, M. R., Pickett, C. B., 1991. The antioxidant responsive element. Activation by oxidative stress and identification of the DNA consensus sequence required for functional activity. J Biol Chem 266, 11632-11639.

Rushmore, T. H., Pickett, C. B., 1990. Transcriptional regulation of the rat glutathione S-transferase Ya subunit gene. Characterization of a xenobiotic-responsive element controlling inducible expression by phenolic antioxidants. J Biol Chem 265, 14648-14653.

Rusznak, C., Mills, P. R., Devalia, J. L., Sapsford, R. J., Davies, R. J., Lozewicz, S., 2000. Effect of cigarette smoke on the permeability and IL-1beta and sICAM-1 release from cultured human bronchial epithelial cells of never-smokers, smokers, and patients with chronic obstructive pulmonary disease. Am J Respir Cell Mol Biol 23, 530-536.

Sarasin, A., 1999. The molecular pathways of ultraviolet-induced carcinogenesis. Mutat Res 428, 5-10.

Saw, C. L., Huang, M. T., Liu, Y., Khor, T. O., Conney, A. H., Kong, A. N., Impact of Nrf2 on UVB-induced skin inflammation/photoprotection and photoprotective effect of sulforaphane. Mol Carcinog.

Schafer, M., Dutsch, S., auf dem Keller, U., Werner, S., Nrf2: a central regulator of UV protection in the epidermis. Cell Cycle 9, 2917-2918.

Schmitz-Hoerner, R., Weissenbock, G., 2003. Contribution of phenolic compounds to the UV-B screening capacity of developing barley primary leaves in relation to DNA damage and repair under elevated UV-B levels. Phytochemistry 64, 243-255.

Seo, W. Y., Goh, A. R., Ju, S. M., Song, H. Y., Kwon, D. J., Jun, J. G., Kim, B. C., Choi, S. Y., Park, J., Celastrol induces expression of heme oxygenase-1 through ROS/Nrf2/ARE signaling in the HaCaT cells. Biochem Biophys Res Commun.

Stewart, M. S., Cameron, G. S., Pence, B. C., 1996. Antioxidant nutrients protect against UVB-induced oxidative damage to DNA of mouse keratinocytes in culture. J Invest Dermatol 106, 1086-1089.

Verjat, T., Dhenaut, A., Radicella, J. P., Araneda, S., 2000. Detection of 8-oxoG DNA glycosylase activity and OGG1 transcripts in the rat CNS. Mutat Res 460, 127-138.

Villeneuve, N. F., Sun, Z., Chen, W., Zhang, D. D., 2009. Nrf2 and p21 regulate the fine balance between life and death by controlling ROS levels. Cell Cycle 8, 3255-3256.

Wang, L., Chen, Y., Sternberg, P., Cai, J., 2008. Essential roles of the PI3 kinase/Akt pathway in regulating Nrf2-dependent antioxidant functions in the RPE. Invest Ophthalmol Vis Sci 49, 1671-1678.

Wild, A. C., Gipp, J. J., Mulcahy, T., 1998. Overlapping antioxidant response element and PMA response element sequences mediate basal and beta-naphthoflavone-induced expression of the human gamma-glutamylcysteine synthetase catalytic subunit gene. Biochem J 332 ( Pt 2), 373-381.

Wu, C., Chen, F., Wang, X., Wu, Y., Dong, M., He, G., Galyean, R. D., He, L., Huang, G., 2007. Identification of antioxidant phenolic compounds in feverfew (Tanacetum parthenium) by HPLC-ESI-MS/MS and NMR. Phytochem Anal 18, 401-410.

Yu, R., Chen, C., Mo, Y. Y., Hebbar, V., Owuor, E. D., Tan, T. H., Kong, A. N., 2000a. Activation of mitogen-activated protein kinase pathways induces antioxidant response element-mediated gene expression via a Nrf2-dependent mechanism. J Biol Chem 275, 39907-39913.

Yu, R., Lei, W., Mandlekar, S., Weber, M. J., Der, C. J., Wu, J., Kong, A. N., 1999. Role of a mitogen-activated protein kinase pathway in the induction of phase II detoxifying enzymes by chemicals. J Biol Chem 274, 27545-27552.

Yu, R., Mandlekar, S., Lei, W., Fahl, W. E., Tan, T. H., Kong, A. N., 2000b. p38 mitogen-activated protein kinase negatively regulates the induction of phase II drug-metabolizing enzymes that detoxify carcinogens. J Biol Chem 275, 2322-2327.

Zhang, Y., Talalay, P., Cho, C. G., Posner, G. H., 1992. A major inducer of anticarcinogenic protective enzymes from broccoli: isolation and elucidation of structure. Proc Natl Acad Sci U S A 89, 2399-2403.

# 25

# Food Factors and Oxidative DNA Damage / DNA Repair Systems

Takeshi Hirano[1] and Kazuyoshi Tamae[2]
[1]*Department of Life and Environment Engineering, Faculty of Environmental Engineering, The University of Kitakyushu,*
[2]*Division of Teacher Training, Faculty of Education and Culture, University of Miyazaki, Japan*

## 1. Introduction

8-Oxoguanine (7, 8-dihydro-8-oxoguanine, abbreviated as 8-oxo-Gua), a form of oxidized guanine, is a mutagenic lesion formed spontaneously in the genomic DNA of aerobic organisms (Fig. 1) and by the actions of exogenous factors, such as ionizing radiation, chemical pollutants, heavy metals, food factors, and bacteria. 8-Oxo-Gua induces GC-to-TA transversion type point mutations [1]. Point mutations generated via oxidative DNA damage are involved in cancer development, because mutations are a common feature of human cancers. Therefore, 8-oxo-Gua is considered to be involved in carcinogenesis. In this context, studies of 8-oxo-Gua have significant implications for understanding the underlying mechanisms of mutation-associated diseases, including cancer [2]. Although 8-oxo-Gua is not necessarily the most abundant form of oxidative DNA damage, it has been the most extensively studied, because it is quite easily measured by a method utilizing HPLC coupled with electrochemical detection in laboratories [3, 4]. The presence of 8-oxo-Gua and 8-oxoadenine (8-oxo-Ade) in mutagenic oxidized DNA products has been extensively studied, and their frequencies of generation in mammalian DNA and degrees of mutagenicity are similar [5-8]. The relative focus-forming activity, which indicates the mutation inducibility, of 8-oxo-Gua and 8-oxo-Ade were reportedly ~1% [7, 8].

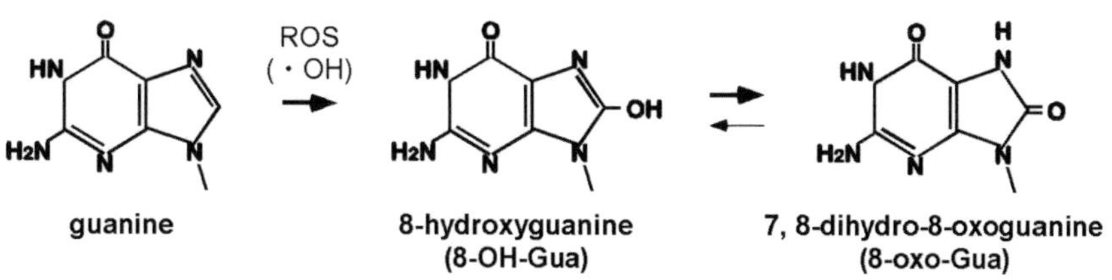


Fig. 1. Structure of 7, 8-dihydro-8-oxoguanine or 8-hydroxyguanine (8-OH-Gua). 8-Oxo-Gua is formed by hydroxylation of guanine at the C-8 position.

Extensive efforts have been made to clone the repair enzymes for 8-oxo-Gua. The first information was obtained from the studies of an enzyme, formamidopyrimidine DNA glycosylase (Fpg or MutM), which excises 8-oxo-Gua, 2, 6-diamino-4-hydroxy-5-formamidopyrimidine (FapyGua), and 4, 6-diamino-5-formamidopyrimidine (FapyAde) from the DNA of *Escherichia coli* [9]. This enzyme has an activity to process the resulting abasic (AP) site, by cleaving both the 3′- and 5′-phosphodiester bonds by successive β- and δ-eliminations [10-12]. In 1996, an Fpg homologue was identified in *Saccharomyces cerevisiae* [13, 14]. This was the first report of an 8-oxoguanine DNA glycosylase 1 (OGG1). In the following year, mammalian (human and other mammals) homologues of OGG1 were identified and cloned [15-21]. 8-Oxo-Gua is efficiently removed from DNA via the short-patch base excision repair (BER) pathway initiated by OGG1.

Among the environmental factors that are related to human diseases, food factors have a large influence on human health. To understand the mechanisms of food-related carcinogenesis, the roles of 8-oxo-Gua have been investigated in relationship with food factors. In this review article, we will focus on and describe the relationship between food factors and 8-oxo-Gua / 8-oxo-Gua repair systems.

## 2. Aminoazo dyes and 8-oxo-Gua / OGG1

Food factors have been extensively investigated in association with oxidative DNA damage and its repair systems. Some food factors, such as aminoazo dyes, are known inhibitors of OGG1 expression. Aminoazo dyes were previously used as artificial color additives to food. Some of them, such as *N*-methyl-4-aminoazobenzene, *N*, *N*-dimethyl-4-aminoazobenzene, and 3′-methyl-4-dimethylaminoazobenzene (3′-MeDAB), are hepato-carcinogenic. We previously analyzed the effects of 3′-MeDAB on 8-oxo-Gua repair systems in rodent livers, and reported that 3′-MeDAB increased 8-oxo-Gua generation and decreased OGG1 expression, possibly by cleaving the protein [22]. These results suggested that the liver carcinogenicity of 3′-MeDAB was due to an increase in 8-oxo-Gua generation via 3′-MeDAB-induced downregulation of OGG1 expression.

The use of 3′-MeDAB as a food additive is now prohibited. However, other types of azo dyes are still being used. Therefore, more research is needed to define the effects of azo dyes on human health.

## 3. Alcohol and 8-oxo-Gua / OGG1

Alcohol consumption has been associated with a variety of human cancers for several centuries. Recent studies revealed that alcohol consumption is associated with an increase in breast cancer incidence in women [23, 24], esophageal cancer [25], and colorectal cancer [26, 27]. On the other hand, the cancer-preventive effects of alcohol drinking have also been reported. It is well known that moderate consumption of wine may prevent some types of cancers [28-30]. These studies concerning wine consumption suggested that anti-oxidant agents, such as polyphenols, including catekin, quercetin and resveratrol, contributed to the cancer–preventive effect of wine [31]. Thus, anti-oxidant agents seem to play a key role in the beneficial effects of wine. It was also suggested that resveratrol could reduce the localized estrogen production that plays a crucial role in the development of breast cancer [32]. On the other hand, for alcoholic beverages other than wine, a cohort study suggested that alcohol (spirits and beer) consumption was associated with a decrease in the risk of renal cell carcinoma in male smokers [33]. A matched case-control study reported a similar result, in which regular, moderate alcohol (beer, wine, and spirits) consumption was associated with a decreased probability of leukoplakia occurrence, with respect to occasional or no alcohol consumption [34]. These results are not conclusive, but suggest that other components of alcoholic beverages (including wine) besides polyphenols may be responsible for the beneficial effects on human health.

The evidence that not only wine but also spirits and beer have cancer-preventive effects prompted us to investigate the molecular mechanisms of these effects of alcohol consumption due to factors other than polyphenols. In fact, recent evidences have suggested that the protective effects of red wine on cancer or cardiovascular diseases were not a consequence of the anti-oxidant capacity of alcohol [35, 36]. Arendt et al. reported the reduction of DNA damage as another mechanism of the cancer-preventive function of wine [35].

In this context, we analyzed the 8-oxo-Gua accumulation level in DNA and its repair ability (8-oxo-Gua nicking activity and mouse OGG1 (mOGG1) expression) in the livers of mice treated with 3′-MeDAB, a well known hepato-carcinogen as described above, and / or ethanol, to examine the effects of alcohol consumption on carcinogenesis (Fig. 2A) [37]. The method used to determine the 8-oxo-Gua nicking activity was described elsewhere [38]. In the study, we found that 12% ethanol reduced the 3′-MeDAB-induced 8-oxo-Gua accumulation (Fig. 2B). Moreover, the 8-oxo-Gua repair activity showed a decreasing tendency in 3′-MeDAB-treated mouse livers with 12% ethanol administration, without any significant differences (Fig. 2C). The decrease in the 8-oxo-Gua repair activity seems to be a reasonable consequence of the lower 8-oxo-Gua levels. Since we speculated that OGG1 fragmentation was a key event for 3′-MeDAB-induced 8-oxo-Gua accumulation [22], we predicted that OGG1 fragmentation might be inhibited by ethanol intake, as in the inhibition of the increase in 8-oxo-Gua levels. However, 12% ethanol intake failed to inhibit the 3′-MeDAB-induced fragmentation of OGG1 (groups D, E, and F in Fig. 2D). The observations indicated that ethanol intake reduced 8-oxo-Gua accumulation, without affecting the function of OGG1. However, since other enzymes besides OGG1 can reportedly repair 8-oxo-Gua [39], we speculate that ethanol consumption might induce these 8-oxo-Gua repair systems to reduce the 8-oxo-Gua level.

## 4. Coffee and 8-oxo-Gua / OGG1

Coffee has been a quite popular beverage in many parts of the world for a long time. However, its effects on human health are not well understood. Some studies suggested that coffee consumption had preventive properties for metabolic diseases, such as type 2 diabetes [40, 41], or cancers, such as hepatocellular carcinoma [42, 43] and colorectal cancer [44, 45], through its content of potentially antimutagenic substances [46]. These findings led to the hypothesis that coffee consumption lowers the risk of some types of cancers.

On the other hand, some studies provided negative conclusions for the effects of coffee consumption on human health. A large cohort study in Sweden and Japan indicated that coffee consumption was not associated with the risk of colorectal cancer [47, 48]. Furthermore, another cohort study indicated that coffee consumption increased the risk of certain cancers, such as gastric cancer [49]. These carcinogenic actions of coffee were supported by evidence that coffee contained numerous substances, such as glyoxal, methylglyoxal, ethylglyoxal, propylglyoxal, diacetyl, and acetol, with potentially genotoxic and mutagenic properties [46, 49-51]. Although the polyphenols in beverages, such as green tea, black tea, and coffee, are antioxidant substances, a recent study indicated the production of hydrogen peroxide, a harmful molecule for living organisms, by polyphenol-rich beverages [52]. Therefore, although numerous studies have been performed, the effects of coffee consumption on human health have remained undefined.

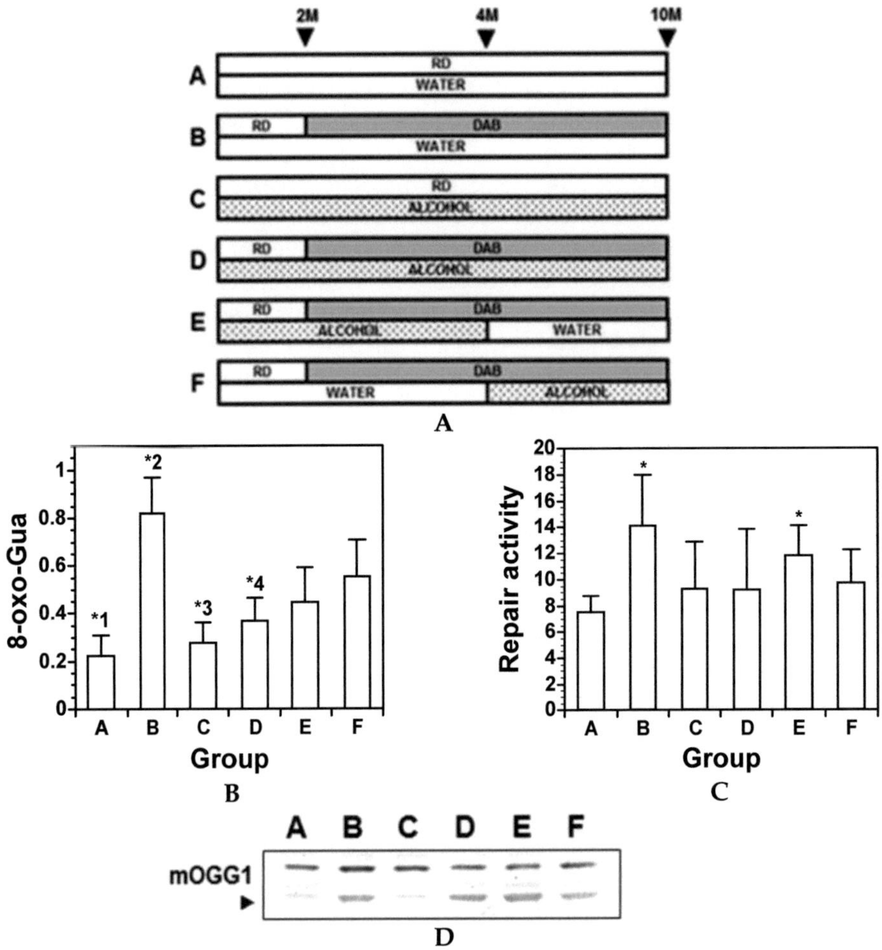


Fig. 2. (A) The experimental protocol. A: control [ND / water] for 10 months; B: [ND / water] for the first 2 months and [0.06% 3′-MeDAB / water] for the last 8 months; C: [ND / alcohol] for 10 months; D: [ND / alcohol] for the first 2 months and [0.06% 3′-MeDAB / alcohol] for the last 8 months; E: [ND / alcohol] for the first 2 months, [0.06% 3′-MeDAB / alcohol] for the next 4 months, and [0.06% 3′-MeDAB / water] for the last 4 months; F: [ND / water] for the first 2 months, [3′-MeDAB / water] for the next 4 months, and [3′-MeDAB / alcohol] for the last 4 months. ND: normal diet, DAB: 3′-MeDAB. (B) The levels of 8-oxo-Gua in the DNA of mouse livers. The 8-oxo-Gua value is expressed as the number of 8-oxo-dG per $10^5$ deoxyguanosine. *1: $P < 0.0005$ *vs.* group B, $P < 0.05$ vs. group E, $P < 0.01$ vs. group F; *2: $P < 0.0001$ vs. group C, $P < 0.005$ vs. group D, $P < 0.01$ vs. group E, $P < 0.05$ vs. group F; *3: $P < 0.05$ vs. group E, $P < 0.005$ vs. group F; *4: $P < 0.05$ vs. group F. (C) 8-Oxo-Gua nicking activity in the mouse livers. The activity was calculated as the ratio of the excised fragment intensity to the total substrate (unexcised substrate intensity plus excised fragment intensity). *: $P < 0.005$ vs. group A. (D) Western blotting of mOGG1 protein in the mouse livers. Mouse livers were removed and homogenized to produce crude extracts. The extracts were electrophoresed and blotted onto a PVDF membrane. A western blot analysis was performed using an anti-mouse OGG1 antibody. The arrowhead indicates fragmented mOGG1. mOGG1: mouse OGG1. This figure was published in reference [37], Copyright Elsevier (license#: 2633951132321).

To address this issue, we focused on the effects of instant coffee consumption on the generation of 8-oxo-Gua. In our previous work, we analyzed the 8-oxo-Gua level and the 8-oxo-Gua repair system in the livers of mice fed with / without a 0.1% instant coffee solution. In addition, we employed an autoclaved diet (low vitamin diet; LV diet) to maintain half of the mice under low vitamin conditions. We found that instant coffee consumption does not alter the 8-oxo-Gua generation level and *OGG1* mRNA expression, although it prevents low-vitamin diet-induced 8-oxo-Gua production [53] (Fig. 3). Our study suggested that daily instant coffee consumption may provide more beneficial effects than detrimental effects. However, we have not examined other types of DNA damage. To clarify the role of coffee consumption on human health, further studies should be performed.

## 5. Urinary 8-oxo-Gua level and food consumption

Urinary 8-oxo-Gua levels are often analyzed, especially as a marker of oxidation [54, 55]. Among the urinary biomarkers of oxidative stresses, 8-oxo-Gua is possibly the most studied. We previously investigated the effects of age, smoking, dietary factors, and other life style factors on urinary 8-oxodeoxyguanosine (8-oxo-dG) levels [56]. Urine samples were collected from healthy employees in a steel-manufacturing company, after obtaining informed consent. The mean level of urinary 8-oxo-dG (μg / g creatinine) in the 361 male subjects was 4.20 ± 1.47 (Table 1). The relationships between 16 categorical lifestyle factors and urinary 8-oxo-dG levels were analyzed by ANOVA. The results revealed that the urinary 8-oxo-dG level was significantly negatively related to fruit consumption ($P = 0.03$) and physical activity ($P = 0.03$). It is noteworthy that, in terms of fruit consumption, the urinary 8-oxo-dG levels of the "rarely" and "two or three times per week" groups were significantly higher than those of the "everyday" group ($P = 0.03$). The results of the Scheffe's test also indicated that fruit consumption significantly reduced the urinary 8-oxo-dG level. Besides urinary analyses, a diet rich in fruit and vegetables was also reportedly effective in the reduction of oxidative stresses [57]. These data indicated that fruit consumption and physical activity reduce oxidative stress generation.

| variables | category | n | % | urinary 8-oxo-dG | *P* |
|---|---|---|---|---|---|
| sleep | deficient | 10 | 2.8 | 4.37 ± 0.25 | 0.53 |
| | slightly deficient | 181 | 50.1 | 4.19 ± 0.12 | |
| | sufficient | 170 | 47.1 | 4.20 ± 0.11 | |
| holiday | little or none | 2 | 0.6 | 5.41 ± 1.20 | 1.00 |
| | once a week | 51 | 14.1 | 3.96 ± 0.21 | |
| | twice a week | 308 | 85.3 | 4.23 ± 0.08 | |
| fatigue | always | 18 | 5.0 | 3.66 ± 0.32 | 0.86 |
| | sometimes | 256 | 70.9 | 4.17 ± 0.09 | |
| | rarely | 87 | 24.1 | 4.39 ± 0.17 | |
| rhythm | irregular | 66 | 18.3 | 4.05 ± 0.19 | 0.25 |
| | mostly regular | 215 | 59.6 | 4.20 ± 0.10 | |
| | regular | 80 | 22.2 | 4.30 ± 0.16 | |
| refreshing | difficult | 13 | 3.6 | 4.40 ± 0.38 | 0.48 |
| | moderate | 255 | 70.6 | 4.13 ± 0.09 | |
| | easy | 93 | 25.8 | 4.33 ± 0.17 | |
| size of a meal | full stomach every time | 24 | 6.6 | 3.87 ± 0.27 | 0.85 |
| | no pattern | 198 | 54.8 | 4.29 ± 0.11 | |
| | moderation every time | 139 | 38.5 | 4.12 ± 0.11 | |

| variables | category | n | % | urinary 8-oxo-dG | *P* |
|---|---|---|---|---|---|
| healthy meal combination | rarely | 46 | 12.7 | 4.25 ± 0.20 | 0.11 |
| | consider sometimes | 187 | 51.8 | 4.33 ± 0.12 | |
| | consider every time | 128 | 35.5 | 3.99 ± 0.11 | |
| skipping meals | one meal every day | 63 | 17.5 | 4.37 ± 0.20 | 0.62 |
| | 2 or 3 meals a week | 103 | 28.5 | 4.09 ± 0.15 | |
| | rarely | 195 | 54.0 | 4.20 ± 0.10 | |
| light-colored vegetable | rarely | 17 | 4.7 | 4.32 ± 0.42 | 0.78 |
| | once a day | 268 | 74.2 | 4.22 ± 0.09 | |
| | each meal | 76 | 21.1 | 4.09 ± 0.14 | |
| green- and yellow-colored vegetables | rarely | 26 | 7.2 | 4.10 ± 0.32 | 0.75 |
| | 2 or 3 times a week | 244 | 67.6 | 4.21 ± 0.10 | |
| | everyday | 91 | 25.2 | 4.18 ± 0.12 | |
| fruit | rarely | 140 | 38.8 | 4.24 ± 0.12 | 0.03 |
| | 2 or 3 times a week | 187 | 51.8 | 4.28 ± 0.11 | |
| | everyday | 34 | 9.4 | 3.57 ± 0.19 | |
| meat, fish, egg, etc. | rarely | 11 | 3.0 | 4.72 ± 0.49 | 0.16 |
| | twice a day | 194 | 53.7 | 4.25 ± 0.11 | |
| | each meal | 156 | 43.2 | 4.09 ± 0.11 | |
| milk | rarely | 118 | 32.7 | 4.32 ± 0.16 | 0.23 |
| | 2 or 3 times a week | 171 | 47.4 | 4.10 ± 0.10 | |
| | everyday | 72 | 19.9 | 4.23 ± 0.15 | |
| oil | rarely | 9 | 2.5 | 4.41 ± 0.58 | 0.55 |
| | 2 or 3 times a week | 192 | 53.2 | 4.15 ± 0.12 | |
| | everyday | 160 | 44.3 | 4.24 ± 0.10 | |
| seaweed | rarely | 58 | 16.1 | 3.99 ± 0.18 | 0.75 |
| | 2 or 3 times a week | 266 | 73.7 | 4.26 ± 0.09 | |
| | everyday | 37 | 10.2 | 4.04 ± 0.21 | |
| physical activity | light | 192 | 53.2 | 4.39 ± 0.11 | 0.03 |
| | moderate | 119 | 33.0 | 4.09 ± 0.12 | |
| | moderately heavy | 12 | 3.3 | 3.85 ± 0.48 | |
| | heavy | 38 | 10.5 | 3.68 ± 0.19 | |

*P*: One-way analysis of variance
Urinary 8-oxo-dG data are expressed as μg / g creatinine ± SE
These data are derived from a report by Tamae et al. [56] with permission from Wiley-Blackwell.

Table 1. The characteristics of categorical lifestyle factors and urinary 8-oxo-dG levels in 361 male subjects

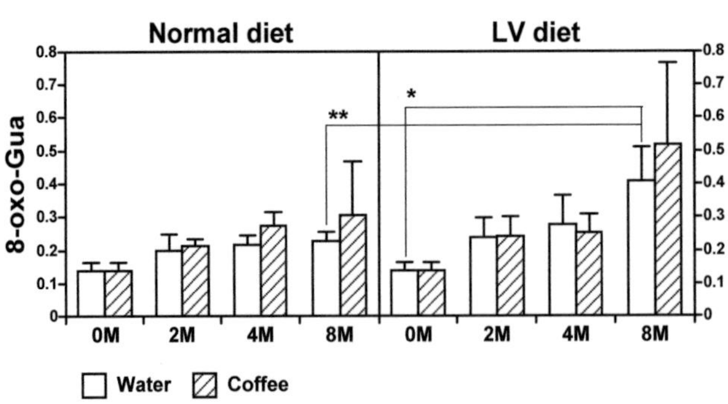


A

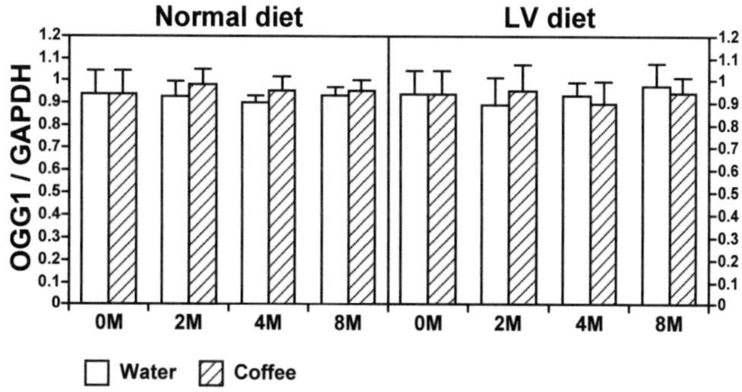


B

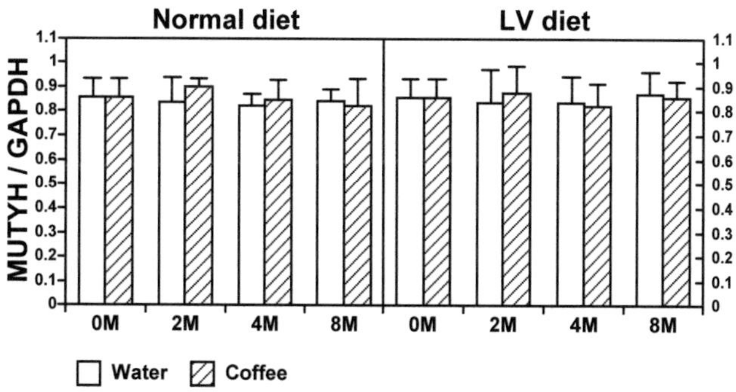


C

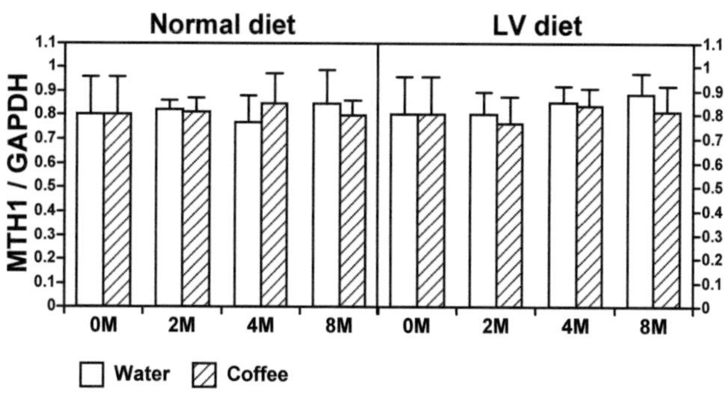


D

Fig. 3. (A) The 8-oxo-dG level in mouse liver DNA. The 8-oxo-dG value is expressed as the number per $10^5$ deoxyguanosine. n=3 for data of 4 and 8 months, n=4 for data of 2 months. (B) *Ogg1* gene expression level. n=4 for LV diet + water for 8 months, n=5 for others. (C) *MUTYH* gene expression level. n=4 for LV diet + water for 8 months, n=5 for others. (D) *MTH1* gene expression level. n=4 for LV diet + water for 8 months, n=5 for others. The *GAPDH* gene was used as an internal standard. The total value of the gene expression level was calculated by the ratio of the expression of each gene to *GAPDH* expression. The values are mean + SD. *P < 0.005, **P < 0.05. LV diet: low vitamin diet. MUTYH: eukaryotic homologue of MutY (mismatched adenine DNA glycosylase), MTH1: eukaryotic homologue of MutT (8-oxo-dGTPase). This figure was published in reference [53], Copyright Blackwell Publishing (license#: 2634430504476).

## 6. Dietary factors and OGG1 polymorphism

Interestingly, Sørensen et al. reported that the effect of vegetable consumption was associated with the *OGG1* Ser326Cys polymorphism [58]. A non-synonymous (associated with an amino acid change) genetic polymorphism at codon 326, Ser326Cys, in the *OGG1* gene is a strong candidate as a genetic factor for cancer risk [59, 60]. In fact, the OGG1 Ser326Cys enzyme exhibited functional defects [61]. OGG1 Ser326Cys excised 8-oxo-Gua from duplex DNA and cleaved abasic sites at rates 2- to 6-fold lower than those of the wild-type enzyme. Yamane et al. reported that 8-oxo-Gua-induced mutations were more efficiently suppressed in OGG1-Ser326 transduced cells than OGG1-Cys326 transduced cells, suggesting that OGG1-Cys326 has reduced ability to prevent mutagenesis by 8-oxo-Gua than OGG1-Ser326 *in vivo* in human cells [62]. Sørensen et al. observed a 54% decrease in lung cancer risk per 50% increase in vegetable intake among homozygous Cys326Cys carriers, and no decrease in risk among carriers of Ser326Ser or Ser326Cys. Therefore, to evaluate the effect of food factors on carcinogenesis, the OGG1 polymorphism should be considered.

## 7. Conclusions

As described above, dietary factors influence 8-oxo-Gua generation and its repair systems in a variety of manners. They may contribute to human diseases, including cancer, by causing DNA damage and affecting DNA repair systems. The effects of food factors on the generation of 8-oxo-Gua and the expression of OGG1 must be further clarified, to reduce the risk of food factor-related diseases, such as cancer or diabetes.

In addition, DNA double-strand break (DAB) is also a well-known DNA damage. Datta *et al.* reported that 8-oxo-formation was associated with $^{125}$I-induced double-strand break (DSB) formation. Therefore, analyses of food factors and DSB formation should be interested as a further study [63].

## 8. Acknowledgements

The authors thank INTECH OPEN ACCESS PUBLISHER, for inviting us to write this review article, and Elsevier LTD, Blackwell Publishing, and Wiley-Blackwell, for permission to reproduce the material in references [37], [53], and [56], respectively.

## 9. References

[1] K.C. Cheng, D.S. Cahill, H. Kasai, S. Nishimura, and L.A. Loeb, "8-Hydroxyguanine, an abundant form of oxidative DNA damage, causes G-T and A-C substitutions," *Journal of Biological Chemistry*, vol. 267, pp. 166-172, 1992.

[2] T. Tsuzuki, Y. Nakatsu, and Y. Nakabeppu, "Significance of error-avoiding mechanisms for oxidative DNA damage in carcinogenesis," *Cancer Sciences*, vol. 98, pp. 465-470, 2007.

[3] L.J. Marnett, "Oxyradicals and DNA damage," *Carcinogenesis*, vol. 21, pp. 361-370, 2000.

[4] R.A. Floyd, J.J. Watson, P.K. Wong, D.H. Altmiller, and R.C. Rickard, "Hydroxyl free radical adduct of deoxyguanosine: sensitive detection and mechanisms of formation," *Free Radical Research Communications*, vol. 1, pp. 163-172, 1986.

[5] Y.J. Wang, Y.S. Ho, M.J. Lo, and J.K. Lin, "Oxidative modification of DNA bases in rat liver and lung during chemical carcinogenesis and aging," *Chemico-Biological Interactions*, vol. 94, 135-145, 1995.

[6] P. Jaruga, and M. Dizdaroglu, "Repair of products of oxidative DNA base damage in human cells," *Nucleic Acids Research*, vol. 24, pp. 1389-1394, 1996.

[7] H. Kamiya, N. Murata-Kamiya, S. Koizume, H. Inoue, S. Nishimura, and E. Ohtsuka, "8-Hydroxyguanine (7, 8-dihydro-8-oxoguanine) in hot spots of the c-Ha-ras gene: effects of sequence contexts on mutation spectra," *Carcinogenesis*, vol. 16, pp. 883-889, 1995.

[8] H. Kamiya, H. Miura, N. Murata-Kamiya, H. Ishikawa, T. Sakaguchi, H. Inoue, T. Sasaki, C. Masutani, F. Hanaoka, S. Nishimura, and E. Ohtsuka, "8-Hydroxyadenine (7, 8-dihydro-8-oxoadenine) induces misincorporation in *in vitro* DNA synthesis and mutations in NIH 3T3 cells," *Nucleic Acids Research*, vol. 23, pp. 2893-2899, 1995.

[9] S. Boiteux, T.R. O'Connor, F. Lederer, A. Gouyette, and J. Laval, "Homogeneous *Escherichia coli* FPG protein," *Journal of Biological Chemistry*, vol. 265, pp. 3916-3922, 1990.

[10] J. Tchou, H. Kasai, S. Shibutani, M.H. Chung, J. Laval, A.P. Grollman, and S. Nishimura, "8-Oxoguanine (8-hydroxyguanine) DNA glycosylase and its substrate specificity," *Proceedings of the National Academy of Sciences of the United States of America*, vol. 88, pp. 4690-4694, 1991.

[11] S. Boiteux, E. Gajewski, J. Laval, and M. Dizdaroglu, "Substrate specificity of the *Escherichia coli* Fpg protein (formamidopyrimidine-DNA glycosylase): excision of purine lesions in DNA produced by ionizing radiation or photosensitization," *Biochemistry*, vol. 31, pp. 106-110, 1992.

[12] M. Bhagwat, and J.A. Gerlt, "3'- and 5'-strand cleavage reactions catalyzed by the Fpg protein from *Escherichia coli* occur via successive beta- and delta-elimination mechanisms, respectively," *Biochemistry*, vol. 35, pp. 659-665, 1996.

[13] P.A. van der Kemp, D. Thomas, R. Barbey, R. De Oliveira, and S. Boiteux, "Cloning and expression in *Escherichia coli* of the OGG1 gene of *Saccharomyces cerevisiae*, which codes for a DNA glycosylase that excises 7,8-dihydro-8-oxoguanine and 2,6-diamino-4-hydroxy-5-N-methylformamidopyrimidine," *Proceedings of the National Academy of Sciences of the United States of America*, vol. 93, pp. 5197-5202, 1996.

[14] H.M. Nash, S.D. Bruner, O.D. Schärer, T. Kawate, T.A. Addona, E. Sponner, W.S. Lane, and G.I. Verdine, "Cloning of a yeast 8-oxoguanine DNA glycosylase reveals the existence of a base-excision DNA-repair protein superfamily," *Current Biology*, vol. 6, pp. 968-980, 1996.

[15] R. Lu, H.M. Nash, and G.L. Verdine, "A mammalian DNA repair enzyme that excises oxidatively damaged guanines maps to a locus frequently lost in lung cancer," *Current Biology*, vol. 7, pp. 397-407, 1997.

[16] T.A. Rosenquist, D.O. Zharkov, and A.P. Grollman, "Cloning and characterization of a mammalian 8-oxoguanine DNA glycosylase," *Proceedings of the National Academy of Sciences of the United States of America*, vol. 94, pp. 7429-7434, 1997.

[17] T. Roldán-Arjona, Y.F. Wei, K.C. Carter, A. Klungland, C. Anselmino, R.P. Wang, M. Augustus, and T. Lindahl, "Molecular cloning and functional expression of a human cDNA encoding the antimutator enzyme 8-hydroxyguanine-DNA glycosylase," *Proceedings of the National Academy of Sciences of the United States of America*, vol. 94, pp. 8016-8020, 1997.

[18] J.P. Radicella, C. Dherin, C. Desmaze, M.S. Fox, and S. Boiteux, "Cloning and characterization of hOGG1, a human homolog of the OGG1 gene of *Saccharomyces cerevisiae*," *Proceedings of the National Academy of Sciences of the United States of America*, vol. 94, pp. 8010-8015, 1997.

[19] M. Bjorås, L. Luna, B. Johnson, E. Hoff, T. Haug, T. Rongnes, and E. Seeberg, "Opposite base-dependent reactions of a human base excision repair enzyme on DNA containing 7, 8-dihydro-8-oxoguanine and abasic sites," *The EMBO Journal*, vol. 16, pp. 6314-6322, 1997.

[20] K, Arai, K. Morishita, K. Shinmura, T. Kohno, S.R. Kim, T. Nohmi, M. Taniwaki, S. Ohwada, and J. Yokota, "Cloning of a human homolog of the yeast OGG1 gene that is involved in the repair of oxidative DNA damage," *Oncogene*, vol. 14, pp. 2857-2861, 1997.

[21] H. Aburatani, Y. Hippo, T. Ishida, R. Takashima, C. Matsuba, T. Kodama, M. Takao, A. Yasui, K. Yamamoto, M. Asano, K. Fukasawa, T. Yoshinari, H. Inoue, E. Ohtsuka, and S. Nishimura, "Cloning and characterization of mammalian 8-hydroxyguanine-specific DNA glycosylase/apurinic, apyrimidinic lyase, a functional mutM homologue," *Cancer Research*, vol. 57, pp. 2151-2156, 1997.

[22] T. Hirano, K. Higashi, A. Sakai, Y. Tsurudome, Y. Ootsuyama, R. Kido, and H. Kasai, "Analyses of oxidative DNA damage and its repair activity in the livers of 3'-methyl-4-dimethylaminoazobenzene-treated rodents," *Japanese Journal of Cancer Research*, vol. 91, pp. 681-695, 2000.

[23] S.A. Smith-Warner, D. Spiegelman, S.S. Yaun, P.A. van den Brandt, A.R. Folsom, A. Goldbohm, S. Graham, L. Holmberg, G.R. Howe, J.R. Marshall, A.B. Miller, J.D. Potter, F.E. Speizer, W.C. Willett, A. Wolk, and D.J. Hunter, "Alcohol and breast cancer in women; A pooled analysis of cohort studies," *JAMA*, vol. 279, pp.535-540, 1998.

[24] R.Z. Stolzenberg-Solomon, S.C. Chang, M.F. Leitzmann, K.A. Johnson, C. Johnson, S.S. Buys, R.N. Hoover, and R.G. Ziegler, "Folate intake, alcohol use, and postmenopausal breast cancer risk in the prostate, lung, colorectal, and ovarian cancer screening trial," *The American Journal of Clinical Nutrition*, vol. 83, pp. 895-904, 2006.

[25] M. Wu, J.K. Zhao, X.S. Hu, P.H. Wang, Y. Qin, Y.C. Lu, J. Yang, A.M. Liu, D.L. Wu, Z.F. Zhang, K.J. Frans, and P. van't Veer, "Association of smoking, alcohol drinking and dietary factors with esophageal cancer in high- and low-risk areas of Jiangsu Province, China," *World Journal of Gastroenterology*, vol. 12, pp. 1686-1693, 2006.

[26] A.L. Klatsky, M.A. Armstrong, and G.D.Friedman, "The relations of alcoholic beverage use to colon and rectal cancer," *American Journal of Epidemiology*, vol. 128, pp. 1007-1015, 1988.

[27] J. Ho, T. Lam, and L. Chiu, "Smoking, drinking and colorectal cancer in Hong Kong Chinese: A case control study," *International Journal of Cancer*, vol. 109, pp. 587-597, 2004.

[28] J.C. Anderson, Z. Alpern, G. Sethi, C.R. Messina, C. Martin, P.M. Hubbard, R. Grimson, P.F. Ells, and R.D. Shaw, "Prevalence and risk of colorectal neoplasia in consumers of alcohol in a screening population," *The American Journal of Gastroenterology*, vol. 100, pp. 2049-2055, 2005.

[29] P.M. Webb, D.M. Purdie, C.J. Bain, and A.C. Green, "Alcohol, wine, and risk of epithelial ovarian cancer," *Cancer Epidemiology, Biomarkers, and Prevention*, vol. 13, pp. 592-599, 2004.

[30] N.C. Briggs, R.S. Levine, L.D. Bobo, W.P. Haliburton, E.A. Brann, and C.H. Hennekens, "Wine drinking and risk of non-Hodgkin's lymphoma among men in the United States: A population-based case-control study," *American Journal of Epidemiology*, vol. 156, pp. 454-462, 2002.

[31] S. Dragoni, J. Gee, R. Bennett, M. Valoti, and G. Sgaragli, "Red wine alcohol promotes quercetin absorption and directs its metabolism towards isorhamnetin and tamarixetin in rat intestine *in vitro*," *British Journal of Pharmacology*, vol. 147, pp. 765-771, 2006.

[32] Y. Wang, K.W. Lee, F.L. Chan, S. Chen, and L.K. Leung, "The red wine polyphenol resveratrol displays bilevel inhibition on aromatase in breast cancer cells," *Toxicological Sciences*, vol. 92, pp. 71-77, 2006.

[33] S. Mahabir, M.F. Leitzmann, M.J. Virtanen, J. Virtamo, P. Pietinen, D. Albanes, and P.R. Taylor, "Prospective study of alcohol drinking and renal cell cancer risk in a cohort of Finnish male smokers," *Cancer Epidemiology, Biomarkers, and Prevention*, vol. 14, pp. 170-175, 2005.

[34] S. Petti and C. Scully, "Association between different alcoholic beverages and leukoplakia among non- to moderate-drinking adults: A matched case-control study," *European Journal of Cancer*, vol. 42, pp. 521-527, 2006.

[35] B.M. Arendt, S. Ellinger, K. Kekic, L. Geus, R. Fimmers, U. Spengler, W.U. Müller, and R. Goerich, "Single and repeated moderate consumption of native or dealcoholized red wine show different effects on antioxidant parameters in blood and DNA strand breaks in peripheral leukocytes in healthy volunteers: a randomized controlled trial (ISRCTN68505294)," *Nutrition Journal*, vol. 14, p. 33, 2005.

[36] R.A.A. Caccetta, V. Burke, V.B. Mori, L.J. Beilin, I.B. Puddey, and K.D. Croft, "Red wine polyphenols, in the absence of alcohol, reduce lipid peroxidative stress

in smoking subjects," *Free Radical and Biological Medicine*, vol. 30, pp. 636-642, 2001.

[37] T. Hirano, A. Sakai, Y. Ootsuyama, and H. Kasai, "Chronic alcohol consumption prevents 8-hydroxyguanine accumulation in 3'-methyl-4-dimethylaminoazobenzene-treated mouse liver," *Biochemical and Biophysical Research Communications*, vol. 387, pp. 316-320, 2009.

[38] T. Hirano, Y. Yamaguchi, H. Hirano, and H. Kasai, "8-Hydroxyguanine levels in nuclear DNA and its repair activity in rat organs associated with age," *Journal of Gerontology*, vol. 51A, pp. B303-B307, 1996.

[39] T.K. Hazra, J.W. Hill, T. Izumi, and S. Mitra, "Multiple DNA glycosylases for repair of 8-oxoguanine and their potential in vivo functions," *Progress in Nucleic Acid Research and Molecular Biology*, vol. 68, pp. 193-205, 2001.

[40] G.B. Keijzers, C.J. Tack, B.E. De Galan, and P. Smits, "Caffeine can decrease insulin sensitivity in humans," *Diabetes Care*, vol. 25, pp. 364-369, 2002.

[41] H. Iso, C. Date, K. Wakai, M. Fukui, A. Tamakoshi, and the JACC Study Group, "The relationship between green tea and total caffeine intake and risk for self-reported type 2 diabetes among Japanese adults," *Annals of Internal Medicine*, vol. 144, pp. 554-562, 2006.

[42] S. Gallus, M. Bertuzzi, A. Tavani, C. Bosetti, E. Negri, C.L. Vecchia, P. Lagiou, and D. Trichopoulos, "Does coffee protect against hepatocellular carcinoma?," *British Journal of Cancer*, vol. 87, pp. 956-959, 2002.

[43] Y. Kurozawa, I. Ogimoto, A. Shibata, T. Nose, T. Yoshimura, H. Suzuki, R. Sakata, Y. Fujita, S. Ichikawa, N. Iwai, and A. Tamakoshi, "Coffee and risk of death from hepatocellular carcinoma in a large cohort study in Japan," *British Journal of Cancer*, vol. 93, pp. 607-610, 2005.

[44] S.R. Brown, P.A. Cann, and N.W. Read, "Effect of coffee on distal colon function," *Gut*, vol. 31, pp. 450-453, 1990.

[45] K.J. Lee, M. Inoue, T. Otani, M. Iwasaki, S. Sasazuki, S. Tsugami, and the JPHC Study Group, "Coffee consumption and risk of colorectal cancer in a population-based prospective cohort of Japanese men and women," *International Journal of Cancer*, vol. 121, pp. 1312-1318, 2007.

[46] A. Nehlig and G. Debry, "Potential genotoxic, mutagenic and antimutagenic effects of coffee: a review," *Mutation Research*, vol. 317, pp. 145-162, 1994.

[47] S.C. Larsson, L. Bergkvist, E. Giovannucci, and A. Wolk, "Coffee consumption and incidence of colorectal cancer in two prospective cohort studies of Swedish women and men," *American Journal of Epidemiology*, vol. 163, pp. 638-644, 2006.

[48] T. Naganuma, S. Kuriyama, M. Akhter, M. Kakizaki, N. Nakaya, K. Matsuda-Ohmori, T. Shimazu, A. Fukao, and I. Tsuji, "Coffee consumption and the risk of colorectal cancer: a prospective cohort study in Japan," *International Journal of Cancer*, vol. 120, pp. 1542-1547, 2007.

[49] M. Nagao, Y. Fujita, K. Wakabayashi, H. Nukaya, T. Kosuge, and T. Sugimura, "Mutagens in coffee and other beverages," *Environmental Health Perspectives*, vol. 67, pp. 89-91, 1986.

[50] B.N. Ames and E.S. Gold, "Environmental pollution, pesticide, and the prevention of cancer: misconceptions," *The FASEB Journal*, vol. 11, pp. 1041-1052, 1997.

[51] S.C. Larsson, E. Giovannucci, and A. Wolk, "Coffee consumption and stomach cancer risk in a cohort of Swedish women," *International Journal of Cancer*, vol. 119, pp. 2186-2189, 2006.

[52] M. Akagawa, T. Shigemitsu, and K. Suyama, "Production of hydrogen peroxide by polyphenols and polyphenol-rich beverages under *quasi*-physiological conditions," *Bioscience, Biotechnology, and Biochemistry*, vol. 67, pp. 2632-2640, 2003.

[53] H. Morii, A. Kuboyama, T. Nakashima, K. Kawai, H. Kasai, K. Tamae, and T. Hirano, "Effects of instant coffee consumption on oxidative DNA damage, DNA repair, and redox system in mouse liver," *Journal of Food Sciences*, vol. 74, pp. H155-H161, 2009.

[54] N. Yoshioka, H. Nakashima, K. Hosoda, Y. Eitaki, N. Shimada, and K. Omae, "Urinary excretion of an oxidative stress marker, 8-hydroxyguanine (8-OH-Gua), among nickel-cadmium battery workers," *Journal of Occupational Health*, vol. 50, 229-235, 2008.

[55] M.C. Cooke, P.T. Henderson, and M.D. Evans, "Sources of extracellular, oxidatively-modified DNA lesions: implications for their measurement in urine," *Journal of Clinical Biochemistry and Nutrition*, vol. 45, pp. 255-270, 2009.

[56] K. Tamae, K. Kawai, S. Yamasaki, K. Kawanami, M. Ikeda, K. Takahashi, T. Miyamoto, N. Kato, and H. Kasai, "Effect of age, smoking and other lifestyle factors on urinary 7-methylguanine and 8-hydroxydeoxyguanosine," *Cancer Sciences*, vol. 100, pp. 715-721, 2009.

[57] S. Guarrera, C. Sacerdote, L. Fiorini, R. Marsala, S. Polidoro, S. Gamberini, F. Saletta, C. Malaveille, G. Talaska, P. Vineis, and G. Matullo, "Expression of DNA repair and metabolic genes in response to a flavonoid-rich diet," *British Journal of Nutrition*, vol. 98, pp. 525-533, 2007.

[58] M. Sørensen, O. Raaschou-Nielsen, R.D. Hansen, A. Tjønneland, K. Overvad, and U. Vogel, "Interaction between the OGG1 Ser326Cys polymorphism and intake of fruit and vegetables in relation to lung cancer," *Free Radical Research*, vol. 40, pp. 885-891, 2006.

[59] T. Kohno, K. Shinmura, M. Tosaka, M. Tani, S.R. Kim, H. Sugimura, T. Nohmi, H. Kasai, and J. Yokota, "Genetic polymorphisms and alternative splicing of the hOGG1 gene, that is involved in the repair of 8-hydroxyguanine in damaged DNA," *Oncogene*, vol. 16, pp. 3219-3225, 1998.

[60] C. Dherin, J.P. Radicella, M. Dizdaroglu, and S. Boiteux, "Excision of oxidatively damaged DNA bases by the human alpha-hOgg1 protein and the polymorphic alpha-hOgg1 (Ser326Cys) protein which is frequently found in human populations," *Nucleic Acids Research*, vol. 27, pp. 4001-4007, 1999.

[61] J.W. Hill and M. Evans, "Dimerization and opposite base-dependent catalytic impairment of polymorphic S326C OGG1 glycosylase," *Nucleic Acids Research*, vol. 34, pp. 1620-1632, 2006.

[62] A. Yamane, T. Kohno, K. Ito, N. Sunaga, K. Aoki, K. Yoshimura, H. Murakami, Y. Nojima, and J. Yokota, "Differential ability of polymorphic OGG1 proteins to suppress mutagenesis induced by 8-hydroxyguanine in human cell *in vivo*," *Carcinogenesis*, vol. 25, pp. 1689-1694, 2004.

[63] K. Datta, P. Jaruga, M. Dizdaroglu, R.D. Neumann, and T.A. Winters, "Molecular analysis of base damage clustering associated with a site-specific radiation-induced DNA double-strand break," *Radiation Research*, vol. 166, pp. 767-781, 2006.

26

# Enhancing DNA Repair by Combining only Dietary Supplement Ingredients that do not Metabolically Compete in Order to Achieve Synergism

Ronald W. Pero
*Section of Immunology, BMC: D14 Lund University, Lund, Sweden*

## 1. Introduction

Here this presentation embraces dietary supplement compositions containing resveratrol material, carotenoid material, nicotinamide material, DMAE material, zinc source material, and qjuinic acid-containing material , where no other known bioactive nutrient agents having competing modes of action to these specified agents are intentionally excluded from mixtures containing at least two of these DNA repair enhancing ingredients. The compositions may be embodied in formulations for oral administration, or alternatively, in formulations for peritoneal administration.

The combined composition may be selected from the group consisting of resveratrol (3, 5, 4'-trihydroxy-stilbene or an equivalent polyphenol in pure chemical form); the carotenoid material may be alpha carotene, beta carotene, canthaxanthin, lycopene and mixtures thereof; the nicotinamide material may be selected from the group consisting of nicotinamide, niacin, and mixtures thereof; the DMAE material selected from a group consisting of other choline analogs that pass the blood brain barrier; the zinc source material may be one or more zinc salts; and the quinic acid-containing material selected from a group consisting of quinic acid compounds that can enhance DNA repair by enhancing the uptake of tryptophan and nicotinamide ingredients (Pero et al 2009b; Pero and Lund 2011).

For human administration, the resveratrol material, carotenoid material, nicotinamide material, zinc source material, DMAE material, and quinic acid material may be present in proportions effective, in combination, to improve resistance to DNA damage, enhance DNA repair capacity, and stimulate immune function in a human subject to whom the composition is administered as a daily dosage (Pero et al 2009b; Pero and Lund 2011).

This formulation named Nutra-Reservatrol (Pero and Garret 2010) also contemplates the provision of a method of treating a human or other animal subject, consisting of administering resveratrol material, carotenoid material, nicotinamide material, DMAE material, zinc source material and quinic acid material to the subject to selectively supplement the subject's dietary intake thereof (i.e. without supplementing the dietary intake of any other active nutrient agents having competing modes of action) and repeating the administration on a substantially daily basis.

Thus, in a particular sense, this dietary supplement combination contemplates the provision of a method of treating a human subject consisting of selectively administering to the subject resveratrol material, carotenoid material, nicotinamide material, DMAE material, zinc source and quinic acid material in daily dosage amounts effective, in combination, to improve resistance to DNA damage, enhance DNA repair capacity, and stimulate immune function. In a specific example of currently preferred dosage range for humans, about 100-500 mg resveratol material, about 100 mg of carotenoid material, about 100 mg of nicotinamide material, about 100-200 mg DMAE material, about 10 mg of zinc source material and between 250-700 mg quinic acid source material are administered daily in this method (Pero and Garret 2010). So far as the author is aware, this particular combination of ingredients devoid of other bioactives has heretofore already been recognized as being synergistic or even effective (Pero 2000, Sheng et al 1998).

The discovery that natural products should not be combined into a natural medicine unless one tests whether each ingredient is additive to the overall desired biological effect, and that one way to accomplish this endpoint is to not combine natural products that have similar modes of action and thus competitive routes of absorption and excretion without first testing the combination for additive effects. That is to say, the present invention avoids inhibited uptake and absorption of natural products, thereby obtaining additive biological effects, by combining only natural products having well defined different, and thus potentially non-competitive modes of action which is, for example, the case with the exclusive combination of carotenoids + nicotinamide + zinc (Pero 2000, Sheng et al 1998).

Diet supplementation of humans or animals for example, by the oral, intraperitoneal, intravenous, subcutaneous or intramuscular routes of administration with the combination of carotenoids + nicotinamide/niacin + an appropriate zinc salt at a dose of this combination that exceeds a normal dietary levels was effective. This practice showed that dietary supplementation containing this combination together with simultaneous supplementation of other nutrients and/or natural products cannot enhance immune function (Payette, H. et al 1990; Zhang et al 1995), but when daily doses of carotenoids (as lycopene at 20 mg and Vitamin E 36 IU), niacin (120 mg) zinc salt (12 mg), reservatol (300 mg) and a quinic acid material (400 mg) were administered in the absence of other known DNA repair enhancers, and above dietary levels, the resistance to oxidative cellular DNA damage, and enhancement of DNA repair and immune function were observed in the clinic (Pero and Lund 2011). These data were taken as proof of concept for this dietary supplement to avoid metabolic competition and synergize DNA repair.

A clinical evaluation already published (Pero 2000, Sheng et al 1998) was also determined by comparing each individual's biological response before and after supplementation. In such a manner, each individual became his own control; e.g. the male subjects were given baseline measurements of resistance to cellular DNA damage, enhancement of DNA repair and stimulation of immune function once a week for 4 weeks, and then they were supplemented daily and the same measurements repeated once a week for the last 5 weeks of a 7 week intervention period. The before measurements (i.e. n = 4) were the baseline biological response parameters to be compared to the after measurements (i.e. n = 5). One individual was not supplemented to provide a control for the supplemented individuals. The data from this experimental design has taught that resistance to cellular DNA damage, enhancement of DNA repair and stimulation of immune function were all significantly modulated by a combination of carotenoids + nicotinamide + zinc when administered as an exclusive drug combination above dietary levels, but not when co-administered together with other additional nutrient or natural product supplements.

The design of this previous study to prove the discovery was based on combining substances with known properties to prevent cancer and stimulate immune function, but with differing mechanisms of action; e.g. carotenoids = electrophilic scavenger of radicals produced endogenously by cells or exogenously by the environment, nicotinamide = amplified source of energy via increased production of NAD or ATP, and zinc = an essential cofactor to antioxidant, replicative and DNA repair enzymes in cells. The hypothesis was that since none of these substances have produced consistent effects in humans as a single administered agent, this shortcoming could be overcome when administered in combination because these substances might produce a consistently additive or synergistic chemo-preventive biological response because of non-competitive modes of action instead of, for example, an inhibited one.

## 2. Scientific history

In 2010 there was an extensive review article published entitled "Historic development of Uncaria preparations and their related bioactive components" (Pero 2010b). This overview has specific relevance to the current review because it was the first recognition of the concept that ingredients could in fact convey properties of enhancement of DNA repair. Before this time, there were no clear cut examples where the process of DNA repair could be shown to be stimulated to higher levels of activity by exogenous nutrients or supplements in our environment. Previously it was believed that DNA repair which regulated our genetic integrity could not afford to be anything less than perfect to satisfy the requirements of orderly evolutionary change. Now it is quite accepted that even genes need to have nutritive treatment, functionality repaired and developed to maturity during life.

Uncaria sp. is a well known herbal medicine used for generations by the Ashinka Indians native to the Amazon basin. There have been two sets of bioactive ingredients for which Uncaria extracts have been developed and standardized. The first are oxindole alkaloids, initially studied and described in 1967; the second are a set of molecules know as Carboxy Alkyl Esters (CAEs ™) first identified and described in 1997 as the bioactive ingredients in AC-11® (Reviewed in Pero 2010b). More recently in 2005 (Sheng et al 2005) it was shown that one of the acid moieties of CAEs is quinic acid, and it is now documented to be one of the more effective DNA repair ingredients found in Uncaria spp, or brightly-colored berry extracts that also contain quinic acid (Stoner et al 2008, Pero 2006), and in turn can enhance DNA repair. It is important to remember that quinic acid is a natural-occurring alpha hydroxy organic acid quite ubiquitous in berries, and also the metabolic source of all other aromatic compound production in plants via the shikimate pathway (Pero 2010a); e.g. the bioactive agents in berries such as hydroxy organic acids (hydroxy benzoic, hydroxy cinnamonic and caffeic acids), flavinoids, and ellagic acid (Stoner et al 2008).

The progression of events that established Cat's Claw extracts as the most consistent and potent DNA repair enhancer of anti-aging effects has become obvious, and signaled why some elements are built of the knowledge of the later events that have happened, to paint a more complete picture of how DNA repair regulates aging. A chronology of events that remain unbroken and additive of each other, that Pero and colleagues have in turn built and learned from are as follows:

1. Specifically Uncaria spp. are an important historical medicine having been used for centuries to treat inflammation and other age-related diseases.
2. When carefully studied, alkaloids were not the main class of bioactive agents, but rather the water soluble carboxy alkyl esters (CAEs) which were only found extracted by water, which explains why indigenous Indians found them useful.
3. Quinic acid containing analogs such as quinic acid esters (QAEs) were identified as the bioactive agents.
4. The mode of action of CAEs/QAEs is via stimulating uptake of tryptophan and nicotinamide (Pero et al 2009b, Pero and Lund 2011). There are no other DNA repair enhancing substances having this mode of action.
5. It became apparent that if a DNA repair enhancer had other non-competitive metabolic modes of action then they would be synergistic to each other.
6. Given that bioactive quinic acid analogs (e.g QAEs) were first discovered in Cat's Claw bark in the 1990's, the bulk of our knowledge that dietary supplements can enhance DNA repair and provide anti-aging properties comes from this plant species (Reviewed in Pero 2010b). There is little doubt that the most extensive documentation of a DNA repair enhancer leading to treatment of anti-aging effects comes from quinic acid analogs and extracts isolated from Uncaria spp. For example, there are voluminous data published establishing Uncaria products can induce (a) DNA repair and anti-aging effects, (b) immune function enhancement, (c) anti-oxidation and (d) neurological effects (Pero 2010b).
7. Based on this historical data, and combined with our background knowledge of the process of excision DNA repair involving at least 5 enzymes each having separate regulatory functional components, it has been fortunate to determine that there exists for many DNA repair enzymes a non-competitive metabolism allowing for a cooperative DNA repair effect that can be synergistic or at least additive. For example, when known DNA repair modulating ingredients were combined to synergize DNA repair, if competing metabolic events were eliminated from these mixtures then metabolic synergism was observed as evidenced by accounting for rehydration properties; i.e thirst quenching, (Pero and Garret 2010) as well as enhanced DNA repair (Pero 2000; Sheng et al 1998, Pero and Lund 2011).
8. After reviewing the Background and Historical Development Sections presented above, it is safe to conclude there have been many milestones achieved documenting the successful development of a dietary supplement that optimally can enhance DNA repair and reduce aging effects from chronic diseases. The learning curve is presented within these 8 points of development, ending up with a synergized combination of the dietary supplements including: resveratrol material, carotenoid material, nicotinamide material, zinc source material, and quinic acid material that is present in proportions effective, in combination, to improve resistance to DNA damage, enhance DNA repair capacity, and stimulate immune function in a human subject to whom the composition is administered as a daily dosage. Any product not encompassing these points of development is by definition an inferior product development.

**Prevalence of DNA repair deficiencies in the general population.** There are now more than 130 DNA repair - regulated genes identified that also can influence individual susceptibility to DNA damage, and as a consequence, the incidence of human diseases. The number has increased dramatically in the last 20 years, and no doubt will continue to increase as the causative importance of this research area to human disease development becomes better known (Wood et al 2001). So far nearly all areas of DNA repair are represented by defective metabolism such as: base excision repair (BER) (glycosylases, endonucleases), PARP (poly ADP ribose polyemerase), direct reversal of damage, repair of DNA protiein crosslinks, mis- matched excision repair (MMR), nucleotide excision repair (NER), homologous recombination, non-homlogous end-joining, modulation of nucleotide pools, DNA polymerase, editing and processing nucleases, Rad 6 pathway, chromatin structure, and genes defective in disease that modulate DNA damage. The mere fact there are so many variant ways to become diseased by defective DNA repair mechanisms is a biologic testimony to the impotance of this pathway to human health.

## 3. A dietary supplement composition that induces rehydration and enhances DNA repair and anti-aging effects

### 3.1 The reservatrol material

The known molecular mechanisms of resveratrol are described herein. The main effects of resveratrol are to regulate cell cycle events that favor growth arrest allowing DNA repair enhancement before cells die from DNA damage blockage of cell replication (Valenzano et al 2006; Gatz et al 2008; Feng et al 2002; Whyte et al 2007). There are changes in both gene and protein expression, such as the up-regulation of p53 and p21 and the down-regulation of cyclin A, chk1, CDC27, and Eg5 (a mitotic motor protein). Resveratrol also alters the intracellular Smad signaling of the TGF-β pathway. Finally, dietary restriction, the best-studied life-extension treatment, causes overexpression of SIRT 1 (Cohen et al. Science 2004), and since these effects are not additive to resveratrol, they suggest that a similar molecular mechanism to dietary restriction.

### 3.2 The carotenoid material

The known molecular mechanisms of carotenoids are described herein. The exact mechanism of action of carotenoids such as beta carotene is not fully understood but it is commonly accepted scientifically that one primary mechanism is to directly scavenge oxygen derived free radicals produced either as by-products of metabolism or from exogenous environmental exposures (Lieber 1993; Bohm et al 1993; Regnault et al 1993; Riso 1999). As a free radical scavenger, carotenoids can be expected to reduce or protect against the chemical damage induced in DNA, RNA and protein of cells by toxic environmental exposures or endogenous cellular metabolic errors that ultimately can result in a disease state. On the other hand, nicotinamide and zinc salts do not possess this chemical property which results in an improved biological cellular function.

### 3.3 The nicotinamide material

The known molecular mechanisms of nicotinamide are described herein. Nicotinamide and its metabolic equivalent nicotinic acid (niacin, vitamin B) or even tryptophan which is the synthetic precursor to niacin is the main precursor for the formation and maintenance of the cellular pool of NAD (Bernofsky 1980; Olsson et al 1993). NAD is essential for cellular ATP production and maintenance of the cell's redox potential, and it is also the substrate for the DNA repair enzyme, poly ADP-ribosyl transferase (ADPRT). Niacin deprivation decreases the NAD pools significantly both in tissue culture cells (Jacobson, E et al 1992) and animal systems (Zhang et al 1993) as well as humans (Fu et al 1989). The depleted cells have an increased sensitivity to DNA damage and the levels of poly (ADP-ribose) production in cultured cells (as cited by Jacobson, E L in Poirier and Moreau (eds) 1992) or in rat liver (Rawling et al 1994) were significantly lower after mild nicotinamide deficiency. On the other hand, when niacin was given as a supplement to ordinary nutrition (i.e. above known dietary levels) the NAD pool increased and the cells were less sensitive to oxygen radicals (Weitberg 1989). Therefore, it is obvious from this review of the prior art that the primary mechanism of action of nicotinamide/niacin differs from carotenoids and zinc in that the cell's potential for energy metabolism is increased by amplifying NAD and ATP pool supplies (i.e. these biochemicals are the energy sources of living organisms) which in turn is useful to cells, tissues and organs to reduce DNA damage, enhance DNA repair (i.e. poly ADP-ribosylation) and stimulate immune function where the relevance to the disease state is apparent (Pero et al 1995).

### 3.4 The zinc material

The known molecular mechanisms of zinc source are described herein. Zinc differs from the resveratrol, carotenoids and nicotinamide with regard to its mechanism of action in that it influences disease development and immune function by being an essential co-factor in several enzyme functions involving replication, DNA repair and antioxidant defense of cells. Zinc is required for cell replication and DNA polymerase activity (Williams, RO et al 1973). There are two zinc fingers in the DNA binding domain of the poly adenosine diphosphate ribosyl transferase (ADPRT) gene and other DNA repair proteins (Dawat, P. et al 1995; Matsuda, T. et al1 1995; Chiriccolo, M. et al 1993) which contain cysteine residues (i.e. an amino acid), and if these cysteine residues are oxidized at their thiol constituents, they would prevent DNA binding and participation in DNA repair (Mazen et al 1989; de Murcia, G. et al 1989; Pero 1995; Althaus et al 1994). Moreover, superoxide dismutase is an antioxidant enzyme protecting cells from the harmful superoxide anion because this radical is a substrate for the enzymatic reaction that also requires zinc as a cofactor (Brunori and Rotilio 1984).

### 3.5 The DMAE material

The known molecular mechanisms of DMAE material is described herein. Dimethylaminoethanol (DMAE) material, also known as deanol, is a naturally occurring substance that has been studied as a possible anti-ageing therapy that can also improve cognitive function, reduce neurological stress, improves immunity and DNA repair especially in skin. It is the precursor to choline and may increase acetylcholine levels (Grossman 2005). While choline is known to be the precursor of acetylcholine, a recognized neurotransmitter, DMAE may also prove to offer a more direct approach to this function by moving into the brain, being acted on by an enzyme (methylation), and thereby undergoing conversion into choline directly where it is needed. DMAE inhibits production of the age-related pigment lipofuscin, which accumulates in all aging tissues. This is significant because cells with increased lipofuscin cause lysosomes to perform poorly, which leads to increased accumulation of poorly functioning mitochondria and increased reactive oxygen species (ROS) production (Terman and Brunk 2006). Evidence also suggests that DMAE decreases the extent of crosslinking of proteins possibly by acting as a free-radical scavenger (Nagy and Nagy 1980).

### 3.6 The quinic acid material

A water extract of Cat's Claw (Uncaria species) called AC-11 or one of its active ingredients quinic acid are also DNA repair enhancers that do not metabolically compete with resveratrol material, carotenoid material, nicotinamide material, DMAE material or zinc material, and as such could be added to the DNA repair mixture without inducing metabolic competition and thus inhibiting DNA repair instead of being synergistic, because the mode of action of AC-11/quinic acid to increasing DNA repair is novel to inducing DNA repair by increasing uptake of urinary tryptophan and nicotinamide (Pero 2008, Pero et al 2009b, Pero and Lund 2009a , 2011). The quinic acid analog being selected for commericial development is from the group consisting of quinic acid salts, chelates, and Uncaria or other plant extracts containing quinic acid analogs (Pero 2001, 2002, 2005, 2006, 2009a, 2009b; Pero and Garret 2010a).

## 4. Discussion

The family of dietary supplements proposed herein; e.g. Nutra-Reservatrol, ReservaQuin, AIO, or carotenoids/nicotinamide/zinc combinations (Pero and Garret 2010, Pero and Lund 2011, Sheng et al 1998) are break through products embedded in the science of synergism, often hypothesized, rarely if ever accomplished. Listed below are 6 ingredients all known to be useful in enhancing DNA repair by independent molecular mechanisms, because their interaction with the DNA repair process results in non-competitive molecular metabolism; i.e. they regulate different pathways essential to mediate successful repair of genetic lesions. In order to achieve synergism of DNA repair, it is necessary to combine at least two of this family of dietary supplements to achieve a synergistic mixture development. This fact in turn provides a great diversity to product development by providing 6 ingredients to choose from and still achieve an increased blend of efficacy for any desired clinical indication. For example, nicotinamide supplies the energy source, zinc helps bind a repair enzyme to the damaged are in DNA, carotenoids help scavenger radicals that in turn damage the DNA in the first place, resveratrol modulates growth arrest and cell survival, DMAE (deanol, dimethylaminoethanol) dietary supplement reduces the harmful health effects of neurological stress, and by increasing critical nutrient uptake such as tryptophan and nicotinamide with quinic acid analogs. The scientific basis for further substantiation can be found in Sections 3.1 to 3.6 of this review.
Most anti-aging products have at least one of the following mechanisms of action that address: Inflammation, Immunity, DNA repair, Nutrition, or Oxidative stress. However, rarely do anti-aging products have most of these known modes of action present and shown to occur by simply avoiding metabolic competition the DNA repair ingredients. The logic in this case is that synergism is hypothesized to come from co-varying lifestyle factors all being simultaneously metabolically regulated by the same dehydration/rehydration properties being induced by non-competitive metabolism of a family of DNA repair enhancing dietary supplements (data in Pero 2000, Pero and Garret 2010, Pero and Lund 2011, ). They are listed below together with optimal dose ranges:

1. NAD (NICOTINAMIDE) INGREDIENT
   (Energy source to Enhance Repair of Cellular Damage to DNA, RNA and protein) (100-200 mg/day)
2. ZINC INGREDIENT
   (Helps Recognize Harmful Lesions in Genetic Material)(10-20 mg/day

3. CAROTENOIDS (CANTAXATHIN) INGREDIENT
   (Powerful water soluble antioxidant carotenoid) (100-200 mg/day)
4. RESERVATROL INGREDIENT
   (Modulates Growth Arrest and Cell Survival and DNA repair) (70-2000 mg/day)
5. DMAE (Deanol) INGREDIENT
   (Reduces Neurological Stress) (100-200 mg/day)
6. QUINIC ACID ANALOG OR EXTRACT INGREDIENTS
   (Enhances DNA repair by increasing tryptophan uptakr, and also providing anti-infective properties (350-700 mg/day)
7. DO SUPRA-PHYSIOLOGIC LEVELS OF DIETARY SUPPLEMENTS AUGMENT DNA REPAIR CAPACITY. The ingredients identified above with the exception of Resveratrol were known to be effective in vivo at the indicated doses above, which were in turn above normal physiologi occurring levels . However, metabolic competition between some agents can seriously alter their bioavailability to the extent that when administered in combination they are no longer efficacious (Sheng et al 1998, Pero 2000). It was hypothesized that this could be the case with resveratrol and the other agents in Nutra-Reveratrol. Hence, they were pre-screened before formulation to avoid any metabolic competition originating from their DNA repair mechanism of action (Pero and Garret 2010).

Weight regulates essentially all aspects of a disease-free life via nutrition and metabolism balances/imbalances that can be estimated reproducibly by assessment of dehydration (Cheuvront et al 2010). Primary causes of everyday ill health from weight gain are bodily fluctuations in water balance (hydration) (Manz 2007). Moreover, it is a very large market since 27% of American adults have metabolic syndrome (i.e. disturbances in hydration), while 85% of overweight people do (Ford et al 2004, Grundy et al 2005). Your lifestyle demands you to react to your environment, and metabolic hydration is the gage of how successful you have managed health risk from exposure to these factors.

Lifestyle factors are key to generation of oxidative stress, aging, and dehydration in turn is the dominant cause behind weight generated ill health, because weight gain also co-varies with the lifestyle changes associated with the obese. Examples are narcotics (smoking, alcohol consumption, drugs, binge over-eating), diet (fats, proteins, carbohydrates, fiber, vitamins, minerals) exercise, weight gain, sleep (psychotropic stress). Hence, treating dehydration with re-hydration, and anti-DNA damaging agent metabolism also optimizes a first good line of defense against age-associated diseases in general.

There is another important link between essential amino acid metabolism and DNA repair capacity. It is based on the discovery of a previously unappreciated metabolic connection between naturally occurring hippuric acid and quinic acid. Hippuric acid is not found in plant material nor is it metabolized by higher plants (Reviewed in Pero 2010b). Hippuric acid is known to be catabolically synthesized from benzene-type aromatic compounds usually believed to be originating from environmental exposures, or from the cyclic sugar type-compound quinic acid. Quinic acid is ubiquitous especially in healthy foodstuffs which in turn can lead to aromatic plant biosynthesis *via* the microbial shikimate pathway existing in the human gastrointestinal tract. Consequently, Pero (2010a) reasoned that if the urinary level of hippuric acid co-varied and increased in proportion with urinary quinic acid levels as they in fact did, then it follows then that the primary levels of these metabolites (i.e hippuric and quinic acids) are coming from the diet and not environmental exposures. Hence, because the GI tract was primarily responsible for this metabolism and not the liver, then there must also be produced large amounts of tryptophan and nicotinamide which becomes immediately available for human absorption and the benefits thereof. In fact this proved to be the case and a direct benefit to stimulation of human DNA repair was established (Pero et al 2009a; 2009b; Pero et al 2011).

Finally the common thread tying this particular dietary supplement development together is the common predominant role of life style factors. First there was the composition itself. Although the DNA repair enhancing ingredients have been studied many times before never in high dose combination with each other. When they were the included DNA repair ingredients they also possessed thirst quenching abilities, never before observed to be associated with DNA repair. This observation was accounted for by the fact that non-metabolic competition between the DNA repair enhancing ingredients could be observed because thirst quenching (i.e. rehydration) was observed whereas as single agents none was. Second, lifestyle factors are key to generation of oxidative stress, aging, and dehydration in turn is the dominant cause behind weight generated ill health, because weight gain also co-varies with the lifestyle changes associated with the obese. Weight regulates essentially all aspects of a disease-free life via nutrition and metabolism balances/imbalances via dehydration/rehyration imbalances.

Thirdly, DNA repair enhancers have also been shown in human studies to be regulated by life style factors that are in turn associated to obesity and lifespan (Banne et al 2004, Pero et al 1985,Pero et al 2000,) and as cited therein for life syle fluctutions and DNA repair capacity) These facts have allowed the development of a proprietary "Wellness Test" that is sensitive to individual fluctuations in life style factors because it can estimate daily changes in urinary nicotinamide and trypotphan and compare them with serum thiol status (Pero 2008). Now success or failure of dietary supplements like Nutra-Reservatrol can be monitored by this functional test to deliver even more accurate health care monitoring.

## 5. References

Althaus, FR, Hofferer L, Kleczkowska, HE, Malanga M, Naegeli H, Panzeter PL, Realini CA. A Histone shuttling by poly ADP-ribosylation. Mol. Cell. Biochem. 138(1-2):53-59, 1994

Banne, A, Amiri, A, Pero, RW. Reduced Level of Serum Thiols in Patients with a Diagnosis of Active Disease. J Anti Aging Med 6(4): 325-32, 2004

Bernofsky. C. Physiology aspects of pyridine nucleotide regulation in mammals. Mol. Cell. Biochem. 33(3): 135-143, 1980

Böhm F, Haley J, Truscott TG, Schalch W. Cellular bound beta-carotene quenches singlet oxygen in man. J Photochem Photobiol *B*, vol. 21(2-3), 219-221, 1993.

Brunori M, and Rotilio G Biochemistry of oxygen radical species. Methods in Enzymology 105: 22-35, 1984

Cheuvront S.N, Ely BR, Kenefick, RW, Sawka MN. Biological variation and diagnostic accuracy of dehydration assessment markers. Am J. Clin. Nutr 92(3): 565-573, 2010

Chiricolo M, Musa AR, Monti D, Zannotti M, Franceschi C. Enhanced DNA repair in lymphocytes of Down syndrome patients: the influence of zinc supplementation. Mutation Res. 295(3):105-111, 1993

Cohen HY, Miller C, Kevin J. Bitterman KJ, Wall NR, Hekking B, Benedikt Kessler B, Howitz KT, Gorospe M, de Cabo R, Sinclair DA. Calorie Restriction Promotes Mammalian Cell Survival by Inducing the SIRT1 Deacetylase Science 305 (5682): 390–392, 2004

Dawat P, de Oliveira R, Ehrlich D, Boiteux, S. Repair of oxidative DNA damage in Gram positive bacteria: the Lactococcus lactis Fpg protein.Microbiol. 141 (Pt 2):411-417, 1995

de Murcia G, Ménissier-de Murcia J, Schreiber V. Poly(ADP-ribose) polymerase: molecular biological aspects. BioEssays: news and reviews in molecular, cellular and developmental biology13 (9):455-62 (1991).

Feng YH , Jian-Ping Z, Xiao-Yu L. Effects of resveratrol and ethanol on production of proinflammatory factors from endotoxin activated murine macrophages Acta Pharmacol Sin 23(10): 893-897, 2002

Ford ED, Giles WH, Mokad AH. Increasing prevalence of the metabolic syndrome among U,S. adult. Diabetes Care 24 (10): 2735-2752, 2004

Fu CS, Swendeid ME, Jacob RA, Mckee YW. Biochemical Markers for Assessment of Niacin Status in Young Men: Levels of Erythrocyte Niacin Coenzymes and Plasma Tryptophan. J. Nutr. 123: 1349-1355, 1993.

Gatz SA , Keimling M, Baumann C, Thilo, Dörk T, Debatin K-M, Fulda S, Wiesmülle, L. Resveratrol modulates DNA double-strand break repair pathways in an ATM/ATR-p53- and -Nbs1-dependent manner. Carcinogenesis 29(3):519-527, 2008

Grossman R. The role of dimethylaminoethanol (DMAE) in cosmetic dermatology. Am J Clin Dermatol 6:39–47, 2005

Grundy SM, Cleeman JI, Daniels SR, Donato KA, Eckel RH, Franklin BA, Gordon DJ, Krauss RM, Savage, PJ, Smith SC jr, Spertus JA, Costa F. Diagnosis and management of metabolic syndrome: An American Heart/National Heart, Lung, and Blood institute scientific statement statement. Circulation 112(17): 2735-2752, 2005

Jacobson, E. et al., IN: ADP-Ribosylation Reactions (Poirier, G. G. and Moreau, P., eds.), pp. 153-162, Springer Verlag, New York, N.Y., 1992

Lieber, DC Antioxidant reactions of carotenoids. Ann. N. Y. Acad. Sci. 691: 20-31, 1993

Manz, F. Hydration and disease. Journal of the American College of Nutrition. 26(9005): 535S-541S, 2007

Matsuda T, Saijo, M, Kuraoka I, Kobatashi T, Nakatsu, Y, Nagal A, Enjoji, T, Massuta C, Sugasawa, K, Hanaoka, F. DNA Repair protein XPA binds replication protein A (RPA). J. Biol. Chem. 270(8):4152-4157, 1995

Mazen A, Menissier-deMurcia J, Molinete M, Simonin F, Gradwohl, G, Poirier, G, deMurcia, G. Poly(ADP-ribose)polymerase: a novel finger protein. Nucleic Acid Res. 17:4689-4698, 1989

Nagy I, Nagy K. On the role of cross-linking of cellular proteins in aging. Mech Ageing Dev 14(1–2):245–251, 1980

Olsson A, Olofsson T, and Pero, RW. Specific binding and uptake of extra cellular nicotinamide in human leukemic K-562 cells. Biochem. Pharmacol. 45(6):1191-1200 (1993)

Payette H, Rola-Pleczcynski, M, Ghadirin P. Nutrition factors in relation to cellular and regulatory immune variables in a free-living elderly population. Am. J. Clin. Nutr. 52:927-932, 1990

Pero, RW. Carotenoid-nicotinamide-zinc compositions and methods of treatment using same. US 6,020,351, Issued Feb. 1, 2000

Pero, RW. Method of preparation and composition of a water soluble extract of the plant species Uncaria. US 6,039,949. Issued Mar. 21, 2000

Pero, RW. Method of preparation and composition of a water soluble extract of the plant species Uncaria for enhancing immune, anti-inflammatory, and anti-tumor processes of warm blooded animals. US 6,238, 675 B1, Issued May 29, 2001

Pero, RW. Method of preparation and composition of a water soluble extract of the plant species Uncaria for enhancing immune, anti-inflammatory, anti-tumor and DNA repair processes of warm blooded animals US 6,361,805 B2 Mar. 26, 2002

Pero, RW. Method of preparation and composition of a water soluble extract of the bioactive component of the plant species Uncaria for enhancing immune, anti-inflammatory, anti-tumor and DNA repair processes of warm blooded animals (Isolation of a quinic acid analog preferably quinic acid lactone) US 6,964,784 . Issued Nov. 15, 2005

Pero, RW. Medicinal compositions of salts, chelates and/or free acids of alpha hydroxyl organic acids and related processes and methods. WO/2006/101922 International filing date 16.03.2006, Publication date 28.09.2006

Pero, RW. A method of increasing tryptohan and nicotinamide levels in vivo. WO/2008/008837. International filing date 11.07.2007, Publication date 17.01.2008

Pero, RW. Method of preparation and composition of a water soluble extract of the bioactive component of the plant species Uncaria for enhancing immune, anti-inflammatory, anti-tumor and DNA repair processes of warm blooded animals (a method of isolating a quinic acid analog). US 7,579,023 B2, Issued Aug. 25, 2009a

Pero, RW. Method of preparation and composition of a water soluble extract of the bioactive component of the plant species Uncaria for enhancing immune, anti-inflammatory, anti-tumor and DNA repair processes of warm blooded animal (a method of isolating a quinic acid salt or chelate or free acid). US 7,595,064 B2, Issued Sept. 29, 2009b.

Pero, RW. Health consequences of catabolic synthesis of hippuric acid. Reviews in Clinical Pharmacology *5:* 67-73, 2010a

Pero, RW. Historic development of Uncaria preparations and their related bioactive components. Chap.9. In Allison E. Thomas (ed). DNA repair, damage repair mechanisms and aging, Nova Science Publishers, ISB 978-1-61668-914-8. pp 223-236, 2010b.

Pero, RW, Garret, S. Nutritional Supplement. US 2010/0215768 A1, filed Feb. 24, 2010, Publication Date Aug. 26, 2010

Pero, RW, Holmgren, K, Persson, L. Gamma-radiation induced ADP-ribosyl tansferase activity and mammalian longevity. Mutation Res 142: 69-73, 1985

Pero, RW, Hoppe, C, Sheng, Y. Serum thiols as a surrogate estimate of DNA repair correlates to mammalian life span. Jour Anti-Aging Med 3 (3): 241-249, 2000

Pero RW and Lund H. In Vivo Treatment of Humans with Quinic Acid Enhances DNA Repair and Reduces the Influence of lifestyle Factors on Risk to Disease. ISSN 0973-2691. Int. J. Biotech. and Biochem. 5 (3): 293–305, 2009a

Pero, RW, Lund H. Dietary quinic acid supplied as the nutritional supplement AIO + AC-11 leads to induction of micromolar levels of nicotinamide and tryptophan in the urine. Phytotherapy Research in press, 2011

Pero RW, Lund H, Leanderson T. Antioxidant metabolism induced by quinic acid. Increased urinary excretion of tryptophan and nicotinamide. Phytotherapy Research 23: 335-346, 2009b

Pero, RW, Olsson, A, Sheng, Y, Hua, J, Moller, C, Kjelle'n, E, Killander, D, Marmor, M. Progress in identifying clinical relevance of inhibition, stimulation and measurements of poly ADP-ribosylation. Biochimie 77:385-393 (1995)

Rawling JM, Jackson TM, Drisscol ER, Kirkland, J. Dietary Niacin Deficiency Lowers Tissue Poly(ADP-Ribose) and NAD+ Concentrations in Fischer 344 Rats J. Nutri. 124:1597-1603, 1994

Regnault C, Postaire ER, Rousse GJ, Bejot M and Hazebroucq, GF Influence of beta carotene, vitamin E, and vitamin C on endogenous antioxidant defenses in erythrocytes Ann. Pharmacotherapy 27(11):1349-1350, 1993

Riso P, Pinder A, Santangelo, A, Porrini, M. Does tomato consumption effectively increase the resistance of lymphocyte DNA to oxidative damage. Am J. Clin Nutr 69(4): 712-718, 1999

Sheng Y., Pero, R.W., Olsson, A.R., Bryngelsson, C. and Hua, J. DNA repair enhancement by a combined supplement of carotenoids, nicotinamide, and zinc. Cancer Det. Prevent. 22(4): 284-292 (1998)

Sheng , Akesson, C. Holmgren K, Bryngelsson C, Giampapa V, Pero, RW. An active ingredient of Cat's Claw water extracts. Identification and efficacy of quinic acid. J Ethanopharmacology 96(3):577-584, 2005

Regnault C, Postaire ER, Rousse GJ, Bejot M and Hazebroucq, GF Influence of beta carotene, vitamin E, and vitamin C on endogenous antioxidant defenses in erythrocytes Ann. Pharmacotherapy 27(11):1349-1350, 1993

Stoner DS, Li-Shu Wang L-S , Casto BC. Laboratory and clinical studies of cancer chemoprevention by antioxidants in berries. Carcinogenesis 29(9): 1665-1674, 2008

Terman A, Brunk UT. Oxidative stress, accumulation of biological "garbage," and aging. Antioxid Redox Signal 8(1–2):197–204, 2006

Weitberg, AB. Effect of nicotinic acid supplementation in vivo on oxygen radical-induced genetic damage in human lymphocytes. Mutational Res. 216:197-201, 1989

Valenzano DR, Terzibasi E,Genade T, Cattaneo A, Domenici L , Cellerino A. Resveratrol Prolongs Lifespan and Retards the Onset of Age-Related Markers in a Short-Lived Vertebrate. Current Biology 16 (3): 296-300, 2006

Whyte L, Huang YY, Torres, K, Mehta, RG. Molecular mechanisms of reservatrol action in lung cancer cells using dual protein and microarray analyses. Cancer Res 67(24): 12007–17, 2007

Williams, RO, Loeb L A. Zinc requirement for DNA replication in stimulated human lymphocytes. J. Cell Biol. 58:594-601, 1973

WIN/NIDDK, Weight-Control Information Network/National Institute of Diabetes, Digestive and Kidney Disease. Do you know the health risks of being over weight. http://win.niddk.nih.gov/publication/health risk.htm. December 31, 2010

Wood, RD, Mitchell, M. , Sqouros, J, Lindahl, T. Human DNA repair genes. Science 16: 291 (5507) : 128 4-9, 2001

Zhang J, Henning, SM, Swendseid AE Poly(ADP-Ribose) Polymerase Activity and DNA Strand Breaks Are Affected in Tissues of Niacin-Deficient Rats. J. Nutri. 123:1349-1355, 1993

Zhang YH, Kramer, TR, Taylor, PR, Li, JY, Blot, WJ, Brown, CC, Guo, W, Dawsey, SM, LI, B. Possible immunologic involvement of antioxidants in cancer prevention. Am. J. Clin. Nutr. 62:1477S-1482S, 1995